WITHDRAWN
WRIGHT STATE UNIVERSITY LIBRARIES

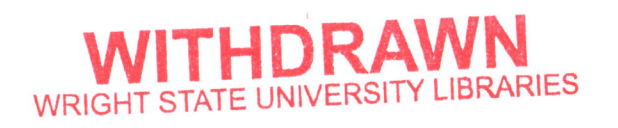

Autoimmune Endocrinopathies

CONTEMPORARY ENDOCRINOLOGY

P. Michael Conn, SERIES EDITOR

21. **Hormones and the Heart in Health and Disease,** edited by LEONARD SHARE, 1999
20. **Endocrinology of Aging,** edited by JOHN E. MORLEY AND LUCRETIA VAN DEN BERG, 1999
19. **Human Growth Hormone:** Research and Clinical Practice, edited by ROY G. SMITH AND MICHAEL O. THORNER, 1999
18. **Menopause:** Endocrinology and Management, edited by DAVID B. SEIFER AND ELIZABETH A. KENNARD, 1999
17. **The IGF System:** Molecular Biology, Physiology, and Clinical Applications, edited by RON G. ROSENFELD AND CHARLES T. ROBERTS, JR., 1999
16. **Neurosteroids:** A New Regulatory Function in the Nervous System, edited by ETIENNE-EMILE BAULIEU, MICHAEL SCHUMACHER, AND PAUL ROBEL, 1999
15. **Autoimmune Endocrinopathies,** edited by ROBERT VOLPÉ, 1999
14. **Hormone Resistance Syndromes,** edited by J. LARRY JAMESON, 1999
13. **Hormone Replacement Therapy,** edited by A. WAYNE MEIKLE, 1999
12. **Insulin Resistance:** The Metabolic Syndrome X, edited by GERALD M. REAVEN AND AMI LAWS, 1999
11. **Endocrinology of Breast Cancer,** edited by ANDREA MANNI, 1999
10. **Molecular and Cellular Pediatric Endocrinology,** edited by STUART HANDWERGER, 1999
9. **The Endocrinology of Pregnancy,** edited by FULLER W. BAZER, 1998
8. **Gastrointestinal Endocrinology,** edited by GEORGE H. GREELEY, JR., 1999
7. **Clinical Management of Diabetic Neuropathy,** edited by ARISTIDIS VEVES, 1998
6. **G Proteins, Receptors, and Disease,** edited by ALLEN M. SPIEGEL, 1998
5. **Natriuretic Peptides in Health and Disease,** edited by WILLIS K. SAMSON AND ELLIS R. LEVIN, 1997
4. **Endocrinology of Critical Disease,** edited by K. PATRICK OBER, 1997
3. **Diseases of the Pituitary:** Diagnosis and Treatment, edited by MARGARET E. WIERMAN, 1997
2. **Diseases of the Thyroid,** edited by LEWIS E. BRAVERMAN, 1997
1. **Endocrinology of the Vasculature,** edited by JAMES R. SOWERS, 1996

AUTOIMMUNE ENDOCRINOPATHIES

Edited by

ROBERT VOLPÉ, MD

University of Toronto, Toronto, Ontario, Canada

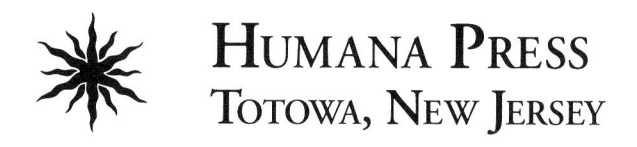

HUMANA PRESS
TOTOWA, NEW JERSEY

© 1999 Humana Press Inc.
999 Riverview Drive, Suite 208
Totowa, New Jersey 07512

For additional copies, pricing for bulk purchases, and/or information about other Humana titles, contact Humana at the above address or at any of the following numbers: Tel: 973-256-1699; Fax: 973-256-8341; E-mail: humana@humanapr.com or visit our website at http://humanapress.com

All rights reserved. No part of this book may be reproduced, stored in a retrieval system, or transmitted in any form or by any means, electronic, mechanical, photocopying, microfilming, recording, or otherwise without written permission from the Publisher.

All articles, comments, opinions, conclusions, or recommendations are those of the author(s), and do not necessarily reflect the views of the publisher.

This publication is printed on acid-free paper. ∞
ANSI Z39.48-1984 (American National Standards Institute)
Permanence of Paper for Printed Library Materials.

Cover caption: Photomicrograph of thyroid showing Hashimoto's (autoimmune) thyroiditis.

Cover design by Patricia F. Cleary.

Photocopy Authorization Policy:
Authorization to photocopy items for internal or personal use, or the internal or personal use of specific clients, is granted by Humana Press Inc., provided that the base fee of US $10.00 per copy, plus US $00.25 per page, is paid directly to the Copyright Clearance Center at 222 Rosewood Drive, Danvers, MA 01923. For those organizations that have been granted a photocopy license from the CCC, a separate system of payment has been arranged and is acceptable to Humana Press Inc. The fee code for users of the Transactional Reporting Service is: [0-89603-680-4/99 $10.00 + $00.25].

Printed in the United States of America. 10 9 8 7 6 5 4 3 2 1

Autoimmune endocrinopathies / edited by Robert Volpé.
    p. cm. — (Contemporary endocrinology ; 15)
   Includes bibliographical references and index.
   ISBN 0-89603-680-4 (alk. paper)
   1. Endocrine glands—Diseases—Immunological aspects.
2. Autoimmune diseases.   I. Volpé, Robert, 1926– . II. Series:
Contemporary endocrinology ; 15.
RC649.A976 1999
616.4' 079—dc21

                                            99-10951
                                              CIP

PREFACE

This preface introduces *Autoimmune Endocrinopathies*, a series of essays on these pathologies and related topics written by experts in the field. This is the fourth volume on this general subject that I have written *(1)* or edited *(2,3)* over 18 years, and given my advanced age, this is undoubtedly the last. Having read the chapters offered by the contributors to the present volume, I hope it will not be unseemly if I make the claim that this last effort is also the best.

Although there are diverse features that distinguish these autoimmune endocrinopathies, there are also certain links of susceptibility and pathogenesis that connect them. Chapters in this volume will attest to the view that the disturbance(s) in immunoregulation that lead to the organ-specific autoimmune endocrine diseases appear to be partly genetic and partly environmental in nature. Autoimmune endocrine diseases (and those nonendocrine autoimmune disorders with which they are associated) (Table 1) tend to aggregate in families, and more than one of these maladies may occur concomitantly within the same patient or her/his family. The modes of inheritance of these disorders do not follow simple genetic rules, and such environmental factors as stress, infection, trauma, drugs, nutrition, smoking, and aging may distort the penetrance and expressivity of these conditions (by their actions on the immune system). Questions related to the pathogenesis and immunogenetics of the autoimmune endocrinopathies are largely dealt with in Chapters 1–5, and are also discussed in relation to the specific entities in the chapters that follow. There tends to be a strong female preponderance in most of these autoimmune diseases that appears to be largely related to hormonal factors, as described in Chapter 7, on sex hormones and autoimmunity. Additionally, as the nature of the autoantigens involved in these diseases became increasingly known (see Chap. 8, Autoantigens in the Autoimmune Endocrinopathies), it became clear that the antigen(s) in each of the entities are distinct from one another, and thus antigenic cross-reactivity was not likely to explain the occasional association of more than one organ-specific autoimmune disease in the same individual; rather, the explanation may lie in closely related genetically induced disturbances in the immune system. The proliferative response of subsets of T lymphocytes to the different autoantigens has been shown to be antigen (disease)-specific. Finally, in experimental animals, the inheritance of insulin-dependent diabetes mellitus can be shown to be separate from that of autoimmune thyroid disease. One thus can only conclude that the autoimmune endocrine diseases are each based on unrelated antigens, and are genetically separate, despite overlapping genetic links. The essays on each of the specific conditions in turn are followed by a chapter on possible preventive measures, as well as new immunomodulatory approaches (Chap. 17).

Certainly, there is much to be learned about the events that lead to the development and progression, as well as the treatment and possible prevention, of these disorders. A number of questions remain unanswered, and form the grist for future studies. For example, the precise genes for each organ-specific autoimmune disease need to be identified and a comparison made between the various entities. Once identified, their actions and interactions will have to be worked out. The antigen-presenting genes are prime suspects for

Table 1
Associated Endocrine and Nonendocrine Organ-Specific Autoimmune Disease

Endocrinopathy	Nonendocrine disease
Hashimoto's thyroiditis (and variants)	Pernicious anemia
Graves' (Parry's, Basedow's) disease	Myasthenia gravis
Insulin-dependent diabetes mellitus	Vitiligo
Autoimmune Addison's disease	Sjögren's syndrome
Autoimmune oophoritis and orchitis	Rheumatoid arthritis
Autoimmune hypoparathyroidism	Idiopathic thrombocytopenic purpura
Autoimmune hypophysitis	Disseminated lupus erythematosus
Infertility due to antisperm antibodies	Chronic active hepatitis
	Malabsorption syndrome
	Primary biliary cirrhosis

this role, but this remains to be proved. If so, what is the nature of the genetic abnormality? Do autoantigens constantly have access to, and activate elements of the immune system, such as regulatory cells, in normal individuals? Can a genetic abnormality in antigen-presenting cells be modified by cytokines or other means? What is the role of the target cell: Is it a passive victim to immunological events? Do mutations of autoantigens, e.g., surface receptors, play any role in inducing autoimmunity? Is there a role for microbes and their antigens in the induction of endocrine autoimmunity? What role, if any, does molecular mimicry play? Though there is no compelling evidence for this notion at present, some workers feel that such a possibility is at least attractive. If there is such a role, can it be modified? What is the nature of the variations of antigenic epitope binding by antibodies and T lymphocytes? Are these of genetic or clinical significance? What role do environmental influences have in inducing endocrine autoimmunity? Which environmental influences? Do these all play on the immune system? If so, where and how? How are cytokines coordinated, by what mechanisms, and what are their roles? What are the roles of other ancillary molecules, e.g., ICAM-l, LFA, HSP, CD40, Ctla-4, etc., and what is the sequence of their appearance? What is the precise role of target cell Class I and II expression? What is the impact of present therapies on the immune system, and the mechanisms thereof? What about future immunotherapies? Gene therapy? These and other important questions will undoubtedly keep investigators occupied for a long time to come.

I want to thank all the chapter authors (selected on the basis of their world-renowned expertise in the field) for their warm cooperation throughout this project, and for the high quality of their contributions. I am also indebted to the overall editor of this series, Dr. Michael Conn, particularly for his forebearance, and to Mr. Paul Dolgert and Ms. Debra Koch of Humana Press, for their attention to detail. I am also grateful to Mrs. Josie Thomson for her excellent secretarial assistance.

Finally, I wish to dedicate this volume to the memory of my dear late wife, Ruth, who died suddenly and unexpectedly in 1997. She was my most dedicated and single-minded loving supporter over my entire career, and her absence leaves a void in my life that made it difficult for me to muster the resources to complete this project.

REFERENCES

1. Volpé R. Autoimmunity in the Endocrine System, Monographs in Endocrinology, No. 20, Springer-Verlag, Heidelberg, New York, 1981.
2. Volpé R. Autoimmunity and Endocrine Disease, Marcel Dekker, New York, 1985.
3. Volpé R. Autoimmune Diseases of the Endocrine System. CRC Press, Boca Raton, FL, 1990.

Robert Volpé, MD

DEDICATION

This volume is dedicated with all my heart to my late wife, Ruth Pullan Volpé (1927–1997).

CONTENTS

Preface v
Dedication viii
Contributors xi

1 Normal Mechanisms for Self-Tolerance 1
   Yoshinori Iwatani and Mikio Watanabe

2 Immunoregulation in Experimental Autoimmune
     Endocrine Disease 31
   Peter McCullagh

3 The Genetic Susceptibility to Type 1 (Insulin-Dependent)
     Diabetes Mellitus and the Autoimmune Thyroid Diseases:
     From Epidemiological Observations to Gene Mapping 57
   Yaron Tomer, David A. Greenberg, and Terry F. Davies

4 Experimental Models for Autoimmune Thyroid Disease:
     Recent Developments 91
   Yi-chi M. Kong

5 Animal Models for Insulin-Dependent Diabetes Mellitus 113
   Sabine Bieg and Åke Lernmark

6 The Epidemiology of Autoimmune Thyroid Disease 141
   Mark P. J. Vanderpump and W. Michael G. Tunbridge

7 Sex Hormones and Immune Responses 163
   William J. Kovacs and Nancy J. Olsen

8 Autoantigens in the Autoimmune Endocrinopathies 183
   Jadwiga Furmaniak, Jane Sanders, and Bernard Rees Smith

9 The Immunology of Human Autoimmune Thyroid Disease 217
   Robert Volpé

10 Thyroid-Associated Ophthalmopathy and Dermopathy 245
   Anthony P. Weetman

11 Postpartum Autoimmune Endocrine Syndromes 271
   Nobuyuki Amino, Hisato Tada, and Yoh Hidaka

12 Etiology and Pathogenesis of Human
      Insulin-Dependent Diabetes Mellitus 293
   Jean-François Bach

13 Autoimmune Adrenocortical Failure 309
   Hemmo A. Drexhage

14 Autoimmune Hypophysitis 337
   Shereen Ezzat and Robert G. Josse

15 The Polyglandular Autoimmune Syndromes 349
   Mark Maes and George S. Eisenbarth

16 Autoimmune Endocrinopathies in Female
   Reproductive Dysfunction 365
   Antonio R. Gargiulo and Joseph A. Hill

17 Immunotherapy and Prevention
   of Autoimmune Endocrinopathies 393
   Parth Narendran, Edwin A. M. Gale, and Colin M. Dayan

Index 419

CONTRIBUTORS

Nobuyuki Amino, MD, *Department of Laboratory Medicine, Osaka University Medical School, Suita, Osaka, Japan*

Jean-François Bach, MD, DSc, *INSERM U 25, Hopital Necker, Paris, France*

Sabine Bieg, PhD, *Department of Medicine, University of Washington School of Medicine, Seattle, WA*

Terry F. Davies, MD, FRCP, *Division of Endocrinology and Metabolism, Mt. Sinai Hospital, New York, NY*

Colin M. Dayan, PhD, FRCP, *Division of Diabetes and Metabolism, Department of Medicine, University of Bristol, Southmead Hospital, Bristol, UK*

Hemmo A. Drexhage, MD, PhD, *Department of Immunology, Erasmus University, Rotterdam, The Netherlands*

George S. Eisenbarth, MD, PhD, *Barbara Davis Center for Childhood Diabetes, University of Colorado Health Sciences Center, Denver, CO*

Shereen Ezzat, MD, FRCP(C), *The Mt. Sinai Hospital, University of Toronto, Toronto, Canada*

Jadwiga Furmaniak, MD, PhD, *Endocrine Immunology Unit, University of Wales School of Medicine, Pentwyn, Cardiff, Wales*

Edwin A. M. Gale, MA, FRCP, *Division of Diabetes and Metabolism, Department of Medicine, University of Bristol, Southmead Hospital, Bristol, UK*

Antonio R. Gargiulo, MD, *Division of Reproductive Medicine, Department of Obstetrics, Gynecology, and Reproductive Biology, Brigham and Women's Hospital, Harvard Medical School, Boston, MA*

David A. Greenberg, PhD, *Division of Endocrinology and Metabolism, Mt. Sinai Hospital, New York, NY*

Yoh Hidaka, MD, *Department of Laboratory Medicine, Osaka University Medical School, Suita, Osaka, Japan*

Joseph A. Hill, MD, *Division of Reproductive Medicine, Department of Obstetrics, Gynecology, and Reproductive Biology, Brigham and Women's Hospital, Harvard Medical School, Boston, MA*

Yoshinori Iwatani, MD, PhD, *Department of Clinical Laboratory Science, School of Allied Health Sciences, Faculty of Medicine, Osaka University, Suita, Osaka, Japan*

Robert G. Josse, MD, FRCP(C), *St. Michael's Hospital, University of Toronto, Toronto, Ontario, Canada*

Yi-Chi M. Kong, PhD, *Department of Immunology, Wayne State University School of Medicine, Detroit, MI*

William J. Kovacs, MD, *Department of Medicine, Vanderbilt University School of Medicine, and Department of Veterans Affairs Medical Center, Vanderbilt University School of Medicine, Nashville, Tennessee*

Åke Lernmark, MD, *Department of Medicine, University of Washington School of Medicine, Seattle, Washington*

MARC MAES, MD, PHD, *Barbara Davis Center for Childhood Diabetes, University of Colorado Health Sciences Center, Denver, CO*

PETER MCCULLAGH, MD, DPHIL, MRCP, *Developmental Physiology Group, John Curtin School of Medical Research, The Australian National University, Canberra, Australia*

PARTH NARENDRAN, BSC, MRCP, *Division of Diabetes and Metabolism, Department of Medicine, University of Bristol, Southmead Hospital, Bristol, UK*

NANCY J. OLSEN, MD, *Department of Medicine, Vanderbilt University School of Medicine, and Department of Veterans Affairs Medical Center, Vanderbilt University School of Medicine, Nashville, Tennessee*

BERNARD REES SMITH, BSC, PHD, DSC, *Endocrine Immunology Unit, University of Wales School of Medicine, Pentwyn, Cardiff, Wales*

JANE SANDERS, BSC, PHD, *Endocrine Immunology Unit, University of Wales School of Medicine, Pentwyn, Cardiff, Wales*

HISATO TADA, MD, *Department of Laboratory Medicine, Osaka University Medical School, Suita, Osaka, Japan*

YARON TOMER, MD, *Division of Endocrinology and Metabolism, Mt. Sinai Hospital, New York, NY*

W. MICHAEL G. TUNBRIDGE, MD, FRCP, *Department of Postgraduate Medical Education, Medical School Offices, John Radcliffe Hospital, Oxford University and Region, Oxford, UK*

MARK P. J. VANDERPUMP, MD, MRCP, *North Middlesex Hospital Trust, London, UK*

ROBERT VOLPÉ, MD, FRCP(C), FACP, FRCP, *Division of Endocrinology, Department of Medicine, The Wellesley Hospital, University of Toronto, Toronto, Ontario, Canada*

MIKIO WATANABE, MD, PHD, *Department of Clinical Laboratory Science, School of Allied Health Sciences, Faculty of Medicine, Osaka University, Suita, Osaka, Japan*

ANTHONY P. WEETMAN, MD, DSC, *University of Sheffield Clinical Sciences Centre, Northern General Hospital, Sheffield, UK*

1 Normal Mechanisms for Self-Tolerance

*Yoshinori Iwatani, MD, PhD,
and Mikio Watanabe, MD, PhD*

CONTENTS
> INTRODUCTION
> IMMUNE SYSTEM
> T-CELL TOLERANCE
> B-CELL TOLERANCE
> AUTOIMMUNITY
> CONCLUSIONS
> REFERENCES

INTRODUCTION

The immune system is confronted with a variety of molecules, and it recognizes them as either self or nonself (foreign), taking action against the latter only. The repertoire of receptors on immune cells that recognize at least more than 10^8 foreign antigens is not destined by the genetic information encoded in the genome. This repertoire is randomly formed by gene rearrangement and so on during the development of immune cells. As a result, an enormously wide repertoire (about 10^{15} diversity) of receptors is acquired *(1,2)*. This random mechanism of gene rearrangement, however, produces many receptors that react with self-antigens. Self-reactive immune cells are eliminated (negatively selected) during the development of T lymphocytes in the thymus and of B lymphocytes in the bone marrow *(3–11)*. Only immune cells that react with foreign antigen strongly, but with self-antigen very weakly are positively selected and compose the repertoire of peripheral immune cells. This is the reason why immune cells do not react with self and only attack nonself. This selection mechanism of immune cells in thymus or bone marrow is termed "central tolerance." The mechanism of central immunological tolerance that deletes self-reactive immune cells is not complete, and a part of self-reactive immune cells escape to the periphery. However, such self-reactive immune cells do not function in the periphery of normal subjects. They are positively managed in the periphery by the fail-safe mechanism against autoimmunity *(12–15)*, and are eliminated *(16–21)*, rendered unresponsive *(22–25)*, or suppressed *(26–35)*. This mechanism is termed "peripheral tolerance." The failure in these mechanisms of immunological self-tolerance may involve the induction of autoimmune disease *(12,14,15)*.

From: *Contemporary Endocrinology: Autoimmune Endocrinopathies*
Edited by: R. Volpe © Humana Press Inc., Totowa, NJ

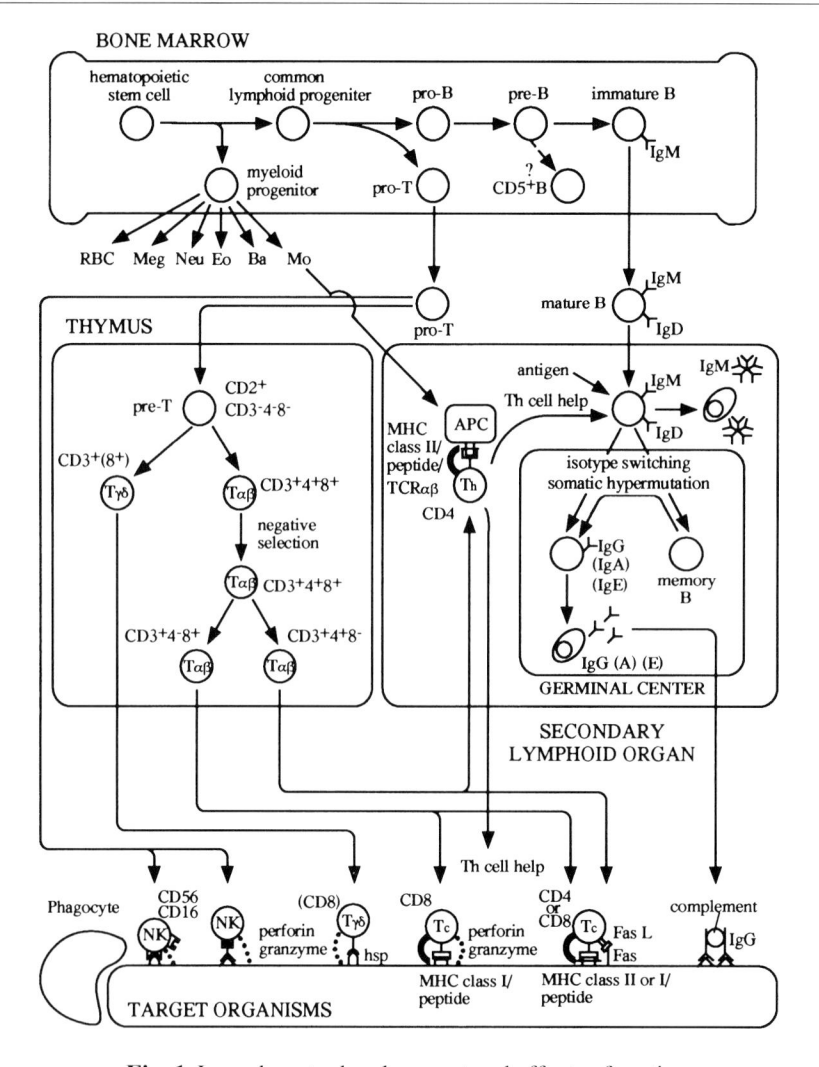

Fig. 1. Lymphocyte development and effector functions.

IMMUNE SYSTEM

Lymphocyte Development and Immune Responses

The immune system is composed of cells within the lymphoreticular organs, which include the primary lymphoid organs, such as bone marrow and thymus, and the secondary lymphoid organs, such as spleen, lymph nodes, and mucosa-associated lymphoid tissues (Fig. 1). T and B lymphocytes are the fundamental and predominant immune cells, and both of them originate from the common lymphoid progenitors that originate from the hematopoietic stem cell, together with the myeloid progenitor *(36)*.

T-lymphocyte precursors (pro-T cells) differentiate in the bone marrow, migrate to the thymus, and undergo the maturation and differentiation within the thymic microenvironment *(37,38)*. At the earliest stages of development, they express several T-cell surface molecules, such as CD2, but still have germline configurations of their T-cell receptor (TCR) genes. Thymocytes destined to become T cells with α/β chains of TCR

(Tαβ cells) pass through a critical CD4⁺CD8⁺ phase, during which self-reactive T cells are deleted by negative selection. Then, CD4⁺CD8⁺ Tαβ cells differentiate into either mature CD4⁺CD8⁻ or CD4⁻CD8⁺ Tαβ cells. A small portion of CD4⁻CD8⁻ thymocytes develops into T cells with γ/δ chains of TCR (Tγδ cells), which can be either CD4⁻CD8⁻ or CD4⁻CD8⁺ *(39)*. Tαβ lymphocytes then emigrate from the thymus, populate the T-cell areas of peripheral lymphoid organs, and exhibit their functions as helper T (Th) cells, cytotoxic T (Tc) cells, and so on.

B lymphocytes (pro-B, pre-B, and immature B cells) mature and differentiate in the bone marrow, and migrate to the B-cell areas of peripheral lymphoid organs *(40)*. Then, a part of mature B lymphocytes are activated, proliferated, and differentiated to become plasma cells producing IgM antibodies on stimulation with antigen and helper factors (Th-cell help). These helper factors are derived from activated CD4⁺ Th cells that are stimulated by professional antigen-presenting cells (APCs), such as macrophages, dendritic cells, and so on *(41)*. Most of the other proliferating B cells that do not differentiate into plasma cells instead revert to the resting state to become memory B cells, and survive for years within lymphoid follicles *(42)*. When memory B cells are further activated and proliferated, two types of genetic processes, that is, isotype switching (class switching) and somatic hypermutation, occur frequently to increase the diversity in effector function and specificity of immunoglobulins, respectively. Then, plasma cells secreting IgG, IgA, or IgE antibodies with higher affinity to their target antigen are produced in the germinal centers of secondary lymphoid organs and migrate to the bone marrow to secrete large amounts of immunoglobulins derived from the same genes *(41)*.

The original role of the immune system is the recognition and disposal of foreign or nonself materials that enter the body, such as life-threatening infectious microbes *(43,44)* (Fig. 1). There are several mechanisms to dispose of or kill such foreign organisms: in innate immunity, phagocytosis by phagocytes, such as neutrophils (Neu), monocytes (Mo), macrophages (Mφ), dendritic cells, and so on, and cytotoxicity by natural killer (NK) cells; and in adaptive immunity, antibody-dependent, complement-mediated cytotoxicity, antibody-dependent, cell-mediated cytotoxicity (ADCC) by NK cells with IgG-Fc receptors (CD16), cytotoxicity by Tγδ cells that recognize heat-shock protein (hsp) on target cells/organisms, and cytotoxicity by CD8⁺ or CD4⁺ Tc cells *(45,46)*. CD8⁺ Tc cells are activated by the recognition of specific antigenic peptides bound to class I major histocompatibility complex (MHC) molecules on target cells/organisms and IL-2 (Th-cell help) from nearby activated CD4⁺ Th cells, and kill the target by either secreting cytotoxins (perforin and granzyme) or by inducing apoptosis through the Fas-FasL contact. CD4⁺ Tc cells are activated by the recognition of specific antigenic peptides bound to class II MHC molecules on the target and IL-2 from nearby activated CD4⁺ Th cells, and kill the target by inducing apoptosis through the Fas-FasL contact. By using these cytotoxic mechanisms, the immune system destroys foreign substances in the body.

Antigen Presentation

Processing and presentation of the foreign antigens to T lymphocytes by APCs is an initial step in adaptive immunity *(47–49)* (Fig. 2). T cells recognize antigenic peptides, which are broken down into short peptides in APCs and are then displayed in association with MHC molecules on their surface. Therefore, this characteristic of T cell recognition is said to be MHC-restricted *(50,51)*. MHC class I molecules present peptides derived from endogenous antigens, such as self-antigens, or pathogens that have access to the

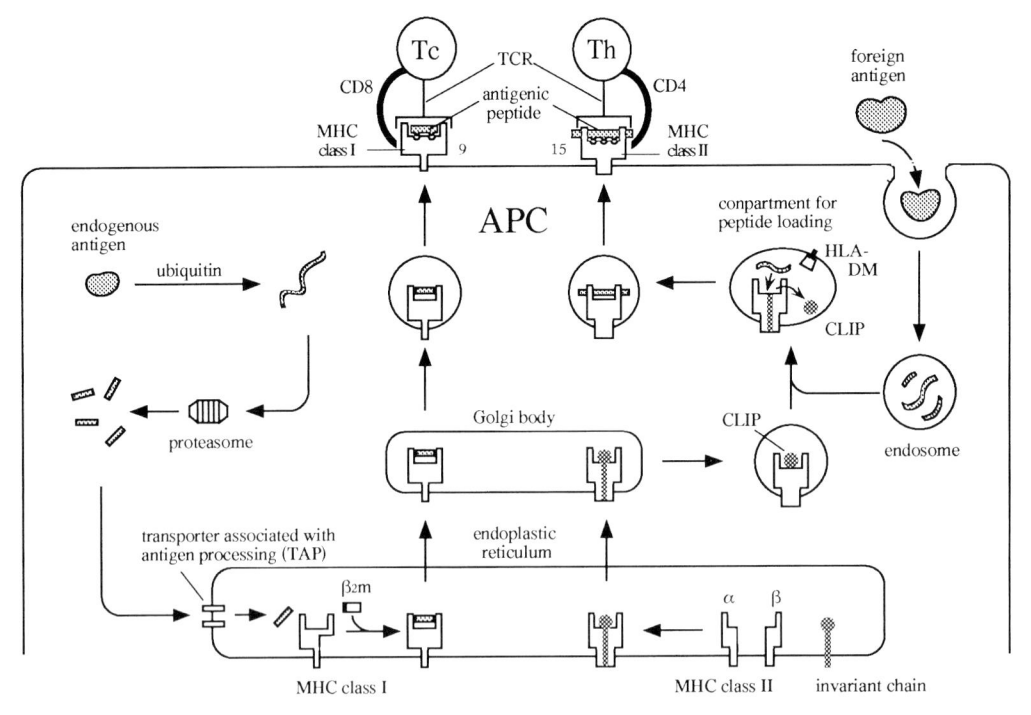

Fig. 2. Antigen presentation.

cytosolic compartment of cells (e.g., viruses), to CD8+ Tc cells, whereas MHC class II molecules present peptides derived from antigens that reside extracellularly and are internalized by endocytosis (e.g., bacteria) to CD4+ Th cells.

Human MHC, which is called human leukocyte antigen (HLA) complex, locates on the short arm of chromosome 6, and divides into three separate regions, class I, class II, and class III genes *(52–54)*. The class I (Ia) region encodes HLA-A, HLA-B, and HLA-C loci, the class Ib region encodes HLA-E, HLA-F, and HLA-G loci, and the class Ic region encodes genes for CD1, FcRn, zinc-α_2-glycoprotein (ZAG), and so on. The class II region encodes HLA-DP, HLA-DQ, and HLA-DR loci, and the genes related to the antigen processing, transport, and presentation, such as proteasome components and transporter associated with antigen processing (TAP). The class III region encodes genes for tumor necrosis factors α and β (TNF-α and TNF-β), complement factors C2, C4, B, and F, hsp, and 21-hydroxylase. Class III products are not involved in antigen presentation to conventional T (T$\alpha\beta$) cells.

Mouse MHC, which is called H-2, locates on chromosome 17, is also divided into three separate regions (class I, class II, and class III genes), and is closely analogous to HLA *(53)*. The class I (Ia) region encodes H-2D, H-2K, and H-2L loci, the class Ib genes map telomerically to the H-2D, H-K, and H-L loci in regions called H-2Q(Qa), H-2T(Tla), and H-2M, and the class Ic genes encode CD1 and FcRn. The class II region encodes I-A and I-E loci, and the genes encoded in the class III region are similar to those in HLA complex. I-A and I-E molecules in mice are similar to HLA-DQ and HLA-DR molecules, respectively, in humans, in molecular homology. However, the relationships in the amounts of their expression on cell surfaces are opposite; I-A > I-E in mice, and DR > DQ in human.

MHC class I (Ia) antigens are found on all somatic cells, whereas MHC class Ib antigens are expressed only on some cell types, e.g., HLA-F on fetal livers, and HLA-G on placenta *(55,56)*. CD1 molecules are expressed on Langerhans cells, dendritic cells, macrophages, and B cells. MHC class II antigens are also constitutively expressed on dendritic cells, macrophages, and B cells, which are called professional APCs. Virtually all types of cells, except mature erythrocytes, express MHC class II antigens under particular conditions, e.g., after stimulation with interferon γ (IFN-γ) *(15,57–59)*.

An endogenous cytosolic protein is coupled covalently to ubiquitin with the sine residue, followed by addition of multiple ubiquitin molecules to the first ubiquitin (Fig. 2). This covalent coupling appears to signal ATP-dependent proteolysis of the target protein by 26S proteasomes to degrade unnecessary proteins roughly *(60–62)*. Then, small polypeptide chains generated seem to be further degraded by PA28 proteasome activator–20S proteasome complexes to peptides with adequate lengths for MHC class I-restricted antigen presentation *(63)*. IFN-γ induces replacements of the proteasomal subunits X, Y, and Z in 26S proteasomes by LMP7, LMP2, and LMP10, respectively, to produce 20S proteasomes that perhaps function more appropriate for the processing of endogenous antigens *(64)*. Furthermore, the PA28 proteasome activator (11S) is also induced greatly by IFN-γ. The 20S proteasome can associate at both ends of the cylindrical structure with the PA28 activator complex that enhances the cleavage of short peptide substrates, but not the cleavage of ubiquitinated proteins *(65)*. Antigenic peptides generated by the PA28-20S proteasome complex are then translocated by TAP to the endoplastic reticulum, where MHC class I molecules await them for binding *(66,67)*. In endoplastic reticulum, the peptides of 8–10 amino acids bind in the binding grooves of newly assembled MHC class I-$β_2$ microglobulin ($β_2$m) dimers *(68–71)*. Then, the MHC class I–peptide complex is transported through the Golgi complex directly to the cell surface for presentation to CD8$^+$ Tc cells *(72,73)*.

A foreign antigen that resides extracellularly is internalized in professional APCs by endocytosis. There are three possible mechanisms involved in the generation of antigenic peptides. First, antigens might be degraded by proteases in the endolysosomes, and the peptides might be transported into the compartments for peptide loading on MHC class II molecules. Second, antigens might be internalized in the compartments for peptide loading directly and be degraded there. Third, antigens might bind to the MHC class II molecules after which degradation by exopeptidases would generate the proper epitopes *(74)*.

The MHC class II molecules consist of an ab heterodimer that assembles in the endoplastic reticulum with a third molecule, the invariant chain (Ii) *(71)*. After transport to the Golgi body, the MHC class II–Ii complex is targeted to the endosome owing to sorting signals present in the Ii cytoplasmic tail *(75)*. In the endosome, an ab heterodimer further makes a complex with an Ii-derived peptide that is termed a class II-associated invariant chain peptide (CLIP). A CLIP is generated by limited proteolysis of Ii. In the compartment for peptide loading that is made up by fusion of endosomes, including the MHC class II–CLIP complex or antigenic peptides, a CLIP is exchanged for antigenic peptides of 10–34 amino acids (mostly 15 amino acids) under the control of HLA-DM molecules *(76,77)*. Peptide binding to MHC class II molecules is fundamentally different from MHC class I peptide binding *(69,78)*. MHC class II-associated peptides extend beyond the binding groove at both ends in MHC class II molecules. The nine residues of the peptide are located within the binding groove *(79)*. MHC class II–peptide complexes are then transported to the cytoplasm membrane, where they can be recognized by CD4$^+$ Th cells.

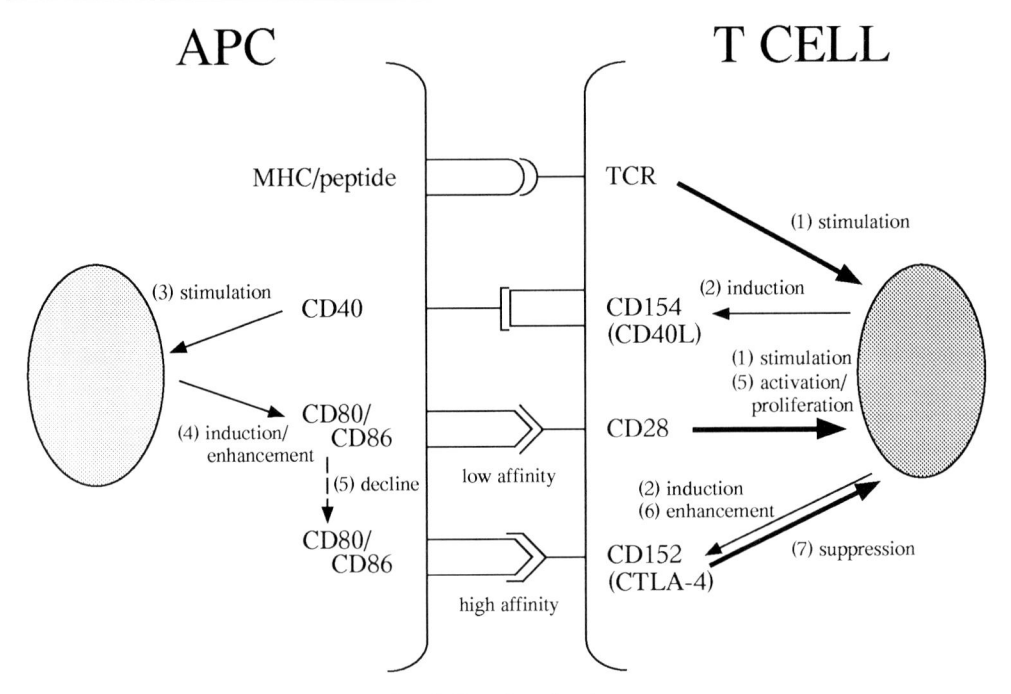

Fig. 3. T-cell activation.

In general, MHC class I molecules present peptides derived from endogenous antigens, such as self-antigens, or pathogens that have access to the cytosolic compartment of cells (e.g., viruses) to $CD8^+$ Tc cells, whereas MHC class II molecules present peptides derived from antigens that reside extracellularly and are internalized by endocytosis (e.g., bacteria), to $CD4^+$ Th cells. However, bone marrow-derived APCs in the regional lymph node can present a "foreign antigen" that is a specific antigen derived from the cell membrane of a nearby differentiated organ, in association with the MHC class I molecules *(80)*. Aggregated proteins *(81)*, proteins that are endocytosed with a large, indigestible particle *(82)*, and proteins that are excessively endocytosed by cytokine stimulation *(83)* are easily presented partially by MHC class I molecules. Furthermore, MHC class II molecules also bind peptides derived from many membrane-bound self-antigens as well as foreign antigens *(69)*. These self-antigenic peptides also form complexes with MHC class II molecules in the compartment for peptide loading *(84)*.

T-Cell Activation

Optimal activation of naive antigen-specific T cells requires at least two signals *(85–87)* (Fig. 3). One is the TCR signal that is provided by the interaction between the T-cell receptors on antigen-specific T cells and the antigenic peptide–MHC complexes on APCs. The other is the costimulatory signal that is delivered by the interaction between the costimulatory molecule CD28 on T cells and its ligands, CD80 (B7, B7-1) and CD86 (B70, B7-2), on APCs *(88–91)*. These two signals induce the activation and proliferation of T cells, the synthesis of interleukin 2 (IL-2) by T cells, and the expression of the anti-apoptotic protein Bcl-xL on T cells *(92)*. CD28 is expressed on the majority of T cells *(88,93)*. CD80 is expressed primarily on dendritic cells, but is expressed at low or undetectable levels on resting APCs and lymphocytes. However, CD86 is constitutively expressed at moderate levels on resting APCs, such as dendritic cells and B cells *(94–96)*. Both CD80 and CD86 molecules are upregulated on activation, but CD86 is upregulated rapidly and maintained strongly from 24 to 96 h after stimulation. On the other hand, the expression time of CD80 is short, between 48 and 72 h after activation *(94–96)*.

Interaction between CD154 (CD40 ligand [CD40L]) on T cells and CD40 on APCs is also important for T-cell activation *(97,98)*. CD154–CD40 interaction (CD40 ligation) induces or enhances the expression of both CD80 and CD86 on APCs *(99,100)*. CD40 ligation of monocytes and dendritic cells also results in the secretion of multiple cytokines, such as IL-1, IL-6, IL-8, IL-10, IL-12, TNF-α, and so on *(101)*. T-cell activation through the CD28 ligation enhances the expression of CD154 on T cells *(102,103)*. CD154 is mainly expressed on activated CD4$^+$ T cells, and also expressed on basophils, eosinophils, activated B cells, and blood dendritic cells *(104)*. CD40 expression is much broader, and found on monocytes, dendritic cells, hematopoietic progenitors, endothelial cells, and epithelial cells *(104)*.

The CD28 homolog cytotoxic T-lymphocyte antigen-4 (CTLA-4, CD152) functions to suppress T-cell responses *(105–109)*. CD152 is expressed at low or undetectable levels on resting T cells, and appears to be upregulated by the CD28 ligation and/or IL-2 *(110,111)*. Its expression peaks at 48–72 h after stimulation *(105,110,111)*. CD28 and CD152 share the same counterreceptors, CD80 and CD86, on APCs. However, CD152 has a 20-fold higher affinity than CD28 for their ligands *(112,113)*. Moreover, CD152 appears to bind CD80 with a higher affinity and a slower off-rate than CD86 *(114)*.

Therefore, the mechanisms for T-cell activation may be summarized as follows (Fig. 3): an antigen-specific signal through the MHC–peptide–TCR interaction with a costimulatory signal of CD28 ligation with CD86 molecules stimulates T cells to induce the expression of CD154 and CD152 on the T cells. Binding of CD154 on T cells with CD40 on APCs induces or enhances the expression of CD80/CD86 molecules on APCs. Then, the CD80/CD86 molecules bind to CD28 on T cells more strongly to activate and proliferate T cells, which function as effector cells. T-cell activation also enhances the expression of CD152 on T cells. Since the avidity of CD152 for CD80/CD86 is higher than CD28, CD80/CD86 molecules bind preferentially to CD152 on activated T cells, which in turn suppresses the function of T cells.

B-Cell Activation

The activation of naive antigen-specific B-cells and their differentiation into antibody-secreting cells also require two signals as well as those of T cells (Fig. 4). Naive B cells are triggered by antigens and also require accessory signals that come from activated Th cells. In some antigens, naive B cells obtain accessory signals directly from antigen constituents. The former type of antigen that stimulates antibody production in the presence of MHC class II-restricted T-cell help is called thymus-dependent (TD) antigen *(41)*. The latter type is called thymus-independent (TI) antigen, which is further divided into two categories, TI type1 (TI-1) and TI type 2 (TI-2) *(115)*. TD antigens consist of soluble proteins or peptides, TI-1 antigens consist of lipopolysaccharides from Gram-negative bacterial cell walls, and TI-2 antigens consist of polysaccharides from bacterial cell wall, or polymeric protein structures.

Th cells also control isotype switching and initiate somatic hypermutation of antibody-variable region genes of B cells *(116,117)*. The interaction between CD40 and

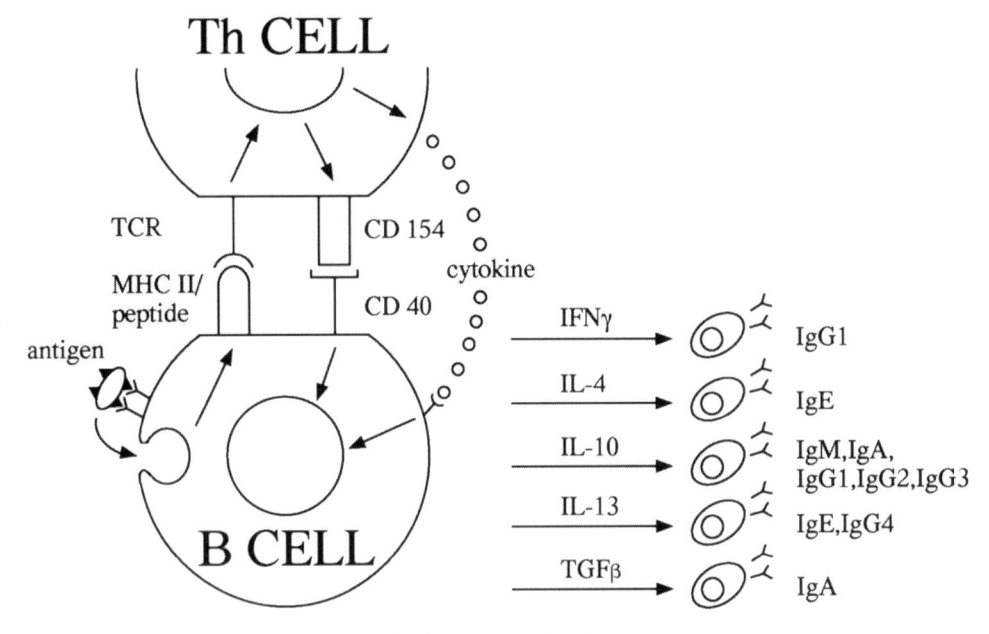

Fig. 4. B-cell activation.

CD154 and the cytokine produced by Th cells are necessary for isotype switching of antibody-producing cells and also for the formation of germinal centers in the secondary lymphoid organs. In human, IFN-γ induces switching to IgG1. IL-4 is a switch factor for the IgE in CD40-activated B cells; IL-10 is for the IgM, IgA, IgG1, IgG2, and IgG3; IL-13 is for the IgE and IgG4; and TGF-β is for the IgA *(118,119)* (Fig. 4). The immunoglobulin isotype switch is critical for the generation of functional diversity of a humoral immune response. Somatic hypermutation, which is an unusually frequent point mutation undergone in the genes of immunoglobulin-variable region during the course of an immune response, is necessary for the affinity maturation of antibodies. Therefore, antibodies produced later in an immune response tend to have higher affinity for the target antigen than those produced earlier.

TI-1 antigens have the property that they activate most of both specific and nonspecific B cells, so they are called polyclonal B-cell activators *(115)*. TI-1 antigens also stimulate macrophages to produce cytokines, such as IL-1 and tumor necrosis factor α (TNF-α), which augment immune responses. TI-2 antigens possess the properties embodied by polysaccharide antigens, such as large molecular weight, repeating antigenic epitopes, ability to activate the complement cascade, poor in vivo degradability, and inability to stimulate MHC class II-dependent T-cell help *(115)*.

T-CELL TOLERANCE

Central T-Cell Tolerance

T lymphocytes develop from bone-marrow-derived pro-T cells that mature in the thymus *(38,120)* (Fig. 5). Early in development, thymocytes (pre-T cells) express pre-TCR and CD2, which are characteristic of the T-cell lineage, but they lack other T-cell-surface molecules, such as CD4 and CD8, and thus, are known as double-

Chapter 1 / Self-Tolerance

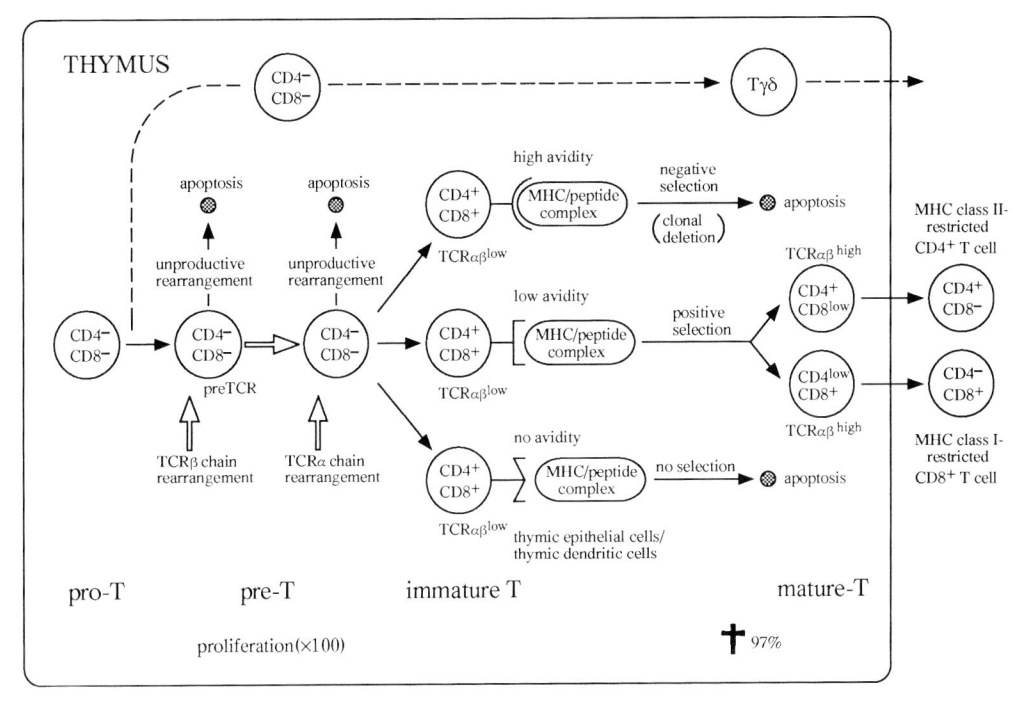

Fig. 5. Central T-cell tolerance.

negative (CD4⁻CD8⁻) thymocytes. Rearrangement of the TCR genes occurs at this double-negative stage. Thymocytes (pre-T cells) that are destined to become Tαβ cells rearrange the TCRβ gene first, and then the α gene. If unproductive rearrangements of TCR genes, which lead to the formation of nonfunctional TCRβ and/or α proteins, occur at this stage, thymocytes are programmed to die by apoptosis *(121–123)*. If rearrangements lead to the formation of functional TCRα and β proteins, thymocytes express TCRαβ, which is a dimer of TCRα and β proteins, and CD3 molecules at low levels on the cell surface. The thymocytes (immature T cells) also express both CD4 and CD8 at this time of development, and are called double-positive (CD4⁺CD8⁺) thymocytes. At the transition stage from double-negative to double-positive thymocytes, they proliferate markedly about 100-fold. Positive and negative selections of thymocytes occur at the stage of double-positive (CD4⁺CD8⁺) T cells on the basis of the avidity of their TCRαβ to recognize antigenic peptides in association with self-MHC molecules (MHC–peptide complexes) on thymic epithelial cells/thymic dendritic cells *(124,125)*. Positive selection occurs in the thymic cortex, where developing CD4⁺CD8⁺ immature thymocytes encounter epithelial cells that express both class I and class II MHC molecules loaded with self-peptides, and induces the differentiation of CD4⁺CD8⁺ immature thymocytes into CD4⁺CD8⁻ or CD4⁻CD8⁺ mature thymocytes that mount immune response on foreign antigenic peptides bound to self-MHC molecules in the periphery *(126–132)*. Negative selection appears to takes place in the thymic medulla, where thymocytes migrate from the cortex. There, CD4⁺CD8⁺ immature thymocytes encounter bone-marrow-derived dendritic cells and macrophages, as well as thymic medullary epithelial cells that express both class I and class II MHC molecules loaded with self-peptides. Then thymocytes bearing TCRs specific for self-peptides bound to self-MHC molecules are deleted

(3–11,133,134). At least 97% of developing T cells undergo apoptosis within the thymus. After the selections, positively selected thymocytes increase the expression of TCRαβ, lose the expression of either CD4 or CD8, and become mature single-positive T cells. Then, T cells with the phenotype of mature peripheral T cells exit the thymus to the periphery. Mature CD4+ T cells are activated in the periphery in an MHC class II-restricted fashion, and CD8+ T cells in an MHC class I-restricted fashion.

The conceptual paradox between positive and negative selection may be explained by a differential avidity model in which the fate of T cells is determined by the cell-surface density of MHC–peptide complexes as well as the intrinsic affinity of TCRs for the ligands *(135–137)*. Therefore, the avidity of T cells to the MHC–peptide complexes on thymic medullary dendritic cells or epithelial cells reflects both the number of TCRs engaged and their affinity for binding the MHC–peptide complex. According to the avidity model, T cells with high avidity to the MHC–peptide complexes would thus be eliminated (negative selection), whereas T cells with low avidity to the MHC–peptide complexes would be positively selected. If the avidity is zero or very low, T cells would not be selected and not have an effective signal to survive. The biochemical factor that constitutes the critical difference between the survival signal delivered by low avidity of TCR binding and the apoptotic signal triggered by high-avidity interactions is still unknown, but considerable evidence for the avidity model is accumulating. The cell-surface density of a single MHC class I–peptide complex affects the fate of CD8+ T cells expressing the transgenic TCR *(136,138)*. Also, the cell surface density of a single MHC class II–peptide complex affects the fate of CD4+ T cells *(139)*. Furthermore, in vitro experiment suggests that the qualitative difference in the recognition of MHC–peptide complex by TCRs, probably owing to the difference in kinetics or conformational change in the interaction, affects the fate of T cells *(138)*. Coreceptors CD4 and CD8 also influence thymic selection *(40)*. In addition, it is possible that costimulatory interactions between CD28 and CD80/CD86 *(141)* and between CD154 (CD40L) and CD40 *(142)* and adhesion molecules, such as lymphocyte function-associated antigen-1 (LFA-1) *(143)*, are also involved in preferential deletion of self-reactive thymocytes (negative selection) in the medullary region of the thymus.

Peripheral T-Cell Tolerance

The diversity of TCRαβ theoretically reaches 10^{15} by random rearrangement of five TCR gene segments and random nucleotide addition *(20)*. Therefore, undesirable T cells with TCRs specific for self-peptides–self-MHC complexes are also produced by the gene rearrangement, but most autoreactive T cells are deleted in the thymic medulla by encountering peptides derived from ubiquitously expressed self-antigens or circulating self-antigens in association with the self-MHC molecules. However, not all of the self-peptides, including those derived from proteins expressed in a highly tissue-specific fashion in organs, such as endocrine organs and nerve tissues, would be presented to thymocytes during their development in the thymus. Furthermore, a threshold in the deletion of autoreactive T cells is dictated with various factors that determine the affinity of the TCR for its MHC–peptide ligand. Some autoreactive T cells that do not reach to the threshold may not be deleted in the thymus. It is known, indeed, that negative selection is not 100% effective and that some potentially autoreactive T cells especially specific for peripheral tissue antigens do escape to the periphery *(144)*. T-cell tolerance is thus

Chapter 1 / Self-Tolerance

Fig. 6. Peripheral T-cell tolerance.

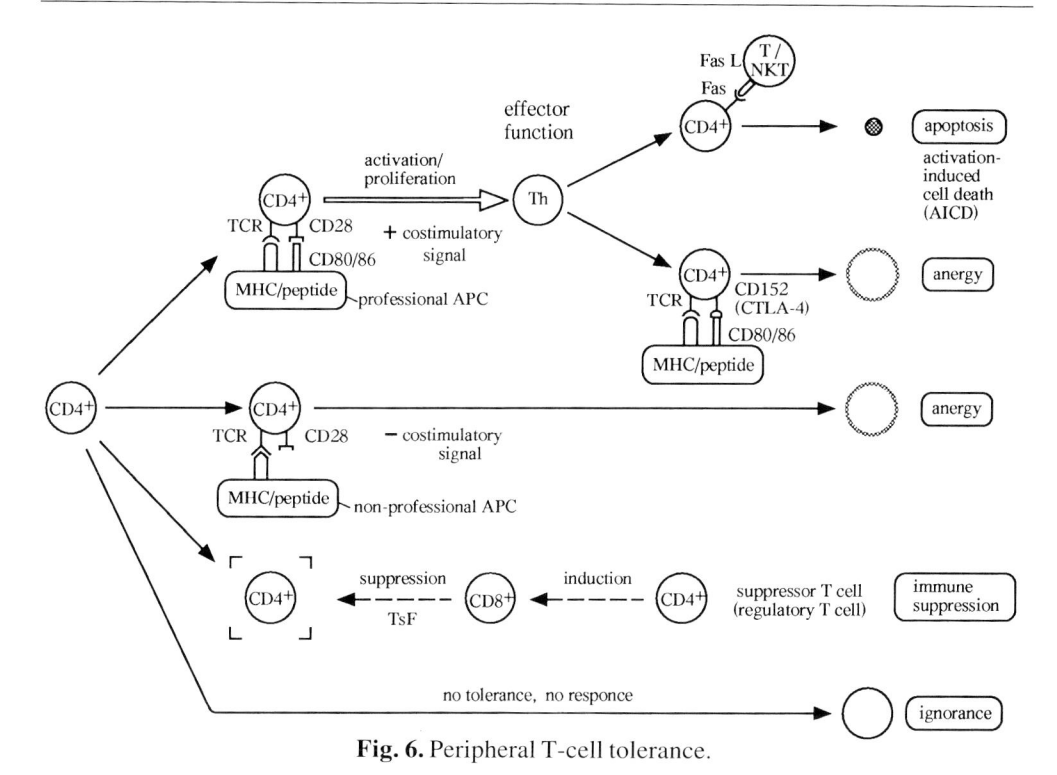

achieved by several complementary mechanisms arranged in a fail-safe manner, not only in the thymus, but also in the periphery. The latter is called peripheral T-cell tolerance.

The peripheral immune system can maintain tolerance to self-antigens through a variety of mechanisms (Fig. 6). Clonal deletion (apoptosis) of autoreactive T cells escaped from the thymus may play an important role in limiting rapidly expanding responses *(20,21)*, but there are many examples where autoreactive T cells still remain. Therefore, peripheral tolerance may be mainly induced or maintained by the induction of unresponsiveness to the self-antigen (anergy) *(22–25)*, or by the induction of regulatory cells, such as suppressor T cells, to suppress the autoimmune reaction (active suppression) *(26–35)*. A part of autoreactive T cells may never encounter the self-antigen, simply because the antigens are few or normally sequestered from the immune system (ignorance) *(145,146)*. Immune deviation, where noninflammatory Th2 responses could suppress inflammatory Th1 responses, may also induce peripheral tolerance.

Clonal deletion and clonal anergy, which are induced by either superantigens or conventional antigens, are followed by T-cell activation and expansion. Peripheral deletion of T cells occur in part through local apoptosis and in part through migration to the gut and liver *(16–21)*. High antigen dose and chronic stimulation favor the peripheral elimination both in CD4⁺ T and CD8⁺ T cells *(20,21,147)*. Furthermore, the frequency of antigen-specific T cells to be made tolerant is also important in the induction of tolerance by peripheral elimination *(148)*. Therefore, autoreactive T cells specific for very rare self-antigens may be difficult to be adequately deleted. Peripheral T cells express Fas (CD95) antigens on their surface rapidly after activation with TCR stimulation, but are not vulnerable to Fas engagement, because the expression of Bcl-xL that protects against Fas ligation is induced by CD28 ligation during activation *(92)*. From several days after activation, when Bcl-xL has declined, T cells become susceptible to the Fas ligation with the Fas ligand (FasL) on activated T cells, NKT cells, and so on, which induces the apoptosis by further stimulation *(149)*. Fas functions mostly to induce this activation-induced cell death (AICD) in CD4+ T cells *(150)*. Therefore, autoreactive T cells specific for peripheral self-antigens might be deleted by apoptosis induced by continuous stimulation with the self-antigens present abundantly in the periphery. Furthermore, the p75 TNF receptor performs a similar role as Fas in $CD8^+$ T cells and downregulates the proliferation of $CD8^+$ T cells by induction of apoptosis *(151)*. Persistent antigen exposure downregulates the expression of CD8 antigen on $CD8^+$ T cells *(20,152)*, and then induces the apoptosis *(152)*.

On the other hand, CD152 (CTLA-4), which is a homolog of CD28 that binds with higher affinity to CD80/CD86, is induced and enhanced by the interactions of MHC–peptide/TCR and CD80/86/CD28, and functions as a negative regulator of immune responses *(105,111)*, as described above (Fig. 3). Recently, it has been reported that in vivo T-cell anergy may be induced as a result of specific recognition of CD80/CD86 molecules by CD152 (CTLA-4) *(153)*.

Professional APCs activate T cells by providing two signals; one is an antigen-specific signal through the interaction of MHC class II molecule–peptide complexes and TCRs, and another is an activating costimulatory signal through the engagement of the CD28 receptor on T cells by CD80/CD86 of APCs (Fig. 3). However, signaling through the TCR alone induces a state of unresponsiveness (anergy) *(22–25)* (Fig. 6). Professional APCs, such as macrophages, dendritic cells, B cells, and Langerhans cells, express CD80/CD86 on their surface, and can provide a costimulatory signal to T cells. In contrast, most nonhematopoietic cells in the tissues, such as epithelial cells, do not express CD80/CD86 molecules on their surfaces, even when they are stimulated by IFN-γ to induce the expression of MHC class II molecules *(25)*. Therefore, these cells, called nonprofessional APCs, cannot provide a costimulatory signal, and induce anergy in T cells. This two-signal model for T-cell activation may explain the fact that T cells are tolerant or unresponsive to self- (or foreign) antigens presented on peripheral tissues. Another mechanism to induce anergy in T cells is a lack of proliferation signals provided by IL-2, IL-4, and IL-7 when T cells are stimulated with both antigen-specific and costimulatory signals *(25)*.

Autoreactive T cells may be silent and never be activated by encountering the self-antigen, if the antigens are few or normally sequestered from the immune system. There is no response and also no induction of tolerance in autoreactive T cells in this situation, which is called immunological ignorance *(154)*.

Active suppression may be the main mechanism for inducing or maintaining peripheral tolerance to autoantigens *(26–35)*. The concept of antigen-specific suppressor T (Ts) cells and suppressor factors (TsF) is too complicated, so it may be dismissed by some as artifact. Recently, however, the concept of antigen-specific TsF has been mostly clarified *(32,33,155–158)*. To summarize *(33)*:

1. TsF and TCRαβ recognizes a common epitope, representing an external structure of antigen.
2. TsF, which is an antigen-specific glycosylation inhibiting factor (GIF), contains the 55-kDa peptide that has both GIF determinant and TCRα determinant, and possesses GIF bioactivity.
3. The 55-kDa GIF is a product of the TCRα chain cDNA.

4. Ovalbumin- (OVA) specific GIF consists of the 55-kDa GIF and a peptide with TCRβ determinant.
5. The 55-kDa GIF can be released from CD8$^+$, I-J$^+$ Ts cells without association of TCRβ chain.
6. The 55-kDa GIF lacks mRNA, indicating that the peptide is a conjugate of the 13-kDa GIF and TCRα chain.
7. Formation of the 55-kDa GIF is unique for Ts cells, which form bioactive 13-kDa GIF.
8. Bioactive GIF peptide is generated from cytosolic, inactive GIF peptide by posttranslational modification.
9. I-J determinant is generated by posttranslational modification of the GIF peptide, and does not represent a portion of primary amino acid sequence.

There are many reports supporting the presence of antigen-specific suppressor T cells *(27,29–31,34,35,155,159–163)*. The phenotypes of suppressor (regulatory) T cells reported are mainly CD4 *(27,30,159,161)*, but there are several reports that both CD4$^+$ and CD8$^+$ cells mediate active suppression *(31,34,35,155,162,163)*. In in vitro experiments on the antigen-specific suppressor circuit, CD4$^+$ suppressor-inducer T cells induce CD8$^+$ Ts cells to suppress the immune response *(163)*. Therefore, CD4$^+$ suppressor-inducer T cells may induce CD8$^+$ Ts cells continuously in vivo, but CD8$^+$ Ts cells, when injected alone in vivo, may not be enough to induce and maintain the peripheral tolerance to the self-antigens. It is thought that Ts cells exert their suppressive activity via antigen-specific TsF molecules *(32,33,155–158)*. Another possibility is via cytotoxicity, but not all of the Ts clones are cytotoxic *(164)*. The requirements for induction of Ts cells in terms of APCs are apparently different from those required for induction of Th cells. The interactions between APCs and Ts cells are restricted by the antigen in association with either I-E in mice *(165)* or HLA-DQ in humans *(160)*. Organ-specific self-reactive CD4$^+$ cells normally escape from the thymus and potentially retain sufficient TCR sensitivity to be reactivated in the discrete organ, so this reactivity may under different circumstances actively reinforce tolerance or provoke autoimmunity *(144)*. Therefore, these findings may also support the possibility for the induction of Ts cells that nonprofessional APCs, such as epithelial cells, expressing MHC class II molecules on their surface by stimulation with IFN-γ, might activate CD4$^+$ suppressor-inducer T cells specific for the self-antigens on the non-APCs to induce specific CD8$^+$ Ts cells, as well as the induction of clonal anergy in CD4$^+$ Th cells specific for the self-antigens *(12–15)*. Indeed, coculture of autologous T cells with gut epithelial cells expressing class II molecules results in the proliferation of CD8$^+$ T cells with suppressor function *(166)*, and CD4$^+$ tissue-specific suppressor T cells involved in self-tolerance are activated extrathymically by self-antigen *(167,168)*.

Based on the patterns of cytokine synthesis, CD4$^+$ T cells can be classified into at least two populations with different immune regulatory functions *(169–171)* (Fig. 7). Th1 cells, producing IL-2 and IFN-γ, are often associated with cell-mediated immune responses that involve macrophages, such as delayed-type hypersensitivity (DTH), whereas Th2 cells, secreting IL-4, IL-5, IL-6, IL-10, and IL-13, usually provide B-cell help and enhance allergic reactions that involve mast cells and eosinophils *(170,171)*. Naive CD4$^+$ T precursors (Thp) produce IL-2, but not IL-4 or IFN-γ, on antigen stimulation. Repeated stimulation in the presence of IL-12, a macrophage-derived cytokine, causes Th cells to differentiate into Th1 cells, which produce IL-2 and IFN-γ. Stimulation in the presence of IL-4 derived from NKT cells *(172–176)*, on the other hand, promotes the development

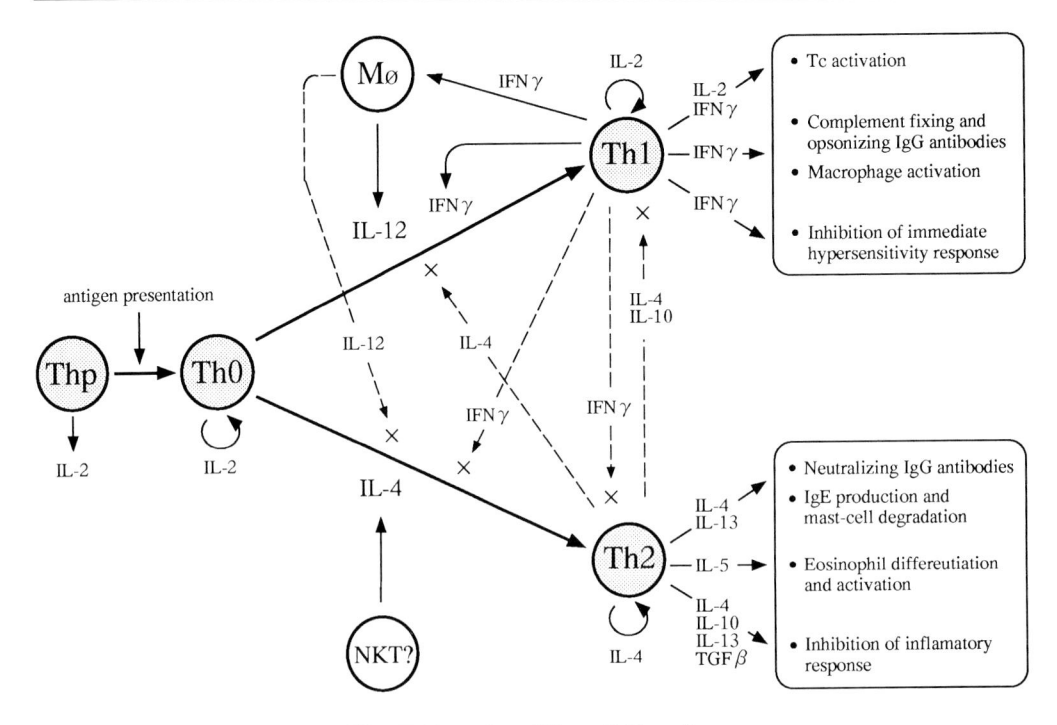

Fig. 7. Type 1 and Type 2 Th cells.

of Th2 cells, which produce IL-4, and so on. The differentiation into either Th1 or Th2 cells probably involves common Th cells (Th0 cells), which produce IL-2, IFN-γ, and IL-4. IFN-γ produced by Th1 cells amplifies Th1 development and inhibits proliferation and function of Th2 cells, whereas IL-4 produced by Th2 cells blocks activation of Th1 cells. IFN-γ produced by Th1 cells stimulates macrophages to produce IL-12, which in turn inhibits proliferation of Th2 cells *(170,171)*. Therefore, Th2 cells regulate the inflammation and tissue injury that may be mediated by Th1 cells and may protect against autoimmune responses *(170,171)*. However, there is a finding that does not support this hypothesis. In NOD mice grafted with skewed Th cell lines derived from mice transgenic for a diabetogenic TCR, Th1 cell lines from these transgenic mice can transfer disease to healthy NOD recipients, but Th2 cell lines derived from these mice are not pathogenic. Cotransfer of Th2 cells with Th1 cells, however, does not protect the recipient mice, even when the Th2 cells are transferred in excess over the Th1 cells *(177)*.

Distinct cytokine patterns have been recently identified in CD8[+] T cells *(178)*. Naive CD8[+] T cells, similar to CD4[+] T cells, can differentiate into at least two subsets of cytolytic effector cells with distinct cytokine patterns: T cytotoxic-1 (Tc1) cells secrete a Th1-like cytokine pattern, including IL-2 and IFN-γ; and Tc2 cells produce Th2 cytokines, including IL-4, IL-5, and IL-10. However, both Tc1 and Tc2 cells induce similar DTH *(179)*.

B-CELL TOLERANCE

Central B-Cell Tolerance

B cells develop from bone-marrow-derived pro-B cells that mature in bone marrow *(40,180,181)* (Fig. 8). Early in development, B cells express pre-B-cell receptor (pre-

Chapter 1 / Self-Tolerance

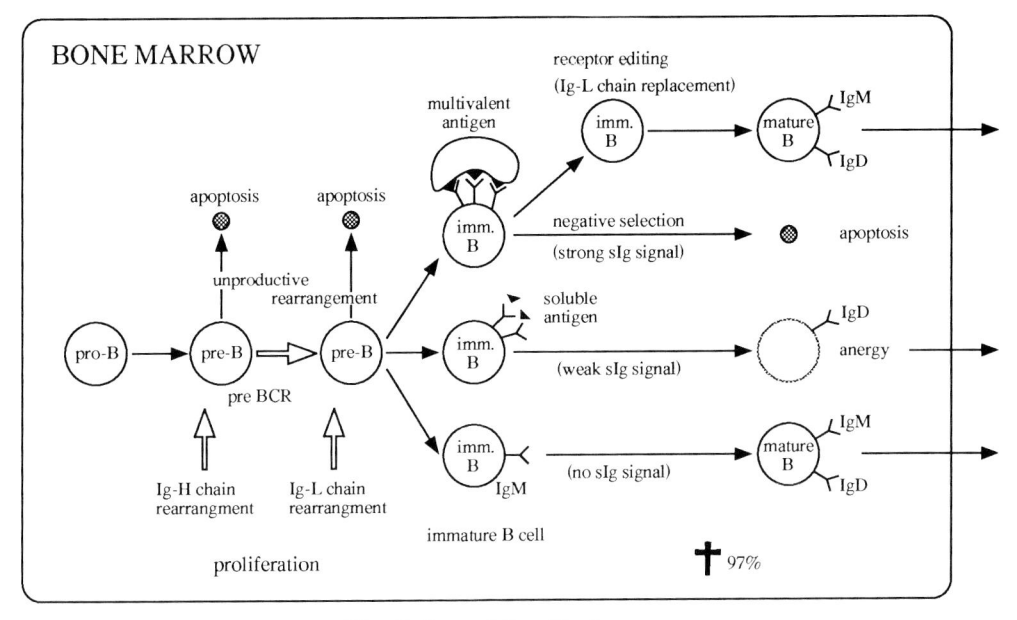

Fig. 8. Central B-cell tolerance.

BCR) and several surface molecules, such as CD19 and CD20, that are characteristic of the B-cell lineage. Rearrangement of the BCR genes occurs at this pre-B-cell stage. Pre-B cells that are destined to become mature B cells rearrange the immunoglobulin-heavy (Ig-H) chain gene first, and then the immunoglobulin-light (Ig-L) chain gene. If unproductive rearrangements of the BCR gene, which lead to the formation of nonfunctional Ig-H and Ig-L chains, occur at this stage, pre-B cells are programmed to die by apoptosis *(182)*. If rearrangement leads to the formation of functional Ig-H and Ig-L chains, pre-B cells become immature B cells expressing IgM, which is a dimer of Ig-H and Ig-L chains, and CD21 on the cell surface. A third of the precursor cells successfully rearrange heavy and light chain genes to become B cells. During rearrangement of Ig-H and Ig-L chains in pre-B cells, they proliferate markedly. However, the random assembly of V, D, and J segments of immunoglobulin genes during B-cell development inevitably produces some B-cell clones whose immunoglobulins recognize self-antigens on normal cells or tissues. Because such autoreactive immunoglobulins are potentially harmful to the self, strict measures are needed to ensure that they are not secreted. Negative selection of autoreactive B cells occurs at the stage of immature B cells on the basis of the avidity of their BCR (surface IgM) to recognize antigens *(10,183,184)*. When immature B cells are specific for multivalent self-antigens present ubiquitously on cell surface, such as MHC class I molecules, immature B cells have high avidity to the antigens, obtain strong signals by crosslinking of the surface immunoglobulin (sIg), and are eliminated by the mechanism of apoptosis (clonal deletion) *(185,186)*. Also, soluble protein antigens, which presumably generate weaker signals through the BCR of a immature B cell, do not cause cell death, but instead make the cell unresponsive to activating stimuli (clonal anergy) *(187,188)*. They migrate to the periphery where they express IgD, but remain anergic. However, anergic B cells can be activated under some circumstances, so clonal anergy is a less absolute mechanism for enforcing tolerance to self. Only immature B cells with no avidity to antigens present in the bone marrow become mature B cells bearing both IgM and IgD on their surface. At least 97% of developing B cells undergo apoptosis or anergy within the bone marrow.

Instead of inducing apoptosis, a part of autoreactive immature B cells resume rearranging their light-chain genes, when their BCRs are strongly crosslinked by multivalent self-antigens on the cell surface (Fig. 8). As a result of this rearrangement, the genes are permanently inactivated, and the autoreactive B cells can then attempt to assemble a new κ or λ gene on one of their other chromosomes. This process has been called receptor editing *(189–191)*. If the original κ chain contributed to recognition of self-antigen, then replacing it with a new light chain may eliminate autoreactivity. In that case, it is believed that the cell can resume maturation, shut off its recombinase activity, and eventually be released from the bone marrow. If receptor editing fails, the autoreactive B cell remains arrested in the undifferentiated state and eventually dies.

Peripheral B-Cell Tolerance

The mechanisms of apoptosis and receptor editing occurring in immature B cells would be effective only for eliminating cells that recognize self-antigens found in the bone marrow, such as serum proteins and ubiquitous cell-surface or extracellular matrix proteins. Many other self-antigens, however, are found only outside the bone marrow, and for these antigens a different mechanism is needed to ensure B-cell tolerance. This mechanism acts only on mature B cells in peripheral tissues and relies on the fact that B-cell activation by most protein antigens requires the participation of Th cells (Fig. 9).

Without an antigenic signal through the BCR, mature B cells are eliminated by activated T cells through the interactions between CD40 and CD154 (CD40L) and between Fas and FasL molecules on their surfaces *(192–194)*. Without appropriate T-cell help, antigenic stimulation through BCR induces either apoptosis or anergy in mature B cells *(195,196)*. The fate of the B cell depends on the physical nature of the antigen involved. Membrane-bound or particulate antigens induce the apoptosis, and soluble protein antigens, which presumably generate weaker signals through the BCR, induce the anergy *(196–198)*. Mature B cells internalize antigen, process it, and present antigenic peptides to T cells in association with MHC class II molecules, thereby activating T cells to induce CD154 (CD40L) on their surface. Before induction of CD154 molecules on an activated T cell, when CD40 ligation with CD154 is absent, a mature B cell becomes a plasma cell producing IgM after stimulation with antigen and cytokine *(199,200)*. In the presence of CD40 ligation with CD154 on an activated T cell, an antigen-stimulated mature B cell becomes a plasma cell producing a different isotype of Ig, such as IgG, IgA, or IgE, in the germinal center of a lymphoid organ under appropriate cytokine stimulation (isotype switching) *(201-203)* (Fig. 4). Furthermore, somatic hypermutation in the Ig variable region genes of such a mature B cell, which changes the affinity and specificity of BCRs, also occurs in the germinal center *(202,204)*. After somatic hypermutation, mutants with low-affinity antigen receptors die by apoptosis owing to their failure to bind antigens on follicular dendritic cells (FDCs). A few mutants with improved high-affinity antigen receptors bind antigen on FDCs. These cells internalize antigen, process it, and present antigenic peptides to T cells in association with MHC class II molecules. Then, T cells are activated and induce the expression of CD154 on their surface *(205)*. Probably before induction of CD154 molecules on an activated T cell, when CD40 ligation with CD154 is absent, a mature B cell becomes a plasma cell producing high-affinity IgG, IgA, or IgE

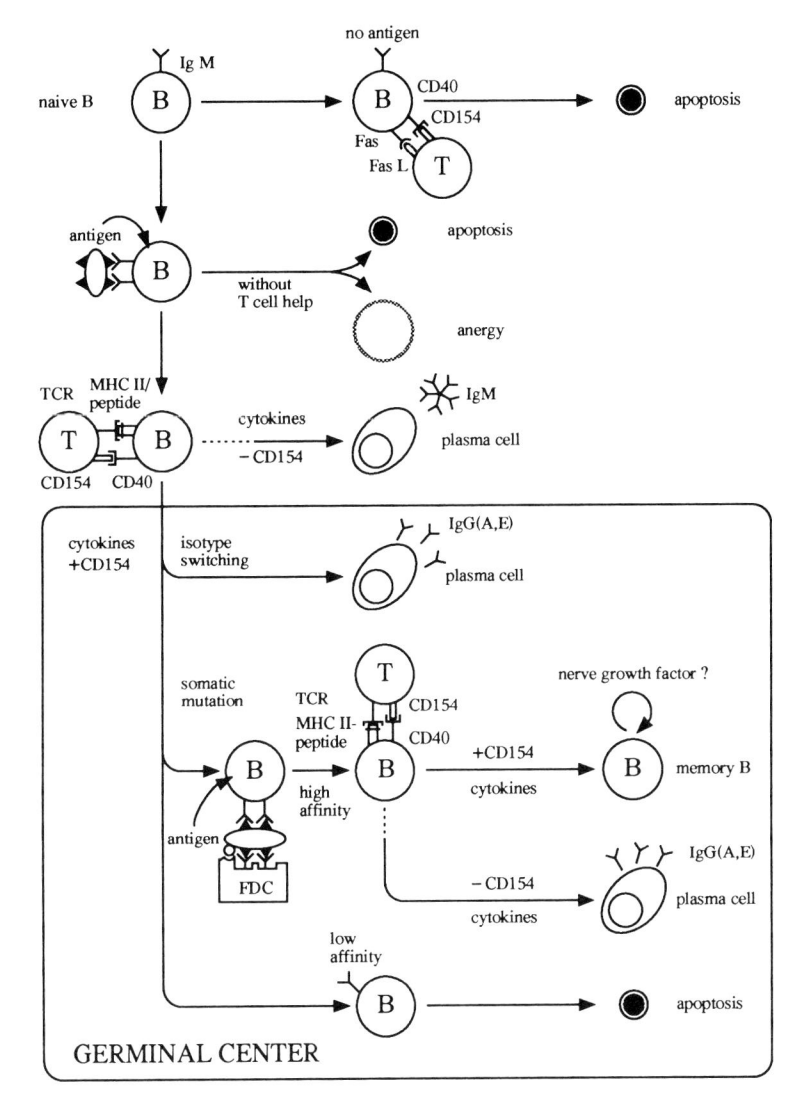

Fig. 9. Peripheral B-cell tolerance.

under stimulation with an appropriate cytokine *(42,206,207)*. In the presence of CD40 ligation with CD154, an antigen-stimulated mature B cell becomes a memory B cell producing autocrine proliferating factor.

AUTOIMMUNITY

Breakdown of T-Cell Tolerance

T-cell tolerance is ensured by several fail-safe mechanisms, but sometimes the breakdown of T-cell tolerance occurs, resulting in the induction of autoimmune phenomenon or autoimmune disease. There are many possible mechanisms to break down the T-cell tolerance (Table 1). In the thymus, a defect of a molecule related to costimulatory signals (CD28, CD154, CD80, or CD86) and an apoptosis-related molecule (Fas or FasL)

Table 1
T-Cell Tolerance and the Breakdown Mechanisms

Tolerance mechanism		Breakdown mechanism of tolerance
Central tolerance	Apoptosis (clonal deletion)	Defect of costimulatory signals (CD28, CD154)
		Defect of apoptosis-related molecules (Fas/FasL)
Peripheral tolerance	Apoptosis (activation-induced cell death: AICD)	Defect of apoptosis-related molecules (Fas/FasL, sFas, CD152)
	Anergy	Defect of anergy induction (aberrant CD80/CD86 expression)
	Ignorance	Release of sequestered antigens
		Appearance of cryptic antigen epitopes
	Active suppression	Defect of suppressor (regulatory) cells (suppressor T cells, NKT cells)
		Defect of suppressor T-cell induction cytokine-induced immune deviation (Th$_1$/Th$_2$ cells)

(208–210) on thymocytes/thymic dendritic cells may not induce apoptosis (clonal deletion) of thymocytes specific for self-peptides. Also, in the periphery, a defect of an apoptosis-related molecule (Fas, FasL, sFas, or CD152) *(107,211,212)* on T cells/APCs may not induce apoptosis (activation-induced cell death) of autoreactive T cells. However, it is difficult to consider that these defects in apoptosis induction cause organ-specific autoimmune diseases. Aberrant expression of CD80/CD86 molecules on nonprofessional APCs, such as epithelial cells, is a possible cause of organ-specific autoimmune disease, but there is no report on such aberrant expression *(213)*. Furthermore, clonal ignorance of T cells cannot be maintained if antigens sequestered from the immune system release in the blood, or if cryptic epitopes of antigens that have never been recognized by the immune system are presented for T-cell recognition by some cause *(214–217)*. As a defect of active suppression, a defect of antigen-specific suppressor T cells *(159,218–222)* and a defect in induction of active suppression or anergy *(12,14,15)* may also cause organ-specific autoimmune disease. Recently, NKT cells *(223–226)* are given attention on the pathogenesis of autoimmune disease, but the significance still remains to be resolved. Furthermore, cytokine-induced immune deviation by abnormal Th1/Th2 cell balance *(170,171,227)* is also a possible cause of autoimmune diseases, but there is a finding that does not support it *(177)*.

Breakdown of B-Cell Tolerance

Autoreactive B cells are deleted or functionally inactivated at several different steps of maturation from immature B cells to antibody-producing cells, as described above. These self-tolerance mechanisms appear to involve B-cell apoptosis or anergy induced by signaling via the BCR (sIg) or Fas. In mice prone to systemic autoimmune diseases, such as bcl-2 transgenic, NZB, or (NZB × NZW) F1 mice, antigen receptor-mediated B-cell apoptosis is defective *(195,228,229)*. In another systemic autoimmunity-prone mouse MRL/lpr, autoantibody production requires defects of Fas in B cells *(230)*. These

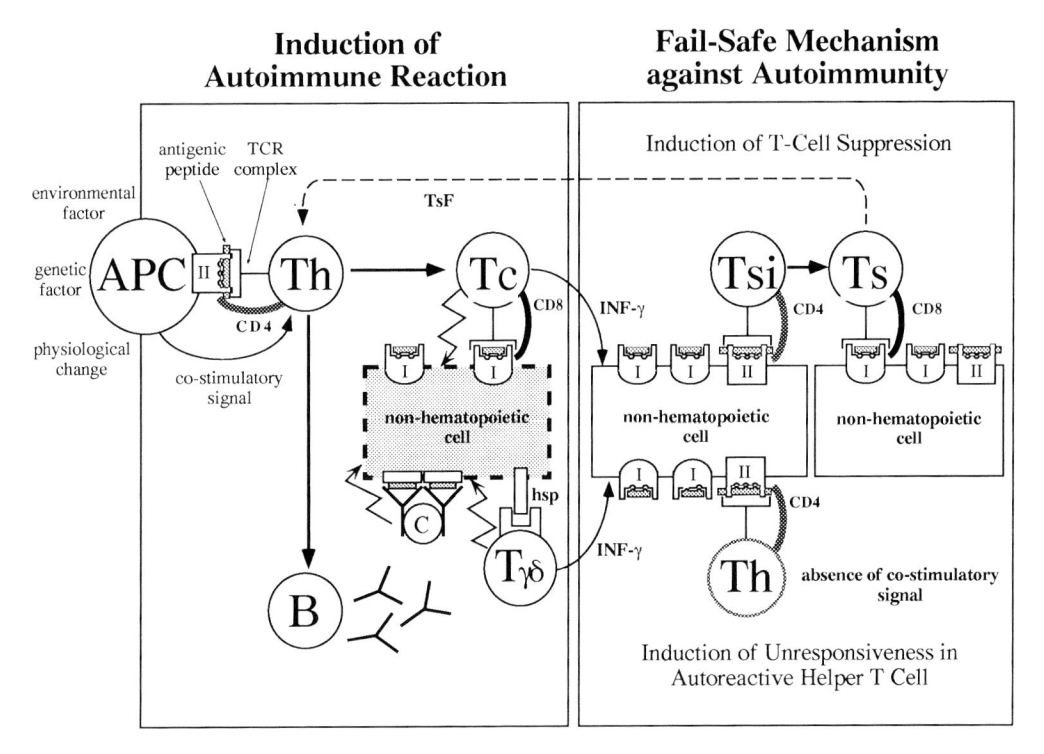

Fig. 10. Fail-safe mechanism against autoimmunity (modified from Iwatani et al. *[15]*).

findings strongly suggest that the defects in B-cell tolerance play an important role in the pathogenesis of systemic autoimmune diseases.

Hypothesis on Organ-Specific Autoimmune Disease (see also Chapter 2)

Organ-specific autoimmune diseases might be caused by a defect in the induction of peripheral tolerance, especially in the induction of active suppression or clonal anergy, which is a fail-safe mechanism against autoimmunity *(12–15,226,231)* (Fig. 10). Even in healthy subjects, autoimmune phenomena occur sometimes under continuous attack by environmental and other factors, which may mimic self-antigenic determinants, alter self-antigens, act as polyclonal immune activators, or induce an idiotype crossreaction to self-antigens. However, IFN-γ produced by autoimmune reaction in the target organ induces expression of MHC class II molecules on the intact target cells near damaged cells, which would then drive the induction of peripheral tolerance to resolve the evoked autoimmune reaction. In that case, the antigen-specific suppressor circuit amplified by this autoimmune reaction would maintain the unresponsiveness to the self-antigen more steadily *(232)*. In patients with a defect in the peripheral tolerance induction, the target cells could not completely suppress the autoimmune reaction by inducing the expression of MHC class II molecules on the cells, resulting in the development of the disease. Autoimmune diseases that are caused by such a defect would progress slowly, because a strong autoimmune reaction induces strong suppression even if the induction of suppressor cells is incomplete. Thus, this hypothesis could explain the prolonged latency period *(233)* and the continuous expression of MHC class II molecules of target cells *(59)* observed in autoimmune diseases.

**Peripheral Self-Tolerance
by a Fail-Safe Machanism against Autoimmunity**

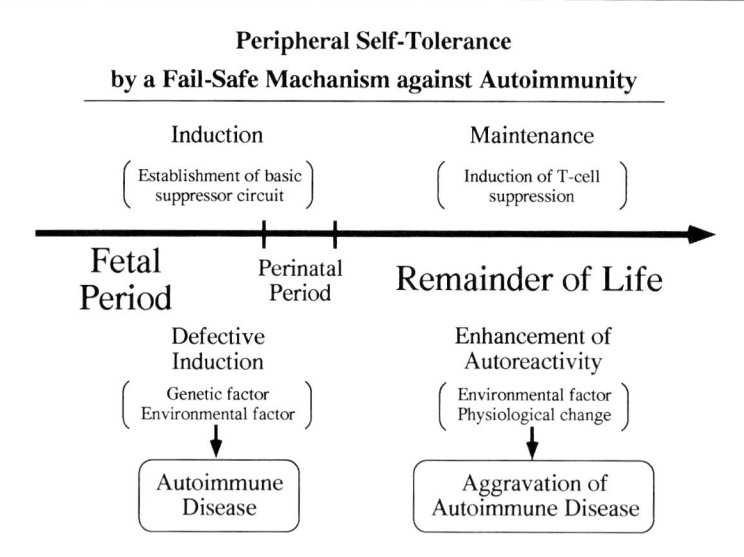

```
                Induction                    Maintenance
        ⎛ Establishment of basic ⎞      ⎛ Induction of T-cell ⎞
        ⎝   suppressor circuit   ⎠      ⎝     suppression     ⎠
    ──────────────────┬──────┬─────────────────────────────────▶
       Fetal        Perinatal        Remainder of Life
       Period        Period
              Defective                 Enhancement of
              Induction                  Autoreactivity
        ⎛   Genetic factor   ⎞      ⎛ Environmental factor ⎞
        ⎝ Environmental factor ⎠    ⎝  Physiological change ⎠
                  ↓                            ↓
              Autoimmune                  Aggravation of
               Disease                  Autoimmune Disease
```

Fig. 11. Hypothesis on peripheral tolerance and organ-specific autoimmune disease (from ref. *15*).

Basic immunological self-tolerance seems to be induced during the fetal or perinatal period, when immature lymphocytes are exposed to self-antigens. Thus, when the first autoreactive T lymphocytes attack target cells at a critical point during the ontogenic development of the immune cells, the cells might induce and establish a basic suppressor circuit that inhibits the autoimmune reaction against them by a fail-safe mechanism against autoimmunity *(12–15)* (Fig. 11). Then, when the autoreactive T cells attack the target cells afterward, the activity of this basic suppressor circuit might be evoked by the fail-safe mechanism, which maintains peripheral tolerance during the remainder of the life of the organism. Therefore, some abnormality of the fail-safe mechanism against autoimmunity in certain cells at this critical point during the fetal or perinatal period might cause a defect in the basic suppressor circuit (including a defect of antigen-specific Ts cells), which results in a defect in the fail-safe mechanism to maintain self-tolerance afterward, giving rise to organ-specific autoimmune disease. One likely abnormality is that self-antigenic determinants in certain cells may not be adequately presented at the critical period of the immune system for some reason, such as the delayed development of a highly differentiated organ *(234,235)*, the transient changes in self-antigenic determinants, or the blocking of the presentation by genetic, environmental, and/or physiological factors.

CONCLUSIONS

Immunological self-tolerance is achieved by variety of mechanisms, such as clonal deletion, clonal anergy, ignorance, and active suppression. In vivo model systems for self-tolerance, which utilize transgenic mice, knockout mice, or mutant mice have clearly shown the presence of clonal deletion, anergy, and ignorance, the importance of the avidity between T cells and APCs, the significance of costimulatory signals, and so on. T-cell-mediated suppression is a well-established phenomenon, as confirmed by adoptive transfer systems in which T cells from tolerant mice transfer tolerance to naive recipient mice. Recent studies have mostly clarified the content of antigen-specific TsF, although the functional mechanism of TsF to induce immune suppression and the induction mechanism of Ts cells still remain to be resolved. Among the mechanisms for self-tolerance, active suppression especially mediated by antigen-specific Ts cells might be most important to induce and maintain the unresponsiveness of autoreactive T cells specific for tissue-specific antigens in the periphery. Therefore, a defect of antigen-specific Ts cells (probably a defect of the Ts cell induction) might be the cause of organ-specific autoimmune disease.

REFERENCES

1. Tonegawa S. Somatic generation of antibody diversity. Nature 1983;302:575–581.
2. Davis MM, Bjorkman PJ. T-cell antigen receptor genes and T-cell recognition. Nature 1988;334: 395–402.
3. Kappler JW, Roehm N, Marrack, P. T cell tolerance by clonal elimination in the thymus. Cell 1987; 49:273–280.
4. Kisielow P, Bluthmann H, Staerz UD, Steinmetz M, von-Boehmer H. Tolerance in T-cell-receptor transgenic mice involves deletion of nonmature $CD4^+8^+$ thymocytes. Nature 1988;333:742–746.
5. MacDonald HR, Schneider R, Lees RK, Howe RC, Acha-Orbea H, Festenstein H, et al. T-cell receptor $V\beta$ use predicts reactivity and tolerance to Mlsa-encoded antigens. Nature 1988;332:40–45.
6. Sha WC, Nelson CA, Newberry RD, Kranz DM, Russell JH, Loh DY. Positive and negative selection of an antigen receptor on T cells in transgenic mice. Nature 1988;336:73–76.
7. Murphy KM, Heimberger AB, Loh DY. Induction by antigen of intrathymic apoptosis of $CD4^+CD8^+TCR^{lo}$ thymocytes in vivo. Science 1990;250:1720–1723.
8. Nemazee DA, Burki K. Clonal deletion of B lymphocytes in a transgenic mouse bearing anti-MHC class I antibody genes. Nature 1989;337:562–566.
9. Erikson J, Radic MZ, Camper SA, Hardy RR, Carmack C, Weigert M. Expression of anti-DNA immunoglobulin transgenes in non-autoimmune mice. Nature 1991;349:331–334.
10. Goodnow CC. Transgenic mice and analysis of B-cell tolerance. Annu Rev Immunol 1992;10:489–518.
11. Okamoto M, Murakami M, Shimizu A, Ozaki S, Tsubata T, Kumagai S, et al. A transgenic model of autoimmune hemolytic anemia. J Exp Med 1992;175:71–79.
12. Iwatani Y, Row VV, Volpe R. What prevents autoimmunity? Lancet 1985;2:839–840.
13. Iwatani Y, Iitaka M, Row VV, Volpe R. Effect of HLA-DR positive thyrocytes on in vitro thyroid autoantibody production. Clin Invest Med 1988;11:279–285.
14. Iwatani, Y, Amino, N, Miyai, K. Fail-safe mechanism against autoimmunity. Lancet 1989;1:1141.
15. Iwatani Y, Amino N, Miyai K. Peripheral self-tolerance and autoimmunity: the protective role of expression of class II major histocompatibility antigens on non-lymphoid cells. Biomed Pharmacother 1989;43:593–605.
16. Jones LA, Chin LT, Longo DL, Kruisbeek AM. Peripheral clonal elimination of functional T cells. Science 1990;250:1726–1729.
17. Webb S, Morris C, Sprent J. Extrathymic tolerance of mature T cells: clonal elimination as a consequence of immunity. Cell 1990;63:1249–1256.
18. Rocha B, von-Boehmer H. Peripheral selection of the T cell repertoire. Science 1991;251:1225–1228.
19. Moskophidis D, Lechner F, Pircher H, Zinkernagel RM. Virus persistence in acutely infected immunocompetent mice by exhaustion of antiviral cytotoxic effector T cells. Nature 1993;362:758–761.
20. Huang L, Soldevila G, Leeker M, Flavell R, Crispe IN. The liver eliminates T cells undergoing antigen-triggered apoptosis in vivo. Immunity 1994;1:741–749.
21. Sprent J, Webb SR. Intrathymic and extrathymic clonal deletion of T cells. Curr Opinion Immunol 1995;7:196–205.
22. Gaspari AA, Jenkins MK, Katz SI. Class II MHC-bearing keratinocytes induce antigen-specific unresponsiveness in hapten-specific Th1 clones. J Immunol 1988;141:2216–2220.
23. Markmann J, Lo D, Naji A, Palmiter RD, Brinster RL, Heber-Katz E. Antigen presenting function of class II MHC expressing pancreatic β cells. Nature 1988;336:476–479.
24. Mueller DL, Jenkins MK, Schwartz RH. Clonal expansion versus functional clonal inactivation: a costimulatory signalling pathway determines the outcome of T cell antigen receptor occupancy. Annu Rev Immunol 1989;7:445–480.

25. Schwartz RH. Models of T cell anergy: is there a common molecular mechanism? J Exp Med 1996; 184:1-8.
26. Tada T, Taniguchi M, Takemori T. Properties of primed suppressor T cells and their products. Transplant Rev 1975;26:106–129.
27. Sakaguchi S, Fukuma K, Kuribayashi K, Masuda T. Organ-specific autoimmune diseases induced in mice by elimination of T cell subset. I. Evidence for the active participation of T cells in natural self-tolerance; deficit of a T cell subset as a possible cause of autoimmune disease. J Exp Med 1985;161: 72–87.
28. Morimoto C, Letvin NL, Distaso JA, Aldrich WR, Schlossman SF. The isolation and characterization of the human suppressor inducer T cell subset. J Immunol 1985;134:1508–1515.
29. Taguchi O, Nishizuka Y. Self tolerance and localized autoimmunity. Mouse models of autoimmune disease that suggest tissue-specific suppressor T cells are involved in self tolerance. J Exp Med 1987; 165:146–156.
30. Sugihara S, Maruo S, Tsujimura T, Tarutani O, Kohno Y, Hamaoka T, et al. Autoimmune thyroiditis induced in mice depleted of particular T cell subsets. III. Analysis of regulatory cells suppressing the induction of thyroiditis. Int Immunol 1990;2:343–351.
31. Chen Y, Inobe J, Weiner HL. Induction of oral tolerance to myelin basic protein in CD8-depleted mice: both CD4$^+$ and CD8$^+$ cells mediate active suppression. J Immunol 1995;155:910 916.
32. Nakano T, Ishii Y, Ishizaka K. Biochemical characterization of antigen-specific glycosylation-inhibiting factor from antigen-specific suppressor T cells. I. Identification of a 55-kilodalton glycosylation-inhibiting factor peptide with TCR α-chain determinant. J Immunol 1996;156:1728–1734.
33. Ishizaka K, Nakano T, Ishii Y, Liu YC, Mikayama T, Mori A. Controversial issues and possible answers on the antigen-specific regulation of the IgE antibody response. Adv Exp Med Biol 1996; 409:317–325.
34. Kong YY, Eto M, Omoto K, Umesue M, Hashimoto A, Nomoto K. Regulatory T cells in maintenance and reversal of peripheral tolerance in vivo. J Immunol 1996;157:5284–5289.
35. Kumar V, Coulsell E, Ober B, Hubbard G, Sercarz E, Ward ES. Recombinant T cell receptor molecules can prevent and reverse experimental autoimmune encephalomyelitis: dose effects and involvement of both CD4 and CD8 T cells. J Immunol 1997;159:5150–5156.
36. Galy A, Travis M, Cen D, Chen B. Human T, B, natural killer, and dendritic cells arise from a common bone marrow progenitor cell subset. Immunity 1995;3:459–473.
37. von-Boehmer H. The developmental biology of T lymphocytes. Annu Rev Immunol 1988;6:309–326.
38. Anderson G, Moore NC, Owen JJ, Jenkinson EJ. Cellular interactions in thymocyte development. Annu Rev Immunol 1996;14:73–99.
39. Havran WL, Boismenu R. Activation and function of γδT cells. Curr Opinion Immunol 1994;6:442–446.
40. Burrows PD, Cooper MD. B cell development and differentiation. Curr Opinion Immunol 1997;9: 239–244.
41. Parker DC. T cell-dependent B cell activation. Annu Rev Immunol 1993;11:331–360.
42. Arpin C, Dechanet J, Van-Kooten C, Merville P, Grouard G, Briere F, et al. Generation of memory B cells and plasma cells in vitro. Science 1995;268:720–722.
43. Berke G. The binding and lysis of target cells by cytotoxic lymphocytes: molecular and cellular aspects. Annu Rev Immunol 1994;12:735–773.
44. Fearon DT, Locksley RM. The instructive role of innate immunity in the acquired immune response. Science 1996;272:50–53.
45. Tschopp J, Nabholz M. Perforin-mediated target cell lysis by cytolytic T lymphocytes. Annu Rev Immunol 1990;8:279–302.
46. Takayama H, Kojima H, Shinohara N. Cytotoxic T lymphocytes: the newly identified Fas (CD95)-mediated killing mechanism and a novel aspect of their biological functions. Adv Immunol 1995; 60:289–321.
47. Cresswell P. Assembly, transport, and function of MHC class II molecules. Annu Rev Immunol 1994; 12:259–93.
48. York IA, Rock KL. Antigen processing and presentation by the class I major histocompatibility complex. Annu Rev Immunol 1996;14:369–396.
49. Watts C. Capture and processing of exogenous antigens for presentation on MHC molecules. Annu Rev Immunol 1997;15:821–850.
50. Zinkernagel RM, Doherty PC. The discovery of MHC restriction. Immunol Today 1997;18:14–17.

51. Parham P. Pictures of MHC restriction. Nature 1996;384:109,110.
52. Bodmer JG, Marsh SG, Albert ED, Bodmer WF, Dupont B, Erlich HA, et al. Nomenclature for factors of the HLA system, 1994. Hum Immunol 1994;41:1–20.
53. Trowsdale J. "Both man & bird & beast": comparative organization of MHC genes. Immunogenetics 1995;41:1–17.
54. Campbell RD, Trowsdale J. Map of the human MHC. Immunol Today 1993;14:349–352.
55. Shawar SM, Vyas JM, Rodgers JR, Rich RR. Antigen presentation by major histocompatibility complex class I-B molecules. Annu Rev Immunol 1994;12:839–880.
56. Stroynowski I, Forman J. Novel molecules related to MHC antigens. Curr Opinion Immunol 1995;7:97–102.
57. Pober JS, Collins T, Gimbrone M, Jr, Cotran RS, Gitlin JD, Fiers W, et al. Lymphocytes recognize human vascular endothelial and dermal fibroblast Ia antigens induced by recombinant immune interferon. Nature 1983;305:726–729.
58. Iwatani Y, Gerstein HC, Iitaka M, Row VV, Volpe R. Thyrocyte HLA-DR expression and interferon-γ production in autoimmune thyroid disease. J Clin Endocrinol Metab 1986;63:695–708.
59. Hanafusa T, Pujol Borrell R, Chiovato L, Russell RC, Doniach D, Bottazzo GF. Aberrant expression of HLA-DR antigen on thyrocytes in Graves' disease: relevance for autoimmunity. Lancet 1983;2:1111–1115.
60. Coux O, Tanaka K, Goldberg AL. Structure and functions of the 20S and 26S proteasomes. Annu Rev Biochem 1996;65:801–847.
61. Koopmann JO, Hammerling GJ, Momburg F. Generation, intracellular transport and loading of peptides associated with MHC class I molecules. Curr Opinion Immunol 1997;9:80–88.
62. Tanaka K, Tanahashi N, Tsurumi C, Yokota KY, Shimbara N. Proteasomes and antigen processing. Adv Immunol 1997;64:1–38.
63. Groettrup M, Soza A, Eggers M, Kuehn L, Dick TP, Schild H, et al. A role for the proteasome regulator PA28α in antigen presentation. Nature 1996;381:166–168.
64. Hisamatsu H, Shimbara N, Saito Y, Kristensen P, Hendil KB, Fujiwara T, et al. Newly identified pair of proteasomal subunits regulated reciprocally by interferon γ. J Exp Med 1996;183:1807–1816.
65. Groll M, Ditzel L, Lowe J, Stock D, Bochtler M, Bartunik HD, et al. Structure of 20S proteasome from yeast at 2.4 A resolution. Nature 1997;386:463–471.
66. Grandea AG 3rd, Androlewicz MJ, Athwal RS, Geraghty DE, Spies T. Dependence of peptide binding by MHC class I molecules on their interaction with TAP. Science 1995;270:105–108.
67. Androlewicz MJ, Cresswell P. How selective is the transporter associated with antigen processing? Immunity 1996;5:1–5 issn: 1074–7613.
68. Germain RN. MHC-dependent antigen processing and peptide presentation: providing ligands for T lymphocyte activation. Cell 1994;76:287–299.
69. Rammensee HG, Friede T, Stevanoviic S. MHC ligands and peptide motifs: first listing. Immunogenetics 1995;41:178–228.
70. Smith KJ, Reid SW, Harlos K, McMichael AJ, Stuart DI, Bell JI, et al. Bound water structure and polymorphic amino acids act together to allow the binding of different peptides to MHC class I HLA-B53. Immunity 1996;4:215–228.
71. Jones EY. MHC class I and class II structures. Curr Opinion Immunol 1997;9:75–79.
72. Garboczi DN, Ghosh P, Utz U, Fan QR, Biddison WE, Wiley DC. Structure of the complex between human T-cell receptor, viral peptide and HLA-A2. Nature 1996;384:134–141.
73. Garcia KC, Degano M, Stanfield RL, Brunmark A, Jackson MR, Peterson PA, et al. An alphabeta T cell receptor structure at 2.5 A and its orientation in the TCR-MHC complex. Science 1996;274:209–219.
74. Rammensee HG. Chemistry of peptides associated with MHC class I and class II molecules. Curr Opinion Immunol 1995;7:85–96.
75. Pieters J. MHC class II restricted antigen presentation. Curr Opinion Immunol 1997;9:89–96.
76. Sanderson F, Kleijmeer MJ, Kelly A, Verwoerd D, Tulp A, Neefjes JJ, et al. Accumulation of HLA-DM, a regulator of antigen presentation, in MHC class II compartments. Science 1994;266:1566–1569.
77. Weber DA, Evavold BD, Jensen PE. Enhanced dissociation of HLA-DR-bound peptides in the presence of HLA-DM. Science 1996;274:618–620.
78. Stern LJ, Brown JH, Jardetzky TS, Gorga JC, Urban RG, Strominger JL, et al. Crystal structure of the human class II MHC protein HLA-DR1 complexed with an influenza virus peptide. Nature 1994;368:215–221.

79. Jardetzky TS, Brown JH, Gorga JC, Stern LJ, Urban RG, Strominger JL, et al. Crystallographic analysis of endogenous peptides associated with HLA-DR1 suggests a common, polyproline II-like conformation for bound peptides. Proc Natl Acad Sci USA 1996;93:734–738.
80. Kurts C, Heath WR, Carbone FR, Allison J, Miller JF, Kosaka H. Constitutive class I-restricted exogenous presentation of self antigens in vivo. J Exp Med 1996;184:923–930.
81. Schirmbeck R, Bohm W, Melber K, Reimann J. Processing of exogenous heat-aggregated (denatured) and particulate (native) hepatitis B surface antigen for class I-restricted epitope presentation. J Immunol 1995;155:4676–4684.
82. Reis-e-Sousa C, Germain RN. Major histocompatibility complex class I presentation of peptides derived from soluble exogenous antigen by a subset of cells engaged in phagocytosis. J Exp Med 1995;182:841–851.
83. Pfeifer JD, Wick MJ, Roberts RL, Findlay K, Normark SJ, Harding CV. Phagocytic processing of bacterial antigens for class I MHC presentation to T cells. Nature 1993;361:359–362.
84. Rudensky AY, Maric M, Eastman S, Shoemaker L, DeRoos PC, Blum JS. Intracellular assembly and transport of endogenous peptide-MHC class II complexes. Immunity 1994;1:585–594.
85. Bretscher P, Cohn M. A theory of self-nonself discrimination. Science 1970;169:1042–1049.
86. Lenschow DJ, Walunas TL, Bluestone JA. CD28/B7 system of T cell costimulation. Annu Rev Immunol 1996;14:233–258.
87. Chambers CA, Allison JP. Co-stimulation in T cell responses. Curr Opinion Immunol 1997;9:396–404.
88. June CH, Ledbetter JA, Linsley PS, Thompson CB. Role of the CD28 receptor in T-cell activation. Immunol Today 1990;11:211–216.
89. Yokochi T, Holly RD, Clark EA. B lymphoblast antigen (BB-1) expressed on Epstein-Barr virus-activated B cell blasts, B lymphoblastoid cell lines, and Burkitt's lymphomas. J Immunol 1982;128:823–827.
90. Freeman GJ, Gray GS, Gimmi CD, Lombard DB, Zhou LJ, White M, et al. Structure, expression, and T cell costimulatory activity of the murine homologue of the human B lymphocyte activation antigen B7. J Exp Med 1991;174:625–631.
91. Azuma M, Ito D, Yagita H, Okumura K, Phillips JH, Lanier LL, et al. B70 antigen is a second ligand for CTLA-4 and CD28. Nature 1993;366:76–79.
92. Boise LH, Minn AJ, Noel PJ, June CH, Accavitti MA, Lindsten T, et al. CD28 costimulation can promote T cell survival by enhancing the expression of Bcl-XL. Immunity 1995;3:87–98.
93. June CH, Bluestone JA, Nadler LM, Thompson CB. The B7 and CD28 receptor families. Immunol Today 1994;15:321–331.
94. Hathcock KS, Laszlo G, Pucillo C, Linsley P, Hodes RJ. Comparative analysis of B7-1 and B7-2 costimulatory ligands: expression and function. J Exp Med 1994;180:631–640.
95. Inaba K, Witmer-Pack M, Inaba M, Hathcock KS, Sakuta H, Azuma M, et al. The tissue distribution of the B7-2 costimulator in mice: abundant expression on dendritic cells in situ and during maturation in vitro. J Exp Med 1994;180:1849–1860.
96. Lenschow DJ, Sperling AI, Cooke MP, Freeman G, Rhee L, Decker DC, et al. Differential up-regulation of the B7-1 and B7-2 costimulatory molecules after Ig receptor engagement by antigen. J Immunol 1994;153:1990–1997.
97. Griggs ND, Agersborg SS, Noelle RJ, Ledbetter JA, Linsley PS, Tung KS. The relative contribution of the CD28 and gp39 costimulatory pathways in the clonal expansion and pathogenic acquisition of self-reactive T cells. J Exp Med 1996;183:801–810.
98. Foy TM, Aruffo A, Bajorath J, Buhlmann JE, Noelle RJ. Immune regulation by CD40 and its ligand GP39. Annu Rev Immunol 1996;14:591–617.
99. Yang Y, Wilson JM. CD40 ligand-dependent T cell activation: requirement of B7-CD28 signaling through CD40. Science 1996;273:1862–1864.
100. Grewal IS, Foellmer HG, Grewal KD, Xu J, Hardardottir F, Baron JL, et al. Requirement for CD40 ligand in costimulation induction, T cell activation, and experimental allergic encephalomyelitis. Science 1996;273:1864–1867.
101. Stout RD, Suttles J. The many roles of CD40 in cell-mediated inflammatory responses. Immunol Today 1996;17:487–492.
102. de-Boer M, Kasran A, Kwekkeboom J, Walter H, Vandenberghe P, Ceuppens JL. Ligation of B7 with CD28/CTLA-4 on T cells results in CD40 ligand expression, interleukin-4 secretion and efficient help for antibody production by B cells. Eur J Immunol 1993;23:3120–3125.

103. Klaus SJ, Pinchuk LM, Ochs HD, Law CL, Fanslow WC, Armitage RJ, et al. Costimulation through CD28 enhances T cell-dependent B cell activation via CD40-CD40L interaction. J Immunol 1994;152:5643–5652.
104. van-Kooten C, Banchereau J. Functions of CD40 on B cells, dendritic cells and other cells. Curr Opinion Immunol 1997;9:330–337.
105. Walunas TL, Lenschow DJ, Bakker CY, Linsley PS, Freeman GJ, Green JM, et al. CTLA-4 can function as a negative regulator of T cell activation. Immunity 1994;1:405–413.
106. Tivol EA, Borriello F, Schweitzer AN, Lynch WP, Bluestone JA, Sharpe AH. Loss of CTLA-4 leads to massive lymphoproliferation and fatal multiorgan tissue destruction, revealing a critical negative regulatory role of CTLA-4. Immunity 1995;3:541–547.
107. Waterhouse P, Penninger JM, Timms E, Wakeham A, Shahinian A, Lee KP, et al. Lymphoproliferative disorders with early lethality in mice deficient in Ctla-4. Science 1995;270:985–988.
108. Walunas TL, Bakker CY, Bluestone JA. CTLA-4 ligation blocks CD28-dependent T cell activation. J Exp Med 1996;183:2541–2550.
109. Krummel MF, Allison JP. CTLA-4 engagement inhibits IL-2 accumulation and cell cycle progression upon activation of resting T cells. J Exp Med 1996;183:2533–2540.
110. Linsley PS, Greene JL, Tan P, Bradshaw J, Ledbetter JA, Anasetti C, et al. Coexpression and functional cooperation of CTLA-4 and CD28 on activated T lymphocytes. J Exp Med 1992;176:1595–1604.
111. Krummel MF, Allison JP. CD28 and CTLA-4 have opposing effects on the response of T cells to stimulation [see comments]. J Exp Med 1995;182:459–465.
112. van-der-Merwe PA, Bodian DL, Daenke S, Linsley P, Davis SJ. CD80 (B7-1) binds both CD28 and CTLA-4 with a low affinity and very fast kinetics. J Exp Med 1997;185:393–403.
113. Greene JL, Leytze GM, Emswiler J, Peach R, Bajorath J, Cosand W, et al. Covalent dimerization of CD28/CTLA-4 and oligomerization of CD80/CD86 regulate T cell costimulatory interactions. J Biol Chem 1996;271:26,762–26,771.
114. Linsley PS, Greene JL, Brady W, Bajorath J, Ledbetter JA, Peach R. Human B7-1 (CD80) and B7-2 (CD86) bind with similar avidities but distinct kinetics to CD28 and CTLA-4 receptors [published erratum appears in *Immunity* 1995;Feb;2(2):following 203]. Immunity 1994;1:793–801.
115. Mond JJ, Lees A, Snapper CM. T cell-independent antigens type 2. Annu Rev Immunol 1995;13: 655–692.
116. Harriman W, Volk H, Defranoux N, Wabl M. Immunoglobulin class switch recombination. Annu Rev Immunol 1993;11:361–384.
117. Wagner SD, Neuberger MS. Somatic hypermutation of immunoglobulin genes. Annu Rev Immunol 1996;14:441–457.
118. Banchereau J, Bazan F, Blanchard D, Briere F, Galizzi JP, van-Kooten C, et al. The CD40 antigen and its ligand. Annu Rev Immunol 1994;12:881–922.
119. Malisan F, Briere F, Bridon JM, Harindranath N, Mills FC, Max EE, et al. Interleukin-10 induces immunoglobulin G isotype switch recombination in human CD40-activated naive B lymphocytes. J Exp Med 1996;183:937–947.
120. Shortman K, Wu L. Early T lymphocyte progenitors. Annu Rev Immunol 1996;14:29–47.
121. Levelt CN, Eichmann K. Receptors and signals in early thymic selection. Immunity 1995;3:667–672.
122. Fehling HJ, Krotkova A, Saint-Ruf C, von-Boehmer H. Crucial role of the pre-T-cell receptor α gene in development of αβ but not γδ T cells. Nature 1995;375:795–798.
123. Penit C, Lucas B, Vasseur F. Cell expansion and growth arrest phases during the transition from precursor (CD4−8−) to immature (CD4+8+) thymocytes in normal and genetically modified mice. J Immunol 1995;154:5103–5113.
124. von-Boehmer H. Positive selection of lymphocytes. Cell 1994;76:219–228.
125. Nossal GJ. Negative selection of lymphocytes. Cell 1994;76:229–239.
126. Bevan MJ. In a radiation chimaera, host H-2 antigens determine immune responsiveness of donor cytotoxic cells. Nature 1977;269:417–418.
127. Zinkernagel RM, Callahan GN, Althage A, Cooper S, Klein PA, Klein J. On the thymus in the differentiation of "H-2 self-recognition" by T cells: evidence for dual recognition? J Exp Med 1978;147:882–896.
128. Kisielow P, Teh HS, Bluthmann H, von-Boehmer H. Positive selection of antigen-specific T cells in thymus by restricting MHC molecules. Nature 1988;335:730–733.
129. Sha WC, Nelson CA, Newberry RD, Kranz DM, Russell JH, Loh DY. Selective expression of an antigen receptor on CD8-bearing T lymphocytes in transgenic mice. Nature 1988;335:271–274.

130. Teh HS, Kisielow P, Scott B, Kishi H, Uematsu Y, Bluthmann H, et al. Thymic major histocompatibility complex antigens and the alpha beta T-cell receptor determine the CD4/CD8 phenotype of T cells. Nature 1988;335:229–233.
131. Benoist C, Mathis D. Positive selection of the T cell repertoire: where and when does it occur? Cell 1989;58:1027–1033.
132. Berg LJ, Pullen AM, Fazekas de St Groth B, Mathis D, Benoist C, Davis MM. Antigen/MHC-specific T cells are preferentially exported from the thymus in the presence of their MHC ligand. Cell 1989;58: 1035–1046.
133. Marrack P, Lo D, Brinster R, Palmiter R, Burkly L, Flavell RH, et al. The effect of thymus environment on T cell development and tolerance. Cell 1988;53:627–634.
134. Laufer TM, DeKoning J, Markowitz JS, Lo D, Glimcher LH. Unopposed positive selection and autoreactivity in mice expressing class II MHC only on thymic cortex. Nature 1996;383:81–85.
135. Janeway C, Jr. Thymic selection: two pathways to life and two to death. Immunity 1994;1:3–6.
136. Ashton-Rickardt PG, Bandeira A, Delaney JR, Van-Kaer L, Pircher HP, Zinkernagel RM, et al. Evidence for a differential avidity model of T cell selection in the thymus. Cell 1994;76:651–663.
137. Kawai K, Ohashi PS. Immunological function of a defined T-cell population tolerized to low-affinity self antigens. Nature 1995;374:68–69.
138. Hogquist KA, Jameson SC, Heath WR, Howard JL, Bevan MJ, Carbone FR. T cell receptor antagonist peptides induce positive selection. Cell 1994;76:17–27.
139. Fukui Y, Ishimoto T, Utsuyama M, Gyotoku T, Koga T, Nakao K, et al. Positive and negative CD4$^+$ thymocyte selection by a single MHC class II/peptide ligand affected by its expression level in the thymus. Immunity 1997;6:401–410.
140. Davis CB, Littman DR. Thymocyte lineage commitment: is it instructed or stochastic? Curr Opinion Immunol 1994;6:266–272.
141. Punt JA, Osborne BA, Takahama Y, Sharrow SO, Singer A. Negative selection of CD4$^+$CD8$^+$ thymocytes by T cell receptor-induced apoptosis requires a costimulatory signal that can be provided by CD28. J Exp Med 1994;179:709–713.
142. Foy TM, Page DM, Waldschmidt TJ, Schoneveld A, Laman JD, Masters SR, et al. An essential role for gp39, the ligand for CD40, in thymic selection. J Exp Med 1995;182:1377–1388.
143. Carlow DA, van-Oers NS, Teh SJ, Teh HS. Deletion of antigen-specific immature thymocytes by dendritic cells requires LFA-1/ICAM interactions. J Immunol 1992;148:1595–1603.
144. Akkaraju S, Ho WY, Leong D, Canaan K, Davis MM, Goodnow CC. A range of CD4 T cell tolerance: partial inactivation to organ-specific antigen allows nondestructive thyroiditis or insulitis. Immunity 1997;7:255-271.
145. Ohashi PS, Oehen S, Buerki K, Pircher H, Ohashi CT, Odermatt B, et al. Ablation of "tolerance" and induction of diabetes by virus infection in viral antigen transgenic mice. Cell 1991;65:305–317.
146. Miller JF, Heath WR. Self-ignorance in the peripheral T-cell pool. Immunol Rev 1993;133:131–150.
147. Renno T, Hahne M, MacDonald HR. Proliferation is a prerequisite for bacterial superantigen-induced T cell apoptosis in vivo. J Exp Med 1995;181:2283–2287.
148. Forster I, Hirose R, Arbeit JM, Clausen BE, Hanahan D. Limited capacity for tolerization of CD4$^+$ T cells specific for a pancreatic β cell neo-antigen. Immunity 1995;2:573–585.
149. Lynch DH, Watson ML, Alderson MR, Baum PR, Miller RE, Tough T, et al. The mouse Fas-ligand gene is mutated in gld mice and is part of a TNF family gene cluster. Immunity 1994;1:131–136.
150. Lynch DH, Ramsdell F, Alderson MR. Fas and FasL in the homeostatic regulation of immune responses. Immunol Today 1995;16:569–574.
151. Zheng L, Fisher G, Miller RE, Peschon J, Lynch DH, Lenardo MJ. Induction of apoptosis in mature T cells by tumour necrosis factor. Nature 1995;377:348–351.
152. Dillon SR, MacKay VL, Fink PJ. A functionally compromised intermediate in extrathymic CD8$^+$ T cell deletion. Immunity 1995;3:321–333.
153. Perez VL, Van-Parijs L, Biuckians A, Zheng XX, Strom TB, Abbas AK. Induction of peripheral T cell tolerance in vivo requires CTLA-4 engagement. Immunity 1997;6:411–417.
154. Schonrich G, Kalinke U, Momburg F, Malissen M, Schmitt-Verhulst AM, Malissen B, et al. Down-regulation of T cell receptors on self-reactive T cells as a novel mechanism for extrathymic tolerance induction. Cell 1991;65:293–304.
155. Nakano T, Liu YC, Mikayama T, Watarai H, Taniguchi M, Ishizaka K. Association of the "major histocompatibility complex subregion" I-J determinant with bioactive glycosylation-inhibiting factor. Proc Natl Acad Sci USA 1995;92:9196–9200.

156. Ishii Y, Nakano T, Ishizaka K. Biochemical characterization of antigen-specific glycosylation-inhibiting factor from antigen-specific suppressor T cells. II. The 55-kDa glycosylation-inhibiting factor peptide is a derivative of TCR α-chain and a subunit of antigen-specific glycosylation-inhibiting factor. J Immunol 1996;156:1735–1742.
157. Ishii Y, Nakano T, Ishizaka K. Cellular mechanisms for the formation of a soluble form derivative of T-cell receptor α chain by suppressor T cells. Proc Natl Acad Sci USA 1996;93:7207–7212.
158. Nakano T, Watarai H, Liu YC, Oyama Y, Mikayama T, Ishizaka K. Conversion of inactive glycosylation inhibiting factor to bioactive derivatives by modification of a SH group. Proc Natl Acad Sci USA 1997;94:202–207.
159. Taguchi O, Takahashi T, Nishizuka Y. Self-tolerance and localized autoimmunity. Curr Opinion Immunol 1989;2:576–581.
160. Salgame P, Convit J, Bloom BR. Immunological suppression by human CD8+ T cells is receptor dependent and HLA-DQ restricted. Proc Natl Acad Sci USA 1991;88:2598–2602.
161. Nabozny GH, Cobbold SP, Waldmann H, Kong YC. Suppression in murine experimental autoimmune thyroiditis: in vivo inhibition of CD4+ T cell-mediated resistance by a nondepleting rat CD4 monoclonal antibody. Cell Immunol 1991;138:185–196.
162. Bloom BR, Salgame P, Diamond B. Revisiting and revising suppressor T cells. Immunol Today 1992;13:131–136.
163. Dorf ME, Kuchroo VK, Collins M. Suppressor T cells: some answers but more questions. Immunol Today 1992;13:241–243.
164. Koide J, Engleman EG. Differences in surface phenotype and mechanism of action between alloantigen-specific CD8+ cytotoxic and suppressor T cell clones. J Immunol 1990;144:32–40.
165. Oliveira DB, Mitchison NA. Immune suppression genes. Clin Exp Immunol 1989;75:167–177.
166. Mayer L, Shlien R. Evidence for function of Ia molecules on gut epithelial cells in man. J Exp Med 1987;166:1471–1483.
167. Taguchi O, Kontani K, Ikeda H, Kezuka T, Takeuchi M, Takahashi T, et al. Tissue-specific suppressor T cells involved in self-tolerance are activated extrathymically by self-antigens. Immunology 1994;82:365–369.
168. Taguchi O, Takahashi T. Mouse models of autoimmune disease suggest that self-tolerance is maintained by unresponsive autoreactive T cells. Immunology 1996;89:13–19.
169. Mosmann TR, Cherwinski H, Bond MW, Giedlin MA, Coffman RL. Two types of murine helper T cell clone. I. Definition according to profiles of lymphokine activities and secreted proteins. J Immunol 1986;136:2348–2357.
170. Mosmann TR, Sad S. The expanding universe of T-cell subsets: Th1, Th2 and more. Immunol Today 1996;17:138–146.
171. Abbas AK, Murphy KM, Sher A. Functional diversity of helper T lymphocytes. Nature 1996;383:787–793.
172. Yoshimoto T, Paul WE. CD4+, NK1.1+ T cells promptly produce interleukin 4 in response to in vivo challenge with anti-CD3. J Exp Med 1994;179:1285–1295.
173. Yoshimoto T, Bendelac A, Watson C, Hu-Li J, Paul WE. Role of NK1.1+ T cells in a TH2 response and in immunoglobulin E production. Science 1995;270:1845–1847.
174. Sabin EA, Kopf MA, Pearce EJ. Schistosoma mansoni egg-induced early IL-4 production is dependent upon IL-5 and eosinophils. J Exp Med 1996;184:1871–1878.
175. Brown DR, Fowell DJ, Corry DB, Wynn TA, Moskowitz NH, Cheever AW, et al. β2-microglobulin-dependent NK1.1+ T cells are not essential for T helper cell 2 immune responses. J Exp Med 1996;184:1295–1304.
176. Szabo SJ, Dighe AS, Gubler U, Murphy KM. Regulation of the interleukin (IL)-12R β2 subunit expression in developing T helper 1 (Th1) and Th2 cells. J Exp Med 1997;185:817–824.
177. Katz JD, Benoist C, Mathis D. T helper cell subsets in insulin-dependent diabetes. Science 1995;268:1185–1188.
178. Sad S, Marcotte R, Mosmann TR. Cytokine-induced differentiation of precursor mouse CD8+ T cells into cytotoxic CD8+ T cells secreting Th1 or Th2 cytokines. Immunity 1995;2:271–279.
179. Li L, Sad S, Kagi D, Mosmann TR. CD8Tc1 and Tc2 cells secrete distinct cytokine patterns in vitro and in vivo but induce similar inflammatory reactions. J Immunol 1997;158:4152–4161.
180. Rajewsky K. Clonal selection and learning in the antibody system. Nature 1996;381:751–758.
181. Papavasiliou F, Jankovic M, Gong S, Nussenzweig MC. Control of immunoglobulin gene rearrangements in developing B cells. Curr Opinion Immunol 1997;9:233–238.

182. Osmond DG, Rico-Vargas S, Valenzona H, Fauteux L, Liu L, Janani R, et al. Apoptosis and macrophage-mediated cell deletion in the regulation of B lymphopoiesis in mouse bone marrow. Immunol Rev 1994;142:209–230.
183. Melchers F, Rolink A, Grawunder U, Winkler TH, Karasuyama H, Ghia P, et al. Positive and negative selection events during B lymphopoiesis. Curr Opinion Immunol 1995;7:214–227.
184. Cornall RJ, Goodnow CC, Cyster JG. The regulation of self-reactive B cells. Curr Opinion Immunol 1995;7:804–811.
185. Nemazee D, Buerki K. Clonal deletion of autoreactive B lymphocytes in bone marrow chimeras. Proc Natl Acad Sci USA 1989;86:8039–8043.
186. Hartley SB, Cooke MP, Fulcher DA, Harris AW, Cory S, Basten A, et al. Elimination of self-reactive B lymphocytes proceeds in two stages: arrested development and cell death. Cell 1993;72:325–335.
187. Nossal GJ, Pike BL. Clonal anergy: persistence in tolerant mice of antigen-binding B lymphocytes incapable of responding to antigen or mitogen. Proc Natl Acad Sci USA 1980;77:1602–1606.
188. Goodnow CC, Crosbie J, Adelstein S, Lavoie TB, Smith-Gill SJ, Brink RA, et al. Altered immunoglobulin expression and functional silencing of self-reactive B lymphocytes in transgenic mice. Nature 1988;334:676–682.
189. Gay D, Saunders T, Camper S, Weigert M. Receptor editing: an approach by autoreactive B cells to escape tolerance. J Exp Med 1993;177:999–1008.
190. Tiegs SL, Russell DM, Nemazee D. Receptor editing in self-reactive bone marrow B cells. J Exp Med 1993;177:1009–1020.
191. Radic MZ, Zouali M. Receptor editing, immune diversification, and self-tolerance. Immunity 1996;5:505–511.
192. Garrone P, Neidhardt EM, Garcia E, Galibert L, van-Kooten C, Banchereau J. Fas ligation induces apoptosis of CD40-activated human B lymphocytes. J Exp Med 1995;182:1265–1273.
193. Schattner EJ, Elkon KB, Yoo DH, Tumang J, Krammer PH, Crow MK, et al. CD40 ligation induces Apo-1/Fas expression on human B lymphocytes and facilitates apoptosis through the Apo-1/Fas pathway. J Exp Med 1995;182:1557–1565.
194. Rathmell JC, Townsend SE, Xu JC, Flavell RA, Goodnow CC. Expansion or elimination of B cells in vivo: dual roles for CD40- and Fas (CD95)-ligands modulated by the B cell antigen receptor. Cell 1996;87:319–329.
195. Tsubata T, Murakami M, Honjo T. Antigen-receptor cross-linking induces peritoneal B-cell apoptosis in normal but not autoimmunity-prone mice. Curr Biol 1994;4:8–17.
196. Parry SL, Hasbold J, Holman M, Klaus GG. Hypercross-linking surface IgM or IgD receptors on mature B cells induces apoptosis that is reversed by costimulation with IL-4 and anti-CD40. J Immunol 1994;152:2821–2829.
197. Parry SL, Holman MJ, Hasbold J, Klaus GG. Plastic-immobilized anti-μ or anti-δ antibodies induce apoptosis in mature murine B lymphocytes. Eur J Immunol 1994;24:974–979.
198. Rathmell JC, Cooke MP, Ho WY, Grein J, Townsend SE, Davis MM, et al. CD95 (Fas)-dependent elimination of self-reactive B cells upon interaction with CD4+ T cells. Nature 1995;376:181–184.
199. Kawabe T, Naka T, Yoshida K, Tanaka T, Fujiwara H, Suematsu S, et al. The immune responses in CD40-deficient mice: impaired immunoglobulin class switching and germinal center formation. Immunity 1994;1:167–178.
200. Renshaw BR, Fanslow WC 3rd, Armitage RJ, Campbell KA, Liggitt D, Wright B, et al. Humoral immune responses in CD40 ligand-deficient mice. J Exp Med 1994;180:1889–1900.
201. Facchetti F, Appiani C, Salvi L, Levy J, Notarangelo LD. Immunohistologic analysis of ineffective CD40-CD40 ligand interaction in lymphoid tissues from patients with X-linked immunodeficiency with hyper-IgM. Abortive germinal center cell reaction and severe depletion of follicular dendritic cells. J Immunol 1995;154:6624–6633.
202. Chu YW, Marin E, Fuleihan R, Ramesh N, Rosen FS, Geha RS, et al. Somatic mutation of human immunoglobulin V genes in the X-linked HyperIgM syndrome. J Clin Invest 1995;95:1389–1393.
203. van-Essen D, Kikutani H, Gray D. CD40 ligand-transduced co-stimulation of T cells in the development of helper function. Nature 1995;378:620–623.
204. Razanajaona D, van-Kooten C, Lebecque S, Bridon JM, Ho S, Smith S, et al. Somatic mutations in human Ig variable genes correlate with a partially functional CD40-ligand in the X-linked hyper-IgM syndrome. J Immunol 1996;157:1492–1498.
205. Kosco MH, Szakal AK, Tew JG. In vivo obtained antigen presented by germinal center B cells to T cells in vitro. J Immunol 1988;140:354–360.

206. Silvy A, Lagresle C, Bella C, Defrance T. The differentiation of human memory B cells into specific antibody-secreting cells is CD40 independent. Eur J Immunol 1996;26:517–524.
207. Bergman MC, Attrep JF, Grammer AC, Lipsky PE. Ligation of CD40 influences the function of human Ig-secreting B cell hybridomas both positively and negatively. J Immunol 1996;156:3118–3132.
208. Herron LR, Eisenberg RA, Roper E, Kakkanaiah VN, Cohen PL, Kotzin BL. Selection of the T cell receptor repertoire in Lpr mice. J Immunol 1993;151:3450–3459.
209. Singer GG, Abbas AK. The fas antigen is involved in peripheral but not thymic deletion of T lymphocytes in T cell receptor transgenic mice. Immunity 1994;1:365–371.
210. Castro JE, Listman JA, Jacobson BA, Wang Y, Lopez PA, Ju S, et al. Fas modulation of apoptosis during negative selection of thymocytes. Immunity 1996;5:617-627.
211. Cheng J, Zhou T, Liu C, Shapiro JP, Brauer MJ, Kiefer MC, et al. Protection from Fas-mediated apoptosis by a soluble form of the Fas molecule. Science 1994;263:1759–1762.
212. Jodo S, Kobayashi S, Kayagaki N, Ogura N, Feng Y, Amasaki Y, et al. Serum levels of soluble Fas/APO-1 (CD95) and its molecular structure in patients with systemic lupus erythematosus (SLE) and other autoimmune diseases. Clin Exp Immunol 1997;107:89–95.
213. Tandon N, Metcalfe RA, Barnett D, Weetman AP. Expression of the costimulatory molecule B7/BB1 in autoimmune thyroid disease. Q J Med 1994;87:231–236.
214. Sercarz EE, Lehmann PV, Ametani A, Benichou G, Miller A, Moudgil K. Dominance and crypticity of T cell antigenic determinants. Annu Rev Immunol 1993;11:729–766.
215. Wekerle H, Bradl M, Linington C, Kaab G, Kojima K. The shaping of the brain-specific T lymphocyte repertoire in the thymus. Immunol Rev 1996;149:231–243.
216. Warnock MG, Goodacre JA. Cryptic T-cell epitopes and their role in the pathogenesis of autoimmune diseases. Br J Rheumatol 1977;36:1144–1150.
217. Djaballah H. Antigen processing by proteasomes: insights into the molecular basis of crypticity. Mol Biol Rep 1997;24:63–67.
218. Volpe R. Immunological aspects of autoimmune thyroid disease. Prog Clin Biol Res 1981;74:1–27.
219. Volpe R. Immunoregulation in autoimmune thyroid disease. N Engl J Med 1987;316:44–46.
220. Volpe R. Suppressor T lymphocyte dysfunction is important in the pathogenesis of autoimmune thyroid disease: a perspective. Thyroid 1993;3:345–352.
221. Arnon R, Sela M, Teitelbaum D. New insights into the mechanism of action of copolymer 1 in experimental allergic encephalomyelitis and multiple sclerosis. J Neurol 1996;243:S8–13.
222. Bergman B, Haskins K. Autoreactive T-cell clones from the nonobese diabetic mouse. Proc Soc Exp Biol Med 1997;214:41–48.
223. Mieza MA, Itoh T, Cui JQ, Makino Y, Kawano T, Tsuchida K, et al. Selective reduction of Vα14+ NK T cells associated with disease development in autoimmune-prone mice. J Immunol 1996;156:4035–4040.
224. Sakamoto A, Sumida T, Maeda T, Itoh M, Asai T, Takahashi H, et al. T cell receptor Vb repertoire of double-negative α/β T cells in patients with systemic sclerosis. Arthritis Rheum 1992;35:944–948.
225. Baxter AG, Kinder SJ, Hammond KJ, Scollay R, Godfrey DI. Association between αβTCR+CD4− CD8− T-cell deficiency and IDDM in NOD/Lt mice. Diabetes 1997;46:572–582.
226. Iwatani Y, Hidaka Y, Matsuzuka F, Kuma K, Amino N. Intrathyroidal lymphocyte subsets, including unusual CD4+ CD8+ cells and CD3^{lo}TCRαβ$^{lo/-}$CD4−CD8− cells, in autoimmune thyroid disease. Clin Exp Immunol 1993;93:430–436.
227. Kroemer G, Hirsch F, Gonzalez-Garcia A, Martinez C. Differential involvement of Th1 and Th2 cytokines in autoimmune diseases. Autoimmunity 1996;24:25–33.
228. Nisitani S, Tsubata T, Murakami M, Okamoto M, Honjo T. The bcl-2 gene product inhibits clonal deletion of self-reactive B lymphocytes in the periphery but not in the bone marrow. J Exp Med 1993;178:1247–1254.
229. Nomura T, Han H, Howard MC, Yagita H, Yakura H, Honjo T, et al. Antigen receptor-mediated B cell death is blocked by signaling via CD72 or treatment with dextran sulfate and is defective in autoimmunity-prone mice. Int Immunol 1996;8:867-875.
230. Sobel ES, Katagiri T, Katagiri K, Morris SC, Cohen PL, Eisenberg RA. An intrinsic B cell defect is required for the production of autoantibodies in the lpr model of murine systemic autoimmunity. J Exp Med 1991;173:1441–1449.
231. Ridgway WM, Fasso M, Lanctot A, Garvey C, Fathman CG. Breaking self-tolerance in nonobese diabetic mice. J Exp Med 1996;183:1657–1662.

232. Flynn JC, Kong YC. In vivo evidence for CD4+ and CD8+ suppressor T cells in vaccination-induced suppression of murine experimental autoimmune thyroiditis. Clin Immunol Immunopathol 1991; 60:484–494.
233. Eisenbarth GS. Type I diabetes mellitus. A chronic autoimmune disease. N Engl J Med 1986;314: 1360–1368.
234. Adams TE, Alpert S, Hanahan D. Non-tolerance and autoantibodies to a transgenic self antigen expressed in pancreatic beta cells. Nature 1987;325:223–228.
235. Eishi Y, McCullagh P. Acquisition of immunological self-recognition by the fetal rat. Immunology 1988;64:319–323.

2 Immunoregulation in Experimental Autoimmune Endocrine Disease

Peter McCullagh, MD, DPHIL, MRCP

CONTENTS

INTRODUCTION
INTERACTION BETWEEN IMMUNE AND ENDOCRINE SYSTEMS
DEVELOPMENT OF CONCEPTS ABOUT ENDOCRINE AUTOIMMUNITY
POTENTIAL MECHANISMS OF REGULATION
 OF ANTIENDOCRINE AUTOIMMUNITY
THE SIGNIFICANCE OF AUTOANTIGEN IN EXPERIMENTAL
 AUTOIMMUNE ENDOCRINE DISEASE
REGULATION IN EXPERIMENTAL MODELS
 OF ENDOCRINE AUTOIMMUNITY
FUTURE DIRECTIONS
ACKNOWLEDGMENT
REFERENCES

Probably the most satisfactory way to look at autoimmune disease is as a failure at some point of the normal homeostatic mechanisms that prevent the emergence of forbidden clones (1).

INTRODUCTION

The proposition of Mackay and Burnet that failure of immune regulation is best envisaged as the central feature of autoimmune disease remains as relevant three decades later as it was in 1964. Nevertheless, views on the precise manner in which immune homeostasis is achieved have changed since then, accompanying changes in perception of the mechanisms mediating immune functions. It is likely that they will be subject to ongoing modification as understanding of the immune system is further refined.

The aim of this chapter is to consider those aspects of the process of immune regulation that are especially exemplified by, and have been found to be operative in, experimental autoimmune endocrine disease. To do this will entail passing over (other than mentioning) those processes of regulation of autoimmunity that have not been specifically associated with experimental autoimmune endocrine disease (*see* Chapter 1). Discussion of a possible role for some mechanisms in regulating autoimmunity has been omitted,

From: *Contemporary Endocrinology: Autoimmune Endocrinopathies*
Edited by: R. Volpe © Humana Press Inc., Totowa, NJ

either because they do not appear to have a central role in experimental endocrine autoimmunity or because the protocols employed to investigate experimental autoimmune endocrine disease are not suited to probing the operation of those types of regulatory process. For example, if clonal deletion has a major role in preventing experimentally induced endocrine autoimmunity, it is evident that any constraints that it imposes have already been circumvented by the procedures adopted in the experimental induction of a specific autoimmune endocrine disease. Consequently, restraints to autoimmunity imposed by clonal deletion will no longer remain susceptible to experimental examination once autoimmune disease has been induced.

Central to this article will be the contention that the most common approach to the exploration of autoimmune disease, namely, as an exclusively immunological problem, has not been conducive to its solution. On the contrary, to perceive autoimmune endocrine disease primarily from either an immunological or an endocrinological perspective is likely to hinder its understanding. The subdivision of different aspects of investigation of a pathological process into separate disciplines has not, of course, been a feature peculiar to autoimmune endocrine disease. Starting with medical curricula that split biology into numerous subdisciplines, which then form the basis for departments, for research programs within those departments and, ultimately, for the thinking within those programs, predisposes to a fragmented approach. In theory, reduction of a problem to its components, which are then addressed in isolation, after which the results are reassembled to provide a comprehensive account of the original problem, may appear logical. However, in the case of a problem, such as autoimmune endocrine disease, which is characterized at every stage by the interweaving of biological processes that are claimed as their own by separate, administratively defined disciplines, a comprehensive understanding as a result of reduction of the problem to its components is likely to remain elusive.

In a prescient comment, Mackay and Burnet opined that endocrine glands "are undoubtedly concerned" in holding autoimmune reactions in check *(1)*. Their conclusion has had little impact on subsequent immunological research. Nevertheless, the possibility that interaction between endocrine and immune systems may fulfill purposes other than merely preventing the outbreak of overt autoimmunity should not be discarded out of hand. Perhaps such interactions could be important in the normal operation of both systems. On the basis of the concerns outlined above, this author's assessment is that a full explanation of autoimmune endocrine disease will only emerge from a full explication of the nature of normal interactions between immune and endocrine systems rather than from a synthesis of data on the deviation from normal function of both systems in the course of autoimmune disease.

INTERACTION BETWEEN IMMUNE AND ENDOCRINE SYSTEMS

Interaction During Development

The thymus, as the central organ in development of the T-lymphocyte component of the immune system, and as the earliest part of that system to become functional during mammalian ontogeny, has been observed on many occasions to exert a substantial influence on the developing endocrine system. However, apart from the use of thymectomy as a stratagem to elicit autoimmune endocrine diseases in experimental animals, as described (*see* Autoimmune Disease Following Elimination of Lymphocytes section), this influence has not had a major impact on research on normal immune–endocrine interaction. Prior to the overwhelming claims for the thymus as part of the immune system, which emerged in response to the description of the dramatic effects of neonatal thymectomy on immune function in some species, the thymus gland was often accorded honorary status as part of the endocrine system. On this basis, early reports of the consequences of thymectomy emphasized its impact on endocrine tissues.

One consequence of thymectomy in early life, namely that of facilitating the subsequent development of autoimmune reactions in endocrine tissue, has been the subject of much investigation. This emphasis on autoimmune disease has tended to overshadow the early reports of sequelae of this procedure in relation to endocrine organs that, from their original description, appear to have been patently nonimmune. Thus, neonatal thymectomy of mice was shown consistently to result in arrested development of the ovary with subsequent sterility *(2)*. The histological changes observed in affected ovaries in the original reports did not suggest any immunological process. Without exception, there was a striking decrease in the numbers of ripening follicles together with the presence of some degenerative follicles. Corpora lutea were lacking, and the ovarian parenchyma consisted almost exclusively of interstitial gland cells. It was suggested that thymectomy had resulted in injury to ovarian follicles at a very early stage of their development. Furthermore, a strong indication of the marked difference between these ovarian changes and those sequelae of thymectomy that have been classified subsequently as autoimmune was provided by the great discrepancy observed between the number of normal mouse spleen cells required to prevent ovarian dysgenesis compared with prevention of immune deficiency. Whereas there was a requirement for 5×10^6 cells for prevention of immunological depression, as few as 15×10^4 cells sufficed to prevent ovarian dysgenesis, suggesting that different processes were involved in the two situations *(3)*. However the likely multifactorial basis of ovarian autoimmunity developing, in addition to arrested development, after thymectomy was strikingly demonstrated when neonatally thymectomized mice were additionally exposed to an increased level of gonadotrophin stimulation. Whereas thymectomy alone led to the failure of formation of ovarian follicles together with hyperplasia of the interstitial cells, gonadotrophin stimulation of these thymectomized mice led to the development of an ovarian lymphocytic infiltrate highly suggestive of autoimmune disease *(4)*. This early suggestion of a requirement for the concurrence of both immunological and endocrinological prerequisites in order for development of autoimmune endocrinopathies was somewhat unexpected. Earlier studies in which ovaries had been removed and heterotopically transplanted to the spleen, resulting in inactivation of their hormonal products draining into the hepatic portal system, had revealed the capacity of excessive gonadotrophin stimulation, in the absence of feedback inhibition, to initiate pathological ovarian changes *(5)*.

Besedovsky and Sorkin have postulated the existence of a "network of immune–neuroendocrine interactions" involved in immunoregulation *(6)*. Furthermore, they suggested that a bidirectional interaction between immune and endocrine systems occurs during ontogeny. In addition to the observations noted above of the occurrence of lymphocytic infiltration in endocrine organs, they cited their earlier demonstrations of degranulation of somatotrophin-producing cells in the pituitary, delayed puberty, persistence of the adrenal reticular zone, hypothyroidism, and alterations in blood levels of gonadal hormones after thymectomy. In view of these consequences, it would be simplistic to regard a neonatally thymectomized mouse as being normal apart from its immune system.

Interaction Evidenced in the Mature Structure and Function of Immune and Endocrine Systems

The anatomical associations between endocrine and immune systems are extraordinarily close and are often, equally extraordinarily, ignored. Some dictionary definitions of endocrine glands, in order to clarify the distinction from exocrine tissue, have specified as their defining attribute the secretion of their products directly into the bloodstream *(7)*. A more accurate, although less concise, description would note that the products of endocrine glands were secreted into the extracellular fluid from which they passed into the bloodstream both directly and via the lymphatic system. The entry of hormonal products into draining lymphatics has been observed in the case of all of the endocrine glands in which it has been sought, and in the case of at least one gland, carriage via local lymphatics appears to account for a substantial part of the hormone output.

To assess the possible biological significance of the carriage of hormones from endocrine glands via lymphatics, it is necessary to consider both the quantity of hormone transported by this route and its concentration in the lymph. Evaluation of the relative importance of removal of any hormone, via lymphatic vessels and veins, for its distribution throughout the body will necessarily be based on the relative quantities of hormone transported by each route. On the other hand, assessment of the possible impact on local lymphoid tissue of a hormone passing to the lymph node(s) draining an endocrine gland via its afferent lymphatic vessels will be dependent on the concentration of that hormone in lymph. This will determine the intensity of exposure to the products of that endocrine gland of cells trafficking through those lymph nodes. Since the rate of lymph flow from an endocrine gland is invariably less than the rate of flow of blood in its draining veins (often by two or more orders of magnitude), comparable concentrations of hormone can readily exist in vein and lymphatic, even though there is a much greater transport of hormone via the former. If the effects of any hormone on its draining lymph node are divided artificially, but conventionally into the "endocrinological" and the "antigenically specific," the magnitude of either could reasonably be expected to be affected by hormone concentration. It would be no less reasonable to anticipate that early and continuing exposure of local draining lymphoid tissue to products released from an endocrine gland would render it more susceptible than the immune system in general to induction of tolerance of those products.

Lymph nodes draining any endocrine gland are likely to be distinguished in a number of ways from the remainder of the immune system. The migration, in the afferent lymph draining to those nodes, of antigen-presenting cells that have been resident in the stroma of the endocrine gland will exert an influence additional to that of any hormonal products free in the lymph plasma. Although the role of antigen-presenting cells in the induction of immune responses has been well recognized, the possibility of their involvement in tolerance induction remains largely unexplored. As a general observation, the significance of the local lymph nodes in regulating any instance of endocrine autoimmunity will likely depend on the relative importance of the alternative mechanisms available to achieve regulation in that instance. If, for example, deletion of specifically reactive clones were to be the major regulatory mechanism, it is difficult to envisage ways in which a single lymph node, or group of nodes, could efficiently purge the entire immune system of antiself-reactivity directed against an endocrine gland in their field of drainage. On the other hand, if positive downregulation of autoimmunity by a specifically reactive subset of T lymphocytes were of major importance, then the local lymph nodes, which were continually exposed to relevant autoantigenic material, could be readily envisaged as the ideal location for generation of these cells and their export throughout the body via the lymphatic system.

With regard to the entry of hormones into lymph, Daniel et al. reported as early as 1961 that a thyroid hormone (measured by its incorporation of radioiodine) was present in lymph draining from the thyroid gland of rabbits, cats, and sheep at a higher concentration than in venous blood from the gland *(8)*. They concluded that a significant proportion of the thyroid hormone output was transported from the gland in its draining lymph. It was also found that the ^{131}I, which could be detected in lymph draining from the thyroid gland of cats and monkeys, represented both thyroxine and thyroglobulin, although the latter had previously been assumed to be a "hidden antigen" to which the immune system was not exposed *(9)*.

Subsequently, examination of lymph draining from the ovary and testis of four species found that the lymph concentration of hormones produced by the gonad exceeded that in the peripheral venous blood. Estimation of corticosteroid levels in lymph draining from the adrenal gland was limited by the need to sample from the cisterna chyli after dilution by intestinal lymph *(10)*, since lymph entering the cisterna chyli has already traversed one or more regional lymph nodes. Depending on their proximity to the adrenal glands, it is inevitable that the concentrations of hormonal products to which those nodes were exposed would have been considerably higher than those measured in the cisterna. Examination of lymph from the testis of sheep revealed that although only a minority of the hormone reached the systemic circulation via lymphatics, concentrations in these local draining lymphatics were two to eight times those of peripheral blood *(11)*. More strikingly, the progesterone concentration in ovarian lymph was more than 200 times greater than that in peripheral blood *(12)*.

Immune–Endocrine Interactions at a Molecular Level

Close comparison of many products of endocrine cells and lymphocytes has increasingly indicated their structural identity. The number of functions that have been documented as being mediated by cytokines and hormones exceeds the number of molecular species, providing a clear indication of multiple actions by single factors. As a consequence, there are an increasing number of reports that products of one system can evoke responses by cells of the other. As implied by this observation, cells of one system may express receptors for the products of the other. Furthermore, in a number of instances, cells of one system have been observed to release molecules identical with products of the other. The inescapable conclusion from this "molecular sharing" is that endocrine and immune systems may be expected to influence each other in a variety of ways, and that this is one aspect of their normal functioning.

Potential immune–endocrine molecular interactions will be summarized into four arbitrary groups, namely:

1. Action of lymphokines on endocrine tissue.
2. Actions of hormones on immune function.
3. Expression of receptors for hormones by lymphocytes.
4. Production of hormones, normally regarded as exclusive products of endocrine tissue, by lymphocytes.

Although numerous instances exist of the release of, or response to, active molecules from one system by the cells of the other, the physiological relevance of associated interactions remains less clear. Such issues as the comparability of concentrations examined in vitro with those occurring in vivo, the persistence of activity in circulation and tissues, and the likelihood of access of the factors under consideration to specific tissues must all be taken into consideration.

Specific indications of immune–endocrine molecular interactions include reports of the action of lymphokines on a number of endocrine glands. Thus, interleukin 1 (IL-1) can act as a glucocorticoid-increasing factor, an effect that appears to be exerted centrally via the hypothalamus rather than directly on the adrenals *(13)*. IL-1 has also been found, at concentrations within the range normally occurring in serum, to stimulate the release of a range of pituitary hormones *(14)*. It is likely that this observation explains the phenomenon of release of hormones from the anterior pituitary gland in response to bacterial endotoxin. Endotoxin has a well-established capacity to sitmulate the production of IL-1 by monocytes. It is likely that the demonstrated IL-1 stimulation of secretion of corticotrophin, luteinizing hormone, growth hormone, and thyrotrophin, but not of prolactin, by rat pituitary cell monolayers represents the mechanism of this endotoxin action. The concentrations of IL-1 required to stimulate pituitary cells in tissue culture fell within the range normally observed in serum. More recently, it has been demonstrated that both IL-1 and interleukin 2 (IL-2) can enhance the expression of pro-opiomelanocortin (POMC) mRNA by pituitary cells *(15)*. IL-1 and IL-2 appear to act in a manner similar to that of corticotrophin-releasing factor to increase POMC mRNA in mouse pituitary tumor cells. It has been speculated that the resulting increased release of corticotrophin would lead to changes in glucocorticoid levels that could, in turn, impact on the immune system to create a potential regulatory loop *(15)*. The impact of thymic products on the immature endocrine system is also thought to be mediated through the pituitary *(16)*. Thus, abnormally low levels of thyroxine and testosterone have been observed during first few days of life of neonatally thymectomized mice. (Similar abnormalities are also observed in nude mice born without a thymus.) The administration of thyrotrophin to mice thymectomized neonatally induces a rapid increase in serum thyroxine levels, implying that the normal effect of an intact thyroid gland is exerted at a hypothalamic level.

Interactions in the other direction, namely of endocrine products on the immune system, have also frequently been detected. Some of these, such as the lympholytic effects of steroids, have been recognized for decades and have provided the basis for therapeutic interference with immune function. Similarly, the existence of pronounced susceptibility, based on gender, to some autoimmune endocrine diseases has been associated with the facilitating influence of hormones. More recently, a number of more subtle influences of other hormones on immune function have been discovered. For example, α-endorphin has been shown to depress the antibody response of peripheral blood lymphocytes, apparently by binding to opioid receptors *(17)*. The dose-response curve of this effect was biphasic with the hemolytic plaque-forming cell response returning to control values at higher concentrations of α-endorphin. In evaluating the physiological significance of this effect, it was considered that although the α-endorphin concentrations used in tissue culture were relatively high by comparison with serum levels, this may have been compatible with the exercise of a paracrine role by α-endorphin secreted by cells of the immune system *(17)*. β-endorphin has been shown to increase the cytolytic activity of natural killer cells as well as interferon production by lymphocytes *(18)*.

POMC-derived peptides have the capacity to increase the production of interleukin 10 (IL-10) by monocytes, an action that may have the effect of suppressing an immune response *(19)*. Since IL-10 can inhibit the production of inflammatory cytokines and has been shown to inhibit both the induction and elicitation of delayed-type hypersensitivity, this effect of α-melanocyte-stimulating hormone could have biological significance. It was notable that it applied to monocytes, but not to T lymphocytes *(19)*. Apart from the occurrence of direct effects of hormones on cells of the immune system in vitro, the migration of lymphocytes can also be affected. Prolactin has been found to increase the selective retention in the mammary gland of migrating IgA-positive cells derived from gut-associated lymphoid tissue *(20)*. Conversely, the administration of testosterone to lactating mice not only inhibited the development of the mammary secretory immune system, but also decreased the migration of lymphocytes from the gut to the mammary gland. Given the central role of lymphocyte migration in immune responses, it would be most surprising if effects of this type did not have substantial implications for immunological function. Subsequently, lymphocytes have been shown to express receptors for prolactin and to be stimulated by the binding of the hormone to these *(21)*. A regulatory role for prolactin has been postulated in both humoral and cell-mediated immune responses. Apart from any actions on lymphocyte migration, serum prolactin levels have been shown to influence lymphocyte reactivity. Thus, interference with prolactin release from the pituitary by means of bromocriptine has been shown to reduce lymphocyte reactivity, both in mixed lymphocyte and graft-vs-host reactions *(22)*.

Apart from the expression of receptors for hormones by lymphocytes and responsiveness of those cells to the appropriate hormone and the capacity of lymphokines to affect the functioning of endocrine tissues, the production of specific hormones by lymphoid cells has been confirmed in a number of instances. A wide range of hormones that have previously been assumed to be exclusively products of the formally defined endocrine system have now been observed also to be produced by lymphocytes. Although the nature of the hormone produced in any situation has been dependent on the type of stimulus, the significance of each hormone in the circumstances surrounding its production is not yet clear. Nevertheless, it is likely that in at least some of these situations, "conventional" hormones produced by lymphocytes may be acting primarily on other lymphocytes to regulate immune responsiveness, further exemplifying the incestuous relationship between immune and endocrine systems.

Paralleling the normal derivation of adrenocorticotrophin (ACTH) and the endorphins from a common precursor molecule in the pituitary, it has been demonstrated that 100% of a population of human peripheral blood lymphocytes infected with Newcastle disease virus were capable of producing both ACTH and γ-endorphin-related substances, apparently associated with interferon α *(23)*. In contrast with this outcome, if lymphocytes of similar origin were exposed to the mitogen staphylococcal enterotoxin A, thyroid-stimulating hormone (TSH) (but not ACTH) was produced *(24)*. Subsequent investigation of the circumstances influencing antibody responses in vitro has revealed that TSH can enhance these *(25)*. This TSH-mediated effect is independent of macrophages, but requires the presence of T cells. It was speculated that TSH produced by lymphocytes might act to promote T-cell growth or differentiation or, less directly, by enhancing the release of other soluble mediators. In light of these reports, the production of TSH by lymphocytes may represent an immunoregulatory mechanism.

An example of production of another hormone by human peripheral blood lymphocytes in response to a third type of immunological stimulus is the release of chorionic gonadotrophin by the participating cells in the course of mixed lymphocyte reactions *(26)*. The production of gonadotrophin in response to confrontation with allogeneic cells has predictably led to the suggestion that this could represent a component of the reaction of the maternal immune system to exposure to the implanting blastocyst, which has the effect of facilitating implantation. There is evidence that at least in some circumstances, recognition of the antigenic foreignness of the blastocyst by the maternal immune system may assist in its survival. Since adequate levels of chorionic gonadotrophin are a prerequisite if implantation is to be successful, the local release of this hormone by lymphocytes in the endometrium at the site of implantation could be advantageous.

Apart from the effects of prolactin on lymphocyte migration and immunological reactivity both in vitro and in vivo, it appears that appropriately stimulated lymphocytes may themselves produce this hormone. Thus, a prolactin-related mRNA, differing from that detectable in pituitary cells, has been detected in murine lymphocytes following stimulation with the mitogen concanavalin A *(22)*. This raises the possibility, already referred to in the case of TSH, of a "conventional" hormone also being utilized as a locally acting factor capable of modulating the immune responsiveness of the lymphocyte population producing it.

Assessment of the biological significance of observations of the type summarized above is less simple than their detection. The specificity of action of cytokines in general is conferred by the close localization of that action to the cell, which has released the cytokine *(27)*. An illustration of the extreme localization of effect to the site of release of a cytokine has been provided by a report that cytokine release could be targeted specifically in the direction of the cell eliciting it *(28)*. In a tissue in which the position of cells is fixed, the action of any cytokine could be as predictable and immutable as the interaction between two neurons fixed on either side of a synapse. However, lymphocytes are not fixed cells. They migrate through almost all tissues in the body with considerable specificity conferred by their antigenic (and autoantigenic) specificity. Consequently, although it is difficult to examine whether interactions between lymphocytes and endocrine cells occur normally in the body, it remains likely that such interactions fulfill a purpose given the extensive sharing of products and the receptors corresponding to them.

It remains likely that, both in the initiation and the progression of autoimmune pathological processes, interactions between lymphocytes and endocrine cells contribute to the outcome and to overt autoimmunity. For example, responsiveness of the hypothalamus of the OS chick to the glucocorticoid-increasing action of IL-1 appears to be impaired. Although lymphocytes from this strain, which is susceptible to spontaneous autoimmune thyroiditis, produce IL-1 in a normal manner when activated, this cytokine fails to affect the neuroendocrine axis as in a normal chick *(13)*. The extent to which this deficiency serves to explain the genetic susceptibility of this strain to autoimmunity remains unknown. Further evidence for an interplay between processes conventionally regarded as "immunological" and "endocrinological" during the development of autoimmune thyroiditis in the OS chick has come with the observation of functional abnormalities in the thyroid gland antedating the onset of the autoimmune process *(29)*. The abnormally high uptake of iodine into the thyroid glands of TSH-suppressed OS chicks occurs also in the Cornell strain from which the OS strain was originally derived. Although Cornell strain chicks do not spontaneously develop thyroiditis, this does occur if they receive autoreactive cells from OS donors. This has suggested that both the abnormality of thyroid metabolism and the genetic predisposition to autoimmunity are required for the development of this form of thyroiditis. (*See* Chapter 4.)

In addition to the likely hypothalamic influences exerted on the immune system by means of endocrine glands, there is ample anatomical evidence for direct access of the nervous system to the organs of the immune system. It is reasonable to anticipate not only that such connections fulfill a role in normal functioning of immune and endocrine systems, but also that they afford a capacity for interaction during the development and resolution of autoimmune pathology. On the basis of anatomical studies, Felten et al. have proposed that norepinephrine, demonstrable in lymphoid tissue, acts as a neurotransmitter *(30)*. The operation of extensions of the sympathetic nervous system within the immune system could explain earlier observations, such as the persistence of changes in immune responsiveness associated with stress in hypophysectomized animals. The apparently selective direction of postganglionic noradrenergic fibers to T-lymphocyte zones supports the existence of a specific role. The entry of these fibres into thymic tissue may also correlate with the demonstration of stimulation of lymphopoiesis in cultivated fetal mouse thymus by phenylephrine *(31)*. Apart from demonstrations of interactions of the types summarized above, between the normally functioning immune and endocrine systems, some examples of deviations of endocrine gland function as a direct consequence of a specific action of the immune system (as distinct from aberrant endocrine function secondary to autoimmune damage) have been recognized. The earliest of these was the observation by Adams of the presence of a serum factor, designated as long-acting thyroid stimulator (LATS) in some cases of hyperthyroidism *(32)*. Subsequent investigations have raised the possibility that LATS was an antibody directed against the TSH receptor on thyrocytes and, therefore, able to bind to and stimulate them (reviewed in *33*; *see also* Chapter 9). Election microscopic examination of thyrocytes exposed to LATS has revealed changes morphologically indistinguishable from those produced by exposure to TSH, although with a different time scale. These include the formation of pseudopods and the appearance of large colloid droplets, fusing with lysosomes to form phagolysosomes *(33)*. Other examples of stimulatory effects on thyroid function initiated by antithyroid autoantibodies have been observed. It has been suggested that at least in one instance, deliberate interference with interaction between a hormone and the receptors for it expressed by lymphocytes may be the basis for a therapeutic effect. Thus, the powerful immunosuppressive agent cyclosporin is known to block the synthetic events that succeed binding of prolactin to lymphocytes and appear to be essential for mediation of the immune stimulation that follows binding *(21)*.

The frequency with which molecules are shared by immune and endocrine systems could suggest that in addition to the close functional interaction that characterizes these systems, they have had a close evolutionary association. Any attempt to test for this would require consideration of associations between endocrine and immunological functioning in less-evolved species and is beyond the scope of this chapter.

DEVELOPMENT OF CONCEPTS ABOUT ENDOCRINE AUTOIMMUNITY

Speculation and assumption about the nature of autoimmunity have followed presumptions and insights about functioning of the immune system as a whole. Clinical and experimental examples of autoimmunity against endocrine tissues have exerted more influence on thinking about autoimmunity than general understanding of the immune system has contributed to elucidating the basis of autoimmune endocrine disease. The first serious attempt to develop an explanation for autoimmunity was associated with Burnet's presentation of the clonal selection theory. It is notable, however, that there had been a presumption, antedating this and probably attributable to Ehrlich's writing on *horror autotoxicus*, that autoimmunity must be inherently bad *(34)*. This presumption that any response on the part of the immune system to an autoantigen is invariably undesirable has directed (and perhaps distorted) thinking about autoimmunity and autoimmune disease. However, in view of the accumulating indications of both autoimmune activity and immune–endocrine interactions in normal subjects, this presumption is now no longer tenable. Burnet envisaged pathological autoimmunity as an inevitable consequence of the persistence of "forbidden clones" of lymphocytes with antiself-reactivity. It was proposed that autoreactive clones did not produce damage in normal animals, either because they had been deleted as a consequence of exposure to their target self-antigens before the development of immune competence or because those target self-antigens remained permanently hidden from the immune system. Unless the possibility of deletion of antiself-reactive clones of lymphocytes remained available throughout life, it would be necessary to postulate that any autoantigens that only appeared for the first time after acquisition of immune competence (such as antigens expressed by cells of the mature gonads) would have to remain "hidden."

Experimental investigation of antiendocrine autoimmunity has been directed by ideas current at any time about immunological function in general. These determined both those experiments that were performed and those that were not. An early example of the latter and, in particular, of acceptance of the notion of hidden antigens as an explanation for regulation of autoimmunity, influenced Triplett in planning an experiment to test whether complete removal of an autoantigen before immunological competence had been attained would curtail the capacity of the immune system to recognize it as self. The thyroid gland was specifically excluded as a tissue to be removed, because thyroglobulin was regarded as a hidden antigen *(35)*. (The outcome and implications of this experiment will be discussed later, but it was anticipated that if thyroglobulin was a completely hidden antigen, the removal of its source would not have any effect on the capacity of the immune system to initiate autoimmune thyroiditis). However, the validity of regarding thyroglobulin as a hidden antigen failed to survive for long after its designation as such, once its entry into the draining lymph was recognized. Demonstration that thyroglobulin not only left the thyroid gland, but did so via lymphatic vessels, with the implications of this for exposure of the local lymphoid tissue to it, effectively excluded any possibility that it was hidden from the immune system.

Recognition that at least some of the autoantigens expressed by tissues that did not fully develop until after immunological maturation had been completed were not sequestrated from the immune system, but nevertheless failed to evoke an autoimmune response, ensured that the concept of "hidden" antigens could not serve as a general explanation for regulation of autoimmunity. An additional obstacle to providing a comprehensive explanation for regulation based exclusively on clonal deletion was the accumulation of reports of the presence of autoreactive lymphocytes in the circulation of normal animals in which there was no suggestion of autoimmune disease affecting the target tissues against which their autoreactivity was directed *(36)*. If only one class of lymphocytes was required to undertake an immune response to completion, and autoreactive cells of that class were detectable, it would be very difficult to explain the lack of overt autoimmunity. However, with recognition of the significance of collaboration between T and B cells in mounting immune responses, reconciliation of the presence of cells capable of producing autoantibodies in normal subjects with the absence of autoimmune disease became feasible. Whereas the presence of autoreactive lymphocytes directed against a tissue or organ that nevertheless remained undamaged is incompatible with deletion of that autoreactive clone as suggested by Mackay and Burnet, the persistence of autoreactive cells of one class could be consistent with the absence of autoimmune damage provided appropriately reactive cells of the other class, which were essential for collaboration, were lacking. An explanation on this basis, which was proposed by Allison et al. could suffice to explain the absence of an autoimmune disease, which was mediated by antibody, despite the presence of antiself-reactive B cells, provided collaborating T cells were unavailable *(37)*. Interruption of the regulation of autoimmunity achieved in this manner was envisaged as a consequence of vicarious stimulation of autoreactive B lymphocytes by a process not dependent on the presence of T lymphocytes with the same antiself-reactivity. In effect, regulation would still be primarily dependent on the absence of autoreactive cells.

Another hypothesis advanced by Allison et al. represented the first suggestion that T lymphocytes might be responsible for direct suppression of autoantibody production by B lymphocytes *(37)*. This proposal was based on the preceding demonstration that such suppression accounted for tolerance of some nonself-antigens. Rather than being dependent on the lack of cooperation from T lymphocytes, it was suggested that self-tolerance could reflect a "specific feedback control" exerted by these cells on autoreactive B cells.

Two recurrent observations derived from clinical and experimental studies of autoimmune endocrine disease have continued to influence the further development of concepts of immune regulation. The first observation concerned the tendency of autoimmunity affecting endocrine glands to pass into spontaneous remission. The second was the tendency of autoimmunity simultaneously to affect more than one endocrine organ, indicating the occurrence of autoreactivity directed against a number of dissimilar autoantigens. Both of these observations have been interpreted as supporting the existence of positive mechanisms (as distinct from merely the absence of specifically reactive cells required for the expression of autoimmunity) that can downregulate autoreactivity.

The tendency for spontaneous remission of autoimmune endocrine disease to occur has led to the inference of the existence of a positive mechanism to maintain self-tolerance on the basis that the downregulation of an established autoimmune process observed in spontaneous remission represented the regaining of ascendancy by the process that was normally responsible for preventing the emergence of overt autoimmunity in the first place. Although this appears to be a reasonable hypothesis, it is not proven. There is no *a priori* reason, apart from biological economy, why any process that evolves in the course of overt autoimmune disease and has the effect of curtailing it should be identical with that process, or processes, originally charged with the prevention of development of disease in a normal subject. However, since the regulatory process that normally prevails, and ensures the absence of autoimmune pathology is not observable (in contrast to the autoimmune events that occur if it is interrupted), it has been logistically simpler to obtain data relating to mechanisms that are superimposed on an existing autoimmune state. Nevertheless, although documentation of the latter may provide clues, it cannot furnish proof about regulatory mechanisms operating in normal subjects.

The second recurrent observation, namely that autoimmune processes often develop simultaneously in more than one endocrine organ, has been considered to favor an (antigenically nonspecific) suspension of normal downregulation in general as the basis for endocrine autoimmune disease. The most common inference has been that an autoantigenically nonspecific stimulus has interrupted the normal regulatory process. This would contrast with the situation in which an abnormal process was triggered by the presentation of an autoantigen to the immune system in circumstances that lead to the activation of specific autoreactive cells as the primary event. (The latter is, incidentally, the presumed mechanism operative in the most common type of model that has been employed to study autoimmunity, namely, the challenge of a normal animal with autoantigen plus an adjuvant.) Both of these types of observations (spontaneous remission and multiple-organ involvement) have exerted considerable influence on subsequent perceptions of the regulation of autoimmune endocrine disease.

Since the subject of this chapter is not experimental autoimmune endocrine disease *per se*, but its regulation, there will be very little discussion of a widely used protocol for induction of autoimmunity, namely the presentation of autoantigen (either intact or modified) together with adjuvant. Although this type of approach affords a readily reproducible means of producing an organ-specific autoimmune disease, it might be increasingly seen as distant from the processes that underlie the spontaneous initiation of autoimmune disease to the extent that these represent an interruption of a normal regulatory mechanism. Attempts to infer the nature of the pre-existing regulation of autoimmunity from the study of autoimmune diseases induced using adjuvants are likely to be bedevilled by the difficulty of distinguishing between adjuvant-initiated processes that are on the direct path to autoimmune disease and other phenomena that represent no more than one of the many incidental and poorly understood side effects of adjuvants.

POTENTIAL MECHANISMS OF REGULATION OF ANTIENDOCRINE AUTOIMMUNITY

Although efforts to explain a phenomenon, such as antiendocrine autoimmunity, and the safeguards normally in place to curtail it have usually commenced with the implicit proposition that a single mechanism would suffice to explain all instances, this has certainly now been recognized as overly simplistic. It has become clear that at least four discrete mechanisms could potentially contribute to preventing the development of endocrine autoimmunity. These may be conveniently summarized as the deletion of autoreactive clones, the lack of presentation of autoantigens in a manner adequate for inducing an immune response (including the seclusion of autoantigens from the immune system), the induction of an autoantigenically specific anergy, and the operation of dominant, or suppressive, mechanisms capable of curtailing the induction of autoimmunity. The following paragraphs provide a brief summary of what it might, and might not, be possible to discover about each of these theoretical mechanisms from study of experimental autoimmune endocrine diseases. Before examining the experimental models that are currently in use to investigate details of these different mechanisms, the likely implications of each mechanism for interpretation of observations obtained from those models will be briefly considered.

The central feature of clonal deletion that bears on its applicability to regulation of autoimmune endocrinopathies is the probable anatomical restriction of this process to the thymus. There have been indications that clonal deletion is possible extrathymically. However, the likely requirements for this to occur, namely, initial stimulation of T lymphocytes by persistent, high antigen concentrations, are unlikely to be readily applicable to endocrine autoantigens *(38)*. Apart from extrathymic elimination of clones, an alternative possibility for permitting clonal deletion of endocrine autoantigens, namely the intrathymic expression of these autoantigens, could be suggested. However, evidence for this remains relatively limited. There have been reports that transgenic "neoantigens" targeted to other tissues have been expressed in the thymus *(39)*. Although these observations certainly carry implications for the interpretation of experiments intended to study the existence of extrathymically induced tolerance of these neoantigens, their implications for the expression of endocrine tissue-specific autoantigens by thymic cells are uncertain. The presence in the thymus of mRNA for normal autoantigens, such as insulin, produced in other tissues, has also been reported and may be more relevant *(40)*. In either of these situations, it would be necessary to envisage clonal deletion as a more extended process than originally proposed by Burnet because of the delay in expression of some endocrine autoantigens until a stage of development considerably later than the timing of maturation of the immune system. That is, an extension of the process of clonal deletion in both time and location would be required.

Apart from the physical elimination of specifically autoreactive cells, evidence has accumulated suggesting that in some situations, such cells may not be destroyed, but may be rendered anergic or unreactive *(41)*. The basis for induction of anergy in T cells is likely to be the normal requirement for contact between molecules on the T-cell surface and corresponding molecules on the antigen-presenting cell, in addition to exposure to the target autoantigen if T-cell activation is to occur. In the absence of these auxiliary processes (for example, if the cells presenting antigen lack the required costimulatory surface molecules), exposure of a T cell to its specific autoantigen is likely to render it anergic. It appears that the molecules required to provide the auxiliary stimulus have to be located on the interacting cells (i.e., antigen-presenting and T cell). Nondeletional types of inactivation have also been demonstrated in the case of B cells. The observed short life-span of anergic B cells suggests that this may represent a stage on the way to deletion *(41)*. Consequently, whether anergy of autoreactive cells necessarily represents a stage in a process of physical deletion or is itself a stable state in which cells may survive indefinitely remains uncertain.

The presentation of endocrine autoantigens in a way that was inadequate to induce autoimmunity might be accomplished by their seclusion from the immune system or by their expression or their exposure to the immune system in circumstances that are unsuitable for its effective stimulation *(42,43)*. The original proposal that some autoantigens might remain permanently "hidden" from the immune system has not gained much experimental support, and it would appear to be difficult confidently to confirm such seclusion, nor is it feasible to specify a threshold of antigenic exposure below which autoantigens would be incapable of stimulating the immune system.

However, if the requirement for an autoantigen to be "hidden" was that no quantity of it whatsoever escaped from the source organ, substantiation of this status would approach the technologically unattainable. Considerable information has accumulated about the requirements for effective antigen presentation to the immune system. As noted above, expression of costimulatory molecules by antigen-presenting cells is essential if they are to stimulate T cells effectively *(42)*. Absence from an endocrine gland of antigen-presenting cells expressing the appropriate molecules could effectively preclude activation of specifically reactive T cells entering that organ. To the extent that inadequate presentation of an autoantigen accounted for the lack of an immune response against it, the expectation would be that the immune system remained neither specifically immune to, nor tolerant of, that antigen. As a consequence, dysregulation, with the resultant development of autoimmunity, should require no more than its effective presentation to the immune system.

Elucidation of the significance of antigen expression by endocrine cells as a possible factor contributing to the initiation of autoimmune disease has been complicated by the occurrence of changes in antigen expression as a consequence of established autoimmune disease. For example, uncertainty remains concerning the role of class II human leukocyte antigen expression by thyrocytes in autoimmune thyroid disease. That such expression occurs in thyroid tissue affected by autoimmunity is well established. What remains in contention is whether this reflects a change that antedates and facilitates the development of thyroiditis *(44)*, or whether it is exclusively a consequence of exposure of thyrocytes to cytokines released by inflammatory cells *(43)*. That cytokines can induce expression of class II antigens need not exclude the possibility that such expression can also occur as an initiating event in antithyroid autoimmunity.

The most basic observable feature of any suppressive mechanism responsible for regulation of endocrine autoimmunity would be its dominance over the autoimmune state. That is, admixture of normal and autoreactive cells, either in vivo or in vitro, could reasonably be expected to result in assertion of the normal, dominant state. Acceptance of the existence of immune suppression has been retarded, perhaps because most experimental efforts have been predominantly addressed to identifying discrete suppressor T lymphocytes with distinctive attributes that distinguished them from cytotoxic T cells with the same antigenic specificity. This approach of attempting to isolate and characterize distinctive suppressor cells rather than examining the process of suppression itself derived from the presumption that elucidation of the process of suppression and the characterization of the attributes of a suppressor cell, irrespective of the circumstances in which it was functioning, were synonymous issues. The approach has been notably unproductive and, as a result, both the existence and significance of suppression itself have been severely questioned. The failure over a prolonged period to identify either cells expressing phenotypes exclusively associated with suppression or cell products with specific suppressor functions led to suggestions that immune suppression lacked biological relevance. However, an alternative explanation for this failure could be that the assumptions underlying what to look for were faulty. In particular, research into regulation of experimental allergic encephalomyelitis (EAE) has pointed to the existence of regulatory T cells that recognize the same autoantigenic epitope as the cytotoxic T cells responsible for EAE *(45)*. Such suppressor cells as these need not be distinguishable from autoreactive cytotoxic cells on the basis of phenotype. In the case of EAE, it appears that their capacity for downregulating cytotoxic cells is dependent on their distinctive pattern of cytokine release (differing from that of cytotoxic cells with the same antigenic specificity) in response to exposure to their specific, shared autoantigen *(46)*.

Being exclusively concerned with experimental models of autoimmune regulation, this chapter will deal only with that potential regulatory mechanism to the understanding of which these models have contributed. Study of clonal deletion, anergy, and autoantigen presentation has, in general, not been pursued in the context of experimental endocrine autoimmunity, whereas data on peripheral downregulation of autoimmunity has been derived from this type of model. Nevertheless, it should be emphasized that the relative lack of data derived from studies of endocrine autoimmunity, and relating to the three former potential mechanisms for autoimmune regulation, cannot be automatically interpreted as implying that they do not fill significant roles in curtailing autoimmune disease. It reflects the lesser suitability of the available experimental endocrine autoimmunity models for examining these mechanisms.

THE SIGNIFICANCE OF AUTOANTIGEN IN EXPERIMENTAL AUTOIMMUNE ENDOCRINE DISEASE

Irrespective of which mechanism of regulation of autoimmunity is operative in any situation, the central regulatory role of the autoantigen itself should be stressed. Apart from the expected requirements for antigen to effect clonal deletion or anergy, its presence has been shown to be essential, together with other factors, for the induction of T cells responsible for downregulation in normal animals, and for the development and maintenance of autoimmunity in genetically predisposed animals. Exemplifying the latter role, it has been shown that spontaneous autoimmune thyroiditis fails to develop in obese strain (OS) chickens if neonatal thyroidectomy has been performed *(47)*. Furthermore, if thyroidectomy is undertaken in mature chicks with established thyroiditis, the autoimmune response is not maintained *(47)*. Similar outcomes have been reported in nonobese diabetic (NOD) mice in that the usual capacity of spleen cells from adult NOD mice to transfer diabetes to irradiated recipients is lost if the donors have been treated with alloxan to destroy their β cells earlier in life *(48)*. Furthermore, not only are β cells required to induce autoimmunity in NOD mice, but their continued presence is necessary if spleen cells from actively diabetic NOD mice are to retain their capacity to transfer anti-β-cell autoimmunity after temporary "parking" in irradiated mice. Thus, alloxan-treated mice are inadequate temporary hosts for the preservation of anti-β-cell autoreactivity *(48)*.

The presence of the appropriate autoantigens is also required for the induction of lymphocytes with specific downregulatory capacity in immature animals. Cells from mice that have been oophorectomized as neonates fail to prevent autoimmune oophoritis in thymectomized recipients *(49)*, whereas fetal lambs require an intact thyroid gland if they are to develop T cells capable of suppressing autoimmune thyroiditis *(50)*.

REGULATION IN EXPERIMENTAL MODELS OF ENDOCRINE AUTOIMMUNITY

Each type of model of experimental autoimmune disease provides some clues about possible regulatory mechanisms. In anticipation of considering them, it can be indicated that taken as a group, they do not clearly indict any single mechanism as a general explanation for regulation of autoimmunity in each situation. The operation of different processes in different experimental autoimmune models suggests that a similar diversity may also apply to human autoimmune endocrine disease.

Of the four most common experimental variants for inducing autoimmunity, the most useful assistance in understanding regulation has come from approaches based on lymphocyte depletion and autoantigen deprivation, because they offer an opportunity to detect what is happening in the immune system before the appearance of disease. The use of adjuvant plus autoantigen to induce autoimmunity lends itself to examination of those processes that are likely to be activated in order to downregulate established autoimmunity. As indicated above, it may be possible to extrapolate from processes that curtail established autoimmune disease to infer what might happen as a preventive process.

Reference has already been made to the multiplicity of factors that have been incriminated in the emergence of frank autoimmune disease in genetically predisposed strains of experimental animals. The example of the OS chick in which susceptibility to development of autoimmune thyroiditis depends both on its abnormal thyroid physiology and the presence of autoreactive lymphocytes emphasizes the likelihood that similarly diverse processes are likely to constitute potential regulatory mechanisms. In considering the regulation of thyroid autoimmunity in these animals, it will be necessary to take account of "nonimmunological" factors that also influence the development of autoimmune pathology. Regulation of the progress of overt autoimmune pathology at any time may be as much dependent on endocrinological as on immunological function. If an appropriate concurrence of both factors is required for development of overt autoimmunity, then it is reasonable to surmise that absence of either could suffice to prevent that development.

Autoimmune Disease Following Elimination of Lymphocytes

That thymectomy, undertaken early in postnatal life, can have a widespread impact on endocrine glands has been recognized for almost three decades. As already mentioned, some of the earliest observations of thymectomy effects related to the failure of endocrine tissue to complete its development normally in the absence of the thymus. However, subsequent demonstration of the liability of neonatally thymectomized animals to develop autoimmune disease affecting a variety of tissues has tended to distract attention from the essentially nonimmunological nature of the sequelae that had originally been described. As already noted, the histological changes produced in the mouse ovary by thymectomy are typical of retarded or failed development, not of lymphocytic attack. As also noted, the development of pathological changes attributable to autoimmunity in these mice is dependent not only on thymectomy, but also on the availability to the target ovary of appropriate hormonal stimulation.

To anticipate some of the conclusions of the following section, the removal or destruction of lymphoid tissue has been observed to produce a variety of autoimmune outcomes. The most significant influences on whether overt autoimmunity develops have been the age at which the experimental procedure (most commonly thymectomy, but also including irradiation of lymphoid tissue, exposure to immunosuppressive agents, and various combinations of these forms of intervention) to eliminate lymphocytes was undertaken, together with the identity of the cell population that is eliminated. Although most examples of this type of protocol that induced autoimmunity have been empirically derived and have not set out to eliminate an identified subpopulation of cells, the efficacy with which more recently developed protocols intended to do just that have achieved autoimmunity strongly suggests that earlier protocols were effective because they achieved selective elimination of relevant subpopulations responsible for downregulation.

Protocols that eliminate a subpopulation of lymphocytes as a strategy for inducing autoimmunity have been, by their nature, autoantigen-nonspecific. The rationale underlying them is to test for the presence of regulatory cells that could be eliminated (it is very difficult to construct any hypothesis according to which elimination of lymphocytes would interfere with self-tolerance achieved by clonal deletion, clonal anergy, or inadequate antigen presentation). Reflecting their antigenically nonspecific nature, similar protocols have evoked autoimmune conditions affecting a variety of endocrine organs and other tissues. Given the other, nonimmunological influences that have been discussed above as affecting the development of endocrine autoimmunity, it would be anticipated that the identity of the target tissue could be decided by factors, such as the level of hormonal activity of individual endocrine glands at the time of experimental interference with immune regulation. Variability in the endocrine gland affected by thymectomy-based protocols has taken the form of autoimmunity involving more than one organ simultaneously.

Autoimmune endocrine diseases have been observed to follow thymectomy undertaken at the appropriate age in strains of mice and rats that do not spontaneously develop these conditions. Both the incidence and speed of development of autoimmune endocrine disease can be increased by ancillary measures that nonspecifically damage the immune system, such as repeated, sublethal irradiation and the administration of some immunosuppressive drugs. All of these measures for inducing autoimmune endocrine disease in normal animals have been shown to accelerate the onset of autoimmune endocrinopathies in abnormal strains that spontaneously develop these conditions *(51)*. This presumably reflects both the multifactorial nature of causation in autoimmune endocrine disease and also the reality that these conditions do not conform to an "all or nothing" pattern. That is, a measure of deviation from normality may occur without the detection of overt autoimmune disease, so that the additional influences required to achieve this may do no more than complement those already present in the apparently unaffected animal. Once again, predisposing factors should be sought in both immunological and endocrinological categories.

Postthymectomy autoimmunity has been described in thyroid, ovary, pancreatic islet, and testis, but the most comprehensive analysis of it has been completed in association with the first two organs. The first description of postthymectomy changes as specifically autoimmune was that of Penhale et al. *(52)*. Rats were subjected to thymectomy at the time of weaning (5 wk), followed by 5 exposures to sublethal irradiation at 2-wk intervals. Exemplifying the tendency, already noted, for autoimmunity to affect more than one target simultaneously, it was observed that in addition to the 60% of animals developing thyroiditis, 10% also had antinuclear serum antibodies. The analysis of the mechanism of development of thyroiditis presented in 1973 by Penhale et al. remains substantially in accord with current interpretations. It took account of the suggestion by Allison et al. relating to downregulation of autoimmunity in normal animals *(37)*, and proposed that thymectomy may have depleted a population of cells normally responsible for downregulating autoreactive T cells. Support for this interpretation was provided subsequently with the demonstration that reconstitution of neonatally thymectomized and irradiated rats with normal lymphoid cells prevented development of thyroiditis *(53)*. Significantly, however, reconstitution had to be undertaken within a short time after the final irradiation, even though autoimmunity required a longer period in which to develop. This would suggest that the thymically derived cells exert their regulatory effect on autoreactive, cytotoxic cells at an early stage of activation of the latter.

A pattern of autoimmune disease development similar to that reported in the thyroid has also been observed in the ovary following thymectomy. Experiments entailing the reconstitution of thymectomized mice with lymphoid cells have confirmed and extended those based on thyroiditis *(49)*. Thus, it was shown that thymectomy, if undertaken in the first 4 d after birth, was followed, in some strains of mice, by the development of autoimmune oophoritis by 2 mo of age. An ip injection of 2×10^7 spleen cells from normal female mice effectively prevented development of oophoritis, provided it was administered within 2 wk of thymectomy. (This contrasts with the much lower dose of cells required to reverse dystrophic changes in the ovaries after thymectomy, referred to above.) However, if spleen cells were collected from female mice aged 14 d or less, they failed to prevent oophoritis when transferred. A reduced capacity to prevent oophoritis was also observed when the spleen cells were harvested from adult females that had been ovariectomized within 24 h of birth. However, if ovariectomy had been deferred until 7 d of age, the spleen cells from donor females that had attained adulthood were as effective in downregulating autoimmunity as cells from intact adult mice *(49)*. These results suggest that the development of cells capable of downregulating ovarian autoimmunity in normal mice can occur provided the immune system is exposed to ovarian autoantigens during the first week of life.

Fractionated irradiation of the major lymphoid tissues of mice has been shown to evoke a number of autoimmune diseases, involving endocrine and other organs, a consequence that could be averted by the infusion of normal spleen, thymus, or bone marrow cells *(54)*. Prevention depended on the presence of T cells in the inocula. Radiation-induced autoimmunity was attributed to the preferential destruction of regulatory T cells. The frequent lack of concordance between development of manifestations of autoimmunity in different organs with this protocol strongly suggests that factors additional to nonspecific interference with acquisition of normal immune regulatory function are also necessary for the development of individual autoimmune manifestations. Thus, the observed discordance between development of thyroiditis and insulin-dependent diabetes mellitus in rats submitted to neonatal thymectomy and irradiation provides a clear indication that organ-specific factors are influential in determining the outcome *(55)*. This was also suggested by the observation that thymectomized and irradiated rats from a conventional colony (that is, animals with a "normal" bacterial flora) were significantly less likely than similarly treated specific pathogen-free rats to develop autoimmune conditions *(55)*. Other influences on the development of thyroiditis, which serve to illustrate again the multifactorial nature of endocrine autoimmunity, included the genetic background of the mice examined and their gender. Diabetes could be prevented by the reconstitution of the immune system of thymectomized, irradiated mice, but as with autoimmune thyroiditis, intervention was only effective if undertaken early.

The identity of the regulatory cell population affected by these interventions has been examined by testing the capacity of various subpopulations of lymphocytes from normal rats to interfere with the development of autoimmunity following their transfusion into thymectomized animals. The precise phenotype of the regulatory cells appears to vary between species: the significant finding, however, is their detection in different situations. In different experimental models, the downregulatory population has been described as having a CD4+ CD25 phenotype in mice *(56)* or a CD4+ CD45RC^{low} one in rats *(57)*.

Identification of the phenotypes of those lymphocyte subpopulations the empirical depletion of which had previously been found to lead to endocrine autoimmunity permitted experiments in which the capacity of subsets of lymphocytes to evoke and to suppress development of autoimmune pathology in recipients of those cells became possible. Such an approach may offer the opportunity to study the effects of nonimmunological variations in the target tissue that cannot readily be achieved by study of the entire process of autoimmunity development in the same animal. When mouse lymph node and spleen cell suspensions were depleted of a subpopulation of T cells expressing IL-2 receptor α chains by incubation with a monoclonal antibody (MAb) and then transferred to nude mice, the recipients developed a variety of autoimmune conditions without further intervention, including several affecting endocrine glands *(58)*. Sakaguchi et al. concluded that the depleted cell populations from normal donors retained pathogenic CD4+, CD25− self-reactive cells, and that in normal mice, their activation or expansion was controlled by other CD4+, CD25+ cells. Although the control mechanism remains unknown, they raised the possibility that the regulatory cells might reduce local levels of IL-2 by binding this cytokine, thereby reducing the extent of activation of cytotoxic cells by it. In accord with some other observations of the stage at which downregulation can be achieved, they noted that supplementation of the recipient nude mice with the depleted CD25+ population had to occur very early if autoimmune damage were to be prevented *(58)*.

This would suggest that the regulatory effect has to be exerted at any early stage of activation of autoreactive cells. Having identified the phenotype of the regulatory cell responsible for curtailing autoimmunity in normal animals, Sakaguchi et al. drew attention to the variation in organ affected by autoimmune disease after depletion of that cell type in genetically different strains of mice, and emphasized that factors other than abnormality of regulatory T cells were crucial in the development of disease *(56)*. They also directed attention to the possibility that concurrent immune responses to bacteria or viruses that nonspecifically induce activation of CD25+ T cells might thereby augment downregulation of dormant autoreactive T cells. An effect of this type could have been responsible for the reversal of diabetes in NOD mice subject to virus infection *(59)*. In this experiment, exposure of NOD mice to a lymphotrophic virus prevented the development of diabetes. That the viral effect had been exerted on lymphocytes was inferred from the failure of these cells from infected mice to transfer diabetes in contrast to the capacity of lymphocytes from control (uninfected) NOD mice to do so.

ANTIGEN-DEPRIVATION MODELS OF AUTOIMMUNE ENDOCRINE DISEASE

Irrespective of the nature of the mechanisms responsible for maintaining self-tolerance in relation to endocrine autoantigens, it has been generally assumed that the establishment of self-tolerance would require exposure of the immune system to those autoantigens. The sole exception to this anticipation would be any instance in which self-tolerance was dependent on permanent and complete seclusion of an autoantigen from the immune system. As already noted, seclusion was originally envisaged as the mechanism responsible for protection of some organs, the autoantigens of which were accordingly referred to as "hidden." Subsequent investigation has raised doubts about the relevance of hidden antigens as a means of protecting endocrine organs from autoimmune attack. Nevertheless, the first attempt to establish experimentally that there was a need for exposure of the immune system to autoantigens in order to induce self-tolerance was influenced by the perception that thyroglobulin was a hidden antigen.

The design of an experiment to test whether autoantigen exposure of the developing immune system was mandatory for induction of self-tolerance entailed the surgical removal of the posterior pituitary gland from a larval tree frog *(35)*, before this organ had differentiated sufficiently to start producing its specific products. This procedure was undertaken on tadpoles, and the extirpated pituitary was implanted into a recipient tree frog at a similar larval stage. The pituitary donors were maintained, with a dietary supplement of thyroid extract to permit metamorphosis, after which the pituitary gland was removed from the first recipient and reimplanted in the donor. Its acceptance was assessed by the darkening of the recipient's skin under the renewed influence of melanophore-stimulating hormone (hypophysectomized animals were very pale). In the event, reimplanted, autologous pituitary tissue was subject to immunological rejection, as indicated by its failure to restore pigmentation to recipients. This observation was interpreted as indicating that self-recognition was a process that had to be learned by exposure to autoantigens. At the time when these experiments were undertaken, the only mechanism to have been inferred for regulation of autoimmunity was the deletion of any clones reactive against autoantigens.

Subsequently, similar experiments with larval frogs called into question the interpretation of Triplett's experiments. Rollins-Smith and Cohen examined the effect of removing either the pituitary or eye anlagen from frog embryos before acquisition of immune competence and returning them to the original donor after this event *(60)*. In contrast to the earlier results of Triplett, it was found that self-implants were never rejected. This was interpreted as indicating that frogs could become tolerant of self organ-specific antigens throughout life. The reasons underlying the divergent outcomes of these two groups of experiments are not completely clear. However, they are likely to depend on factors, such as the extent to which the recipients in each experiment had either begun to acquire self-tolerance before the time of tissue extirpation or, on the other hand, might still have remained susceptible to tolerance induction, because of their immaturity, at the time of reimplantation. Another factor could be the extent to which contaminating cells derived from the intermediate host in which the tissue had sojourned while the donor underwent metamorphosis might have triggered rejection. The possibility of sharing of autoantigens between the extirpated organ and other tissues that had not been removed and the extent to which this could have sufficed to induce tolerance of its autoantigens in its absence had also to be taken into account.

More recently, repetition of Triplett's experiments, and their extension, using fetuses of two mammalian species, rather than amphibians, has confirmed that exposure of the developing immune system to an autoantigen is necessary for tolerance induction and has also shed some light on the mechanisms responsible for normal maintenance of self-tolerance to thyroid autoantigens. Despite some substantial differences between the techniques incorporated in the two projects, the results of experiments in fetal rats and sheep have been highly consistent. Thyroid tissue removed from fetal rats and lambs before maturation of the immune system is subject to autoimmune thyroiditis when replaced *(61,62)*. In the case of rats, thyroid tissue was ablated by injection of ^{131}I at 17 d gestation (the stage at which the fetal thyroid gland first has the capacity to concentrate iodine) and the exposed animals received grafts of syngeneic thyroid tissue in their subsequent postnatal life *(62)*. The experiments with fetal lambs entailed surgical removal of the fetal thyroid one-third of the way through gestation (within 1 or 2 d of the age at which iodine is first concentrated by the gland) followed by its "storage" in the subcutaneous tissue of an athymic nude mouse and its reintroduction into the original donor during the last third of gestation after immunological maturation had occurred. (The immune system of the nude mouse lacks the capacity to reject allografts or xenografts.) The possibility that the immune attack observed on reimplanted autologous sheep thyroids actually represented a xenograft reaction against "passenger" cells derived from the nude mouse rather than an autoimmune reaction was excluded by demonstrating the lack of lymphocytic infiltration of single thyroid lobes reimplanted in hemi-thyroidectomized fetal lambs following a period of storage in nude mice. Hemi-thyroidectomized recipients, not having been deprived of thyroid autoantigens, had acquired normal self-tolerance of them *(61)*.

The dominant nature of the normal, self-tolerant state over the antithyroid autoimmune condition in thyroid-deprived animals was demonstrated in later experiments by surgically parabiosing syngeneic rats, one of which was normal, whereas the other had developed antithyroid autoimmunity following loss of its thyroid gland during fetal life. Junction with the normal rat effectively reversed autoimmune thyroiditis in this latter animal, except in those instances in which the normal rat had been exposed to sublethal irradiation before surgery *(63)*. This experiment was interpreted as indicating the presence, in normal rats, of a migratory radiosensitive cell capable of downregulating antithyroid autoimmunity. The results obtained were incompatible with explanations of self-tolerance of thyroid autoantigens based on clonal deletion, anergy, or ineffective antigen presentation. The dominance of normal self-tolerance over autoimmunity in both rat and sheep models was examined further using cultivated thyrocytes. Populations of lymphocytes collected from animals that had been deprived of exposure to thyroid autoantigens during fetal life produced damage in autologous thyrocyte monolayers in tissue culture *(51,64)*. However, this damage could be curtailed if lymphocytes from normal syngeneic (in the case of rats) *(64)* or normal autologous (identical twin) fetal lambs *(50)* were also added to the thyrocyte monolayers. In an observation reminiscent of those reported in relation to the interception of autoimmune thyroiditis *(53)*, oophoritis *(49)*, and diabetes *(55)*, in thymectomized animals, it was found that prevention of autoimmune cytotoxicity directed against cultivated thyrocyte monolayers required the introduction of a normal regulatory population of lymphocytes at the earliest stage *(50,64)*. The regulatory effect of lymphocyte populations from normal fetal lambs was attributable to CD8$^+$ T cells.

It has also been found that the induction of self-tolerance of thyroid autoantigens required their presentation on cells that shared histocompatibility determinants with the fetal lamb to be tolerized. Thus, thyroid glands from unrelated fetal lambs, if substituted for the autologous gland before immunological maturation, failed to induce tolerance of thyroid-specific antigens *(65)*. An incidental observation from this experiment provided another indication of the potential for the concurrent exposure to an immune response and hormonal stimulation to produce outcomes not found in endocrine tissue exposed to only one of these influences. Allografted thyroid rudiments implanted in thyroidectomized fetal lambs were subject simultaneously to TSH stimulation and coexistence with an immune system with which they were histoincompatible. Although the immaturity of the thyroidectomized fetal host precluded allograft rejection, fetal thyroid allografts were subject to grossly aberrant morphological development together with lymphocytic infiltration as they matured (65). This outcome recalls the synergistic effects, noted above, of thymectomy and gonadotrophin in mice (3).

More recent investigations using fetal lambs suggest that overt antithyroid autoimmunity does not develop automatically as a result of thyroid deprivation during development of the immune system, but follows challenge of the immune system (either in the intact fetal lamb or in the form of its lymphocytes in cultivation) with autologous thyroid tissue (66). Examination of the specific antithyroid autoantigen reactivity of both T and B lymphocytes in thyroid-deprived fetal lambs did not reveal any evidence of sensitization, and consequently, it has been inferred that the primary abnormality in these fetuses was an inadequate development of regulatory cell populations (as distinct from an excessive development of the corresponding autoreactive cell populations) (66). This interpretation of the experimental situation in thyroid-deprived fetal lambs would have occurred with the impaired reactivity of thyroid-autoantigen-specific suppressor T lymphocytes that has previously been reported in patients with autoimmune thyroiditis (67).

Since the specific thyroid autoantigens targeted in the fetal rat and lamb models of autoimmune thyroiditis have not been identified, the nature of the suppressor mechanism operating in normal animals remains speculative. However, the demonstration noted above, that the T cells responsible for downregulating the antimyelin basic protein (MBP) cytotoxic cells responsible for EAE recognize an epitope identical to that to which the cytotoxic cells react (45), encourages some speculation about a possible similar mechanism for regulation for autoimmune endocrine disease. Regulatory and cytotoxic cells with identical reactivity against an epitope on MBP have distinct patterns of cytokine secretion in response to activation after recognition of that epitope. Miller et al. have reported that the release of tumor growth factor β (TGF-β) from suppressor cells mediates downregulation of the corresponding cytotoxic cells (46). This suggests the possibility of a mechanism, whereby recognition of an identical epitope by autoreactive and regulatory subpopulations of T lymphocytes in fetal sheep could lead to the cytokine-mediated suppression of the former by the latter (68). The results of deprivation of exposure to thyroid-derived autoantigens in fetal life would be to impair the expansion or appearance of regulatory subpopulations with the outcome that the autoreactive subpopulation would not be curtailed.

If release of cytokines (without specifying their identity) is a major factor in determining whether efficient downregulation or overt autoimmunity eventuates, the capacity for interactions, at a molecular level, between endocrine and immune systems could be of considerable relevance. For example, as already indicated, lymphocytes stimulated by the appropriate mitogen can secrete TSH. Apart from its stimulatory effects on thyrocytes targeted in autoimmune thyroiditis, TSH is known to augment antibody production by B lymphocytes. Consequently, it would be reasonable to anticipate that the processes influencing the outcome during an autoimmune reaction against any endocrine tissue, such as the thyroid gland, are likely to be multifactorial and, leaving aside the question of antigenic specificity, will vary in significant details, such as cytokine profiles, from one endocrine to another.

FUTURE DIRECTIONS

Ideally, in attempting to describe any phenomenon, one starts with the simplest hypotheses, which are most likely to have wide applicability. If and when these become inapplicable, it becomes necessary to postulate more complex processes, any one of which may be applicable only to relatively restricted situations. Several decades of investigation of self-tolerance and autoimmunity in general have provided data to support the existence of several discrete processes that are potentially capable of establishing and preserving self-tolerance. Since in explaining any individual example of autoimmunity it is necessary to distinguish between what could happen and what actually does happen in that situation, it would seem intuitively improbable if each of the variety of candidate mechanisms for maintaining self-tolerance did not fulfill a role in some circumstances.

The complexity introduced into understanding regulation of autoimmunity by the number of available mechanisms is likely to be further compounded in the case of endocrine autoimmunity by the unique opportunities available for interaction between endocrine and immune systems. As indicated in the course of this chapter, the potential for interaction during normal function is apparent in areas as diverse as gross anatomy and molecular structure. As also suggested in introducing the subject, study of these normal interactions may offer the best opportunity for understanding the abnormal. Several variant approaches to exploring endocrine autoimmunity could be worth examination.

The possibility that the induction and maintenance of regulation of autoimmunity of endocrine tissue and its products are dependent on responses in the local immune system, that is, the lymph nodes draining specific endocrine glands, merits more serious attention than it has so far received. Study of such events as the migration of antigen-presenting cells from an endocrine gland to its local node via the afferent lymphatic vessels is indicated as is study of the capacity of these cells to induce either autoimmunity or self-tolerance on arrival there. Detailed understanding of the specific microenvironment of lymph nodes draining endocrine tissue is likely to be essential for explaining the likely variation in reactivity to endocrine autoantigens of cells in local and distant nodes. Experimental approaches that could shed light on whether regulatory lymphocytes are generated in proximity to the source of endocrine autoantigens to which they relate include examination of lymphocytes isolated from within endocrine tissue and emigrating from its primary draining lymphoid tissue. A possible stratagem to facilitate the latter approach might include the preliminary heterotopic transplantation of an endocrine gland to a location drained by lymphoid tissue, the efferent lymphatic vessels from which were more easily accessible.

In view of the likelihood that the release of lymphokines and of "conventional" hormones and neurotransmitters, which then act in a paracrine fashion, may determine the outcome within endocrine tissue that is the subject of an autoimmune process, there are strong indications to attempt to simulate in vitro the microenvironments that develop within those tissues.

An indication of the potential complexity of processes involved in regulation of antiendocrine autoimmunity and, potentially, a clue to a possible approach to investigating this has been provided by a report suggesting that some unidentified feature of the target endocrine tissue in animals that have recovered from autoimmune disease confers resistance to a further autoimmune episode affecting that tissue. Specifically, it has been found that although the ovaries of mice that have recovered from autoimmune oophoritis are resistant to reinduction of this condition, ovaries from normal donors implanted into these mice may be concurrently affected by oophoritis *(69)*. The basis for this target organ resistance is unknown.

The proposition that one or more attributes of the target endocrine organ might determine susceptibility to autoimmune aggression or the duration of this process recalls the concept of graft adaptation. This arose from the common observation that allografts that had survived on a histoincompatible host for a certain period became increasingly likely to achieve indefinite survival and, in some instances, survived after retransplantation to a second histoincompatible host, genetically identical with the first host and not conditioned to accept that graft. Although the observations have never been comprehensively explained, an exchange of the original donor passenger leukocyte population for similar cells derived from the first recipient is generally considered to have been more likely than any modification of graft antigenicity. Although the basis for the alteration in target organ susceptibility is not yet known, modification of the reactivity of passenger leukocytes that could act as antigen-presenting cells in the ovary is a possible explanation. Certainly, neither a reduction in T-cell autoantigen response nor the occurrence of T-suppressor cells in resistant mice could be demonstated *(69)*. Pathogenic T cells could be isolated from resistant mice, as also could specific autoantigens.

Taken together with the capacity for decidedly nonimmunological factors to influence the outcome for potential target endocrine tissue confronted with an autoimmune response, to which reference has already been made *(29)*, the demonstration that apparently intrinsic target tissue properties can affect susceptibility to rechallenge serves to re-emphasize the multifactorial nature of endocrine autoimmunity.

ACKNOWLEDGEMENT

Critical reading of the manuscript by Wes Whitten is gratefully acknowledged.

REFERENCES

1. Mackay IR, Burnet, FM. Autoimmune diseases: pathogenesis, chemistry and therapy. C.C. Thomas. Springfield IL, 1964.
2. Nishizuka Y, Sakakura T. Thymus and reproduction: sex-linked dysgenesia of the gonad after neonatal thymectomy in mice. Science 1969;166:753–755.
3. Sakakura T, Nishizuka Y. Thymic control mechanism in ovarian development: reconstitution of ovarian dysgenesis in thymectomized mice by replacement with thymic and other lymphoid tissues. Endocrinology 1972;90:431–437.
4. Nishizuka Y, Sakakura T. Ovarian dysgenesis induced by neonatal thymectomy in the mouse. Endocrinology 1971; 89:886–893.
5. Biskind MS, Biskind GR. Development of tumors in rat ovary after transplantation into spleen. Proc Soc Exp Biol Med 1994;55:176–179.
6. Besedovsky H, Sorkin E. Network of immune neuroendocrine interactions. Clin Exp Immunol 1977; 27:1–12.
7. Jones HW, Hoerr NL, Osol A. Blakiston's New Gould Medical Dictionary. Blakiston, Philadelphia, PA, 1951.
8. Daniel PM, Excell BJ, Gale MM, Pratt OE. The drainage of thyroid hormone by the lymphatics of the thyroid gland. J Physiol 1961;160:6–7P.
9. Daniel PM, Gale MM, Pratt OE. Radioactive iodine in the lymph leaving the thyroid gland. Q J Exp Phyiol 1963;48:138–145.
10. Daniel PM, Gale MM, Pratt OE. Hormones and related substances in the lymph leaving four endocrine glands-the testis, ovary, adrenal and thyroid. Lancet 1963;i:1232–1234.
11. Lindner HR. Partition of androgen between the lymph and venous blood of the testis in the ram. J Endocrinol 1963;25:483–494.
12. Lindner HR, Sass MB, Morris B. Steroids in the ovarian lymph and blood of conscious ewes. J Endocrinol 1964;30:361–376.
13. Brezinschek HP, Faessler R, Klocker H, Kroemer G, Sgonc R, Dietrich H, et al. Analysis of the immune-endocrine feedback loop in the avian system and its alteration in chickens with spontaneous autoimmune thyroiditis. Eur J Immunol 1990;20:2155–2159.

14. Bernton EW, Beach JE, Holaday JW, Smalbridge RC, Fein HG. Release of multiple hormones by a direct action of interleukin-1 on pituitary cells. Science 1987;238:519–521.
15. Brown SL, Smith LR, Blalock JE. Interleukin 1 and interleukin 2 enhance propiomelanocortin gene expression in pituitary cells. J Immunol 1987;139:3181–3183.
16. Pierpaoli W, Besedovsky HO. Role of the thymus in programing of neuroendocrine functions. Clin Exp Immunol 1975;20:323–338.
17. Heijnen CJ, Bevers C, Kavelaars A, Ballicux RE. Effect of α-endorphin on the antigen-induced primary antibody response of human blood B cells in vitro. J Immunol 1986;136:213–216.
18. Mandler RN, Biddison WE, Mandler R, Serrate SA. β-endophin augments the cytolytic activity and interferon production of natural killer cells. J Immunol 1986;136:934–939.
19. Bhardwaj RS, Schwarz A, Becher E, Mahnke K, Aragane Y, Schwarz T, et al. Pro-opiomelanocortin-derived peptides induce IL-10 production in human monocytes. J Immunol 1996;156:2517–2521.
20. Weisz-Carrington P, Roux ME, McWilliams M, Phillips-Quagliata JM, Lamm ME. Hormonal induction of the secretory immune system in the mammary gland. Proc Natl Acad Sci USA 1978;75:2928–2932.
21. Larson DF. Mechanism of action: antagonism of the prolactin receptor. Prog Allergy 1986;38:222–238.
22. Hiestand PC, Mekler P, Nordmann R, Grieder A, Permmongkol C. Prolactin as a modulator of lymphocyte responsiveness provides a possible mechanism of action for cyclosporine. Proc Natl Acad Sci USA 1986;83:2599–2603.
23. Smith EM, Blalock JE. Human lymphocyte production of corticotrophin and endorphin-like substances: association with leukocyte interferon. Proc Natl Acad Sci USA 1981;78:7530–7534.
24. Smith EM, Phan M, Kruger TE, Coppenhaver DH, Blalock JE. Human lymphocyte production of immunoreactive thyrotrophin. Proc Natl Acad Sci USA 1983;80:6010–6013.
25. Kruger TE, Blalock JE. Cellular requirements for thyrotrophin enhancement of in vitro antibody production. J Immunol 1986;137:197–200.
26. Harbour-McMenamin D, Smith EM, Blalock JE. Production of immunoreactive chorionic gonadotrophin during mixed lymphocyte reactions: a possible selective mechanism for genetic diversity. Proc Natl Acad Sci USA 1986;83:1834–1838.
27. Paul WE, Seder RA. Lymphocyte responses and cytokines, Cell 1994;76:241–251.
28. Poo W-J, Conrad L, Janeway CA. Receptor-directed focusing of lymphokine release by helper T cells. Nature 1988;332:378–380.
29. Roitt IM, Hutchings PR, Dawe KJ, Sumar N, Bodman KB, Cooke A. The forces driving autoimmune disease. J Autoimmunity 1992;5(Suppl A):11–26.
30. Felten DL, Felten SY, Bellinger DL, Carlson SZ, Ackerman KD, Madden KS, et al. Noradrenergic sympathetic neural interaciton with the immune system: structure and function. Immun Rev 1987;100:225–260.
31. Singh U. Effect of catecholamines on lymphopoiesis in fetal mouse thymic explants. J Anat 1979;129:279–292.
32. Adams DD. The presence of an abnormal thyroid-stimulating hormone in the serum of some thyrotoxic patients. J Clin Endocrinol Metab 1958;18:699–712.
33. Pinchera A, Fenzi GF, Macchia E, Bartalena L, Mariotti S, Monzani F. Thyroid-stimulating immunoglobulins. Hormone Res 1982;16:317–328.
34. Ehrlich P. On immunity with special reference to cell life. Proc Roy Soc 1900;66:424–448.
35. Triplett EL. On the mechanism of immunologic self recognition. J Immunol 1962;89:505–510.
36. Bach J-F. Insulin-dependent diabetes mellitus as a β-cell targeted disease of immunoregulation. J Autoimmunity 1995;8:439–463.
37. Allison AC, Denman AM, Barnes RD. Cooperating and controlling functions of thymus-derived lymphocytes in relation to autoimmunity. Lancet 1971; ii:135–140.
38. Webb S, Morris C, Sprent J. Extrathymic tolerance of mature T cells: clonal elimination as a consequence of immunity. Cell 1990;63:1249–1256.
39. Morahan G, Allison J, Miller JFAP. Tolerance of class 1 histocompatibility antigens expressed extrathymically. Nature 1989;339:622–624.
40. Jolicoeur C, Hanahan D, Smith K. T-cell tolerance toward a transgenic β cell antigen and transcription of endogenous pancreatic genes in thymus. Proc Natl Acad Sci USA 1994;91:6707–6711.
41. Nossal GJV. Negative selection of lymphocytes. Cell 1994;76:229–239.
42. Janeway CA, Bottomly K. Signals and signs for lymphocyte responses. Cell 1994;76:275–285.
43. Weetman AP. Antigen presentation in the pathogenesis of autoimmune endocrine disease. J Autoimmunity 1995;8:305–312.

44. Todd I, Bottazzo GF. On the issue of inappropriate HLA class II expression on endocrine cells: an answer to a sceptic. J Autoimmunity 1995;8:313–322.
45. Chen Y, Kuchroo VK, Inobe J, Hafler DA, Weiner HL. Regulatory T cell clones induced by oral tolerance: suppression of autoimmune encephalomyelitis. Science 1994;265:1237–1240.
46. Miller A, Lider O, Roberts AB, Sporn MB, Weiner HL. Suppressor T cells generated by oral tolerization to myelin basic protein suppress both *in vitro* and *in vivo* immune responses by the release of transforming growth factor β after antigen-specific triggering. Proc Natl Acad Sci USA 1992;89:421–425.
47. Pontes de Carvalho LC, Templeman J, Wick G, Roitt IM. The role of self-antigen in the development of autoimmunity in obese strain chickens with spontaneous autoallergic thyroiditis. J Exp Med 1982;155:1255–1265.
48. Larger E, Becourt C, Bach JF, Boitard C. Pancreatic islet β cells drive T cell-immune responses in the nonobese diabetic mouse model. J Exp Med 1995;181:1635–1642.
49. Sakaguchi S, Takahashi T, Nishizuka Y. Study on cellular events in post-thymectomy autoimmune oophoritis in mice. II Requirement of Lyt-1 cells in normal female mice. J Exp Med 1982;156:1577–1586.
50. Chen X, Shelton J, McCullagh P. Suppression of anti-thyrocyte autoreactivity by the lymphocytes of normal fetal lambs. J Autoimmunity 1995;8:539–559.
51. Welch P, Rose NR, Kite JH. Neonatal thymectomy increases spontaneous autoimmune thyroiditis. J Immunol 1973;110:575–577.
52. Penhale WJ, Farmer A, McKenna RP, Irvine WJ. Spontaneous thyroiditis in thymectomized and irradiated Wistar rats. Clin Exp Immunol 1973;15:225–236.
53. Penhale WJ, Irvine WJ, Inglis JR, Farmer A. Thyroiditis in T cell-depleted rats: supression of the autoallergic response by reconstitution with normal lymphoid cells. Clin Exp Immunol 1976;25:6–16.
54. Sakaguchi N, Miyai K, Sakaguchi S. Ionizing radiation and autoimmunity. Induction of autoimmune disease in mice by high dose fractionated total lymphoid irradiation and its prevention by inoculating normal T cells. J Immunol 1994;152:2586–2596.
55. Stumbles PA, Penhale WJ. IDDM in rats induced by thymectomy and irradiation. Diabetes 1993;42:571–578.
56. Sakaguchi S, Toda M, Asano M, Itoh M, Morse SS, Sakaguchi N. T cell-mediated maintenance of natural self-tolerance: its breakdown as a possible cause of various autoimmune diseases. J Autoimmunity 1996;9:211–220.
57. Fowell D, McKnight AJ, Powrie F, Dyke R, Mason D. Subsets of CD4+ T cells and their roles in the induction and prevention of autoimmunity. Immunol Rev 1991;123:37–63.
58. Sakaguchi S, Sakaguchi N, Asano M, Itoh M, Toda M. Immunologic self-tolerance maintained by activated T cells expressing IL-2 receptor α-chains (CD25). Breakdown of a single mechanism of self-tolerance causes various autoimmune diseases. J Immunol 1995;155:1151–1164.
59. Oldstone MBA. Prevention of type 1 diabetes in nonobese diabetic mice by virus infection. Science 1988;239:500–502.
60. Rollins-Smith LA, Cohen N. Self-pituitary grafts are not rejected by frogs deprived of their pituitary anlagen as embyos. Nature 1982;299:820–821.
61. McCullagh P. Interception of the development of self tolerance in fetal lambs. Eur J Immunol 1989;19:1387–1392.
62. Eishi Y, McCullagh P. Acquisition of immunological self-recognition by the fetal rat. Immunology 1988;64:319–323.
63. McCullagh P. Curtailment of autoimmunity following parabiosis with a normal partner. Immunology 1990;71:595–597.
64. Chen X, McCullagh P. Expression and regulation of anti-thyroid autoimmunity directed against cultvated rat thyrocytes. J Autoimmunity 1995;8:521–538.
65. McCullagh P. The inability of thyroid allografts to induce self tolerance of organ-specific antigens in fetal lambs. Immunology 1991;72:405–410.
66. King KJ, Hagan RP, Mieno M, McCullagh P. Cellular interactions during the development of autoimmunity in a fetal lamb model of self-antigen deprivation. Clin Immunol Immunopath 1997;88:56–64.
67. Yoshikawa N, Morita T, Reseltkova E, Arreanza G, Carayon P, Volpe R. Reduced activation of suppressor T lymphocytes by antigens in autoimmune thyroid disease. J Endocrinol Invest 1993;16:609–617.
68. McCullagh P. The significance of immune suppression in normal self tolerance. Immunol Rev 1996;149:127–153.
69. Lou Y-H, McElveen F, Adams S, Tung KSK. Altered target organ. A mechanism of postrecovery resistance to murine autoimmune oophoritis. J Immunol 1995;155:3667–3673.

3

The Genetic Susceptibility to Type 1 (Insulin-Dependent) Diabetes Mellitus and the Autoimmune Thyroid Diseases

From Epidemiological Observations to Gene Mapping

Yaron Tomer, MD, David A. Greenberg, PhD, and Terry F. Davies, MD, FRCP

CONTENTS

INTRODUCTION
EPIDEMIOLOGICAL EVIDENCE FOR A GENETIC SUSCEPTIBILITY
    TO IDDM AND THE AITDs
ANIMAL MODELS
TOOLS USED IN GENE MAPPING STUDIES
THE ROLE OF HLA CANDIDATE GENES IN THE SUSCEPTIBILITY
    TO IDDM AND THE AITDs
NON-HLA CANDIDATE GENES
WHOLE-GENOME SCREENING IN IDDM AND THE AITDs
MECHANISMS OF DISEASE INDUCTION BY SUSCEPTIBILILTY GENES
CONCLUSIONS
ACKNOWLEDGMENTS
REFERENCES

INTRODUCTION

The autoimmune endocrine diseases are disorders in which a perturbation of immune regulation results in immune attack on endocrine glands. Autoimmune disorders affect almost all of the endocrine glands, such as the pituitary (autoimmune hypophysitis), the thyroid (autoimmune thyroid diseases), the pancreas (autoimmune diabetes), the adrenal glands (autoimmune Addison's disease), and the gonads (autoimmune oophoritis causing premature menopause). By far the most common autoimmune endocrine diseases are the autoimmune thyroid diseases (AITDs) and autoimmune diabetes (insulin-dependent diabetes mellitus [IDDM], or Type 1). (*See also* Chapters 9 and 12.) The genetic susceptibility to these diseases has been extensively studied and will be the focus of this chapter.

From: *Contemporary Endocrinology: Autoimmune Endocrinopathies*
Edited by: R. Volpe © Humana Press Inc., Totowa, NJ

We will show how epidemiologic and genetic techniques for studying the inheritance of complex diseases have begun to be applied in the search for the susceptibility genes for IDDM and the AITDs.

The AITDs and IDDM appear to develop as a result of a complex interaction between inherited predisposing genes *(1)* and environmentally encountered triggering agents *(2)*. Thus, the lack of a Mendelian pattern of inheritance and the possibility of an environmental influence have grouped AITDs and IDDM as complex multifactorial diseases. Moreover, it is highly probable that not only are environmental triggers involved in the development of the disease, but that more than one gene is involved. They are "oligogenic" and are believed to be caused by several genes of variable effect. However, the mode of inheritance of these diseases remains unknown. New developments in genetic mapping techniques have made the identification of susceptibility genes in complex diseases a virtual certainty. Moreover, as discussed below, the mechanisms for the development of IDDM and the AITDs will be unraveled by the discovery of new susceptibility genes for these disorders.

EPIDEMIOLOGICAL EVIDENCE FOR A GENETIC SUSCEPTIBILITY TO IDDM AND THE AITDS

Epidemiology is the study of the distribution and spread of disease within populations. Such studies are essential to understanding how a disease develops, and can provide useful data on the relative contributions of genes and environment to disease development.

Secular Trends in the Incidence of IDDM

Most of the reliable epidemiologic data on the pathogenesis of IDDM was obtained in the 1980s after the standardization of the criteria for the diagnosis of diabetes by the WHO in 1980 *(3)*. Moreover, the development of better tools for differentiating IDDM from noninsulin-dependent diabetes mellitus (NIDDM) (such as measurement of islet cell autoantibodies and C-peptide levels) has enabled more accurate epidemiologic data to be collected. IDDM is one of the most common chronic diseases of childhood with a prevalence of about 0.26% by age 20 in Caucasians *(4)*. The average annual incidence of IDDM is 10–20/100,000 *(5)*. However, the incidence of IDDM shows wide variations in different countries. The highest prevalence is observed in Finland and in Sardinia, and the lowest prevalence is seen in Japan *(6,7)*. The geographic variations in the risk for IDDM may reflect genetic or environmental differences between these populations. Supporting, although not proving, a genetic influence are studies showing different incidence rates among various ethnic groups living in the same geographic regions. Thus, in the US, the risk of IDDM in Caucasians is 50% greater than that in African Americans or Hispanics *(8,9)*. If genetic effects account for the varying incidence of IDDM in different populations, this effect could be explained in two ways: (1) the frequency of the same IDDM susceptibility genes is different in the different ethnic populations, or (2) different susceptibility genes exist in different populations. Data on the prevalence of HLA in different populations support the former hypothesis *(see below) (10)*. Another important clue to the relative contribution of genetic susceptibility and environment to the development of a disease comes from studies of the incidence of the disease over time. In the past 30 years, there has been a threefold increase in the incidence of IDDM in many countries *(11)*. This observation supports an environmental effect, since it would seem unlikely that genetic effects could change over such a short period of time. However, males and females have a similar risk for IDDM, but in lower-risk populations (e.g., in Japan) there is a small female excess, whereas in high-risk groups, there is a male preponderance *(9)*.

Secular Trends in the Incidence of the AITDs

A well-designed epidemiological survey in the town of Whickham in the northeastern part of England *(12)* found the prevalence of thyrotoxicosis from any cause to be 27/1000 in women, and 10-fold less in men (1.6–2.3/1000). In a 20-yr follow-up survey of these subjects, the mean incidence of hyperthyroidism was 0.8/1000 in women and was negligible in men *(13)*. In contrast to IDDM, the annual incidence of Graves' disease in different populations is similar and ranges from 0.22 to 0.27/1000 *(14–20; see also* Chapter 6).

A similar pattern was observed for Hashimoto's thyroiditis (HT). In the Whickham survey, the prevalence of spontaneous hypothyroidism was 15/1000 in females (1.5%) compared with <1/1000 in males *(12; see also* Chapter 6). The mean annual incidence of spontaneous hypothyroidism in women was 3.5/1000 and in men was 0.6/1000 *(13)*. The mean age at diagnosis was 57 yr (range 30–76) *(12)*. In a study from Oakland California using the free thyroxine index (FTI) as the basic screening test, the overall prevalence of hypothyroidism was 5/1000, and the overall incidence was 0.8/1000 *(21)*. These incidence rates are similar to those reported in Finland *(22)*, Japan *(23)*, and Sweden *(24)*. The comparable prevalence and incidence of the AITDs in ethnically different populations suggest a significant genetic effect on the development of the AITDs. Moreover, it may imply that in different countries, identical genes with similar population frequencies cause the genetic susceptibility to the AITDs. Therefore, for the AITDs linkage studies, using families from different ethnic groups are feasible, since it is possible that similar genetic variations cause susceptibility to the AITDs across different ethnic backgrounds.

Thyroid Autoantibodies

Autoantibodies to thyroglobulin and thyroid peroxidase (the microsomal antigen) have been widely used to show the population at most risk for the development of the AITDs. Of course, the prevalence of such autoantibodies is entirely dependent on the sensitivity of the assays used for their detection. Data based on the early insensitive hemagglutination assays (which should no longer be used) showed a much lower population rate (10%) compared to the more sensitive immunoassay techniques now in widespread use (demonstrating a 20% prevalence) *(12,25,26)*. Recent evidence suggests that the development of thyroid autoantibodies is a Mendelian dominant trait *(27)*. However, the genetic contribution of the propensity to develop thyroid autoantibodies to the pathogenesis of the AITDs remains to be determined. The Whickham survey also addressed the important issue of the risk of developing overt hypothyroidism in individuals with thyroid autoantibodies. In females who were positive for antithyroid antibodies, the annual risk of developing hypothyroidism was 2.1%, and if both increased TSH and antithyroid antibodies were present, the annual risk of developing hypothyroidism was 4.3% *(13)*. These data further emphasize the use of thyroid autoantibodies in the identification of at-risk individuals.

Variation in Incidence of IDDM with Age

The age-specific incidence rates of diseases can give useful information on the genetic and environmental contributions to disease development. For example, the incidence of malignant diseases associated with exposure to carcinogens rises steadily with age as the length of exposure rises.

The incidence of IDDM in Caucasians begins to increase at about 1 yr of age and peaks at age 12–14 yr *(28)*. Thereafter, the incidence declines, but never reaches 0. The age distribution of IDDM onset is similar across geographic areas and ethnic groups *(29)*. These data suggest that genetically susceptible individuals encounter a common environmental factor early in life causing the incidence of IDDM to rise sharply beginning at 1 yr of age. Since the age variation is similar in different countries, it can be speculated that the environmental agent involved is ubiquitous and that most children are exposed to it. After most susceptible individuals have developed the disease, the incidence decreases starting at age 12–14.

Variations in Incidence of the AITDs with Age

Several studies have reported the incidence of the AITDs in different age groups. Volpe *(30)* showed peaking of the incidence of both Graves' disease and HT in the fifth decade of life in both males and females with subsequent declines to a zero incidence in the eighth decade. Similar results were obtained by Burch and Rowell *(31)*. These data suggested, as with IDDM, that in the genetically predisposed individuals, the probability of developing the disease increased rapidly with age until 80 yr when all the susceptible people will have developed the disease. These data also suggested that the lifetime penetrance of the disease approached 100%, thus causing the incidence to decrease dramatically once all the genetically predisposed individuals had developed their disease. In view of these data, Volpe has offered the hypothesis that Graves' disease and HT developed at random in a genetically predisposed population *(30)*. However, other interpretations of the data are possible (e.g., an environmental effect peaking at the fifth decade of life).

Familial Clustering of IDDM

Although clustering of disease in families suggests a genetic influence on the development of the disease, environmental factors can have a similar influence. According to Risch *(32)*, the degree of clustering in families can be calculated from the ratio of the prevalence of the disease among siblings of patients and the population prevalence of the disease (λ_s). If this ratio is close to 1.0, there is no familial clustering of the disease, and the higher the λ_s value, the stronger the evidence for familial clustering and possible genetic susceptibility to the disease. In IDDM, the population prevalence is approx 0.4% by age 50 *(5)*, and the risk for siblings of an IDDM patient is estimated at 6% giving a λ_s value of 15 *(32)*. Interestingly, offspring of IDDM fathers are at much higher risk for IDDM than are the offspring of IDDM mothers *(33)*. Recent data suggest that exposure to a diabetic environment (or islet cell antibodies and T cells) *in utero* may have a protective effect on the offspring perhaps by inducing immunological tolerance to the antigens involved in the autoimmune process affecting the β cells *(34)*.

Islet cell antibodies often precede the development of IDDM. Several studies have shown a 5–13% prevalence of islet cell antibodies in first-degree relatives of patients with IDDM compared with a population prevalence of 0.2–4.4% *(35)*. Such data depend on the population studied, the age of the subjects, and the assay used to determine Islet cell antibody levels *(36)*. This again provides indirect evidence for a strong genetic predisposition for the development of IDDM. It is possible that the development of islet cell antibodies is a marker for a genetically susceptible individual, since almost all patients with IDDM have islet cell antibodies, even though not all individuals with islet cell antibodies eventually develop IDDM.

Familial Clustering of the AITDs

The familial occurrence of the AITDs has been recognized by investigators for many years. Bartels found evidence of a familial predisposition in 60% of cases with Graves' disease *(37)*. Martin *(38)* found that 20 of 90 (22%) patients with Graves' disease had relatives with Graves' disease. Even though the λ_s value for the AITDs has not been calculated directly, it can be determined for Graves' disease from published data. In different studies, 10–15% of siblings of Graves' disease patients were found to have Graves' disease *(39,40)*, whereas the population prevalence was reported as 0.3–0.5% *(12,17–20)*. Thus, the λ_s value for Graves' disease can be estimated to be at least 20. Even though this is only a crude estimate, it is notable that the value may be higher than that for IDDM, suggesting a greater genetic contribution to the development of Graves' disease when compared to IDDM.

Similar to the finding of islet cell antibodies in relatives of IDDM patients, an increased prevalence of thyroid autoantibodies has been reported in relatives of patients with the AITDs *(41–43)*. Antithyroid autoantibodies (antithyrogloblin and antithyroid peroxidase) have been found in up to 50% of the siblings of patients with the AITDs *(30,42,44)*, in contrast to a prevalence of 7–20% in the general population *(12)*. A large study from Japan found thyroglobulin antibodies in 26% of siblings and microsomal antibodies in 32% of siblings of probands with thyroid antibodies. In contrast, only 11% of siblings of probands who did not have thyroid antibodies were found to have thyroglobulin or microsomal antibodies *(45)*. Hall and Stanbury *(39)* found clinical thyroid disease in 33% of siblings of patients with AITD. In addition, 56% of siblings of patients with AITD were positive for antithyroid antibodies, and in almost all cases, there was an abnormality (AITD or presence of antithyroid antibodies) in one of the parents of an affected individual *(39)*. These data suggested an inherited influence on the production of antithyroid antibodies and are compatible with dominant inheritance *(39)*. Indeed, segregation analyses in a panel of families with the AITDs has suggested a Mendelian dominant pattern of inheritance for the tendency to develop antithyroid antibodies *(27)*.

Twins in Research

Investigating twins is a classical method of studying the genetics of human diseases. Twin studies can provide information concerning the inheritance of a disease and may yield certain quantitative evaluations of the role of heredity in relation to exogenous factors. The twin method is based on comparison of concordance (simultaneous occurrence) of a given disease among monozygotic (MZ) twins with concordance among dizygotic (DZ) twins to avoid conflicting environmental influences. MZ twins have identical genetic makeup, whereas DZ twins share an average of ½ of the genes (like siblings) Therefore, if concordance is higher in the MZ twins when compared to the DZ twins, it suggests that the disease has an inherited component. Any discordance among the MZ twin pairs is usually interpreted to mean that the gene or genes concerned show reduced penetrance, i.e., certain events must occur or certain environmental factors must be present before the disease becomes manifest. The concordance rate in MZ twins is taken as an estimate of the penetrance of the disease up to the ages examined. This information is helpful for studies of multifactorial diseases, such as IDDM and the AITDs, in which reduced penetrance must be assumed in a linkage analysis. Because both of the MZ twins inherit the same genetic material, assuming they are truly identical *(46)*, the discordance among them demonstrates that the gene or genes concerned are insufficient alone to cause the disease, i.e., certain environmental factors must be present, or have been present, before the disease becomes manifest. For example, if the concordance rate among the MZ twins is 50%, this is taken to mean that the penetrance of the disease genes is approx 50%. However, this assumes no genetic heterogeneity, i.e., that the same genetic variations cause the same phenotype in all individuals.

Twins in IDDM Research

Twin studies in IDDM have shown a concordance rate of 30–50% in MZ twins and about 5–10% in DZ twins *(47,48)*. These results supported the notion of a significant genetic contribution to the pathogenesis of IDDM. Moreover, the concordance rate in MZ twins gave a rough estimate of the penetrance of IDDM susceptibility genes, which could be assumed to be 30–50%. However, the relatively high (more than 50%) discordance rate among MZ twins suggests that environmental factors must also play an important role in the development of IDDM *(2)*.

Twins in AITD Research

Unlike in IDDM, there is a surprising sparsity of twin studies performed in the AITDs. In the largest twin study of hyperthyroidism (assumed to be primarily Graves' disease), performed in Denmark, the concordance rate was 76% (16/21) for MZ twins and 11% (4/37) for DZ twins *(49)*. In subsequent studies of the same population, the concordance rate for Graves' disease in MZ twins was found to be lower (approx 30–50%), but the concordance rate in DZ twins was reported to be about 3–9% *(50,51)*. Even though large twin studies of HT have not been performed, there have been individual reports of MZ twins with HT *(52)*, identical triplets with HT *(53)*, and MZ twins in whom one twin was affected by Graves' disease and the other by HT *(54)*.

ANIMAL MODELS

Animal models of complex human diseases are useful tools for understanding the pathogenesis of disease. Mapping the genes responsible for a murine disease, for example, is easier than mapping the human genes because of the investigator's control of mating and environment. Therefore, it was hoped that such information would help map the homologous human genes. Such an approach has proven useful in identifying the obesity genes *(55)*. However, as outlined below, using animal models for identifying the genetic susceptibility to IDDM and the AITDs has proven difficult.

Animal Models of IDDM

The nonobese diabetic (NOD) mouse is thought to be the most useful animal model of IDDM. The mice develop a disease that has many similarities to human IDDM. Spontaneous onset of the disease in mice is accompanied by islet cell infiltrates, selective β-cell destruction, and the presence of islet cell- (specifically GAD) reactive T cells, and autoantibodies in the serum *(56)*. The disease in NOD mice has been shown to be tightly linked to the major histocompatibility complex (MHC) *(57,58)*. This locus has been

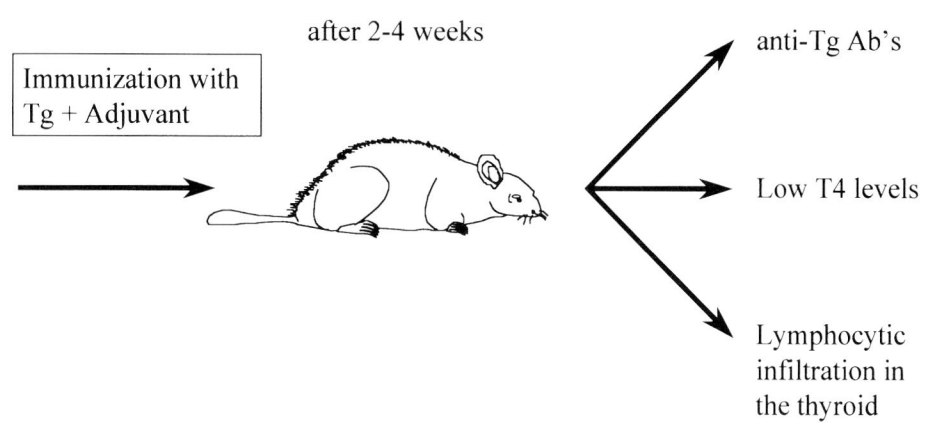

Fig. 1. Experimental autoimmune thyroiditis is induced in certain strains of mice (e.g., mice bearing H-2^k and H-2^s MHC haplotypes) by immunizing them with thyroglobulin (Tg) mixed with an adjuvant. Approximately 2–4 wk after immunization, the mice develop antithyroglobulin antibodies and lymphocytic infiltration of the thyroid, which may be accompanied by low thyroid hormone levels.

labeled Idd-1. Likewise, as will be discussed below, HLA is the major susceptibility gene in human IDDM, supporting the similarity between NOD mice and human IDDM. Whole-genome screening of NOD mice has been completed, and more than 10 loci outside the MHC locus have been identified as conferring susceptibility to diabetes *(59,60)*. These loci are distributed throughout the mouse genome, but the specific genes in these loci have yet to be identified. Initially, it was hoped that the identification of the mouse Idd loci would help map the human IDDM genes. However, after the human IDDM whole-genome screen was completed, it was found that with the exception of the MHC complex, none of the NOD Idd loci corresponded with the human IDDM loci. These results demonstrated the limitations of using mouse models for identifying human susceptibility genes. However, they also underscored the importance of MHC genes in the development of autoimmune diabetes. (*See* Chapter 5.)

Mouse Models of Autoimmune Thyroiditis

Autoimmune thyroiditis can develop spontaneously in certain strains of animals (e.g., the obese strain of chickens), or after immunization with thyroglobulin (experimental autoimmune thyroiditis) (*see* Chapter 4). Experimental autoimmune thyroiditis (EAT) is often used as a model for HT *(61)*, and is characterized by production of antithyroglobulin antibodies, cytotoxic T cells, lymphocytic infiltration of the thyroid gland, follicular destruction, and may be accompanied by a reduction in serum thyroid hormone concentrations (Fig. 1) *(61)*. However, induction of thyroid autoimmunity by immunizing with thyroglobulin could be achieved only in genetically susceptible strains of mice *(62,63)*. Genetic analysis of the susceptible strains showed that the initiation of thyroid autoimmunity was controlled by the H-2 genotype (the mouse MHC region). Mice bearing H-2^k and H-2^s haplotypes displayed the highest incidence of severe disease, whereas strains bearing other H-2 haplotypes, such as H-2^b or H-2^d, were relatively resistant to the induction of EAT *(62)*. Genetic analyses using intra- H-2 recombinants mapped the major gene controlling susceptibility to EAT to the I-A subregion, which corresponds to the D region of human HLA *(64)*. Further studies by Beisel et al. *(65)*

showed that genes at the D end of the mouse H-2 region modified the severity of thyroid infiltration. Similarly, studies in intra-H-2 recombinants and mutant strains pointed to the involvement of the K region in the effector phase of EAT *(66)*. In order to explain these findings, Rose and Burek *(64)* proposed two levels of genetic control of EAT. The first involved the induction of the immune response and was encoded primarily at the I-A region. The second level of genetic control determined the development of the effector response, as manifested by the severity of the thyroid infiltration, and was influenced by the D and K loci. Rose and Burek have proposed *(64)* that the I-A region controls the response of the T-helper cells to immunization with thyroglobulin, whereas the D and K loci control the cytotoxic T-cell response manifested by the infiltration of the thyroid.

Even though the major genetic control of EAT is linked to the H-2 region, there are additional data suggesting that genes outside the H-2 region also influence the development of EAT. Beisel et al. *(67)* found significant differences in the anti-Tg response of congenic mouse strains carrying similar H-2 haplotypes, thus suggesting that non H-2 genes influenced EAT. Recently, Kuppers et al. *(68)* have shown that the IgG2a antibody response to thyroglobulin was linked to the IgH locus in the mouse. Additionally, we have shown that the anti-Tg response, but not the T-cell infiltration of the thyroid, was dependent on idiotype/antiidiotype interactions in mouse strains that were not susceptible to EAT by the H-2 genes *(69)*. We have also reported rat strain-related differences in susceptibility to MHC class 2 antigen expression on thyroid cells *(70)*. These results suggested that the autoantibody response to thyroglobulin and a host of additional important components of the immune response are controlled by genes outside the MHC complex in mice.

Mouse Models of Graves' Disease

Graves' disease is a uniquely human disease, and there have been no examples of an autoimmune-based hyerthyroidism described in any animals. However, there have been many attempts to induce Graves' disease in rabbits, rats, and mice. With the cloning of the (thyroid stimulating hormone) TSH receptor, the major Graves' antigen became available for immunization. A number of studies have been reported using recombinant TSH receptor ectodomain as immunogen, but only TSH receptor-blocking antibodies were induced rather than TSH receptor-stimulating antibodies *(71,72)*. Although the TSH receptor antibody response has been reported to be associated with the MHC gene complex, with H-2d mice being one of the good responder strains, it appears that thyroidits was induced rather than GD *(73)*. More recently, Shimojo et al. *(74)* and our laboratory have reported the induction of thyroid-stimulating antibodies and hyperthyroidism in H-2k mice using TSH receptor-transfected fibroblasts spontaneously expressing MHC class I and II antigens *(75)*. This model also may be MHC-dependent. We need to learn a great deal more about this model, since only 25% of the immunized mice develop the disease, suggesting non-MHC genetic influences.

TOOLS USED IN GENE MAPPING STUDIES

Based on the abundant epidemiologic evidence for a strong genetic effect on the development of IDDM and the AITDs, searches for the susceptibility genes were initiated. The basic strategies used for mapping complex disease genes include association studies and linkage studies of candidate genes and of previously unknown gene loci

THE PRINCIPLE OF LINKAGE

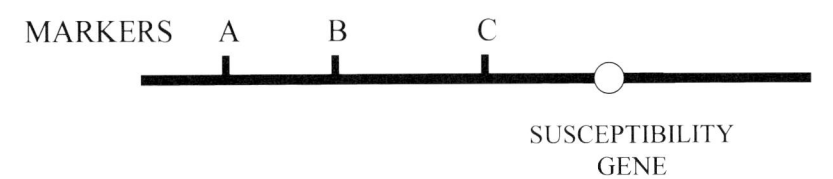

Fig. 2. The principle of linkage analysis is based on the fact that if two genes are close together on a chromosome, they will segregate together. In the figure, marker C will cosegregate more often with the disease than marker B, which in turn, will cosegregate more often with the disease than marker A.

identified by whole-genome screening. These tools have proven successful in the mapping of classical Mendelian disorders and are currently being employed in most searches for the susceptibility genes for complex diseases. It is beyond the scope of this chapter to review these methods in depth, and we will give only a brief overview of these methods.

Association Studies

Association studies are very sensitive and can locate susceptibility genes. These genes are not necessary for the development of the disease, but inheriting these genes puts the individual at a greater risk. Association studies are based on comparisons of the frequencies of specific alleles of marker loci in patients and controls in an ethnically similar population. If the frequency of the tested allele is significantly higher in the affected individuals, it is concluded that the allele is associated with the disease. The strength of the association is measured by the relative risk (RR), which is calculated by multiplying the ratio of patients with the marker to normals with the marker by the ratio of normals without the marker to patients without the marker (Woolf's formula) *(76)*. Other techniques to test for association include the haplotype relative risk *(77)* and transmission disequilibrium tests *(78)*. This approach to genetic analysis is very sensitive, and association studies may detect genes contributing <5% of the total genetic contribution to the disease *(79)*. However, this can also limit the usefulness of association studies if the goal of gene mapping is to find the major contributing genes for a complex disease. Another limiting factor, in using association studies, is that they cannot be utilized easily in a whole-genome screening strategy *(see below)* and are, therefore, most useful in studying candidate genes.

Linkage Analysis

Genetic linkage techniques, as distinct from association, are powerful tools in analyzing complex disease-related genes, because they are known to detect genes that are more directly involved in the pathogenesis of a disease, i.e., they are more likely to detect genes that are more often required (although not necessarily sufficient) for the development of a disease *(80)*. The consequence is that linkage studies are less sensitive than association studies, since they only detect genes contributing approx >10% of total genetic susceptibility *(80)*.

The principle of linkage analysis is based on the fact that if two genes are close together on a chromosome, they will segregate together. Therefore, if a tested marker is close to a disease susceptibility gene, it will cosegregate with the disease in families (Fig. 2). The LOD score is the measure of the likelihood of linkage between a disease and a genetic marker *(81)*. An LOD score of >3 is considered strong evidence for linkage and an LOD score of >2.0 is suggestive of linkage *(82)*. An LOD score of −2.0 is used to exclude linkage. Two analytical approaches can be taken. The parametric approach (standard LOD score analysis) and the nonparametric approach (affected sib-pair analysis or NPL). The parametric approach may be statistically more powerful, since it has the advantage of allowing the investigator to test for genetic heterogeneity within families, and to deduce the mode of inheritance and penetrance of the disease *(83)*.

Analysis of Candidate Genes

Candidate genes are genes of known sequence and location that could, theoretically, be involved in disease pathogenesis. For example, such candidate genes may be involved in the pathological manifestations of the disease. If a candidate locus is the cause of the disease, then markers close to that locus should segregate with the disease within a family, making their identification possible. The candidate gene approach has already been used successfully in a number of diseases, most notable maturity-onset diabetes of the young (MODY *[84]*).

Since the basic abnormality in the autoimmune endocrine diseases is an immune response against endocrine tissues, candidate genes for IDDM and the AITDs include genes that control antibody responses (e.g., the immunoglobulin gene complexes and genes responsible for B-cell growth factors), genes that control T-cell responses (e.g., the HLA region, the T-cell receptor genes, and genes responsible for T-cell growth factors), and genes encoding the target autoantigens in IDDM (e.g., insulin, GAD-65) and the AITDs (thyroglobulin, thyroid peroxidase, and TSH receptor). Many of these genes have now been studied for their possible role in the genetic susceptibility to IDDM and the AITDs.

Whole-Genome Screens

Linkage studies can now be used for genome-wide genetic screening utilizing polymorphic markers that span the whole human genome. These markers span the whole genome at distances that will enable detection of linkage to susceptibility genes located between any two of them. The main obstacle to performing such genome-wide screens has been the lack of easy-to-analyze polymorphic markers that span the whole human genome. The discovery of microsatellite markers *(85)* made the whole-genome screening approach feasible. Microsatellites are regions in the genome that are composed of short repetitive units, from 1 to 5 bp. The most common microsatellites are the 2-base CA-repeats $(dC-dA)_n$. Microsatellite loci are highly polymorphic (i.e., have many alleles), because the number of repeats in each individual is variable; usually, there are 5–15 alleles/locus in the population being studied (Fig. 3). Microsatellites are extremely abundant and uniformly distributed throughout the genome at distances of <1 million bp *(85)* and serve as excellent markers in linkage studies designed to search for unknown disease susceptibility genes. A set of 300 microsatellite markers is now commercially available, each spaced at distances of approx 10 cM (0.1 recombination fraction units). Once a suspected gene region is located, it can be further narrowed using markers that are more closely spaced, and the gene region identified.

It is difficult to perform whole-genome screening in complex diseases, such as IDDM and the AITDs, because the gene penetrance may be relatively low and late in time. It

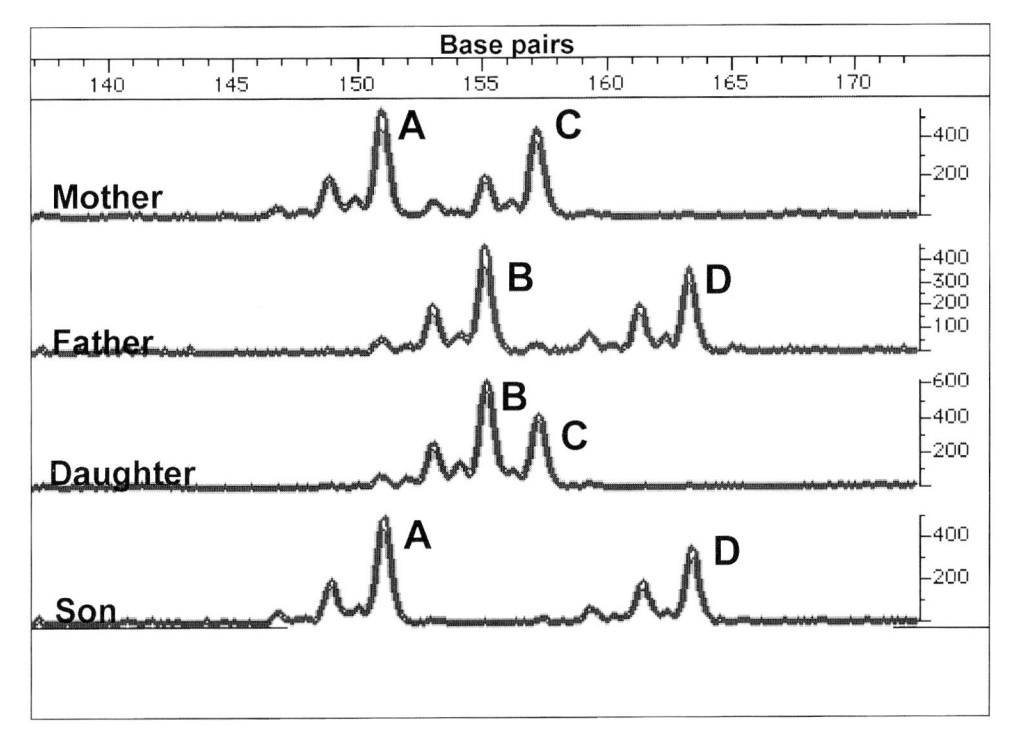

Fig. 3. Microsatellite markers can be analyzed using fluorescent-labeled primers. After PCR amplification, the labeled PCR products (which represent the alleles for that locus for the individual tested) can be separated on a gel and the fluorescence graphed as the intensity vs the size (electropherogram). A family is illustrated in which both the father and the mother are heterozygotes for the tested marker.

would, therefore, be unclear who in the family has yet to develop the disease. Similarly, the gene being studied may be present in healthy persons, since it may not be an obligatory gene. Moreover, in complex diseases, the phenotype definitions can be complicated, and there is a possibility of genetic heterogeneity, i.e., different genotypes causing a similar phenotype (e.g., in MODY). Therefore, in order to identify complex disease genes, it has been necessary to use large numbers of families and to be make a series of assumptions. For example, in the identification of a Crohn's disease locus on chromosome 16, 78 families with at least 2 affected siblings were typed with 270 markers. Linkage analysis revealed an LOD score of 2.04 *(86)*.

THE ROLE OF HLA CANDIDATE GENES IN THE SUSCEPTIBILITY TO IDDM AND THE AITDS

The MHC region, encoding the HLA glycoproteins, consists of a complex of genes located on chromosome 6p21 (Fig. 4). The MHC region also encodes various additional proteins, most of which are associated with immune responsiveness. The MHC locus itself encodes genes that are grouped into three classes:

1. Class I genes include the HLA antigens A, B, and C.
2. The class II genes include the HLA-DR, DP, and DQ genes.
3. The class III genes include several complement components (e.g., C4), tumor necrosis factor α (TNF-α), heat-shock protein 70, and several other genes *(87,88)*.

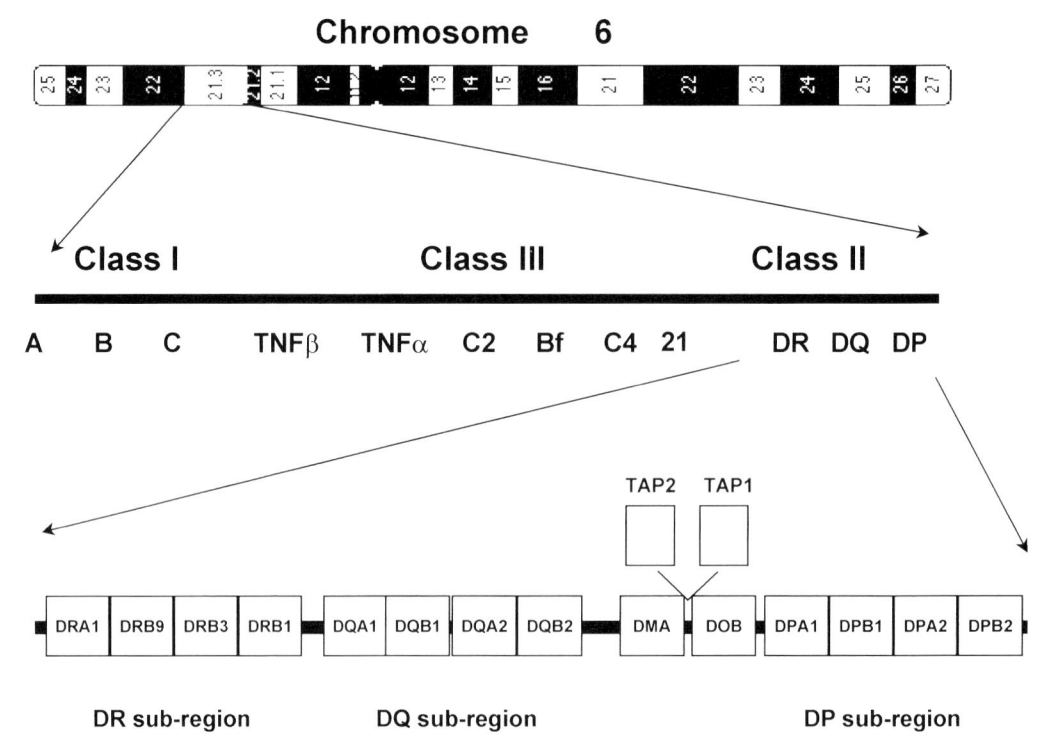

Fig. 4. The HLA region is located on chromosome 6p21. It is a complex genetic region, which consists of several loci, all of which code for proteins that influence the different arms of the immune system. Depicted are the major loci.

Since the HLA region is highly polymorphic and contains many immune response genes, it was the first candidate genetic region to be studied for association and linkage with IDDM and the AITDs.

Association and Linkage of HLA with IDDM

The first evidence for a strong HLA influence on the development of IDDM came from the observation that the risk for developing IDDM in HLA identical siblings was 12.9% compared with a risk of 0.5% in the general population (89). Since the risk in identical twins was about 35% (47), it was estimated that the HLA region contributed 30–40% to the overall genetic susceptibility to IDDM. Thus, HLA genes are the major contributing genes to the development of IDDM. A positive association was first directly observed between IDDM and HLA-B8 (90). This association was later shown to be owing to linkage disequilibrium between these class I alleles and class II alleles. About 95% of Caucasian diabetics were HLA-DR3 and/or DR4, compared to 45–55% of matched controls (91,92). The relative risk for a DR3/DR3-positive individual was 9.8, and for a DR3/DR4 individuals, it was 8.3 (93). Recent analyses have shown that DR4-DQA1*0301-DQB1*0302 and DR3-DQA1*0501-DQB1*0201 are most strongly associated with IDDM. On the other hand, DR15-DQA1*0102-DQB1*0602 demonstrated a strong negative association with IDDM (94). The sequencing of HLA alleles showed that if an aspartic residue occupied position 57 in both alleles of that chain, autoimmune diabetes was unlikely to occur (95,96). Full susceptibility required both alleles to be

Asp[57]-negative; the relative risk for individuals in whom both alleles were non-aspartic acid was 107 *(93)*. Furthermore, in studies of different populations, a linear relationship was found between the incidence of IDDM and the estimated gene frequency of homozygous absence of aspartic acid at position 57 in the population being studied *(97)*. It is hypothesized that an aspartic acid at position 57 on the β chain influences the antigen binding properties of the HLA-DQαβ heterodimer *(see below) (96,98)*. Recently, the presence of arginine at position 52 of the DQα chain has also been shown to confer increased risk for IDDM *(99)*. This risk was additive with the increased risk conferred by the absence of aspartic acid at position 57 of the DQβ chain *(99)*.

In addition to these associations between HLA and IDDM, several studies have also been performed, which have confirmed linkage of HLA-DR to IDDM assuming a recessive mode of inheritance *(100)*. Thus, the confirmation in studies of both linkage and association of HLA genes with IDDM indicates that they are major genes contributing significantly to the overall susceptibility to IDDM. The HLA locus is now designated as the insulin-dependent diabetes mellitus-1 (IDDM-1) susceptibility locus.

Association of HLA with Graves' Disease

Graves' disease was initially found to be associated with HLA-B8 in Caucasians *(101)*. This finding was then confirmed in a great number of studies, mostly examining populations of Caucasian origin. In these early studies, HLA-B8 was associated with relative risks for Graves' disease ranging from 1.5 to 3.5. Subsequently, it was found that Graves' disease was more strongly associated with HLA-DR3, which is now known to be in linkage disequilibrium with HLA-B8 *(102,103)*. The frequency of DR3 in Graves' disease patients was 50–56%, and in the general population, 18–26%, giving a relative risk for people with HLA-DR3 of 2.1–3.7 *(50,103)*. Even though the frequency of HLA-DR3 was increased in Caucasians with Graves' disease, there were also HLA-DR3-negative associations with Graves' disease, and the HLA associations were found to be different in other ethnic groups. In the Japanese population, Graves' disease was associated with HLA-B35 *(104)*, and in the Chinese population, an increased frequency of HLA-Bw46 has been reported *(105)*. In African-Americans, no overall susceptibility could be associated with any DR allele, although subdivision of the patients revealed that DRw6 was associated with thyroid antibody formation *(106)*. Among Caucasians, HLA-DQA1*0501 has recently been described as conferring a risk for Graves' disease over and above that of HLA-DR3 (relative risk 3.8) *(107,108)*. However, the risk of developing Graves' disease in HLA-identical siblings was only 7%, which was not significantly different from the general risk in siblings. Furthermore, this was much lower than the 30–50% concordance for MZ twins described earlier *(109)*. Therefore, it seemed that the HLA genes were not the primary disease genes, and merely conferred a small increase in risk for the development of Graves' disease. These results suggested that other genes outside the HLA region must confer most of the genetic susceptibility to Graves' disease.

The role of HLA polymorphism on the clinical expression of Graves' disease has also been explored. McGregor et al. *(110)* reported an association between the likelihood of relapse of Graves' disease and HLA DR3, but several other workers studying correlations between HLA alleles and Graves' disease severity were unable to demonstrate a higher risk of relapse in Graves' disease patients that carried the HLA-DR3 allele *(111–113)*. It was also possible that rather than conferring general susceptibility to Graves' disease, the HLA genes may have increased the risk for developing certain phenotypes of Graves' disease. The most important clinical phenotype of Graves' disease that can result in severe morbidity is ophthalmopathy, which is closely associated with Graves' disease (in 90% of the cases), and is much less frequently seen with HT *(114)*. The severe form of ophthalmopathy occurs in <10% of Graves' disease patients *(114)*. Studies of HLA associations in GO have so far produced conflicting results. Schleusener et al. *(115)* reported a significantly higher prevalence of HLA-B8 and DR3 in patients with GO and/or TSH receptor antibodies (TSHR-Ab) compared to Graves' disease patients, who had neither ophthalmopathy nor TSHR-Ab. In the same study, the patients without TSHR-Ab and eye signs who relapsed had a significantly higher prevalence of HLA-DR5 than the control group *(115)*. Similarly, Farid et al. *(116)* reported a higher incidence of HLA-DR3 in Graves' disease patients with GO. In two studies performed in Hungary and Newfoundland, Canada, Frecker et al. *(117,118)* reported that HLA-DR7 enhanced the risk for ophthalmopathy in the presence of B8, but had a protective influence in its absence *(117)*. In contrast, others have found no difference in the distribution of HLA-DR alleles between Graves' disease patients with and without ophthalmopathy *(101,116, 119–122)*. Likewise, no difference in the DR3 frequency was found in Graves' disease patients with and without pretibial myxedema *(116)*.

Another subtype of Graves' disease, which typically occurs in Asian populations, is thyrotoxic periodic paralysis (TPP). TPP manifests by episodes of flaccid proximal muscle weakness predominantly of the lower limbs, accompanied by hypokalemia *(123)*. The paralytic episodes occur exclusively during hyperthyroid states *(123)*. The incidence of TPP is 1.8–8.8% in thyrotoxic Japanese patients *(124,125)*, 1.9% in Chinese patients *(126)*, and 0.1–0.2% in hyperthyroid patients in the US *(127)*. In one HLA association study from Japan, an increased incidence of HLA-DRw8 was found in TPP patients when compared to controls and thyrotoxic patients who did not have periodic paralysis *(128)*. However, other studies did not demonstrate a specific association of TPP with any HLA allele in Chinese patients *(129,130)*.

In summary, although certain HLA alleles have been consistently shown to be elevated in Graves' disease patients (mainly HLA-DR3 and DQA1*0501 in Caucasians) compared to control populations, there is no consistent association between HLA polymorphisms and any of the known clinical phenotypes of Graves' disease.

Association of HLA with HT

Data on HLA haplotypes in HT are less definitive than in Graves' disease. A general methodological problem is that although the diagnosis of Graves' disease is relatively straightforward, the definition of HT has been more controversial. This reflects the fact that the disease encompasses a spectrum of manifestations, ranging from the simple presence of thyroid autoantibodies with focal lymphocytic infiltration, which may be of no functional consequence, to the presence goitrous or atrophic thyroiditis, characterized by gross thyroid failure. Since the "disease phenotype" definition assumes particular importance in genetic studies, it is obvious that discordant studies may be explained by problems with disease heterogeneity. Although initial studies failed to demonstrate HLA associations *(131)* for any A- B- or C- antigens, an association with HLA DR5 was observed in goitrous HT (RR = 3.1) *(132)* and with DR3 (RR = 5.1) in atrophic HT *(133)*. These data were confirmed in subsequent studies *(134,135)*, all in Caucasian populations. More recently, an association has been reported between HT and HLA-DQw7 (DQB1*0301) with a relative risk of 4.7 *(134,136)*. Associations of HT with other HLA

LOD SCORES VS. RF FOR TNFA

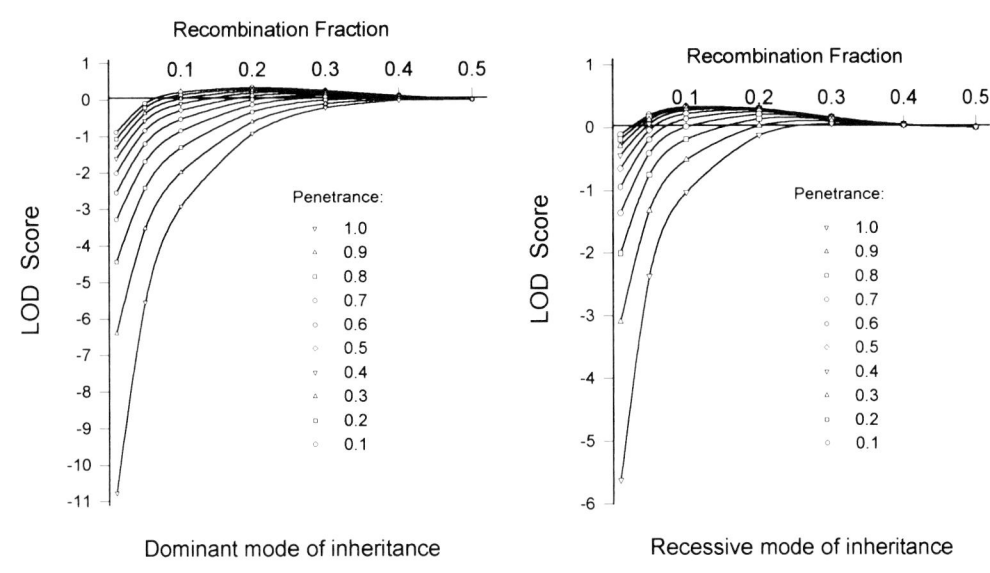

Fig. 5. LOD score results for TNF-α at different assumed penetrances and recombination fractions. Note that under assumed recessive mode of inheritance, slightly positive LOD scores are noted for TNF-α, maximal at a recombination fraction (θ) of 0.1 (LOD score 0.328).

haplotypes have also been reported in different ethnic populations, e.g., HLA-DRw53 in Japanese, and HLA-DR9 in Chinese (for a review *see 137*).

HLA Linkage Studies in the AITDs

Studies in HT have not demonstrated evidence for linkage to HLA genes. Farid et al. *(138)* were unable to find a linkage between Hashimoto's disease and the HLA antigens, and Bode et al. *(139)* also could not demonstrate linkage of familial thyroiditis with any HLA genes. Similarly, in 10 Graves' disease families from Hong Kong, no linkage was demonstrated between HLA alleles and Graves' disease *(140)*. In contrast to these reports, Payami et al. *(141)* found evidence for linkage of Graves' disease to HLA using the sib-pair method. However, the number of sib-pairs used was small and the selection method may have been biased, since these sibs were pooled from previous smaller studies.

We have performed linkage studies between the HLA region and the AITDs using a variety of techniques. In all of these studies, we were able to reject linkage between the AITDs and HLA genes. In our early studies, we tested 27 families for linkage of the AITDs (i.e., Graves' disease or HT) with HLA alleles using both traditional HLA serotyping *(142)* and DNA restriction fragment-length polymorphisms (RFLPs) *(143)*. The results showed negative LOD scores for both recessive and dominant modes of inheritance at various penetrances *(142,143)*. Recently, we also performed a linkage study between the HLA region and the AITDs in 19 families (107 individuals, 14 with Graves' disease, and 32 with HT) using the microsatellite TNF-α, which is located inside the HLA region *(144)*. Our study excluded linkage for penetrances of 0.4 and higher under an assumed dominant mode of inheritance, and for penetrances of 0.8 and higher under an assumed recessive mode of inheritance (Fig. 5). This allowed us to conclude that although certain HLA genes conferred an increased risk of developing one of the

AITDs, as shown by the many association studies, these genes were likely to account for <5% of the genetic contribution. Moreover, as discussed earlier, the concordance rate for the AITDs in HLA-identical siblings was low (7%) confirming the relative importance of non-HLA-related genes in genetic susceptibility to human AITD *(109)*.

NON-HLA CANDIDATE GENES

As mentioned earlier, the HLA genes contribute approx 40% to the genetic susceptibility to IDDM and insignificantly to the susceptibility to the AITDs. Therefore, both in IDDM and in the AITDs, other candidate genes have been sought. In view of the fact that both IDDM and the AITDs are autoimmune diseases, most of the candidate genes studied have been immune response-related genes.

Non-HLA Candidate Genes in IDDM

The first locus outside the HLA region that was consistently found to be associated with IDDM was the insulin gene region on chromosome 11p15. This region was first implicated when a polymorphic region near the insulin gene was discovered, and studies reported that the insulin gene region polymorphisms conferred a risk that was independent of HLA genotype *(145–149)*. The disease-associated locus has recently been mapped to a 4.1-kb region encompassing the insulin gene *(148)*, and it was designated IDDM-2 *(150)*. This region was found to contain 10 polymorphic sites. It is now known that the polymorphism conferring the susceptibility to IDDM *(151)* was the presence of a variable number of tandem repeats (VNTR). Population studies reported an association with class I alleles in this region, which have a smaller number of tandem repeats compared to the class III alleles. The VNTR polymorphisms are located adjacent to defined regulatory DNA sequences and influence insulin gene expression *(152)*. Therefore, it was postulated that the biologically important polymorphisms were actually within the VNTR. Indeed, it has now been shown that the VNTR can influence insulin gene expression in vitro *(153)*, as well as in vivo *(154) (see below)*.

The CTLA-4 gene was a candidate gene in IDDM because of its cardinal role in T-cell interactions with antigen-presenting cells (APCs) *(155)*. Several studies have reported a weak association between the CTLA-4 gene and IDDM (as well as the AITDs described below), which has been designated IDDM-12, even though the association was confined to specific populations. Nistico et al. *(156)* reported linkage and association of a microsatellite marker locus within 1 cM of the CTLA-4 gene in Italian and Spanish families, but not in families from the US and the UK *(156)*. Moreover, in a large study from Germany, a more direct association was found between a polymorphism inside the CTLA-4 gene (either threonine or alanine in position 49 of the protein) and IDDM *(157)*. The phenotypic frequency of the Ala(G)-positive patients (69%) was significantly higher than the frequency in the controls (58%) giving a relative risk of 1.6 *(157)*. Two recent studies using different techniques and populations have now confirmed these results. In a study of 525 Caucasian IDDM patients fro the Belgian Diabetes Registry, an association was found between the Ala(G)-positive polymorphism and IDDM with a relative risk of 1.5, similar to that reported in the German population *(157,158)*. Similarly, Marron et al. found a significant association of the A/G polymorphism of the CTLA-4 gene with IDDM using a multiethnic collection of families and applying the transmission disequilibrium test for association (tdt) *(159)*. In summary, apart from the HLA genes and the insulin VNTR polymorphism, the CTLA-4 gene is the only gene that has been consistently found to be associated with IDDM.

Several other candidate genes have been studied, but the results remain inconsistent (for another review, *see 160*). The recognition and response of T cells to foreign antigens is achieved via the interaction of the T-cell receptor (TCR) with the antigen and class II HLA molecules on APCs. Since the initiation of IDDM may involve abnormalities in T-cell recognition of self-antigens, the TCR has been considered an important candidate gene for susceptibility to IDDM. The TCR is composed of two chains, α and β, each containing constant and variable regions. Both the TCRα and the TCRβ gene regions (on chromosomes 14q and 7q, respectively) have been studied for associations with IDDM. Although no study found an association between the TCRα gene and IDDM *(160,161)*, the results for the TCRβ gene were inconsistent with a positive association *(160,162)* and no association *(160,163)*. In reviewing these data on the TCR, it would seem that TCR polymorphisms are unlikely to confer an important genetic susceptibility to IDDM *(160,164)*.

The immunoglobulin G (IgG) heavy-chain gene complex is located on chromosome 14q. This genetic region has produced generally negative results in patients with IDDM *(160,165)*. Recently, Monos et al. *(166)* reported a strong association between a TNF polymorphism and IDDM in Caucasians giving a relative risk of 53! However, since the TNF gene is inside the HLA region, it is not known whether this is an independent effect or whether it results, more likely, from linkage disequilibrium with the DR3 HLA haplotype *(166)*. Another candidate gene recently found to be associated with IDDM is the interleukin 1 receptor (IL-1R) gene *(167)*. A polymorphism at the IL-1R gene was associated with IDDM (relative risk 2.51) in patients from the UK, but not from Finland or India *(167)*. These studies all need to be validated by other groups in order to determine their contribution to the genetic susceptibility to IDDM.

Non-HLA Candidate Genes Associated with the AITDs

As with IDDM, candidate genes outside the HLA region likely to be important in the AITDs include genes that control antibody response (e.g., the IgH gene complex), genes that control TCRs (e.g., the TCR genes), and genes encoding major disease-specific autoantigens (i.e., thyroglobulin, thyroid peroxidase, and the TSH receptor). Most of these genes have now been studied for their possible role in susceptibility to the AITDs. In addition, the AITDs are associated with several conditions for which the genetic abnormalities are known. For example, it has long been observed that patients with Down syndrome (DS) have an increased incidence of autoimmune hypothyroidism *(168,169)* and possibly Graves' disease *(170)*. Since DS patients have three copies of chromosome 21, it is possible that chromosome 21 may harbor a gene contributing to the susceptibility to the AITDs.

One of the first immune-response genes studied was the IgG heavy-chain gene (IgH). Several reports found an association between the IgG heavy-chain Gm allotypes and Graves' disease, mainly in the Japanese population *(171)*. However, and as discussed later, we were unable to find linkage between the IgH gene and either Graves' disease or HT *(144)*. An RFLP of the TCR β chain was reported to be associated with HT *(172)* and Graves' disease *(173)*. However, these results were not confirmed by other investigators *(103,174)*, although geographical variation may have been responsible. Another study showed a significant association between the presence of anti-Tg antibodies and the TCR β genes *(175)*.

Table 1
Characteristics of the Current Study Sample

Group	Females	Males	Total	F:M
Total affected	108 (56%)	16 (14%)	124 (40%)	6.8:1
Graves' disease	44 (23%)	10 (9%)	54 (18%)	4.4:1
HT	64 (33%)	6 (5%)	70 (22%)	10.7:1
Unaffected	86 (44%)	98 (86%)	184 (60%)	0.9:1
Total	194 (100%)	114 (100%)	308 (100%)	1.7:1

As mentioned earlier, CTLA-4 was consistently found to be associated with IDDM. Similarly, there have been several reports demonstrating an association between the CTLA-4 gene and the AITDs *(156,157,176,177)*. Earlier studies found an association between a microsatellite marker located near the CTLA-4 gene and Graves' disease. The frequency of allele 106 of the microsatellite was 23.4–26.7% in patients with Graves' disease and 12.6–13.5% in controls *(176,177)*, giving a relative risk of 2.1–2.8. With the identification of the alanine/threonine (G/A) polymorphism inside the CTLA-4 leader peptide, this polymorphism was tested for association with the AITDs. Similar to the findings in IDDM, the Ala(G) polymorphism was found to be associated with Graves' disease with a higher relative risk than in IDDM (RR = 2.0) *(157)*. These reports have been consistent in several populations *(156,157,176,177)*, and there is now evidence that the CTLA-4 gene is also associated with autoimmune hypothyroidism *(177)*. However, it is unlikely that the CTLA-4 gene is a major susceptibility gene for AITD, since we found no evidence for linkage (*see* Table 3).

Two studies have also examined possible associations between the IL-R antagonist gene and Graves' disease, and have produced conflicting results *(178,179)*. The different thyroid autoantigens have also now been studied as possible candidates for conferring susceptibility to the AITDs. Pirro and colleagues studied the allelic distribution of a newly identified microsatellite located inside the TPO gene *(180)*. They found no difference in the distribution of the 7 alleles of the TPO microsatellite when comparing 93 patients with Graves' disease, 57 patients with autoimmune thyroiditis, and 121 healthy controls *(180)*. A polymorphism in the ectodomain of the TSH receptor (TSHR) in codon 52 (coding for either threonine of proline) has been described *(181)*. However, despite early reports of an association between this polymorphism and Graves' ophthalmopathy *(182)*, later studies have demonstrated no association between this polymorphism and Graves' disease *(183,184)*.

Non-HLA Candidate Gene-Linkage Studies in the AITDs

The first study in AITD families that examined linkage to loci outside the HLA region was performed by Prentice et al. *(185)*. They tested for linkage between thyroid autoantibodies and several candidate genes, including the IgH gene, TCR-α gene, the IDDM 11q gene, and microsatellites on chromosome 21 (examined because of the reported association between the AITDs and DS *[168,169]*). No linkage was found between the development of thyroid autoantibodies and any of these candidate genes.

Recently, we have examined several candidate genes for linkage with the AITDs using microsatellite marker analysis *(144)*. Forty-eight multiplex families (308 individuals) were recruited for the study and used for analyzing linkage to candidate genes. Table 1

Table 2
Candidate Genes Studied on the Current Study Sample

Gene	Chromosomal location	Marker name, primers
HLA	6p	TNF-α (TNFA2/TNFA3)
IgH	14q32.33	IgH@ (490/491)
TCRα	14q11-12	TCRA
TCRβ	7q35	R-G
CTLA-4	2q33	CTLA-4 (+)
TPO	2p24-25	TPO(+) (sRA-1F/sRA-1R)
Thyroglobulin	8q24	cMYC
IDDM-4	11q	FGF-3
IDDM-5	6q	ESR (ER-1/ER-2)

Table 3
LOD Scores Calculated for Different
Candidate Genes in Patients with the AITDs

Candidate gene	Marker	Maximum LOD score	Lowest LOD score
HLA region	TNF-α	0.278	–10.768
Tg	cMYC	0	–12.017
TPO	TPO(+)	0.420	–6.558
IgH	IgH@	0.078	–7.688
CTLA-4	CTLA-4(+)	0.169	–3.768
IDDM-4	FGF 3	0.038	–7.490
IDDM-5	ESR	0	–8.264

shows the clinical characteristics of the families. Of the 48 families, 10 (21%) had family members affected with Graves' disease only, 21 (44%) had HT-affected family members, and 17 (35%) were mixed having both Graves' disease- and HT-affected family members. Of the clinically and biochemically euthyroid family members, 36% were thyroid antibody-positive, a frequency similar to that reported in previous studies *(44,45)*. The affected female-to-male (F:M) ratio (6.8:1) was also in accord with that reported in the literature.

We have studied three categories of candidate genes (Table 2):

1. Genes related to the immune response (HLA, IgH, TCR, CTLA-4).
2. Genes coding for the thyroid autoantigens targeted by the autoimmune response (TPO, Tg).
3. Some of the newly discovered IDDM loci *(150)*, in view of the known association between the AITDs and IDDM *(186)*.

The TSHR, which is located on chromosome 14q31, was analyzed as part of the screening of chromosome 14 *(see below)*. It should be noted that some of the candidate genes (HLA, Tg, TPO, IDDM-4 and 5) were studied using only the first 19 families collected (107 individuals), but these results have been confirmed using the whole data set of families recruited. Table 3 summarizes the maximum and minimum LOD scores calculated under assumed recessive and dominant modes of inheritance. None of the candidate genes studied have been found to be linked to the AITDs. Linkage was excluded to the HLA region, the IgH gene, the TCR genes, the CTLA-4 genes, the TPO and thyroglobulin genes, and the IDDM-4 and 5 loci. As in our previous studies using serological markers and RFLPs *(142,143)*, we again excluded linkage of the AITDs with the HLA region. The slightly positive LOD scores noted for HLA (0.328) may have reflected the effects of the association between HLA region genes and the AITDs *(80)*. Slightly positive LOD scores were also noted for TPO (0.420). This may need to be investigated further. The negative LOD scores for IDDM-4 and IDDM-5 argued against a common genetic susceptibility to IDDM and the AITDs conferred by these loci.

WHOLE-GENOME SCREENING IN IDDM AND THE AITDS

The availability of microsatellite markers spanning the whole human genome has enabled investigators to screen the genome for linkage with a variety of complex diseases *(187)*. The first successful genome-wide screen was performed in IDDM.

Genome-Wide Screen in IDDM

The HLA and insulin region-associated genes could not completely explain the genetic susceptibility to IDDM. Moreover, studies in NOD mice have suggested the existence of additional susceptibility genes *(59,96)*. Therefore, several independent groups utilized a genome-wide screen for susceptibility genes for IDDM using affected sib-pairs *(149,150)*. With this approach, the central role of the HLA (IDDM-1) and insulin gene (IDDM-2) regions in genetic susceptibility to IDDM was confirmed by demonstrating linkage of IDDM to these loci *(188)*. As mentioned earlier, these loci were previously shown to be associated with IDDM. In addition, whole genome screens using microsatellites yielded evidence for the existence of other susceptibility loci, including IDDM-3 (15q26) *(189)*, IDDM-4 (11q13), IDDM-5 (6q), IDDM-6 (18q) *(149,150)*, IDDM 7 (2q31) *(190)*, and at least five more loci *(188,191,192)*. All of these loci have been mapped, and for each there is evidence for linkage. However, it is important to note that except for IDDM-1 (HLA) and IDDM-2 (insulin VNTR), only three of the newly mapped loci have been confirmed by independent studies using different data sets. The confirmed loci include IDDM-4 (on 11q13), IDDM-5 (on 6q25), and IDDM-8 (on 6q27) *(149,150,193,194)*.

These data confirmed earlier predictions based on simulation analyses that the genetic susceptibility to IDDM was probably influenced by shared alleles at several loci across the genome. It will only be after the IDDM susceptibility genes are cloned that the way they confer increasing susceptibility to IDDM will be understood. It is likely that different individuals with IDDM inherit different combinations of the susceptibility genes conferring different disease prognoses. However, as mentioned earlier, most IDDM patients inherit HLA susceptibility alleles, because they are the major susceptibility genes for IDDM.

Genome-Wide Screening in the AITDs

Recently we *(144)* and others *(195,196)* have initiated whole-genome searches for the susceptibility genes for the AITDs. Preliminary data are now available while these screens are being completed. It is expected that with the completion of the whole-genome screening for the AITDs by several independent groups, important information on the genetics of the AITDs will be revealed.

Chapter 3 / Genetics

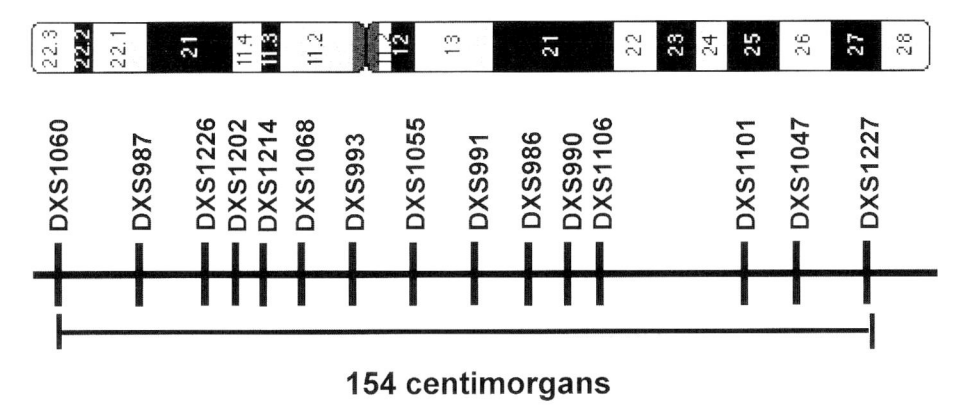

Fig. 6. Map of chromosome X. The markers shown are taken from the published Genethon maps. The average distance between each two markers is approx 10 cM (1 cM = 0.01 recombination fractions).

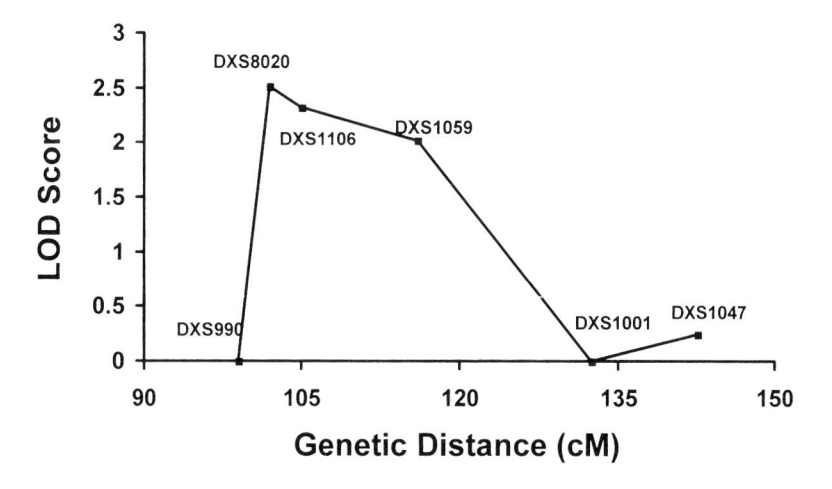

Fig. 7. Maximum LOD score results for markers on chromosome X assuming Graves' disease as affected. Positive LOD scores were obtained in the chromosomal region Xq21-22, with the maximum LOD score (MLS) at marker DXS8020 (MLS = 2.5).

In our study sample (Table 1), the X-chromosome was chosen to test whether genes located on it contribute to the significant female preponderance among patients with AITD. Chromosome 21 was selected because of the known association between DS and the AITDs *(168,169)*, and chromosome 14 was chosen because it contained several important candidate genes (e.g., the TSHR, and IgH genes) *(197)*. Each chromosome was analyzed when considering Graves' disease, HT, or both (the AITDs) as affected. Screening chromosome 21 for the 48 families studied excluded linkage to any of the markers spanning chromosome 21 for affectedness status of Graves' disease, HT, and the AITDs (data not shown).

Figure 6 shows the markers analyzed for screening the X-chromosome. For chromosome X, positive LOD scores were obtained in the region of Xq21-22 when considering Graves' disease as affected (Fig. 7). Using a multipoint analysis, the maximum LOD score was 2.5 (Fig. 7), thus suggesting that a gene participating in the expression of

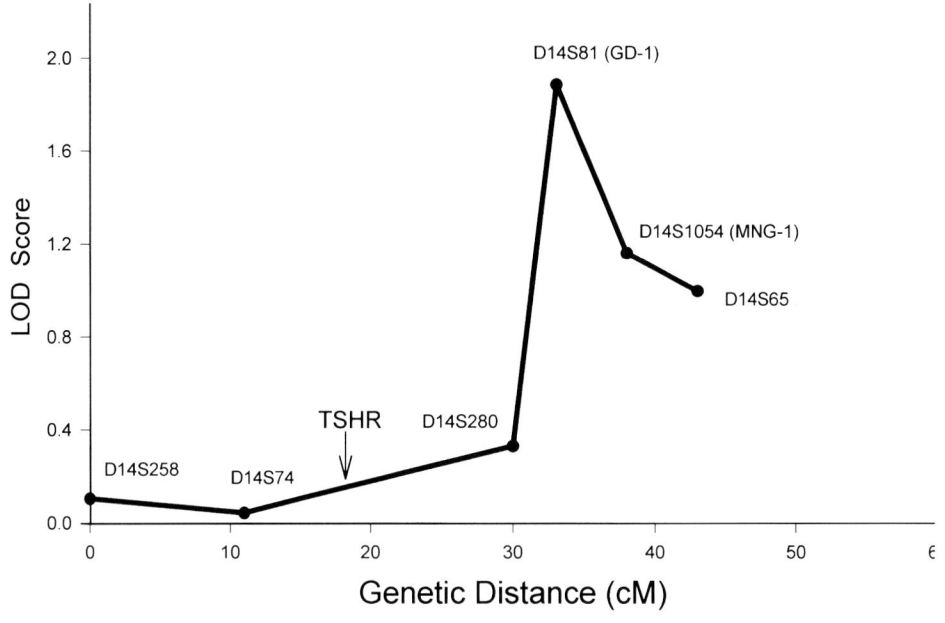

Fig. 8. Maximum LOD score results for markers on chromosome 14q31 when considering Graves' disease as affected. Some markers in this region showed positive LOD scores, the maximum being for the marker D14S81 (MLS = 2.1).

Graves' disease is located in this region. An X-chromosome susceptibility gene for GD can theoretically explain the female preponderance of the disease. This is because females are twice as likely to inherit the gene as males, since females have two X-chromosomes, whereas males have one. Studying additional families for this region as well as denser markers will enable us to determine the importance of this locus in the susceptibility to Graves' disease.

A similar analysis has been performed for chromosome 14. Negative LOD scores were obtained for affectedness status AITD and HT. Positive LOD scores were obtained in the region of 14q31 when considering Graves' disease as affected (Fig. 8). Marker D14S81 (Graves' disease-1) gave the maximum LOD score of 2.1 for recessive mode of inheritance, at a penetrance of 0.3 *(144)*. Moreover, as shown in Fig. 8, the LOD scores of other markers in the region of D14S81 were positive in a geographically logical sequence. A recent study using simulated data has shown that for whole-genome screening with markers spaced at 10 cM, one can expect a maximum of only 1 false peak giving LOD scores of 2 *(82)*. Thus, our results may imply that a gene participating in the expression of Graves' disease is localized in the vicinity of D14S81. Interestingly, this locus is located 5 cM from the recently discovered MNG-1 locus, which was linked to multinodular goiter *(198)* and 13 cM from IDDM-11 *(192)* (Fig. 9). This marker is also located ~20 cM from the TSH receptor gene *(199)* (Fig. 9). However, two recent studies failed to find linkage between markers inside the TSHR gene and Graves' disease *(195,196)*, but they did not examine the surrounding region *(195)*. Likewise, in our studies, we found no linkage between TSHR markers and Graves' disease (data not shown). In summary, we have found preliminary evidence for linkage of Graves' disease to marker D14S81 on chromosome 14q31. This marker is close to the recently discovered MNG-1 locus linked with multinodular goiter.

MAP OF CHROMOSOME 14q31

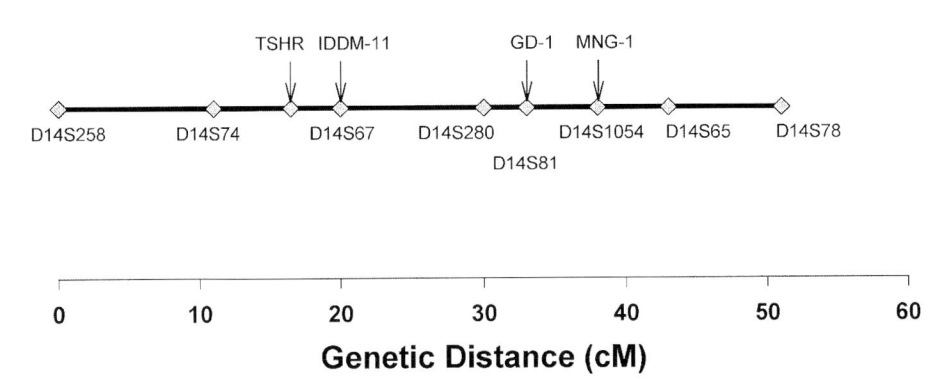

Fig. 9. Map of chromosome 14q31. The markers shown are taken from the published Genethon maps. The MNG-1 locus is ~5 cm telomeric to Graves' disease-1(GD-1), and the IDDM-11 and TSHR loci are approx 15 and 20 cM centromeric to Graves' disease-1, respectively.

MECHANISMS OF DISEASE INDUCTION BY SUSCEPTIBILITY GENES

One of the main reasons for mapping susceptibility genes for complex diseases is to understand their pathogenesis better. Indeed, the recent mapping of several new susceptibility genes in IDDM and the AITDs (e.g., the HLA CTLA-4 and insulin gene VNTR) has already helped unravel some of the mechanisms involved in the development of IDDM, the AITDs, and other autoimmune conditions.

HLA-Related Susceptibility to IDDM and the AITDs

The mechanism by which HLA associations confer disease susceptibility in IDDM are now much better understood, and HLA haplotypes are no longer just undefined genetic markers. For T cells to recognize and respond to an antigen requires the recognition of a complex between the antigenic peptide and HLA molecule *(200)*. The polymorphisms of the HLA antigens are critical for the high-affinity recognition of autoantigens (e.g., isle cell antigens) by TCRs *(87)*. It is thought that lack of aspartic acid at position 57 on the DQβ chain and the presence of arginine at position 52 of the DQα chain permit the autoantigen to fit in the antigen binding groove inside the HLA molecule and to be recognized by the TCR *(201)*. In contrast, the presence of aspartic acid at position 57 of the DQβ chain and absence of arginine at position 52 of the DQα chain prevent the autoantigen from fitting and, therefore, prevent autoantigen presentation to the TCR *(201)*. Thus, the susceptibility to IDDM conferred by the lack of aspartic acid at position 57 of DQβ and the presence of arginine at position 52 of DQα is a result of enhanced ability of APCs to stimulate T cells when presenting them with an autoantigen. However, autoantigen presentation is a physiological process. Why should autoantigens be presented to T cells in association with HLA molecules?

The presentation of autoantigens to T cells is also a normal physiological process that maintains tolerance for all self-proteins. However, the influence of the presentation process may change if the cells that manufacture the autoantigen acquire the functions of professional APCs, thus presenting themselves in large amounts. Unlike normal thyroid cells, thyroid epithelial cells from patients with Hashimoto's disease and Graves' disease and islet cells from patients with IDDM have been shown to express HLA class II antigen molecules, which are normally expressed only on APCs, such as macrophages and dendritic cells *(202–205)*. Given the role of HLA class II molecules in the antigen presentation process *(87)*, it has been proposed that aberrant expression of these molecules, for example, on thyroid cells, could initiate thyroid autoimmunity via direct thyroid autoantigen presentation *(203)*. Indeed, coculture of peripheral blood mononuclear cells (PBMC) from Graves' disease patients with homologous thyrocytes induced T-cell activation *(206)* as well as interferon-γ (IFN-γ) production and thyroid cell HLA class II antigen expression *(207)*. The trigger for MHC class II antigen expression on normal tissue cells may be trauma or a viral infection *(208–210)*. Supporting the role of HLA expression of thyroid cells in the induction of the AITDs have been studies *(74)* showing that immunization of mice with fibroblasts, engineered to express both the TSHR and MHC class II molecules, induced a disease similar to human Graves' disease in the recipient animals *(74)*. The immunized mice developed hyperthyroidism, goiter, and TSHR antibodies *(74)*. The fibroblast is not a professional APC, but appeared to provide the factors necessary for the initiation of the autoimmune process.

Mechanisms of CTLA-4 Participation in the Development of IDDM and the AITDs

As described earlier, the activation of T cells by APCs requires the presentation to the TCR of an antigenic peptide bound to an HLA class II surface protein. However, this signal alone is not sufficient for T-cell activation. A second signal is required, and these costimulatory signals are also provided by APCs *(155)*. Thus, in addition to expressing HLA molecules, APCs express on their surface a family of proteins (e.g., B7-1, B7-2) that interact with molecules (CD28 and CTLA-4) on the surface of CD4$^+$ T lymphocytes during antigen presentation *(155)*. Whereas the binding of B7 to CD28 on T cells costimulates T-cell activation, the binding of B7 to CTLA-4 is thought to downregulate T-cell activation and induce tolerance. The suppressive effects of CTLA-4 on T-cell activation have raised the possibility that mutations altering CTLA-4 function could lead to the development of autoimmunity. Indeed, treatment of female NOD mice at the onset of insulitis (2–4 wk of age) with anti-CTLA-4 (a soluble CD28 antagonist) or a monoclonal antibody (MAb) specific for B7-2 (a CD28 ligand) suppressed the development of diabetes *(211)*. Costimulatory molecules may also influence the resulting Th1 or Th2 T-cell phenotype helping to direct the pattern of the autoimmune reaction *(212,213)*. B7-1 has been reported on thyroid cells in HT, but not in normal thyroid cells, as has CD-40, another costimulatory molecule *(214)*. Therefore, it is likely that both thyroid epithelial cells and professional APCs participate in initiating thyroid autoimmunity *(215)*.

The HLA region harbors several important immune regulatory genes (Fig. 4). It is therefore possible that the HLA susceptibility to IDDM and the AITDs and other autoimmune conditions is mediated by non-HLA immune regulatory genes in this complex genetic region. Evidence for such a mechanism has recently been published. The TAP1 and TAP2 genes are located near the HLA DQB region. These genes encode molecules that transport peptides across membranes and are intimately involved in antigen processing. The TAP molecules function to transport peptides across the endoplasmic reticulum membrane, where the peptides associate with HLA molecules *(216)*. Recently, polymorphisms at the TAP1 gene were shown to be associated with IDDM, suggesting that the susceptibility conferred by this region may be mediated by these genes *(216)*. Additionally, it has been found that the HLA-DQ genes harbor long-terminal repeat (LTR) elements of the human endogenous retrovirus HERV-K. These LTRs were recently shown to be in linkage disequilibrium with HLA-DQA1*0301-DQB1*0302, the haplotype known to confer susceptibility to IDDM *(217)*. Thus, it is possible that the LTR genes in the HLA-DQ region are involved in the susceptibility to IDDM, since the LTRs are believed to be involved in transcriptional activation of adjacent genes. One possibility is that these HLA-DQ LTRs act as enhancers in the transcription of the HLA-DQ locus, thus enhancing its contribution to the susceptibility to IDDM *(217)*.

In summary, since we have obtained a better understanding of the MHC gene complex, the mechanisms by which it operates to confer susceptibility to IDDM have become better understood.

Insulin Gene VNTR and the Susceptibility to IDDM

One of the more interesting areas of research on the pathogenesis of IDDM has been the involvement of the insulin gene VNTR in the susceptibility to the disease. The VNTR is located 365 bp upstream from the initiation of transcription of the insulin gene. The polymorphism arises from a variable number of 14-bp oligonucleotide repeats. Based on the number of repeats, the length of the VNTR can be divided into three classes: class I (~570 bp), class II (~1640 bp), and class III (~2400 bp) *(154,156)*. It has been shown by several independent groups that the class I alleles are associated with IDDM *(154)*. Since the VNTR is located adjacent to regulatory DNA sequences affecting insulin gene expression *(152)*, it was postulated that the polymorphism confers susceptibility to IDDM by influencing insulin gene expression. Indeed, the VNTR was shown to influence insulin gene expression in vitro *(153)*, as well as in vivo *(154)*, with class I alleles being associated with a 1.5- to 3-fold increase in insulin gene transcription in the pancreas. However, it was difficult to reconcile lower insulin mRNA levels in the pancreas (associated with class III alleles) with a dominantly protective effect on IDDM development. Recently, two groups have reported that class III VNTR alleles were associated with significantly higher insulin mRNA levels in human fetal thymus *(218,219)*. The authors postulated that higher levels of thymic insulin expression in individuals with class III alleles promoted the negative selection of insulin-specific T lymphocytes, thus facilitating immune tolerance induction and protection from IDDM *(218,219)*. These findings, if confirmed, may represent a general principle in autoimmunity and may apply to other autoimmune conditions.

CONCLUSIONS

Genetic susceptibility plays an important role in the development of IDDM and the AITDs. Until recently, most studies on the genetics of IDDM and the AITDs were epidemiological in nature. However, in the past decade, the loci conferring susceptibility for IDDM have been mapped, and research is in progress to identify the AITD susceptibility loci. The two major genes contributing approx 50–60% of the overall genetic susceptibility to IDDM are the MHC region and the insulin gene VNTR (IDDM-1 and

IDDM-2, respectively). These genes have been sequenced, and the mechanisms by which they induce autoimmunity are now thought to be understood. Although the HLA region is the most important locus conferring susceptibility to IDDM, it probably makes only a minor contribution to the genetic susceptibility to AITD. Similarly, the CTLA-4 locus, which is associated with IDDM and the AITDs, makes only a minor contribution to their overall susceptibility. In contrast to IDDM, the major susceptibility genes for the AITDs have yet to be identified. It is hoped that the genetic studies on IDDM and the AITDs will better our understanding of the common denominator in these and other autoimmune conditions.

ACKNOWLEDGMENTS

Supported in part by DK35764, DK45011, and DK52464 from NIDDKD (to T. F. D.), DK31775, NS27941, and MH48858 (to D. A. G.), and DK02498 from NIDDKD (to Y. T.).

REFERENCES

1. Tomer Y, Barbesino G, Greenberg DA, Davies TF. The immunogenetics of autoimmune diabetes and autoimmune thyroid disease. Trends Endocrinol Metab 1997;8: 63–70.
2. Tomer Y, Davies TF. Infections and autoimmune endocrine disease. Baillière's Clin Endocrinol Metab 1995;9:47–70.
3. World Health Organization. WHO Expert Committee on Diabetes Mellitus: second report. World Health Organ Tech Rep Ser 1980;646:1–80.
4. LaPorte RE, Fishbein HA, Drash AL, et al. The Pittsburgh Insulin-dependent diabetes mellitus (IDDM) registry. The incidence of insulin-dependent diabetes mellitus in Allegheny County, Pennsylvania (1965–1976). Diabetes 1981;30:279–284.
5. Melton LJ, Palumbo PJ, Chu CP. Incidence of diabetes mellitus by clinical type. Diabetes Care 1983; 6:75–86.
6. Patrick SL, Moy CS, LaPorte RE. The world of insulin-dependent diabetes mellitus: what. Diabetes Metab Rev 1989;5:571–578.
7. LaPorte RE, Tuomilehto J. The DiaMond Project. Practica Diabetes Int 1995;12:93–98.
8. West KM. Epidemiology of Diabetes and Its Vascular Lesions. Elsevier, New York, 1978, pp. 292–293.
9. Diabetes Epidemiology Research International Group. Geographic patterns of childhood insulin-dependent diabetes mellitus. Diabetes Epidemiology Research International Group. Diabetes 1988; 37:1113–1119.
10. Dorman JS, LaPorte RE, Stone RA, Trucco M. Worldwide differences in the incidence of type I diabetes are associated with amino acid variation at position 57 of the HLA-DQ beta chain. Proc Natl Acad Sci USA 1990;87:7370–7374.
11. Krolewski AS, Warram JH, Rand LI, Kahn CR. Epidemiologic approach to the etiology of type I diabetes mellitus and its complications. N Engl J Med 1987;317:1390–1398.
12. Tunbridge WMG, Evered DC, Hall R, et al. The spectrum of thyroid disease in a community: the Whickham survey. Clin Endocrinol (Oxford) 1977;7:481–493.
13. Vanderpump MPJ, Tunbridge WMG, French JM, et al. The incidence of thyroid disorders in the community: a twenty-year follow-up of the Whickham survey. Clin Endocrinol (Oxford) 1995;43: 55–68.
14. Furszyfer J, Kurland LT, McConahey WM, Elveback LR. Graves' disease in Olmsted County, Minnesota, 1935 through 1967. Mayo Clin Proc 1970;45:636–644.
15. Mogensen EF, Green A. The epidemiology of thyrotoxicosis in Denmark. Incidence and geographical variation in the Funen region 1972–1974. Acta Med Scand 1980;208:183–186.
16. Berglund J, Christensen SB, Hallengren B. Total and age-specific incidence of Graves' thyrotoxicosis, toxic nodular goitre and solitary toxic adenoma in Malmo 1970–74. J Intern Med 1990;227:137–141.
17. Phillips DI, Barker DJ, Rees Smith B, Didcote S, Morgan D. The geographical distribution of thyrotoxicosis in England according to the presence or absence of TSH-receptor antibodies. Clin Endocrinol (Oxford) 1985;23:283–287.

18. Mogensen EF, Green A. The epidemiology of thyrotoxicosis in Denmark. Incidence and geographical variation in the Funen region 1972–1974. Acta Med Scand 1980;208:183–186.
19. Haraldsson A, Gudmundsson ST, Larusson G, Sigurdsson G. Thyrotoxicosis in Iceland 1980–1982. An epidemiological survey. Acta Med Scand 1985;217:253–258.
20. Brownlie BE, Welsh JD. The epidemiology of thyrotoxicosis in New Zealand: incidence and geographical distribution in north Canterbury, 1983–1985. Clin Endocrinol (Oxford) 1990;33:249–259.
21. dos Remedios LV, Weber P, M., Feldman R, Schurr DA, Tsoi TG. Detecting unsuspected thyroid dysfunction by the free thyroxine index. Arch Intern Med 1980;140:1045–1049.
22. Gordin A, Heinonen OP, Saarinen P, Lamberg BA. Serum thyrotropohin in symptomless autoimmune thyroiditis. Lancet 1972;1:551–554.
23. Okamura K, Ueda K, Sone H, et al. A sensitive thyroid stimulating hormone assay for screening of thyroid functional disorder in elderly Japanese. J Am Geriatr Soc 1989;37:317–322.
24. Nystrom E, Bengtsson C, Lindquist O, Lindberg S, Lindstedt G, Lundberg PA. Serum triiodothyronine and hyperthyroidism in a population sample of women. Clin Endocrinol (Oxford) 1984;20:31–42.
25. Kohno T, Tsunetoshi Y, Ishikawa E. Existence of anti-thyroglobulin IgG in healthy subjects. Biochem Biophys Res Commun 1988;155:224–229.
26. Ericsson UB, Christensen SB, Thorell J. A high prevalence of thyroglobulin autoantibodies in adults with and without thyroid diesase as measured with a sensitive solid-phase immunosorbent radioassay. Clin Immunol Immunopathol 1985;37:154–162.
27. Phillips DIW, Prentice L, McLachlan SM, Upadhyaya M, Lunt PW, Rees Smith B. Autosomal dominant inheritance of the tendency to develop thyroid autoantibodies. Exp Clin Endocrinol 1991;97:170–172.
28. Christau B, Kromann H, Christy M, Andersen OO, Nerup J. Incidence of insulin-dependent diabetes mellitus (0–29 years at onset) in Denmark. Acta Med Scand Suppl 1979;624:54–60.
29. Rewers M, Stone RA, LaPorte RE, et al. Poisson regression modeling of temporal variation in incidence of childhood insulin-dependent diabetes mellitus in Allegheny County, Pennsylvania, and Wielkopolska, Poland, 1970–1985. Am J Epidemiol 1989;129:569–581.
30. Volpe R. Autoimmune thyroid disease. In: Volpe R, ed. Autoimmunity and Endocrine Disease. Marcel Dekker, New York, 1985, pp. 109–285.
31. Burch PRJ, Rowell NR. Autoimmunity: aetiological aspects of chronic discoid and systemic lupus erythematosus, systemic sclerosis and Hashimoto's thyroiditis: Some immunological complications. Lancet 1963;2:507–515.
32. Risch N. Assessing the role of HLA-linked and unlinked determinants of disease. Am J Hum Genet 1987;40:1–14.
33. Warram JH, Krolewski AS, Gottlieb MS, Kahn CR. Differences in risk of insulin-dependent diabetes in offspring of diabetic mothers and diabetic fathers. N Engl J Med 1984;311:149–152.
34. Warram JH, Martin BC, Krolewski AS. Risk of IDDM in children of diabetic mothers decreases with increasing maternal age at pregnancy. Diabetes 1991;40:1679–1684.
35. Rewers M, Norris JM. Epidemiology of type I diabetes. In: Eisenbarth GS, Lafferty KJ, eds. Type I Diabetes: Molecular, Cellular, and Clinical Immunology. Oxford University Press, London, 1995, pp. 373–400.
36. Pilcher CC, Dickens K, Elliott RB. ICA only develop in early childhood. Diabetes Res Clin Pract 1991;14:S82
37. Bartels ED. Twin Examinations: Heredity in Graves' Disease. Munksgaad, Copenhagen, 1941, pp. 32–36.
38. Martin L. The heredity and familial aspects of exophathalmic goitre and nodular goitre. Q J Med 1945;14:207–219.
39. Hall R, Stanbury JB. Familial studies of autoimmune thyroiditis. Clin Exp Immunol 1967;2:719–725.
40. Vyse TJ, Todd JA. Genetic analysis of autoimmune disease. Cell 1996;85:311–318.
41. Tamai H, Ohsako N, Takeno K, et al. Changes in thyroid function in euthyroid subjects with family history of Graves' disease; a followup study of 69 patients. J Clin Endocrinol Metab 1980;51:1123–1128.
42. Chopra IJ, Solomon DH, Chopra U, Yodhihara E, Tersaki PL, Smith F. Abnormalities in thyroid function in relatives of patients with Graves' disease and Hashimoto's thyroiditis: lack of correlation with inheritance of HLA-B8. J Clin Endocrinol Metab 1977;45:45–54.
43. Tamai H, Kumagai LF, Nagataki S. Immunogenetics of Graves' disease. In: McGregor AM, ed. Immunology of Endocrine Diseases. MTP, Lancaster, UK, 1986, pp. 123–141.

44. Burek CL, Hoffman WH, Rose NR. The presence of thyroid autoantibodies in children and adolescents with AITD and in their siblings and parents. Clin Immunol Immunopathol 1982;25:395–404.
45. Aho K, Gordin A, Sievers K, Takala J. Thyroid autoimmunity in siblings: a population study. Acta Endocrinol 1983;Suppl 251:11–15.
46. Hall JG. Twinning: mechanisms and genetic implications. Curr Opinion Genet Dev 1996;6:343–347.
47. Barnett AH, Eff C, Leslie RDG, Pyke DA. Diabetes in identical twins. A study of 200 pairs. Diabetologia 1981;20:87–93.
48. Tattersall RB, Pyke DA. Diabetes in identical twins. Lancet 1972;2:1120–1125.
49. Harvald B, Hauge M. A catamnestic investigation of Danish twins. Danish Med Bull 1956;3:150–158.
50. Volpe R. Immunology of human thyroid disease. In: Volpe R, ed. Autoimmunity in Endocrine Disease. CRC, Boca Raton, 1990, pp. 73–92.
51. Brix TH, Christensen K, Holm NV, Harvald B, Hegedus L. Genetic versus environment in Graves' disease—a population based twin study. Thyroid 1997;7(Suppl 1):S–13.
52. Irvine WJ, McGregor AG, Stuart AE, Hall GH. Hashimoto's disease in uniovular twins. Lancet 1961; 2:850–853.
53. McGregor AG, Roberts DF, Hall R. A study of triplets with Hashimoto's thyroiditis. Postgrad Med J 1979;55:894–896.
54. Chertow BS, Fidler WJ, Fariss BL. Graves' disease and Hashimoto's thyroiditis in monozygotic twins. Acta Endocrinol 1973;72:18–24.
55. Zhang Y, Proenca R, Maffei M, Barone M, Leopold L, Friedman JM. Positional cloning of the mouse obese gene and its human homologue. Nature 1994;372:425–432.
56. Prochazka M, Leiter EH, Serreze DV, Coleman DL. Three recessive loci required for insulin-dependent diabetes in nonobese diabetic mice. Science 1987;237:286–289.
57. Livingstone A, Edwards CT, Shizuru JA, Fathman CG. Genetic analysis of diabetes in the nonobese diabetic mouse. I. MHC and T cell receptor beta gene expression. J Immunol 1991;146:529–534.
58. Miyazaki T, Uno M, Uehira M, et al. Direct evidence for the contribution of the unique I-ANOD to the development of insulitis in non-obese diabetic mice [see comments]. Nature 1990;345:722–724.
59. Todd JA, Aitman TJ, Cornall RJ, et al. Genetic analysis of autoimmune type 1 diabetes mellitus in mice. Nature 1991;351:542–547.
60. Ghosh S, Palmer SM, Rodrigues NR, et al. Polygenic control of autoimmune diabetes in nonobese diabetic mice. Nat Genet 1993;4:404–409.
61. Charreire J. Immune mechanisms in autoimmune thyroiditis. Adv Immunol 1989;46:263–334.
62. Vladutiu AO, Rose NR. Autoimmune murine thyroiditis: relation to histocompatibiltiy (H-2) type. Science 1971;174:1137–1139.
63. Rose NR, Twarog FJ, Crowle AJ. Murine thyroiditis: importance of adjuvant and mouse strain for the induction thyroid lesions. J Immunol 1971;106:698–704.
64. Rose NR, Burek CL. The genetics of thyroiditis as a prototype of human autoimmune disease. Ann Allergy 1985;54:261–269.
65. Beisel K, David CS, Giraldo AA, Kong Y, M., Rose NR. Regulation of experimental autoimmune thyroiditis: Mapping of susceptibility to the I-A subregion of the mouse H-2. Immunogenetics 1982; 15:427–430.
66. Maron R, Klein J, Cohen IR. Mutations at H-2K or H-2D alter immune response phenotype of autoimmune thyroiditis. Immunogenetics 1982;15:625–627.
67. Beisel KW, Kong Y, M., Babu KS, David CS, Rose NR. Regulation of experimental autoimmune thyroiditis: influence of non H-2 genes. J Immunogenetics 1982;9:257–265.
68. Kuppers RC, Epstein LD, Outschoorn IM, Rose NR. The IgG2a antibody response to thyroglobulin is linked to the Igh locus in mouse. Immunogenetics 1994;39:404–411.
69. Tomer Y, Gilburd B, Sack J, et al. Induction of thyroid autoantibodies in naive mice by idiotypic manipulation. Clin Immunol Immunopathol 1996;78:180–187.
70. Neufeld DS, Davies TF. Strain-specific determination of the degree of thyroid cell MHC class II antigen expression: evaluation of established Wistar and Fisher rat thyroid cell lines. Endocrinology 1990;127:1254–1259.
71. Costagliola M, Many C, Stalmans-Falys M, Tonacchera M, Vassart G, Ludgate M. Recombinant thyrotropin receptor and the induction of autoimmune thyroid disease in BALB/c mice: a new animal model. Endocrinology 1994;135:2150–2159.
72. Vlase H, Nakashima M, Graves PN, Tomer Y, Morris J, Davies TF. Defining the major antibody epitopes on the human TSH receptor in immunized mice. Endocrinology 1995;136:4415–4423.

73. Costagliola M, Many C, Stalmans-Falys M, Vassart G, Ludgate M. The autoimmune response induced by immunizing female mice with recombinant human TSH receptor varies with the genetic background. Mol Cell Endocrinol 1995;115:199–206.
74. Shimojo N, Kohno Y, Yamaguchi K, et al. Induction of Graves-like disease in mice by immunization with fibroblasts transfected with the thyrotropin receptor and a class II molecule. Proc Natl Acad Sci USA 1996;93:11,074–11,079.
75. Kita M, Ahmad L, Marians R, Graves PN, Davies TF. Thyrotoxic death in mice with Graves' disease. The 70th Annual Meeting of the American Thyroid Association, Colorado Springs, CO, 1997 (Abstract).
76. Woolf B. On estimating the relation between blood group and disease. Ann Hum Genet 1955;19:251–253.
77. Falk CT, Rubinstein P. Haplotype relative risks: an easy and reliable way to construct a proper control sample for risk calculations. Ann Hum Genet 1987;51:227–233.
78. Spielman RS, McGinnis RE, Ewens WJ. Transmission test for linkage disequilibrium: the insulin gene region and insulin-dependent diabetes mellitus. Am J Hum Genet 1993;52:506–516.
79. Risch N, Merikangas K. The future of genetic studies of complex human diseases. Science 1996;273:1516,1517.
80. Greenberg DA. Linkage analysis of "necessary" loci versus "susceptibility" loci. Am J Hum Genet 1993;52:135–143.
81. Ott J. Analysis of Human Genetic Linkage. Johns Hopkins University Press, Baltimore, 1996.
82. Lander E, Kruglyak L. Genetic dissection of complex traits: guidelines for interpreting and reporting linkage results. Nature Genet 1995;11:241–247.
83. Greenberg DA, Hodge SE, Vieland VJ, Spence MA. Affecteds-only linkage methods are not a panacea. Am J Hum Genet 1996;58:892–895.
84. Permutt MA, Chiu KC, Tanizawa Y. Glucokinase and NIDDM. A candidate gene that paid off. Diabetes 1992;41:1367–1372.
85. Weber JL. Human DNA polymorphisms based on length variations in simple-sequence tandem repeats. Genome Analysis 1990;1:159–181.
86. Hugot JP, Lauren-Puig P, Gower-Rousseau C, et al. Mapping of a susceptibility locus for Crohn's disease on chromosome 16. Nature 1996;379:821–823.
87. Nelson JL, Hansen JA. Autoimmune disease and HLA. CRC Crit Rev Immunol 1990;10:307–328.
88. Campbell RD, Trowsdale J. Map of the human MHC. Immunol Today 1993;14:349–352.
89. Thomson G, Robinson WP, Kuhner MK, et al. Genetic heterogeneity, modes of inheritance, and risk estimates for a joint study of Caucasians with insulin-depenedent diabtetes mellitus. Am J Hum Genet 1988;43:799–816.
90. Singal DP, Blajchman MA. Histocompatibility (HL-A) antigens, lymphocytotoxic antibodies and tissue antibodies in patients with diabetes mellitus. Diabetes 1973;22:429–432.
91. Spielman RS, Baker L, Zmijewski CM. Gene dosage and susceptibility to insulin-dependent diabetes. Ann Hum Genet 1980;44:135–150.
92. Nerup J, Mandrup-Poulsen T, Molvig J. The HLA-IDDM association: implications for etiology and pathogenesis of IDDM. Diabetes Metab Rev 1987;3:779–802.
93. Morel PA, Dorman JS, Todd JA, McDevitt HQ, Trucco M. Aspartic acid at position 57 of the HLA-DQ beta-chain protects against type I diabetes: a family study. Proc Natl Acad Sci USA 1988;85:8111–8115.
94. Kockum I, Wassmuth R, Holmberg E. HLA-DQ protection and HLA-DR susceptibility in Type 1 (insulin-dependent) diabetes studied in population-based affected families and controls. Am J Hum Genet 1993;42:150–167.
95. Todd JA, Bell JI, McDevitt HO. HLA-DQ beta gene contributes to susceptibility and resistance to insulin-dependent diabetes mellitus. Nature 1987;329:599–604.
96. Aitman TJ, Todd JA. Molecular genetics of diabetes mellitus. Baillière's Clin Endocrinol Metab 1995;9:631–656.
97. Dorman J, LaPorte R, Stone R, et al. Worldwide differences in the incidence of type I diabetes are associated with amino acid variation at position 57 of the HLA-DQ beta chain. Proc Natl Acad Sci USA 1990;87:7370–7374.
98. Brown JH, Jardetzky T, Gofga JC, et al. Three-dimensional structure of the human class II histocompatibility antigen HLA-DR1. Nature 1993;364:33–39.
99. Khalil I, d'Auriol L, Gobet M. A combination of HLA-DQ beta Asp 57-negative and HLA-DQ alpha Arg 52 confers susceptibility to insulin-dependent diabetes mellitus. J Clin Invest 1990;85:1315–1319.

100. Rich SS, Green A, Morton NE, et al. Combined segregation and linkage analysis of insulin-dependent diabetes mellitus. J Hum Genet 1987;40:237–249.
101. Bech K, Lumholtz B, Nerup J, et al. HLA antigens in Graves' disease. Acta Endocrinol 1977;86:510–516.
102. Farid NR, Sampson L, Noel EP, et al. A study of human D locus related antigens in Graves' disease. J Clin Invest 1979;63:108–113.
103. Mangklabruks A, Cox N, DeGroot LJ. Genetic factors in autoimmune thyroid disease analyzed by restriction fragment length polymorphisms of candidate genes. J Clin Endocrinol Metab 1991;73:236–244.
104. Kawa A, Nakamura S, Nakazawa M, et al. HLA-BW35 and B5 in Japanese patients with Graves' disease. Acta Endocrinol (Copenh) 1977;86:754–757.
105. Chan SH, Yeo PP, Lui KF, et al. HLA and thyrotoxicosis (Graves' disease) in Chinese. Tissue Antigens 1978;12:109–114.
106. Sridama V, Hara Y, Fauchet R, DeGroot LJ. HLA immunogentic heterogeny in Black American pateitns with Graves' disease. Arch Intern Med 1987;147:229–231.
107. Barlow ABT, Wheatcroft N, Watson P, Weetman AP. Association of HLA-DQA1*0501 with Graves' disease in English caucasian men and women. Clin Endocrinol 1996;44:73–77.
108. Yanagawa T, Mangklabruks A, Chang YB, et al. Human histocompatibility leukocyte antigen-DQA1*0501 allele associated with genetic susceptibility to Graves' disease in a caucasian population. J Clin Endocrinol Metab 1993;76:1569–1574.
109. Stenszky, V, Kozma L, Balazs C, Rochlitz S, Bear JC, Farid NR. The genetics of Graves' disease: HLA and disease susceptibility. J Clin Endocrinol Metab 1985;61:735–740.
110. McGregor A, Rees Smith B, Hall R, Petersen M, Miller M, Dewar P. Prediction of relapse in hyperthyroid Graves' disease. Lancet 1980;I:1101–1103.
111. Schleusener H, Schwander J, Fischer C, et al. Prospective multicentre study on the prediction of relapse after antithyroid drug treatment in patients with Graves' disease. Acta Endocrinol (Copenh) 1989;120:689–701.
112. Dahlberg PA, Holmlund G, Karlsson FA, Safwenberg J. HLA-A, -B, -C and -DR antigens in patients with Graves' disease and their correlation with signs and clinical course. Acta Endocrinol (Copenh) 1981;97:42–47.
113. McKenna R, Kearns M, Sugrue D, Drury MI, McCarthy CF. HLA and hyperthyroidism in Ireland. Tissue Antigens 1982;19:97–99.
114. Weetman AP. Thyroid-associated ophthalmopathy. Autoimmunity 1992;12:215–222.
115. Schleusener H, Schernthaner G, Mayr WR, et al. HLA-DR3 and HLA-DR5 associated thyrotoxicosis-two different types of toxic diffuse goiter. J Clin Endocrinol Metab 1983;56:781–785.
116. Farid NR, Stone E, Johnson G. Graves' disease and HLA: clinical and epidemiologic associations. Clin Endocrinol (Oxford) 1980;13:535–544.
117. Frecker M, Stenszky V, Balazs C, Kozma L, Kraszits E, Farid NR. Genetic factors in Graves' ophthalmopathy. Clin Endocrinol (Oxford) 1986;25:479–485.
118. Frecker M, Mercer G, Skanes VM, Farid NR. Major histocompatibility complex (MHC) factors predisposing to and protecting against Graves' eye disease. Autoimmunity 1988;1:307–315.
119. Allannic H, Fauchet R, Lorcy Y, Gueguen M, Le Guerrier AM, Genetet B. A prospective study of the relationship between relapse of hyperthyroid Graves' disease after antithyroid drugs and HLA haplotype. J Clin Endocrinol Metab 1983;57:719–722.
120. Kendall-Taylor P, Stephenson A, Stratton A, Papiha SS, Perros P, Roberts DF. Differentiation of autoimmune ophthalmopathy from Graves' hyperthyroidism by analysis of genetic markers. Clin Endocrinol (Oxford) 1988;28:601–610.
121. Weetman AP, So AK, Warner CA, Foroni L, Fells P, Shine B. Immunogenetics of Graves' ophthalmopathy. Clin Endocrinol 1988;28:619–628.
122. Weetman AP, Ratanachaiyavong S, Middleton GW, et al. Prediction of outcome in Graves' disease after carbimazole treatment. Q J Med 1986;59:409–419.
123. Ober KP. Thyrotoxic periodic paralysis in the United States. Report of 7 cases and review of the literature. Medicine 1992;71:109–120.
124. Okinaka S, Shizume K, Lino S, et al. The association of periodic paralysis and hyperthyroidism in Japan. J Clin Endocrinol Metab 1957;17:1454–1459.
125. Satoyoshi E, Murakami K, Kowa H, Kinoshita M, Nishiyama Y. Periodic paralysis in hyperthyroidism. Neurology 1963;13:746–752.

126. McFadzean AJ, Yeung R. Periodic paralysis complicating thyrotoxicosis in Chinese. Br Med J 1967; 1:451–455.
127. Kelley DE, Gharib H, Kennedy FP, Duda RJ, McManis PG. Thyrotoxic periodic paralysis. Report of 10 cases and review of electromyographic findings. Arch Intern Med 1989;149:2597–2600.
128. Tamai H, Tanaka K, Komaki G, et al. HLA and thyrotoxic periodic paralysis in Japanese patients. J Clin Endocrinol Metab 1987;64:1075–1078.
129. Hawkins BR, Ma JT, Lam KS, Wang CC, Yeung RT. Association of HLA antigens with thyrotoxic Graves' disease and periodic paralysis in Hong Kong Chinese. Clin Endocrinol (Oxford) 1985;23: 245–252.
130. Yeo PP, Chan SH, Lui KF, Wee GB, Lim P, Cheah JS. HLA and thyrotoxic periodic paralysis. Br Med J 1978;2:930.
131. Irvine WJ, Gray RS, Morris PJ, Ting A. HLA in primary atrophic hypothyroidism and Hashimoto goitre. J Clin Lab Immunol 1978;3:193–195.
132. Farid NR, Sampson L, Moens H, Barnard JM. The association of goitrous autoimmune thyroiditis with HLA-DR5. Tissue Antigens 1981;17:265–268.
133. Moens H, Farid NR, Sampson L, Noel EP, Barnard JM. Hashimoto's thyroiditis is associated with HLA-DRw3. N Engl J Med 1978;299:133–134.
134. Badenhoop K, Schwartz G, Walfish PG, Drummond V, Usadel KH, Bottazzo GF. Susceptibility to thyroid autoimmune disease: molecular analysis of HLA-D region genes identifies new markers for goitrous Hashimoto's thyroiditis. J Clin Endocrinol Metab 1990;71:1131–1137.
135. Tandon N, Zhang L, Weetman AP. HLA associations with Hashimoto's thyroiditis. Clin Endocrinol (Oxford) 1991;34:383–386.
136. Wu Z, Stephens HAF, Sachs JA, et al. Molecular analysis of HLA-DQ and -DP genes in caucasoid patients with Hashimoto's thyroiditis. Tissue Antigens 1994;43:116–119.
137. Weetman AP. In: Autoimmune Endocrine Disease. Cambridge University Press, Cambridge, 1991, pp. 66–162.
138. Farid NR, Barnard JM, Marshall WH, Woolferey I, O'Driscoll RF. Thyroid autoimmune disease in a large Newfoundland family: the influence of HLA. J Clin Endocrinol Metab 1977;45:1165–1171.
139. Bode HH, Dorf ME, Forbes AP. Familial lymphocytic thyroiditis: analysis of linkage with histocompatibility and blood group. J Clin Endocrinol Metab 1973;37:692–697.
140. Hawkins BR, Ma JT, Lam KS, Wang CC, Yeung RT. Analysis of linkage between HLA haplotype and susceptibility to Graves' disease in multiple-case Chinese families in Hong Kong. Acta Endocrinol (Copenh) 1985;110:66–69.
141. Payami H, Joe S, Thomson G. Autoimmune thyroid disease in Type 1 diabetes. Genet Epidemiol 1989; 6:137–141.
142. Roman SH, Greenberg DA, Rubinstein P, Wallenstein S, Davies TF. Genetics of autoimmune thyroid disease: lack of evidence for linkage to HLA within families. J Clin Endocrinol Metab 1992;74:496–503.
143. O'Connor G, Neufeld DS, Greenberg DA, Concepcion L, Roman SH, Davies TF. Lack of disease associated HLA-DQ restriction fragment length polymorphisms in families with autoimmune thyroid disease. Autoimmunity 1993;14:237–241.
144. Tomer Y, Barbesino G, Keddache M, Greenberg DA, Davies TF. Mapping of a major susceptibility locus for Graves' disease (GD-1) to chromosome 14q31. J Clin Endocrinol Metab 1997;82:1645–1648.
145. Bell GI, Horita S, Karam JH. A polymorphic locus near the human insulin gene is associated with insulin-dependent diabetes mellitus. Diabetes 1984;33:176–183.
146. Bain SC, Prins JB, Hearne CM, et al. Insulin gene region-encoded susceptibility to type 1 diabetesis not restricted to HLA-DR4-positive individuals. Nature Genet 1992;2:212–215.
147. Van der Auwera B, Heimberg H, Schrevens AF, Van Wayenberge C, Flament J, Schuit FC. 5' insulin gene polymorphism confers risks to IDDM independently of HLA class II susceptibility. Diabetes 1993;42:851–854.
148. Lucassen AM, Julier C, Beressi JP, et al. Susceptibility to insulin-dependent diabetes mellitus maps to a 4.1 kb segment of DNA spanning the insulin gene and associated VNTR. Nat Genet 1993;4:305–310.
149. Hashimoto L, Habita C, Beressl JB, et al. Genetic mapping of a susceptibility locus for insulin-dependent diabetes mellitus on chromosome 11q. Nature 1994;371:161–164.
150. Davies JL, Kawauchi Y, Bennet ST, et al. A genome-wide search for human type1 diabetes susceptibility genes. Nature 1994;371:130–136.
151. Undlien DE, Bennet ST, Todd JA, et al. Insulin gene region-encoded susceptibility to IDDM maps upstream of the insulin gene. Diabetes 1995;44:620–625.

152. Docherty K. The regulation of insulin gene expression. Diabetic Med 1992;9:792–798.
153. Kennedy GC, German MS, Rutter WJ. The minisatellite in the diabetes susceptibility locus IDDM2 regulates insulin transcription. Nat Genet 1995;9:293–298.
154. Bennett ST, Lucassen AM, Gough SCL, et al. Susceptibility to human type 1 diabetes at IDDM2 is determined by tandem repeat variation at the insulin gene minisatellite locus. Nat Genet 1995;9:284–292.
155. Reiser H, Stadecker MJ. Costimulatory B7 molecules in the pathogenesis of infectious and autoimmune diseases. N Engl J Med 1996;335:1369–1377.
156. Nistico L, Buzzetti R, Pritchard LE, et al. The CTLA-4 gene region of chromosome 2q33 is linked to, and associated with, type 1 diabetes. Belgian Diabetes Registry. Hum Mol Genet 1996;5:1075–1080.
157. Donner H, Rau H, Walfish PG, et al. CTLA4 alanine-17 confers genetic susceptibility to Graves' disease and to type 1 diabetes mellitus. J Clin Endocrinol Metab 1997;82:143–146.
158. Van der Auwera BJ, Vandewalle CL, Schuit FC, et al. CTLA-4 gene polymorphism confers susceptibility to insulin-dependent diabetes mellitus (IDDM) independently from age anf from other genetic or immune disease markers. Clin Exp Immunol 1997;110:98–103.
159. Marron MP, Raffel LJ, Garchon HJ, et al. Insulin-dependent diabetes mellitus (IDDM) is assocaited with CTLA4 polymorphisms in multiple ethnic groups. Hum Mol Genet 1997;6:1275–1282.
160. Field LL. Non-HLA region genes in insulin dependent diabetes mellitus. Baillière's Clin Endocrinol Metab 1991;5:413–438.
161. Hoover ML, Angelini G, Ball E, et al. HLA-DQ and T-cell receptor genes in insulin-dependent diabetes mellitus. Cold Spring Harbor Symp Quant Biol 1986;51 Pt 2:803–809.
162. Millward BA, Welsh KI, Leslie RD, Pyke DA, Demaine AG. T cell receptor beta chain polymorphisms are associated with insulin- dependent diabetes. Clin Exp Immunol 1987;70:152–157.
163. Concannon P, Wright JA, Wright LG, Sylvester DR, Spielman RS. T-cell receptor genes and insulin-dependent diabetes mellitus (IDDM): no evidence for linkage from affected sib pairs. Am J Hum Genet 1990;47:45–52.
164. Field LL, Stephure DK, McArthur RG. Interaction between T cell receptor beta chain and immunoglobulin heavy chain region genes in susceptibility to insulin dependent diabetes mellitus. Am J Hum Genet 1991;49:627–634.
165. Bertrams J, Baur MP. No interaction between HLA and immunoglobulin IgG heavy chain allotypes in type I diabetes. J Immunogenetics 1985;12:81–86.
166. Monos DS, Kamoun M, Udalova IA. Genetic polymorphism of the human tumor necrosis factor region in insulin-dependent diabetes mellitus. Hum Immunol 1995;44:70–79.
167. Metcalfe KA, Hitman GA, Pociot F, et al. An association between type 1 diabetes and the interleukin-1 type 1 gene. Hum Immunol 1996;51:41–48.
168. Baxter RG, Larkins RG, Martin FI, Heyma P, Myles K, Ryan L. Down syndrome and thyroid function in adults. Lancet 1975;2:794–796.
169. Percy ME, Dalton AJ, Markovic VD, et al. Autoimmune thyroiditis associated with mild "subclinical" hypothyroidism in adults with Down syndrome: a comparison of patients with and without manifestations of Alzheimer disease. Am J Med Genet 1990;36:148–154.
170. Rudberg C, Johansson H, Akerstrom G, Tuvemo T, Karlsson FA. Graves' disease in children and adolescents. Late results of surgical treatment. Eur J Endocrinol 1996;134:710–715.
171. Nakao Y, Matsumoto H, Miyazaki T, et al. IgG heavy chain allotypes (Gm) in atrophic and goitrous thyroiditis. Clin Exp Immunol 1980;42:20–26.
172. Ito M, Tanimoto M, Kamura H, et al. Association of HLA antigen and restriction fragment length polymorphism of T cell receptor beta-chain gene with Graves' disease and Hashimoto's thyroiditis. J Clin Endocrinol Metab 1989;69:100–104.
173. Demaine A, Welsh KI, Hawe BS, Farid NR. Polymorphism of the T cell receptor beta-chain in Graves' disease. J Clin Endocrinol Metab 1987;65:643–646.
174. Weetman AP, So AK, Roe C, Walport MJ, Foroni L. T-cell receptor alpha chain V region polymorphism linked to primary autoimmune hypothyroidism but not Graves' disease. Hum Immunol 1987;20:167–173.
175. Demaine AG, Ratanachaiyavong S, Pope R, Millward BA, McGregor AM. Thyroglobulin antibodies in Graves' disease are associatied with T-cell receptor beta chain and major histocompatibility comples loci. Clin Exp Immunol 1989;77:21–24.
176. Yanagawa T, Hidaka Y, Guimaraes V, Soliman M, DeGroot LJ. CTLA-4 gene polymorphism associated with Graves' disease in a caucasian population. J Clin Endocrinol Metab 1995;80:41–45.

177. Kotsa K, Watson PF, Weetman AP. A CTLA-4 gene polymorphism is associated with both Graves' disease and autoimmune hypothyroidism. Clin Endocrinol 1997;46:551–554.
178. Blakemore AIF, Watson PF, Weetman AP, Duff GW. Association of Graves' disease with an allele of the interleukin-1 receptor antagonist gene. J Clin Endocrinol Metab 1995;80:111–115.
179. Cuddihy RM, Bahn RS. Lack of an association between alleles of interleukin-1 alpha and interleukin-1 receptor antagonsit genes and Graves' disease in a north American Caucasian population. J Clin Endocrinol Metab 1996;81:4476–4478.
180. Pirro MT, De Filippis V, Di Cerbo A, Scillitani A, Liuzzi A, Tassi V. Thyroperoxidase microsatellite polymorphism in thyroid disease. Thyroid 1995;5:461–464.
181. Bohr URM. A heritable point mutation in an extracellular domain of the TSH receptor involved in the interaction with Graves' disease. Biochem Biophys Acta 1993;1216:504–508.
182. Bahn RS, Dutton CM, Heufelder AE, Sarkar G. A genomic point mutation in the extracellular domain of the TSH receptor in patients with Graves' ophthalmopathy. J Clin Endocrinol Metab 1994;78:256–260.
183. Ahmad MF, Stenszky V, Juhazs F, Balzs G, Farid NR. No mutations in the translated region of exon 1 in the TSH receptor in Graves' thyroid glands. Thyroid 1994;4:151–153.
184. Watson PF, French A, Pickerill AP, McIntosh RS, Weetman AP. Lack of association between a polymorphism in the coding region of the thyrotropin receptor gene and Graves' disease. J Clin Endocrinol Metab 1995;80:1032–1035.
185. Prentice L, Phillips DIW, Premawardhana LDKE, Rees Smith B. Genetic linkage analysis of thyroid autoantibodies. Autoimmunity 1993;15:225–229.
186. Torfs CP, King M, Bing H, Malmgren J, Grumet FC. Genetic interrelationship between insulin-dependent diabetes mellitus, the autoimmune thyroid diseases, and rheumatoid arthritis. Am J Hum Genet 1986;38:170–187.
187. Kahn P. Gene hunters close in on elusive prey. Science 1996;271:1352–1354.
188. Todd JA. Genetic analysis of type 1 diabetes using whole genome approaches. Proc Natl Acad Sci USA 1995;92:8560–8565.
189. Field LL, Tobias R, Magnus T. A locus on chromosome 15q26 (IDDM3) produces susceptibility to insulin-dependent diabetes mellitus. Nature Genet 1994;8:189–194.
190. Copeman JB, Cucca F, Hearne CM, et al. Linkage disequilibrium mapping of type 1 diabetes susceptibility gene (IDDM 7) to chromosome 2q31-2q33. Nat Genet 1995;9:80–85.
191. Julier C, Hyer RN, Davies J. Insulin-IGF2 region on chromosome 11p encodes a gene implicated in HLA-DR4-dependent diabetes susceptibility. Nature 1991;354:155–159.
192. Field LL, Tobias R, Thomson G, Plon S. Susceptibility to insulin-dependent diabetes mellitus maps to a locus (IDDM-11) on human chromosome 14q24.3-q31. Genomics 1996;33:1–8.
193. Luo DF, Bui MM, Muir A, Maclaren NK, Thomson G, She JX. Affected sibpair mapping of a novel susceptibility gene to insulin-dependent diabetes mellitus (IDDM8) on chromosome 6q25-27. Am J Hum Genet 1995;57:911–919.
194. Luo DF, Buzzetti R, Rotter JI, et al. Confirmation of three susceptibility genes to insulin-dependent diabetes mellitus: IDDM4, IDDm5 and IDDM8. Hum Mol Genet 1996;5:693–698.
195. De Roux N, Shields DC, Misrahi M, Ratanachaiyavong S, McGregor AM, Milgrom E. Analysis of the thyrotropin receptor as a candidate gene in familial Graves' disease. J Clin Endocrinol Metab 1996;81:3483–3486.
196. Imrie H, Perros P, Young ET, et al. Affected sibling-pair analysis of the thyrotropin receptor gene in Graves' disease. Thyroid 1997;7(Suppl 1):S–76.
197. Libert F, Passage E, Lefort A, Vassart G, Mattei M. Localization of human thyrotropin receptor gene to chromosome 14q31 by in situ hybridization. Cytogen Cell Genet 1991;54:82,83.
198. Bignell GR, Canzian F, Shayeghi M, et al. A familial non-toxic multinodular thyroid goiter locus maps to chromosome 14q but does not account for familial non-medullary thyroid cancer. Am J Hum Genet 1997;61:1123–1130.
199. De Roux N, Misrahi M, Chatelain N, Gross B, Milgrom E. Microsatellites and PCR primers for genetic studies and genomic sequencing of the human TSH receptor gene. Mol Cell Endocrinol 1996;117:253–256.
200. Buus S, Sette A, Grey HM. The interaction between protein-derived immunogenic peptides and Ia. Immunol Rev 1987;98:115–141.
201. Faas S, Trucco M. The genes influencing the susceptibility to IDDM in humans. J Endocrinol Invest 1994;17:477–495.

202. Londei M, Lamb JR, Bottazzo GF, Feldmann M. Epithelial cells expressing aberrant MHC class II determinants can present antigen to cloned human T cells. Nature 1984;312:639–641.
203. Hanafusa T, Pujol Borrell R, Chiovato L, Russell RC, Doniach D, Bottazzo GF. Aberrant expression of HLA-DR antigen on thyrocytes in Graves' disease: relevance for autoimmunity. Lancet 1983; 2:1111–1115.
204. Davies TF. Co-culture of human thyroid monolayer cells and autologous T cells: impact of HLA class II antigen expression. J Clin Endocrinol Metab 1985;61:418–422.
205. Hirose W, Lahat N, Platzer M, Schmitt S, Davies TF. Activation of MHC-restricted rat T cells by cloned syngeneic thyrocytes. J Immunol 1988;141:1098–1102.
206. Davies TF, Bermas B, Platzer M, Roman SH. T-cell sensitization to autologous thyroid cells and normal non-specific suppressor T-cell function in Graves' disease. Clin-Endocrinol (Oxford) 1985; 22:155–167.
207. Eguchi K, Otsubo T, Kawabe K, et al. The remarkable proliferation of helper T cell subset in response to autologous thyrocytes and intrathyroidal T cells from patients with Graves' disease. Isr J Med Sci 1987;70:403–410.
208. Neufeld DS, Platzer M, Davies TF. Reovirus induction of MHC class II antigen in rat thyroid cells. Endocrinology 1989;124:543–545.
209. Parkkonen P, Hyoty H, Koskinen L, Leinikki P. Mumps virus infects beta cells in human fetal islet cell cultures upregulating the expression of HLA class I molecules. Diabetologia 1992;35:63–69.
210. Tomer Y, Davies TF. Infection, Thyroid disease and autoimmunity. Endocr Rev 1993;14:107–120.
211. Lenschow DJ, Ho SC, Sattar H, et al. Differential effects of anti-B7-1 and anti-B7-2 monoclonal antibody treatment on the development of diabetes in the nonobese diabetic mouse. J Exp Med 1995; 181:1145–1155.
212. Lenschow DJ, Herold KC, Rhee L, et al. CD28/B7 regulation of Th1 and Th2 subsets in the development of autoimmune diabetes. Immunity 1996;5:285–293.
213. Abbas AK, Murphy KM, Sher A. Functional diversity of helper T lymphocytes. Nature 1996;383: 787–793.
214. Giordano C, Stassi G, De-Maria R, et al. Potential involvement of Fas and its ligand in the pathogenesis of Hashimoto's thyroiditis. Science 1997;275:960–963.
215. Tandon N, Metcalfe RA, Barnett D, Weetman AP. Expression of the costimulatory molecule B7/BB1 in autoimmune thyroid disease. Q J Med 1994;87:231–236.
216. Jackson DG, Capra JD. TAP1 alleles in insulin-dependent diabetes mellitus: a newly defined centromeric boundary of disease susceptibility. Proc Natl Acad Sci USA 1993;90:11,079–11,083.
217. Badenhoop K, Tonjes RR, Rau H, et al. Endogenous retroviral long terminal repears of the HLA-Dq regions are associated with susceptibility to insulin-dependent diabetes mellitus. Hum Immunol 1996; 50:103–110.
218. Vafiadis P, Bennett ST, Todd JA, et al. Insulin expression in human thymus is modulated by INS VNTR alleles at the IDDM2 locus. Nat Genet 1997;15:289–292.
219. Puglise A, Zeller M, Fernandez Jr. A, et al. The insulin gene is transcribed in the human thymus and transcription levels correlate with allelic variation at the INS VNTR-IDDM2 susceptibility locus for type 1 diabetes. Nat Genet 1997;15:293–297.

4

Experimental Models for Autoimmune Thyroid Disease
Recent Developments

Yi-chi M. Kong, PhD

CONTENTS

INTRODUCTION
GENETIC REGULATION OF SUSCEPTIBILITY AND RESISTANCE
THYROID AUTOANTIGENS AND PATHOGENIC PEPTIDES
PATHOGENIC MECHANISMS
REGULATORY MECHANISMS
RELEVANCE FOR HUMAN DISEASE
ACKNOWLEDGMENTS
REFERENCES

INTRODUCTION

Studies in autoimmune thyroid disease have entered a new and exciting era as a consequence of the rapid progress in recent years in cellular and molecular biology, together with knowledge gained in T-cell recognition, differentiation, and interaction with other cell types. The application of tools, such as transgenic technology and gene cloning and sequencing, shows promise in increasing our understanding of genetic control of susceptibility and autoreactivity to thyroid autoantigens. Since there have been a number of reviews on experimental models of autoimmune thyroid disease, both induced and spontaneous *(1–6)*, this chapter will concentrate on the past five years, primarily in the mouse and rat, where major developments have furthered our understanding. *See also* Chapter 9 for discussion of human autoimmune thyroid disease.

GENETIC REGULATION OF SUSCEPTIBILITY AND RESISTANCE

Major Histocompatibility Complex (MHC) Class II Genes

Although the linkage of autoimmune thyroiditis to the MHC is well known in experimental autoimmune thyroiditis (EAT) in the mouse and rat *(2)*, association of Hashimoto's thyroiditis (HT) or Graves' disease (GD) with human leukocyte antigen (*HLA*), the human MHC, is controversial. In addition to diversity contributed by ethic differences,

From: *Contemporary Endocrinology: Autoimmune Endocrinopathies*
Edited by: R. Volpe © Humana Press Inc., Totowa, NJ

Table 1
Transfer of Murine or Human Class II Genes Renders EAT Susceptibility to Resistant Mice

Expt.	Antigen	Transgene expression	mTg antibody, mean log$_2$ titer ± SE	0	>0–10	>10–20	>20–40	>40–80
1[a]	mTg	H2A^{k+}	10.4 ± 1.0	2	—	1	2	2
		H2A^{k-}	5.5 ± 2.5	1	1	—	—	—
		B10.M	6.8 ± 1.7	4	—	—	—	—
2[b]	mTg	HLA-DR3$^+$	13.2 ± 1.0	1	—	—	4	—
		HLA-DR3$^-$	9.0 ± 1.5	4	—	—	—	—
	hTg	HLA-DR3$^+$	20.0 ± 0.9	—	—	2	3	—
		HLA-DR3$^-$	20.2 ± 2.3	2	2	—	—	—

Column header for right side: *Thyroiditis, no. mice with % thyroid involvement*

[a]Resistant B10.M (*H2^f*) mice with or without murine transgene were immunized sc with 60 µg mTg in CFA on days 0 and 7, and assayed on day 28; adapted from Kong et al. *(7)*.

[b]Resistant B10.M (*H2^f*) mice with or without *HLA-DRB1*0301* (DR3) transgene expression were immunized with 40 µg mTg or 100 µg hTg and 20 µg LPS iv 3 h later on days 0 and 7, and assayed on day 28; adapted from Kong et al. *(8)*.

identification of *HLA* association with HT or GD in patient populations is further complicated by linkage disequilibrium between *DR* and *DQ* genes. To determine if transgenic technology could help decipher the role of *HLA* class II genes in HT susceptibility, we first tested it in murine EAT. Class II genes from a susceptible haplotype, *H2A^k*, were introduced into resistant *H2^f* mice, and the animals were immunized with mouse (m) thyroglobulin (Tg) *(7)*. As shown in Table 1 (Expt. 1), in the presence of the transgene, resistant mice became susceptible to EAT induction, displaying up to 80% thyroid inflammation. Although mTg-immunized resistant mice usually produce autoantibody, a nonpredictor of thyroid involvement, and autoantibody production in H2A^{k-} or the prototype B10.M mice was somewhat expected, the introduction of the transgene also increased mTg autoantibody titers.

HLA-DRB1*0301 (DR3) class II genes were then introduced into the same resistant strain, and the animals were immunized with either mTg or human (h) Tg. The DR3$^+$ B10.M mice showed up to 40% thyroid involvement (*8*; Table 1, Expt. 2) and autoantibody titers in mTg-immunized mice were higher in DR3$^+$ than in DR3$^-$ mice. No differences in titers were observed in hTg-immunized mice, because HTg contains additional foreign epitopes to which resistant B10.M mice readily respond. To focus on the role of DR3 molecules and eliminate the possible contribution of murine class II genes, the DR3 transgene was introduced into class II-negative Ab^0 mice, which have a mutant *H2Ab* (β-chain) gene and a nonfunctional *H2Ea* (α-chain) gene, and thus, do not express any class II molecules. Only DR3$^+$ mice showed thyroid inflammation of 20–80% *(8)*. Similar thyroid involvement was seen in hTg-immunized DR3$^+$Ab^0 mice. To verify that the DR3 molecules served as antigen presenters in vivo, thereby shaping the autoreactive T-cell receptor (TCR) repertoire for both mTg and hTg, we showed that anti-DR3 antibodies blocked the in vitro T-cell proliferative response of mTg- and hTg-primed cells to Tg. Thus, DR3 molecules present Tg both in vivo and in vitro as expected of murine class II molecules. These studies support the implication of HLA-DR3 association with HT, reported for some patient studies (cited in *8*). They show further that Tg may be more than just a diagnostic antigen and may indeed serve as a pathogen, as has been long observed in models of both EAT and spontaneous autoimmune thyroiditis (SAT) (*see* Tg and Conserved Peptides). It is thus possible that Tg may serve as an initiator pathogen in the human.

Table 2
HLA-DRB1 Polymorphism Is a Determinant in Susceptibility
to mTg-Induced EAT in Murine Class II-Negative H2Ab⁰ Mice[a]

Transgene expression	mTg antibody,[b] OD at 1:800	Thyroiditis,[b] no. mice with % thyroid involvement				
		0	>0–10	>10–20	>20–40	>40–80
DR3⁺ E⁺	0.95 ± 0.20	—	2	2	3	2
DR3⁻ E⁺	<0.2	6	1	—	—	—
DR2⁺ E⁺	0.29 ± 0.11	7	—	—	—	—
DR2⁻ E⁺	<0.2	5	1	—	—	—

[a]Adapted from Kong et al. *(8)*.
[b]H2Ab⁰ mice introduced with *HLA-DRB1*0301* (DR3) or *HLA-DRB1*1502* (DR2) class II transgene were immunized with 40 µg mTg and 20 µg LPS iv 3 h later on days 0 and 7, and assayed on day 28.

In other experiments, an *H2Ea* transgene was introduced to provide Eα chains, which would compete with DRα chains for the host's Eβ chains *(8)*. Table 2 shows that the resultant expression of H2E molecules had little effect on susceptibility; all DR3⁺ mice displayed thyroid infiltration after mTg immunization. Since H2E molecules were not involved in susceptibility to mTg-induced EAT, we were able to test *HLA-DRB1*1502* (DR2) transgenic, class II-negative mice that expressed the DR2β chain with the aid of the H2Eα chain, a homolog of DRα, provided by an *H2Ea* transgene *(8)*. Table 2 shows that the DR2 molecules were not permissive for mTg-induced EAT, in contrast to DR3 molecules; antibody titers were also negative in most mice when retested at a 1:100 dilution. Thus, *HLA-DRB1* polymorphism is a determinant of mTg-induced EAT.

It is clear that the use of individual *HLA* class II transgene permits the identification of susceptible vs resistant alleles. We have begun to test *HLA-DQ* genes in transgenic mice. *HLA-DQB1*0601* (DQ6b) transgene in resistant B10.M mice did not afford susceptibility to mTg-induced EAT *(7)*. Since DR3 molecules can present both hTg and mTg, the thyroiditogenic epitopes are most likely shared or even conserved. Also, since DR2 molecules are not permissive for mTg immunization, it would have been of great interest to determine if hTg could induce EAT in DR2 transgenic mice. However, the presence of the *Ea^k* transgene with attendant H2E (Eα^k Eβ^b) expression posed a problem for such studies, because H2E molecules in normal *H2^k* strains have been shown to present hTg *(9)* and a 17-mer Tg epitope *(10)*. Indeed, recent preliminary data showed that the expression of Eα^k Eβ^b molecules in otherwise class II-negative Ab⁰ mice resulted in susceptibility to EAT induced with hTg *(11)*. In contrast, mTg was not capable of inducing EAT in such mice. Since the *Ea* gene, homologous to the *DRa* gene, is conserved in the mouse, susceptibility is encoded by the *Eb* gene of the *b* haplotype. Thus, for the first time, susceptibility to hTg induction can be distinguished from mTg, paving the way for identifying hTg-unique epitopes.

We recently examined the immunogenicity of 12-mer Tg epitopes derived from the primary hormonogenic sites at amino acid positions 5, 2553, and 2567, which are 100% identical between hTg and mTg *(12,13)*. The most antigenic epitope is T4(2553) *(14,15)*, but its antigenicity did not depend on the presence of the four iodine residues and it was not immunodominant *(15; see* Tg and Conserved Peptides). In the event that the lack of immunodominance was the result of the use of one particular susceptible *k* haplotype, we also compared the peptides in another susceptible *s* haplotype, including their MHC-

Table 3
MHC Influence on EAT Susceptibility
to T0- or T4-containing Peptides of Tg After Vigorous Immunization[a]

	$H2^k$		$H2^s$	
	CBA	C57BR	A.SW	SJL
	thyroiditis	thyroiditis	thyroiditis	thyroiditis
Antigen[b]	incidence, %	incidence, %	incidence, %	incidence, %
mTg	100[c]	75[d]	80[d]	100[c]
hT0(5)	71[e]	40[e]	0	17[e]
hT4(5)	43[e]	40[e]	0	0
hT0(2553)	0	20[e]	0	17[e]
hT4(2553)	33[d]	0	0	0

[a]Adapted from Wan et al. (16).
[b]Mice were immunized with 50 mg mTg or peptide + CFA on days 0 (tail base) and 7 (hindfootpads) and were examined on day 28.
[c]Thyroid involvement >40–80%.
[d]Thyroid involvement >20-40%.
[e]Thyroid involvement >10-20%.

identical strains, C57BR and SJL, respectively, which have 50% genomic deletion of TCR Vβ genes (16). Table 3 shows that whereas MTg induced EAT with substantial thyroid inflammation in all four strains, only the *k* strains were susceptible to peptide-induced EAT. Even after relatively vigorous immunization, only mild thyroid involvement of 10–20% was observed. As discussed previously (15) and seen in Table 3, antigenicity did not depend on iodine residues on the thyroxine (T4). Not included here is peptide T4(2567), which is devoid of thyroiditogenicity in either *k* or *s* strains (16).

The importance of MHC class II haplotype in susceptibility to SAT was recently shown in the nonobese diabetic (NOD) mouse in which the incidence of SAT moderately increased in NOD.H2^k mice with the wild-type class II genes $H2A^{g7}$ replaced by breeding (17). Similarly, NOD.H2^{h4} mice, expressing the *k* allele at the *IA* region, also showed increased incidence and accelerated SAT following 8 wk of dietary iodine treatment (18). As we have indicated earlier (2) and reported by Damotte et al. (17), the NOD mouse is highly susceptible to EAT induction, a trait evidently influenced by background genes (*see* Other Genetic or Environmental Influences).

To summarize, MHC class II genes continue to be the primary determinant in EAT susceptibility, a role extendible to humans. The secondary role played by iodine residues in Tg immunogenicity will enable us to determine the involvement of any particular *HLA* transgene without undue concern for the variations in the extent of iodination of Tg molecules in different Tg preparations. However, it should be noted that, in polygenic humans, the multiple class II genes and interactions will ultimately influence susceptibility. We therefore plan to study EAT susceptibility in *DR/DR* and *DR/DQ* double transgenic mice.

MHC Class I Genes

One major advance in T-cell immunobiology is the gradual understanding of the important role MHC class II and class I genes play in shaping the TCR repertoire of CD4$^+$ and CD8$^+$ T cells, respectively, during T-cell development (19). The impact of clonal selection and deletion on self-tolerance and autoreactive T cells is obvious. In murine

Table 4
Protective Effect of Murine Class II Ea^k Transgene on EAT Susceptibility in E⁻ B10.S Mice[a]

Transgene expression	mTg antibody,[b] mean log₂ titer ± SE	Thyroiditis,[b] no. mice with % thyroid involvement			
		0	>0–10	>10–20	>20–40
+	1.6 ± 0.4	3	3	4	—[c]
−	3.5 ± 0.6	—	—	2	2[c]

[a]Adapted from Kong et al. (7).
[b]H2E⁺ mice and their E⁻ sibs were immunized iv with 40 µg mTg and LPS on days 0 and 7, and assayed on day 28.
[c]$p < 0.025$.

EAT, CD8⁺ cells are not needed to initiate autoimmunity at the time of active immunization with mTg *(20)* or adoptive transfer of mTg-activated cells *(21)* as shown by T-cell depletion studies and by the susceptibility of CD8-deficient (β2m −/−) mice *(22)*. However, CD8⁺ T cells are active participants in thyroid pathogenesis *(20,21)*, displaying cytotoxicity in vitro for thyroid epithelial cells *(23,24)*. Although the precise link has not been studied, the *H2K* region exerts some effect on reducing autoantibody level and the incidence or severity of thyroiditis *(3)*, and the *H2D*-end has even stronger moderating influence, depending on the *H2A/D* combination *(25)*. For example, the high incidence and severity in $A^k D^k$ mice were reduced by substituting D^k with the D^b gene. Interestingly, a recent model of SAT in NOD.H2^h4 mice harboring the $A^k D^b$ combination showed no diabetes, but increased mTg autoantibody levels and incidence of thyroiditis, compared with NOD mice, particularly after 8 wk of dietary iodine treatment *(18)*. Whether the D^b gene has a modifying influence on SAT development in this model is unknown, since this complex strain also has background genes contributing to autoimmunity.

Protective Influence of MHC Molecules

In polygenic humans, codominance of MHC class II and class I genes provides ample opportunity for mutual influences, directly or indirectly, leading to diverse immune responses. EAT susceptibility is dominant as seen by early studies in F₁ mice *(3)* and by *H2 (7)* or *HLA (8)* class II gene transfer of susceptibility traits into resistant mice (*see* Major Histocompatibility Complex [MHC] Class II Genes). However, this susceptibility trait can be modified by the presence of class II transgene from a different locus. For example, when *H2Ea^k* transgene was introduced into normally E⁻-susceptible B10.S mice, resulting in the expression of stable $Eα^k Eβ^s$ molecules, the incidence and severity of thyroiditis were significantly reduced, similar to several autoimmune disease models *(7;* Table 4). In early studies mentioned above on *H2D*-end downregulation of autoimmune responses *(25)*, we noted that recombinant strains with different *H2A/E* combinations showed a range of incidence, some highly reduced. In view of the transgenic experiments, these differences could partly be explained by the extent of interplay between these MHC class II genes. Furthermore, these differences were probably not owing to clonal deletion of particular Vβ⁺ T cells, since the TCR repertoire for EAT susceptibility is highly flexible (*see* Flexibility of Thyroiditogenic TCR Repertoire). Further study will be required to determine if the combined effects of *A/E* genes are applicable to *DQ/DR* genes. The possible consequences of coexisting *DQ/DR* genes in human autoimmune diseases have gained investigative attention in recent years *(26)*.

Table 5
Moderating Influence of Heterozygosity
on EAT Development in CBA-Vβ8.2 Transgenic Mice[a]

H2 type	Transgene expression	mTg antibody,[b] mean log$_2$ titer ± SE	Thyroiditis,[b] no. mice with % thyroid involvement		
			0–20	>20–40	>40–80
k/q	+	11.6 ± 2.0	4	1	—[c]
k/q	−	21.2 ± 1.6	—	2	3[c]
k/k	+	10.8 ± 0.8	2	5	1
k/k	−	14.8 ± 0.8	2	3	—

[a]Adapted from Lomo et al. *(27)*.
[b]CBA-Vβ8.2 mice harboring the irrelevant ovalbumin-specific transgene on either k/k or k/q background were immunized with 40 μg mTg and 20 μg LPS iv 3 h later on days 0 and 7, and killed on day 28.
[c]$p < 0.02$.

Downregulation of the autoimmune response could also be seen in heterozygous mice, a normal situation in the human. We introduced an irrelevant antiovalbumin transgene into susceptible CBA mice on either a *k/k* or *k/q* background with the expressed purpose of skewing the TCR repertoire. The mice expressed about 76 and 90% of this Vβ8.2 transgene, respectively, in the CD4⁺ and CD8⁺ T-cell subset *(27)*. The data in Table 5 show that only in *k/q* mice were the incidence and severity of thyroiditis significantly reduced. Although the reduction in mTg autoantibody titers was seen in transgenic mice of both strains, autoantibody levels in EAT do not correlate with the extent of thyroid inflammation, and are usually present in both susceptible and resistant strains. Whether the downregulation on thyroid inflammation is related specifically to the *q* haplotype, which is intermediate in EAT susceptibility *(7)*, is unknown. Such heterozygous effects may be beneficial in diminishing the host's capacity to recognize multiple thyroiditogenic epitopes while retaining responses to foreign invaders.

Flexibility of Thyroiditogenic (TCR) Repertoire

As described above, it is clear that as long as the appropriate MHC class II genes encoding susceptibility are present, skewing the TCR repertoire has minimal effects on thyroid infiltration. In addition, we have tested mice with different genomic TCR Vβ gene deletions. Table 3 has shown in the *k* haplotype that C57BR mice with about 50% TCR Vβ gene deletion responded to EAT induction as CBA mice with the usual TCR Vβ gene repertoire. However, these strains are not congenic. To study further the plasticity of the TCR repertoire, we produced congenic B10.K (Vβ^b) mice with 50% (Vβ^a) or 70% (Vβ^c) genomic deletion, and found no diminution in thyroid involvement after mTg immunization *(28)*. Furthermore, CD8-deficient (β2m −/−) mice also responded to EAT induction with thyroid involvement of 35–40%, comparable to wild-type B10.K mice *(22)*. One possibility for the marked response in antiovalbumin-transgenic (Table 5) and CD8-deficient (Table 6) mice could stem from the use of intact mTg molecule containing sufficient epitopes to which different remaining T cells could respond. mTg does not seem to be endowed with any immunodominant epitopes, and both conserved and unique epitopes contribute to its total thyroiditogenicity *(15; see* Tg and Conserved Peptides).

Table 6
Flexibility of Thyroiditogenic T-Cell Repertoire Reflected
in Adoptive Transfer of EAT by mTg- or Peptide-Activated Cells
in β2m –/– (CD8-Deficient), B10.K-Vβ^c (70% TCR-Depleted), or B10.K Mice[a]

Mouse strain	In vitro activator	No. cells, ($\times 10^{-7}$), transferred	Thyroiditis incidence,[b] % positive
β2m –/–	mTg	2.7	100
(k/k)	T4(5)	4.0	100
	T4(2553)	4.0	50
B10.K-Vβ^c	mTg	2.0	100
	T4(5)	3.4	100
	T4(2553)	3.8	100
B10.K	mTg	2.0	100
	T4(5)	4.0	100
	T0(2553)	4.0	75
	T4(2553)	4.0	100

[a]Adapted from Lomo et al. (22).
[b]Recipient mice received syngeneic, mTg-primed spleen cells activated in vitro for 3 d with 20 μg/mL mTg, 20 μg/mL T4(5), 10 μg/mL T0(2553) or 5 μg/mL T4(2553). Thyroids were removed on day 14 for histologic evaluation.

To reduce the number of epitopes involved, we employed the 12-mer conserved peptides from the primary hormonogenic sites to activate mTg-primed cells to determine if there were T cells remaining to recognize these small peptides (22). Table 6 shows that recipients of activated cells developed thyroiditis, regardless of whether the hosts were CD8-deficient (β2m–/–) or 70% TCR Vβ gene-deficient (Vβ^c), or whether the transferred cells were T4(5)- or T4(2553)-activated. These different approaches confirm the highly flexible nature of the thyroiditogenic TCR repertoire.

Other Genetic or Environmental Influences

The mouse and rat models of SAT in recent use were derived from spontaneous diabetic strains. These strains with their autoimmune endocrinopathies are particularly prone to environmental influences, probably because non-MHC background genes contribute to susceptibility, similar to the obese strain (OS) chicken (5,29). These unidentified factors, which may include diet and animal husbandry, are illustrated by the greatly varied incidence of thyroiditis from NOD colony to colony (2,17), whereas in induced EAT, only the constant use of mouse breeder chow has been reported to reduce the incidence and severity of EAT (30). By substituting the MHC class II genes in NOD.H2^{h4} (18) and NOD.H2^k strains (17) or developing lymphocytic thyroiditis-prone sublines in BB/Wor (BioBreeding/Worcester) rat (31), susceptibility to SAT and diabetes can be segregated and increased incidence of thyroiditis observed. The continued development of SAT without substituting the MHC genes in the rat or with substituting the MHC genes in the mouse clearly indicates the contribution of non-MHC genes, similar to wild-type diabetes. As noted above, the *IA^k* genes in NOD.H2^{h4} and NOD.H2^k mice could result in enhancement of SAT or inhibition of diabetes. In mTg-induced EAT, the introduction of the *IA^k* transgene into *H2^q* mice intermediate in susceptibility enhanced thyroiditis severity, emphasizing the role of class II genes (7). Clearly, in addition to the *IA^k* class II genes, the non-MHC genes play a role in exacerbating SAT development.

In the NOD.H2^k strain, mTg-induced lesions were reportedly slow to resolve, compared with CBA mice *(17)*, an indication of background gene influence observed by these workers. However, in our earlier study *(32)*, CBA mice showed severe lesions for at least 18 mo. Reasons for the discrepancy are unknown, and may be related to the protocol of immunization and the adjuvant used.

Non-MHC genes may also contribute to the influence of dietary iodine as seen in the OS chicken *(29)*. After prolonged treatment, both NOD.H2^{h4} mice *(18)* and BB/Wor rat subline *(31)* displayed accelerated incidence of SAT. Recently, the development of SAT in MRL-lpr/lpr mice used as a lupus model has been described *(33)*. Interestingly, this highly abnormal mouse strain, which also expresses H2A^k, develops a high incidence of thyroiditis with age and symptoms of hypothyroidism, including increased thyroid-stimulating hormone (TSH) and decreased T4 level, as well as autoantibodies to Tg and thyroid peroxidase (TPO). Confirmation of these studies and the extent of contribution by background genes associated with the lupus abnormality will be needed to determine how closely this strain reflects a particular population of HT patients. A similar question may also be posed for the OS chicken with its highly abnormal genetic traits, including a hyperactive target organ and abnormal iodine metabolism *(29)*.

THYROID AUTOANTIGENS AND PATHOGENIC PEPTIDES

Tg and Conserved Peptides

Tg has been a prototype autoantigen for >30 yr, and has paved the way for our understanding of MHC linkage with autoimmune disease in both animal and human models. Its potential as an initiator pathogen has regained recognition owing to recent studies from two directions. First, similar to the OS chicken, SAT models derived from the NOD mouse *(17,18)*, and the BB/Wor rat *(34)* produce antibodies and autoreactive T cells to Tg. In the NOD.H2^k mouse, anti-Tg levels can be correlated with thyroiditis *(17)*. Manipulation followed by adoptive transfer of certain T-cell subset into T-cell-depleted mice results in the development of Tg-reactive T cell lines and clones, and thyroiditis *(35)*. Regarding anti-TPO production, it is still unclear in the OS chicken because of anti-Tg in the sera in earlier assays. No anti-TPO has been observed even with prolonged iodine administration to accelerate murine SAT *(18)*. Second, HLA-DR3 transgenic mice respond to both mTg and hTg immunization, correlating with some clinical patient studies on *HLA* association with HT *(8)*.

What shared epitopes between hTg and mTg are presented by HLA-DR3 are yet undetermined. It is known, however, that shared epitopes are important contributors to thyroiditogenicity in mTg-induced EAT and certainly in heterologous Tg-induced EAT in susceptible strains, and that they can expand sufficient T cells to mediate adoptive transfer and cytotoxicity for thyroid monolayers *(3)*. The observations of two identical TCR CDR3 motifs in the Vβ13$^+$ T-cell subset of the thyroidal infiltrate after either hTg *(36)* or mTg *(37)* induction further suggest the involvement of shared epitopes. In addition, although cross-stimulation and cross-tolerance studies with mTg, hTg, and porcine Tg have confirmed the presence of mTg-unique epitopes *(3)*, no immunodominant epitopes have emerged from studies in several laboratories *(38)*. Clearly, shared/conserved and mTg-unique epitopes contribute to the total thyroiditogenicity of mTg. The identification of mTg-unique epitopes is now possible with the completed sequencing of mTg, which can be compared with complete sequences of hTg and bovine Tg *(13)*.

Moreover, our recent data demonstrating the induction of EAT with hTg, but not mTg, in *H2Ea* transgenic mice expressing EαEβ^b molecules open the door to the study of hTg-unique epitopes (*11; see* Major Histocompatibility Complex [MHC] Class II Genes). Thus, the study of Tg epitopes has entered a new era.

Since Tg is an inducing antigen for both SAT and EAT models, it is not too surprising that excessive and prolonged intake of dietary iodine, related to enhancement of Tg immunogenicity, could lead to increased incidence or severity of thyroiditis *(14,18, 31,39)*. However, in thyroiditis-prone BB/Wor rat, Tg-reactive T cells recognize Tg regardless of iodine content *(40)*. Most iodine intake in humans is normally incorporated into the four primary hormonogenic sites on Tg *(41)*. As discussed recently *(3,42)*, retrospective epidemiological studies of necropsy materials from whites, black Americans, and Japanese in three continents have demonstrated that distinct genetic and ethnic differences are primary determinants of susceptibility and are little influenced by environmental factors. In particular, whites with high iodine intake in the US showed comparable incidence/severity as those with low intake in the UK, and high iodine intake in coastal regions of Japan did not result in greater incidence/severity than the low intake in mountainous regions *(43,44)*. In studies using conserved, synthetic peptides with or without tyrosine or with uniodinated tyrosine, thyroiditogenicity has been demonstrated in EAT *(6,38)*.

Since none of the conserved synthetic peptides is immunodominant and the T cells recognizing them cannot be expanded by intact Tg, the importance of iodination is best tested by using peptides to expand either mTg- or peptide-primed T cells, and the most iodinated peptides are from the primary hormonogenic sites. Their thyroiditogenicity can then be determined by adoptive transfer of the activated T cells into normal recipient mice. One such 12-mer peptide from the site at position 2553, T4(2553), was first determined not to be thyroiditogenic, unless the tyrosine residue had been substituted with T4 *(14)*. However, on testing in parallel, we found also thyroiditogenic the noniodinated thyronine- (T0) substituted peptide, T0(2553) *(15)*. We also tested the other two conserved 12-mer peptides at hormonogenic sites 5 and 2567 with either T0 or T4 substitution of the tyrosine residue. T0(2567) and T4(2567) lack immunogenicity, and T0(5) and T4(5) are very weakly immunogenic in the same *H2^k* strain. As nonimmunodominant contributor after active immunization, T0(5), T4(5), and particularly T0(2553) and T4(2553), can expand mTg-primed T cells to transfer thyroiditis, provided large numbers of in vitro-expanded T cells have been used (Table 6) *(15,16,22)*. In contrast, all three pairs of peptides display little immunogenicity in another susceptible *s* haplotype (Table 3) *(16)*. We conclude from these findings that: (1) iodination plays a secondary role to the primary and intrinsic role of amino acid composition in immunogenicity for a given epitope, and (2) the most important determinant in immunogenicity for any Tg epitope rests with the appropriate class II gene in antigen presentation and selection of the T-cell repertoire.

Reciprocal priming and stimulation experiments between T0(2553) and T4(2553), the most antigenic peptide from the three hormonogenic sites, has suggested that the presence of iodine residues increases binding affinity in vitro *(15)*. Given the observed difference in in vitro proliferative response, it is not surprising that hybridoma can be selected to respond only to T4, but not T0-containing peptide, which was not used for priming *(45)*. Recently, we determined their capacity to generate cytotoxic T cells as well as serve as target antigens *(46)*. Lymph node cells from mTg-immunized mice cultured with mTg or hTg developed cytotoxicity for T4(2553)-, T0(2553)-, or T4(5)-labeled, but

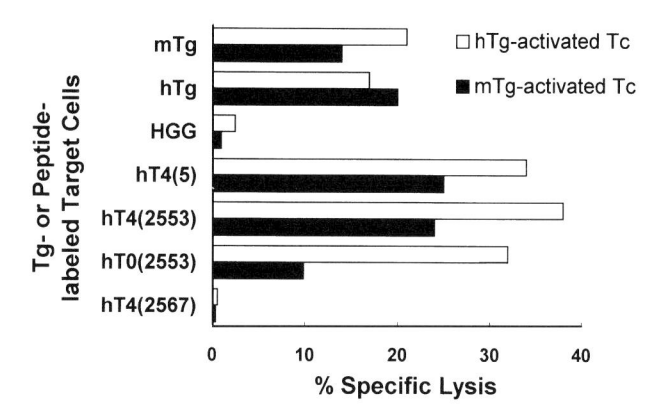

Fig. 1. Specific hormonogenic site peptides as target epitopes for Tg-generated Tc. Effector lymph node cells from CBA mice immunized with 100 µg mTg in CFA were cultured in vitro for 3 d with 40 µg/mL mTg (black bar) or hTg (white bar) plus equal numbers of irradiated normal spleen cells. 10^4/Well BW5147 lymphoma cells loaded with peptide, T4(5), T4(2553), T0(2553), or T4(2567), at 20 µg/mL, or mTg, hTg, or hGG at 40 µg/mL served as target cells; effector:target ratio = 50:1; reproduced from Wan et al. *(46)*.

Table 7
Cytotoxicity Generated by T0- or T4-Containing Peptide Derivative
from Tg Hormonogenic Site at Amino Acid Position 2553[a]

In vitro activator	Stimulation index	% Specific lysis of peptide-labeled target cells[b]			
		T0(2553)	T4(2553)	T0(2567)	T4(2567)
T0(2553)	1.2	17	44	0	4
T4(2553)	12.7	17	55	9	12

[a]Adapted from Wan et al. *(46)*.
[b]See Fig. 1 legend for protocol.

not T4(2567)-labeled target cells, indicating that the antigenic peptides can serve as target antigen (Fig. 1). T0(2553) and T4(2553) can also generate cytotoxic T cells with reciprocal specificity for T0(2553)- and T4(2553)-labeled target cells (Table 7). T4(2553) is highly reactive, stimulating mTg-primed cells to mediate strong cytotoxicity at a dose high for this peptide, at times with some bystander cytotoxicity (although this is unusual) for T4(2567)-labeled target cells. T4(2553) is also a reactive target for T0(2553)-generated effector cells. Thus, this peptide, a weak and nonimmunodominant inducer of EAT, can show high reactivity in vitro not seen with other T4-containing peptides.

To summarize, T4(5) and T4(2553), but not T4(2567), from the primary hormonogenic sites, now known to be 100% identical between hTg and mTg as well as rat Tg *(12,13)*, are thyroiditogenic by adoptive transfer and cytotoxicity assays in *H2^k* mice *(15,46)*, with iodine at the four sites playing only a secondary role, if any. The 12-mer peptide from the fourth primary hormonogenic site 2746 at the C-terminus is quite heterogeneous among mammalian species and cannot be considered a *bona fide* self-peptide. This should be kept in mind while studying its immunogenicity. Still to be determined are the shared epitopes between hTg and mTg presented by DR3 molecules and the mTg- and hTg-unique epitopes using *H2* and *HLA* transgenic mice.

Thyroid Peroxidase and Thyroid-Stimulating Hormone Receptor (TSHR)

Interests in using TPO and TSHR as thyroid autoantigens in animal models are natural with the hope of perturbing thyroid function to simulate hypothyroidism and/or hyperthyroidism. Porcine (p) TPO has been reported to induce thyroiditis in $H2^b$ mice, a haplotype resistant to EAT induction by Tg *(47)*. To our knowledge, this finding has not been confirmed. Purified hTPO from thyroids is often contaminated with hTg, and even with recombinant technology, animal studies require large amounts of purified hTPO and mTPO, both of which are not yet available. Mice are not very sensitive to perturbation of thyroid function and generally do not exhibit consistent symptoms of hypothyroidism after EAT induction. There is yet no reliable assay for mTSH, and their T4 levels often fluctuate and show large biologic variations even within inbred strains *(48)*. Moreover, despite prolonged oral treatment with iodine resulting in accelerated SAT in autoimmune-prone NOD.H2^{h4} mice, no TPO antibodies have been detected *(18)*. Thus, establishing a murine model with TPO may be difficult.

The severe combined immunodeficient mouse strain has served primarily as an in vivo test tube to study the interactions of GD cells and tissues *(49,50)*. Thus, there have been many attempts to produce GD models with various preparations of hTSHR in different strains, but with limited success, as reviewed recently *(51)*. Repeated immunizations with hTSHR or peptides resulted in antibody production, transient variations in T3 levels, and thyroiditis in $H2^q$ and $H2^s$, but not $H2^d$ mice *(52)*. Others observed thyroiditis, which can be transferred in BALB/c ($H2^d$) and NOD mice after the injection of recombinant (r) hTSHR extracellular domain (ECD) produced in bacteria as a fusion protein *(53)*. The use of rTSHR-ECD from insect cells evoked the production of antibodies blocking TSH binding, but not thyroiditis in several strains, with BALB/c mice displaying increased T4 levels *(51,54)*. Recently, GD-like features were observed in ~20% of AKR ($H2^k$) mice repeatedly immunized with an $H2A^k$-expressing fibroblast line transfected with hTSHR *(55)*. In a follow-up study, the importance of the MHC class II molecules over background genes on immunizing transfected cells was affirmed, particularly for the induction of stimulating TSHR antibodies *(56)*. The increase in T4 levels was correlated with the stimulating antibodies, but the incidence remained ~20%. Stimulating antibodies were not detected unless the TSH binding inhibitory antibodies were also present. It would be of interest to determine if mTSHR-transfected cells would produce similar symptoms and incidence, and if the T- and B-cell epitopes are shared or distinct between hTSHR and mTSHR.

Very recently, two different methods produced thyroiditis rather than GD-like symptoms in BALB/c mice. One was by repeated immunizations with a truncated rTSHR-ECD fragment 43-282 deleted of immunodominant B-cell epitopes or with a longer, related fragment 43-316; the same pattern of antibody profile was observed in both groups, but some mice immunized only with fragment 43-282 also exhibited lymphocytic infiltration *(57)*. The antibody profiles were distinct from those produced after immunization with the whole ECD. Whether the thyroiditogenic T-cell epitopes will turn out to be conserved is unknown. The recent production of rmTSHR-ECD from insect cells *(58)* should greatly enhance studies of the T-cell epitopes involved in pathogenesis. The second method was to immunize with plasmid DNA harboring hTSHR cDNA. Both TSH binding and blocking antibodies as well as thyroid inflammation were detected, but T4 levels remained unchanged *(59)*. These interesting studies show additional, promising approaches to provide further insights into the antigenicity of hTSHR in mice. How closely these features simulate GD in the human remains to be determined.

PATHOGENIC MECHANISMS

TCR Gene Usage

Studies with genomic deletions of 50–70% of TCR Vβ genes have revealed the flexibility of the T-cell repertoire (*see* Flexibility of Thyroiditogenic TCR Repertoire). Thus, the absence of specific TCR Vβ$^+$ T cells did not diminish the incidence or severity of EAT for a given susceptible haplotype *(28)*, nor did severely skewing the T-cell repertoire with an irrelevant transgene restrict thyroid involvement *(27)*. Similarly, the presence of a particular Vβ phenotype in the thyroid does not necessarily signify antigen-specific usage. For example, Vβ8$^+$ T cells are abundant in CBA mice, representing up to 30% of total T cells. They are reputed to mediate many autoimmune diseases and are frequently found in the thyroidal infiltrate. However, we did not find any significant involvement of Vβ8$^+$ T cells in EAT, even when the intact mTg molecule was used for induction *(60)*. Their presence in the thyroid, as confirmed by others *(61)*, could stem from the recruitment of bystander T cells.

On the other hand, we have observed Vβ13$^+$ T cells undergoing clonal expansion within the thyroid after either active immunization with mTg *(62)* or adoptive transfer of mTg-primed T cells following in vitro activation with mTg *(37)* or staphylococcal enterotoxin A (Qiang Wan et al., unpublished data). As mentioned in Tg and Conserved Peptides, although their antigenic specificity has not been determined, two CDR3 motifs identical to those found after hTg immunization *(36)* were among the clonally expanded Vβ13$^+$ T-cell subset in the thyroid, suggesting shared epitope specificity. This subset was not prominent in another report where thyroids were pooled *(61)* rather than examined individually. Given the plasticity of the TCR repertoire, it is perhaps not surprising to find such discrepancies. Even using 12-mer peptides, adoptive transfer is readily shown in Vβ^c mice missing ~70% TCR Vβ genes (Table 6). In SJL mice with ~50% genomic deletion, T cells responding to a 9-mer peptide were found to contain at least three different Vβ T-cell subset *(63)*. Unless more Tg epitopes are identified, the use of Vα genes would be even more difficult to pinpoint. Taken together, the results from animal experiments emphasize the flexibility of the TCR repertoire despite development under a homozygous MHC umbrella, in contrast to polygenic humans, and even after selection by 9- to 12-mer peptides in the context of the same MHC.

Effector T-Cell Mechanisms

Both CD4$^+$ and CD8$^+$ T-cell subsets are found in the thyroidal infiltrate after active immunization and adoptive transfer, with CD4$^+$ cells showing an early influx and predominance and CD8$^+$ T-cells subsequently establishing its presence, as reviewed elsewhere *(3,6)*. Sequential analysis of the kinetics of infiltration by *in situ* immunohistochemistry reveals cyclic variations in percentage of CD8$^+$ T cells, but the ratio of CD4:CD8 remains between 2.4 and 3.0 for up to 6 wk *(64)*. By day 70, the ratio is about 2 in a total of thyroidal T cells of about 30%, with macrophages at 30–35%, and B cells at <2–6% *(20,65)*. Chronic thyroid inflammation shows little change up to 18 mo after EAT induction in CBA mice *(32)*.

After adoptive transfer of activated T cells, which contain a high number of CD4+ cells from the brief 3-d culture period, the initial influx of total thyroidal T cells could reach 56% *(65)*. CD8+ cells then establish themselves, reaching a CD4:CD8 ratio of about 1.7, with some cyclic variations in CD8 percentage as seen after active immunization. In contrast, a reverse CD4:CD8 ratio determined by flow cytometry of pooled thyroid suspension at a later interval after transfer was reported *(66)*. These workers also reported the same reverse ratio in their transfer granulomatous model derived by including MAb to interleukin (IL) 2 receptor or interferon (IFN) γ during in vitro activation *(67,68)*. The differences observed could be owing to MAbs with different affinities being used and *in situ* analysis vs pooled suspension at a later time-point. Despite such discrepancies, any shift in ratio is still best examined within the target organ rather than using peripheral blood leukocytes.

A T-cell-mediated disease is likely to evoke a number of mechanisms resulting in damage, including the production of proinflammatory cytokines not unlike other autoimmune diseases. These mechanisms are not mutually exclusive, and compensatory mechanisms exist, replacing a particular cytokine with another. In EAT, cytotoxic T cells described in Tg and Conserved Peptides have been demonstrated among mTg- or peptide-activated T cells (Fig. 1; Table 7). *In situ*, these CD8+ T cells are likely recruited, as the macrophages, by CD4+ T cells and their cytokines. That cytotoxic T cells are not required for thyroid damage is seen when CD8-deficient (β2m–/–) mice were used (Table 6) *(22)*. Although we do not know if these CD4+ T cells are also cytolytic, the cytokines they produce are sufficient to mediate severe thyroiditis. Indeed, MAb immunotherapy has previously shown that each subset in the thyroid is independent, remaining after the other has been depleted, whether thyroiditis has been induced by active immunization *(20)* or adoptive transfer *(21)*. Such effector function of CD8+ T cells is in contrast to another report *(66)*. The presence of macrophages, however, is dependent on both T-cell subsets, disappearing if both subsets have been depleted by combined CD4 and CD8 MAb therapy (*see* Effects of Immunotherapy).

Regarding proinflammatory cytokines, both CD4+ and CD8+ T-cell clones propagated from the T-cell depletion model produce IFN-γ and tumor necrosis factor (TNF), in addition to IL-2 *(35,69)*. Thyroid pathology and a cytotoxic T-cell phenotype were diminished in porcine Tg-induced EAT by anti-IFN-γ treatment *(70)*. Two other proinflammatory cytokines important for Th-1 phenotype activation are IL-1 and IL-12. IL-1 can serve as an adjuvant for EAT induction with mTg, similar to lipopolysaccharide (LPS), and given at a critical time, IL-1 can interfere with mTg activation of CD4+ suppressor T cells (Ts) *(71*; *see* Induction of Resistance with Tg and TSH). Recently, we have obtained preliminary data to show that IL-12 also prevents tolerance induction with mTg *(72)*. Thus, more than one cytokine can participate in EAT pathogenesis, and their particular role is likely to depend on the stage of EAT development.

Effects of Immunotherapy

The long- and short-term effects of anti-CD4 and anti-CD8 MAb therapy have been reviewed recently *(3,6)*. Briefly, using highly efficient, synergistic pairs of CD4 and/or CD8 MAbs to deplete the subsets, we show that anti-CD4 is efficacious in inhibiting EAT induction at the initiation stages after mTg immunization, but has no effect on the CD8 subset in the thyroid when given later during EAT development *(20)*. Anti-CD8 has neither a preventative nor an enhancing effect on induction, but reduces infiltration when given later by eliminating CD8⁺ T cells and leaving the CD4 subset *in situ*. Their notable independence in the thyroid necessitates the depletion of both by combined therapy. Interestingly, a regimen of only two anti-CD4 and anti-CD8 injections, 4 d apart, results in complete clearance of all infiltrating cells, including macrophages, suggesting that the role of macrophages is dependent on T-cell presence *(20)*. The clearance is long-lasting, despite the continued presence of autoantibodies and T-cell recovery from the thymus. After a second immunization, thyroid pathology resembles a first immunization *(73)*. Although immunotherapy is not required to treat HT normally, the efficiency in treating autoimmune thyroiditis could serve as an example for other autoimmune diseases. On the other hand, the use of nondepleting anti-CD4 and anti-CD8 was ineffective in ameliorating thyroiditis severity at advanced stages. Evidently, it is necessary to eliminate memory T cells with thyroiditogenic specificity.

Treatment with anti-CD40L MAb to block the help of costimulatory molecules brought about by the interactions between CD40L on activated CD4⁺ T cells with CD40 molecules on antigen-presenting cells and B cells reduced thyroid infiltration, as reflected by diminished IFN-γ release in vitro *(74)*. It is more difficult to block the effects of costimulatory molecules, cytokines, and adhesion molecules, all of which continuously evolve during development. Thus, repeated doses of anti-CD40L MAb were applied. Other studies using multiple injections of anti-IFN-γ in mice *(70)*, and anti-intercellular adhesion molecule-1 (ICAM-1) and antilymphocyte function-associated antigen-1 (LFA-1) in rats *(75)* also showed diminished thyroiditis. Treating with the immunosupressive agent, FK 506, reduced ICAM-1 expression and thyroid pathology in rats thymectomized and irradiated to induce thyroiditis *(76)*. On the other hand, anti-ICAM-1 administration had no effect on murine transfer EAT, whereas anti-α4 (VCAM) integrin lowered thyroid inflammation *(77)*. Treatment with multiple rhIL-10 doses, considered a cytokine that could inhibit proinflammatory cytokine function, during mTg immunization moderated thyroid infiltration in association with apoptotic T-cell death and reduced cytotoxicity without lowering antibody titers *(78)*. The need for repeated doses obviously makes such treatments unsuitable for chronic human conditions.

REGULATORY MECHANISMS

Induction of Resistance with Tg and TSH

Several protocols have been used to induce tolerance to EAT induction, as reviewed in some detail recently *(3,6)*. The three protocols we have used all share the common characteristics of increasing circulatory Tg levels for ≥2–3 d and activating an antigen-specific subset of CD4⁺ Ts, i.e., cells with suppressor function for other autoreactive T cells. These protocols are:

1. Two 100-μg doses of deaggregated (d) mTg *(48,71)*.
2. 20 μg LPS 24 h before two subtolerogenic, 20-μg doses of dMTg *(79)*.
3. TSH infusion for 3–4 d *(48,79)*.

After challenge, the pretreated mice display either no thyroid infiltration, T-cell proliferative response to mTg, and mTg autoantibody production, or markedly diminished levels in all three parameters. As discussed elsewhere *(48)*, endogenously released Tg by TSH, which may contain low iodine content, is nevertheless efficient in inducing T-cell tolerance, but less effective for B-cell tolerance owing to the low levels of circulatory Tg that can be achieved with TSH infusion via an osmotic pump. This T-cell tolerance, mediated by CD4+ Ts, suppresses immunization with thyroidal Tg with higher iodine content, another indication that iodination plays a secondary role in Tg immunogenicity (*15*; *see* Tg and Conserved Peptides). That Tg with low iodine content can induce tolerance was also observed in the OS chicken (*80*). However, the OS chicken has very abnormal thyroid metabolism, and its SAT apparently is markedly dependent on the presence of iodine residues.

The ability of pretreated animals to withstand immunogenic challenge indicates a heightened level of self-tolerance in susceptible mice, well above the normal level of unresponsiveness to immunization with mTg without adjuvant. Thus, the normal dominance of regulatory T cells has been raised by further expansion and/or differentiation into CD4+ Ts, which require 2–3 d to become fully activated after dmTg pretreatment (*48,81*). Once established, resistance to EAT induction is durable, lasting for at least 2–3 mo (*82*). It is transferable to normal recipient mice with CD4+ Ts (*81,83*). Moreover, resistance cannot be rescued by the administration of IL-2 (*71*) or overcome by the infusion of immunocompetent cells (one spleen equivalent) (*84*), suggesting that anergy does not play any major role. Suppressor function is abrogated only by depleting CD4+, but not CD8+, Ts; the loss of tolerance is demonstrable by the response to EAT induction of subsequently infused immunocompetent cells (*84*).

Others have induced suppression by oral administration of heterologous hTg (*85*) or pTg (*86*) in repeated mg doses and challenging the animals with hTg or mTg (*85,86*). Since heterologous Tgs possess foreign epitopes, hyporesponsiveness rather than strong suppression to hTg-induced EAT was observed (*85*), and only T-cell proliferation but not anti-mTg production was reduced in pTg-treated mice immunized with mTg (*86*). After inducing tolerance by injecting hTg (*87*), pTg, or hTg + pTg (*88*) and challenging with mTg, we too observed reduced proliferation to the shared epitopes, but thyroiditis subsequently developed, most likely owing to T cells recognizing mTg-unique, thyroiditogenic epitope(s). Thus, heterologous Tgs induce incomplete tolerance. It would be more difficult to induce tolerance once symptoms of HT have appeared, since the chance of further sensitizing rather than tolerizing would have increased. The cells mediating oral tolerance have not been delineated.

Induction of Resistance with Idiotype-Specific T Cells

After in vivo triggering of autoreactive T cells by thyroid autoantigens, idiotype-bearing T cells expressing specific CDR3 regions expand and differentiate; thyroid dysfunction may or may not result, as seen in humans. To determine if such T cells can induce anti-idiotype regulatory T cells, we have used irradiated, mTg-primed and activated spleen cells (*89*), and others have utilized an mTg-derived thyroiditogenic cell line (*90*) and a pTg-derived, cytotoxic CD8+ hybridoma (*91*) to vaccinate mice. In addition to reduced thyroiditis as seen by others, we also observed lowered antibody levels (*89*). Although vaccination can be achieved with irradiated CD4+ T cells, full protection requires both CD4+ and CD8+ Ts. The possible mechanisms are discussed in Regulatory T-Cell Mechanisms.

Regulatory T-Cell Mechanisms

General acceptance of regulatory T cells with suppressor function appears cyclic, but Ts have recently regained status, partly because CD4+ T cells, in addition to CD8+ T cells, have been found by many to be involved and partly because cytokines with inhibitory effects on pathogenic T cells have been well described. The mechanisms by which CD4+ Ts prevent EAT induction have been under study and could involve a number of different avenues, depending on the mode of activation. As mentioned above, both IL-1β *(71)* and IL-12 *(72)* can inhibit tolerance induction with dmTg, but the timing is critical and must occur prior to the establishment of tolerance, which takes 2–3 d. For example, IL-1β must be administered within 24 h of dmTg injection, with a 3-h interval being superior to a 24-h interval *(71)*. However, the 3-h interval must be after dmTg and not before, probably because of the short t½, a general feature of cytokines. The limited time span for IL-1β effectiveness demonstrates that, to divert the tolerogenic signal from Ts activation toward a commitment to pathogenic T cells, timing of the second signal is critical.

Since physiologic manipulation by TSH infusion leading to a transient and gradual increase of circulatory Tg level, peaking within the same interval of 2–3 d, also activates CD4+ Ts, and since this increase could occur periodically in vivo, we have hypothesized that tolerogenic signals are normally dominant *(48,79)*. Indeed, when we examined this window for the role of CD4 molecules in activation of Ts, using a nondepleting MAb, which modulates surface CD4 molecules, dmTg-induced tolerance was unaffected *(92)*. However, this low level of CD4 molecules is sufficient to interfere with the suppressive action toward autoreactive T cells at the time of challenge. It is unknown if the interference is owing to blocking of costimulatory signals. Using the same nondepleting MAb, but at high doses, another group reported the interference of mTg immunization resulting in a Ts subset *(93)*. It appears that to block immunization with adjuvant so that a tolerogenic signal is rendered, very high doses of anti-CD4 are required to induce Ts. The mechanisms by which these Ts exert their action are unknown.

The CD4+ suppressive action induced by dmTg lends itself to an examination of the role of Th2-like cytokines, such as IL-4 and IL-10; IL-10 administration has been shown to moderate EAT development *(78)*. However, when we administered anti-IL-4 and anti-IL-10, separately or together, at the time of dmTg injection, the induction of Ts was unabated *(72)*. Since the anti-IL-4 used has relatively low affinity, we also injected anti-IL-10 into IL-4 knockout mice, and again dmTg-induced tolerance became well established. Thus, IL-4 and IL-10 do not seem to play a role in dmTg-induced resistance. Whether T-cell-transforming growth factor-β (TGF-β) plays any role in the action of Ts is under study. Both IL-4 and TGF-β as well as an enriched CD8+ subset have been implicated in the hTg-induced oral tolerance cited above *(85)*. A recent study implicated many cytokines in dmTg-treated mice; reduced gene transcription was observed in the spleen for IFN-γ, IL-4, IL-10, TNF-α, and TGF-β *(94)*. The finding of both Th1 and Th2 cytokine production is probably related to the protocol of tolerance induction and immunization, interspersing tolerogenic and immunogenic doses. In our hands, tolerance induction is not complete until a second dose is also given 7 d later, prior to immunization *(81)*. Thus, the animals were immunized before tolerance induction had been fully established *(94)*, making it difficult to differentiate the cytokines involved in resistance and pathogenesis. Further studies will be required to determine what cytokines, if any, are involved in dmTg-induced resistance.

Other observations illustrate further that the mechanisms involved may depend on the mode of resistance induction. Anti-idiotype antibodies are implicated in protecting mice vaccinated with pTg-derived hybridoma against pTg-induced EAT *(95)*, and we have found both CD4+ and CD8+ Ts involved in vaccination with idiotype-specific

T cells *(89; see* Induction of Resistance with Idiotype-Specific T Cells). Interestingly, a synergistic, protective effect was observed when subtolerogenic doses of both dmTg and irradiated, mTg-activated cells were given to the same mice *(96)*. However, dmTg doses must precede the irradiated cells, indicating that anti-idiotype stimulation from the irradiated cells, when given first, diminished or neutralized the activation of Ts by dmTg. It is possible that both mechanisms operate in vivo, with normally low circulating mTg maintaining $CD4^+$ Ts dominance, and if there is triggering of autoreactive cells, $CD4^+$ and $CD8^+$ Ts with anti-idiotype activity may offer a second level control.

RELEVANCE FOR HUMAN DISEASE

This chapter primarily covers studies over the past five years, and the major advances in rodent models for autoimmune thyroid disease have dovetailed developments in molecular and transgenic technology and T-cell immunobiology. These advances have propelled us into a new and exciting arena. The major observations are:

1. *HLA-DRB1* polymorphism is a determinant of EAT susceptibility to mTg induction as shown in class II transgenic mice.
2. The permissiveness of HLA-DR3 molecules for hTg-induced EAT not only correlates with some clinical observations of *HLA* association with HT, but also demonstrates the potential of Tg as an initiator and relevant pathogen, a possibility supported by Tg as the antigen thus far recognized in SAT models.
3. The protective influence of different class II transgenes shows the relevance of studying *HLA* double-transgenic interactions.
4. The complete sequencing of mTg will permit a determination of the shared/conserved epitopes between hTg and mTg presented by HLA-DR3 molecules and those unique to hTg presented by $H2E^b$ molecules and other class II genes being identified.
5. The lack of immunodominant Tg epitopes and the demonstrated flexibility of the thyroiditogenic TCR repertoire could in part explain the discrepancies in establishing *HLA* association with HT; the secondary role of iodination in Tg immunogenicity, supported by retrospective human necropsy surveys in three continents, illustrates that variations in iodine residues in Tg preparations would not influence the study in transgenic mice to determine susceptible and protective genes.
6. The increase in circulatory Tg level owing to exogenous dmTg administration or endogenous release by TSH activates $CD4^+$ regulatory T cells to maintain resistance, and the cytokines IL-4 and IL-10 appear not to be involved.
7. The recent reports of GD-like symptoms in mice immunized with hTSHR-transfected cells also under MHC control, and thyroid infiltration in mice immunized with a truncated TSHR-ECD show promising approaches in developing GD-associated models and future testing in *HLA* transgenic mice.

Clearly, the relationship of experimental animal models to human thyroid disease has never been closer. As a result, their relevance has never been greater.

ACKNOWLEDGMENTS

The author gratefully acknowledge the fruitful collaborations and ever-stimulating dialogues with Alvaro A. Giraldo and Chella S. David, who have made the ongoing research pleasurable, and for the help of Qiang Wan in manuscript preparation. This work was supported by the National Institute of Diabetes, and Digestive and Kidney Diseases, DK 45960.

REFERENCES

1. Kong YM, Lewis, M. Animal models of autoimmune diseases: diabetes and thyroiditis. In: Volpé, R, ed. Autoimmune Diseases of the Endocrine System. CRC, Boca Raton, FL, 1990, pp. 23–50.
2. Kong YM, Giraldo AA. Experimental autoimmune thyroiditis in the mouse and rat. In: Cohen IR, Miller A, eds. Autoimmune Disease Models: A Guidebook. Academic, San Diego, 1994, pp. 123–145.
3. Kong YM. Regulatory mechanisms in autoimmune thyroiditis: recent lessons from a murine model. Fundam Clin Immunol 1994;2:199–213.
4. Weetman AP, McGregor AM. Autoimmune thyroid disease: further developments in our understanding. Endocr Rev 1994;15:788–830.
5. Wick G, Cole R, Dietrich H, Maczek Ch, Muller P-U, Hala K. The obese strain of chicken with spontaneous autoimmune thyroiditis as a model for Hashimoto disease. In: Cohen IR, Miller A, eds. Autoimmune Disease Models: A Guidebook. Academic, San Diego, 1994, pp. 107–122.
6. Kong YM. Animal models of autoimmune thyroiditis: recent advances. In: Weetman, AP, ed. Endocrine Autoimmunity and Associated Conditions. Kluwer, Dordrecht, The Netherlands, 1998, pp. 1–23.
7. Kong YM, David CS, Lomo LC, Fuller BE, Motte RW, Giraldo AA. Role of mouse and human class II transgenes in susceptibility to and protection against mouse autoimmune thyroiditis. Immunogenetics 1997;46:312–317.
8. Kong YM, Lomo LC, Motte RW, Giraldo AA, Baisch J, Strauss G, et al. HLA-DRB1 polymorphism determines susceptibility to autoimmune thyroiditis in transgenic mice: definitive association with HLA-DRB1*0301 (DR3) gene. J Exp Med 1996;184:1167–1172.
9. Krco CJ, Gores A, David CS, Kong YM. Immunogenetic aspects of human thyroglobulin-reactive T cell lines and hybridomas. J Immunogenet 1990;17:361–370.
10. Chronopoulou E, Carayanniotis G. H-2E^k expression influences thyroiditis induction by the thyroglobulin peptide (2495-2511). Immunogenet 1993;38:150–153.
11. Wan Q, McCormick DJ, Shah R, Giraldo AA, David CS, Kong YM. Induction of autoimmune thyroiditis by unique human thyroglobulin epitopes in H2E transgenic mice. FASEB J 1998;12:A1051.
12. Kuppers RC, Hu Q, Rose NR. Mouse thyroglobulin: conservation of sequence homology in C-terminal immmunogenic regions of thyroglobulin. Autoimmunity 1996;23:175–180.
13. Caturegli P, Vidalain PO, Vali M, Aguilera-Galaviz LA, Rose NR. Cloning and Characterization of Murine Thyroglobulin cDNA. Clin Immunol Immunopathol 1997;85:221–226.
14. Hutchings PR, Cooke A, Dawe K, Champion BR, Geysen M, Valerio R, et al. A thyroxine-containing peptide can induce murine experimental autoimmune thyroiditis. J Exp Med 1992;175:869–872.
15. Kong YM, McCormick DJ, Wan Q, Motte RW, Fuller BE, Giraldo AA, et al. Primary hormonogenic sites as conserved autoepitopes on thyroglobulin in murine autoimmune thyroiditis: secondary role of iodination. J Immunol 1995;155:5847–5854.
16. Wan Q, Motte RW, McCormick DJ, Fuller BE, Giraldo AA, David CS, et al. Primary hormongenic sites as conserved autoepitopes on thyroglobulin in murine autoimmune thyroiditis: role of MHC class II. Clin Immunol Immunopathol 1997;85:187–194.
17. Damotte D, Colomb E, Cailleau C, Brousse N, Charreire J, Carnaud C. Analysis of susceptibility of NOD mice to spontaneous and experimentally induced thyroiditis. Eur J Immunol 1997; 27:2854–2862.
18. Rasooly L, Burek CL, Rose NR. Iodine-induced autoimmune thyroiditis in NOD-H2^{h4} mice. Clin Immunol Immunopathol 1996;81:287–292.
19. Kotzin BL, Leung DYM, Kappler J, Marrack P. Superantigens and their potential role in human disease. Adv Immunol 1993;54:99–166.
20. Kong YM, Waldmann H, Cobbold S, Giraldo AA, Fuller BE, Simon LL. Pathogenic mechanisms in murine autoimmune thyroiditis: short- and long-term effects of in vivo depletion of CD4$^+$ and CD8$^+$ cells. Clin Exp Immunol 1989;77:428–433.
21. Flynn JC, Conaway DH, Cobbold S, Waldmann H, Kong YM. Depletion of L3T4$^+$ and Lyt-2$^+$ cells by rat monoclonal antibodies alters the development of adoptively transferred experimental autoimmune thyroiditis. Cell Immunol 1989;122:377–390.
22. Lomo LC, Zhang FS, McCormick DJ, Giraldo AA, David CS, Kong YM. Flexibility of the thyroiditogenic T cell repertoire for murine autoimmune thyroiditis in CD8-deficient (β2m–/–) and T cell receptor-Vβ^c congenic mice. Autoimmunity 1998;27:127–133.
23. Creemers P, Rose NR, Kong YM. Experimental autoimmune thyroiditis: in vitro cytotoxic effects of T lymphocytes on thyroid monolayers. J Exp Med 1983;157:559–571.
24. Salamero J, Charreire J. Syngeneic sensitization of mouse lymphocytes on monolayers of thyroid epithelial cells. VII. Generation of thyroid-specific cytotoxic effector cells. Cell Immunol 1985;91:111–118.

25. Kong YM, David CS, Giraldo AA, ElRehewy M, Rose NR. Regulation of autoimmune response to mouse thyroglobulin: influence of *H-2D*-end genes. J Immunol 1979;123:15–18.
26. Zanelli E, Gonzalez-gay MA, David CS. Could HLA-DRB1 be the protective locus in rheumatoid arthritis? Immunol Today 1995;16:274–278.
27. Lomo LC, Motte RW, Giraldo AA, Nabozny GH, David CS, Rimm IJ, et al. Vβ8.2 transgene expression interferes with development of experimental autoimmune thyroiditis in CBA k/q but not k/k mice. Cell Immunol 1996;168:297–301.
28. Fuller BE, Giraldo AA, Motte RW, Wang C, Nabozny GH, David CS, Kong YM. T cell receptor Vβ gene usage in experimental autoimmune thyroiditis. Ann NY Acad Sci 1995;756:450–452.
29. Wick G. The role of the target organ in the development of autoimmune diseases exemplified in the obese strain (OS) chicken model for human Hashimoto disease. Exp Clin Endocrinol Diabetes 1996; 104(Suppl. 3):1–4.
30. Bhatia SK, Rose NR, Schofield B, Lafond-Walker A, Kuppers RC. Influence of diet on the induction of experimental autoimmune thyroid disease. Proc Soc Exp Biol Med 1996;213:294–300.
31. Allen EM, Braverman LE. The biobreeding worcester rat—a model of organ-specific autoimmunity. Exp Clin Endocrinol Diabetes 1996;104(Suppl. 3):7–10.
32. Okayasu I, Hatakeyama S, Kong YM. Long-term observation and effect of age on induction of experimental autoimmune thyroiditis in susceptible and resistant mice. Clin Immunol Immunopathol 1989;53:254–267.
33. Green LM, LaBue M, Lazarus JP, Colburn KK. Characterization of autoimmune thyroiditis in MRL-lpr/lpr mice. Lupus 1995;4:187–196.
34. Allen EM, Thupari JN. The pathogenicity of spontaneously-occurring thyroglobulin-reactive T lymphocytes from BB/WOR rats. Autoimmunity 1996;23:35–44.
35. Sugihara S, Fujiwara H, Shearer GM. Autoimmune thyroiditis induced in mice depleted of particular T cell subsets: characterization of thyroiditis-inducing T cell lines and clones derived from thyroid lesions. J Immunol 1993;150:683–694.
36. Matsuoka N, Unger P, Ben-Nun A, Graves P, Davies TF. Thyroglobulin-induced murine thyroiditis assessed by intrathyroidal T cell receptor sequencing. J Immunol 1994;152:2562–2568.
37. Nakashima M, Kong YM, Davies TF. The role of T cells expressing TcR Vβ13 in autoimmune thyroiditis induced by transfer of mouse thyroglobulin-activated lymphocytes: identification of two common CDR3 motifs. Clin Immunol Immunopathol 1996;80:204–210.
38. Carayanniotis G, Rao VP. Searching for pathogenic epitopes in thyroglobulin: parameters and caveats. Immunol Today 1997;18:83–88.
39. Sundick RS, Bagchi N, Brown TR. The obese strain chicken as a model for human Hashimoto's thyroiditis. Exp Clin Endocrinol Diabetes 1996;104(Suppl. 3):4–6.
40. Allen EM, Thupari JN. Thyroglobulin-reactive T lymphocytes in thyroiditis-prone BB/Wor rats. J Endocrinol Invest 1995;18:45–49.
41. Stenszky V, Balazs C, Kraszits E, Juhasz F, Kozma L, Balazs G, et al. Association of goitrous autoimmune thyroiditis with HLA-DR3 in eastern Hungary. J Immunogenet 1987;14:143–148.
42. Kong YM. Recent developments in the relevance of animal models to Hashimoto's thyroiditis and Graves' disease. Curr Opinion Endocrinol Diabetes 1997;4:347–353.
43. Okayasu I, Hatakeyama S, Tanaka Y, Sakurai T, Hoshi K, Lewis PD. Is focal chronic autoimmune thyroiditis an age-related disease? Differences in incidence and severity between Japanese and British. J Pathol 1991;163:257–264.
44. Okayasu I, Hara Y, Nakamura K, Rose NR. Racial and age-related differences in incidence and severity of focal autoimmune thyroiditis. Am J Clin Pathol 1994;101:698–702.
45. Dawe KI, Hutchings PR, Geysen M, Champion BR, Cooke A, Roitt IM. Unique role of thyroxine in T cell recognition of a pathogenic peptide in experimental autoimmune thyroiditis. Eur J Immunol 1996; 26:768–772.
46. Wan Q, McCormick DJ, David CS, Kong YM. Thyroglobulin peptides of specific primary hormonogenic sites can generate cytotoxic T cells and serve as target autoantigens in experimental autoimmune thyroiditis. Clin Immunol Immunopathol 1998;86:110–114.
47. Kotani T, Umeki K, Yagihashi S, Hirai K, Ohtaki S. Identification of thyroiditogenic epitope on porcine thyroid peroxidase for C57BL/6 mice. J Immunol 1992;148:2084–2089.
48. Lewis M, Giraldo AA, Kong YM. Resistance to experimental autoimmune thyroiditis induced by physiologic manipulation of thyroglobulin level. Clin Immunol Immunopathol 1987;45:92–104.
49. Volpe R. Graves' disease/model of SCID mouse. Exp. Clin. Endocrinol Diabetes 1996;104(Suppl. 3): 37–40.

50. Martin A, Matsuoka N, Zhang J, Zhou A, Nakashima M, Unger P, et al. Preservation of functioning human thyroid "organoids"in the *scid* mouse. IV. *In vivo* selection of an intrathyroidal T cell receptor repertoire. Endocrinology 1997;138:4868–4875.
51. Prabhakar BS, Fan JL, Seetharamaiah GS. Thyrotropin-receptor-mediated diseases: a paradigm for receptor autoimmunity. Immunol Today 1997;18:437–442.
52. Marion S, Braun JM, Ropars A, Kohn LD, Charreire J. Induction of autoimmunity by immunization of mice with human thyrotropin receptor. Cell Immunol 1994;158:329–341.
53. Costagliola S, Many M-C, Stalmans-Falys M, Vassart G, Ludgate M. Transfer of thyroiditis, with syngeneic spleen cells sensitized with the human thyrotropin receptor, to naive BALB/c and NOD mice. Endocrinology 1996;137:4637–4643.
54. Banga JP. Immunopathogenicity of thyrotropin receptor—ability to induce autoimmune thyroid disease in an experimental animal model. Exp Clin Endocrinol Diabetes 1996;104(Suppl 3):32–34.
55. Shimojo N, Kohno Y, Yamaguchi KI, Kikuoka SI, Hoshioka A, Niimi H, et al. Induction of Graves-like disease in mice by immunization with fibroblasts transfected with the thyrotropin receptor and a class II molecule. Proc Natl Acad Sci USA 1996;93:11,074–11,079.
56. Yamaguchi KI, Shimojo N, Kikuoka S, Hoshioka A, Hiraj A, Tahara K, et al. Genetic control of antithyrotropin receptor antibody generation in H-2k mice immunized with thyrotropin receptor-transfected fibroblasts. J Clin Endocrinol Metab 1997;82:4266–4269.
57. Wang SH, Carayanniotis G, Zhang Y, Gupta M, McGregor AM, Banga JP. Induction of thyroiditis in mice with thyrotropin receptor lacking serlogically dominant regions. Clin Exp Immunol 1998;113:119–125.
58. Vlase, H, Matsuoka, N, Graves, PN, Magnusson, RP, Davies, TF. Folding-dependent binding of thyrotropin (TSH) and TSH receptor autoantibodies to the murine TSH receptor ectodomain. Endocrinology 1997;138:1–9.
59. Costagliola S, Rodien P, Many MC, Ludgate M, Vassart G. Genetic immunization against the human thyrotropin receptor causes thyroiditis and allows production of monoclonal antibodies recognizing the native receptor. J Immunol 1998;160:1458–1465.
60. Fuller BE, Giraldo AA, Motte RW, Nabozny GH, David CS, Kong YM. Noninvolvement of Vβ8+ T cells in murine thyroglobulin-induced experimental autoimmune thyroiditis. Cell Immunol 1994;159:315–322.
61. McMurray RW, Hoffman RW, Tang H, Braley-Mullen H. T cell receptor Vβ usage in murine experimental autoimmune thyroiditis. Cell Immunol 1996;172:1–9.
62. Nakashima M, Kong YM, Wan Q, Davies TF. Prospective study of T cell receptor utilization following the induction of murine thyroiditis. Exp Clin Endocrinol Diabetes 1996;104(Suppl 4):46–51.
63. Rao VP, Russell RS, Carayanniotis G. Recruitment of multiple Vβ genes in the TCR repertoire against a single pathogenic thyroglobulin epitope. Immunology 1997;91:623–627.
64. Conaway DH, Giraldo AA, David CS, Kong YM. *In situ* kinetic analysis of thyroid lymphocyte infiltrate in mice developing experimental autoimmune thyroiditis. Clin Immunol Immunopathol 1989;53:346–353.
65. Conaway DH, Giraldo AA, David CS, Kong YM. *In situ* analysis of T cell subset composition in experimental autoimmune thyroiditis after adoptive transfer of activated spleen cells. Cell Immunol 1990;125:247–253.
66. McMurray RW, Sharp GC, Braley-Mullen H. Intrathyroidal cell phenotype in murine lymphocytic and granulomatous experimental autoimmune thyroiditis. Autoimmunity 1994;18:93–102.
67. Braley-Mullen H, Sharp GC, Bickel JT, Kyriakos M. Induction of severe granulomatous experimental autoimmune thyroiditis in mice by effector cells activated in the presence of anti-interleukin 2 receptor antibody. J Exp Med 1991;173:899–912.
68. Stull SJ, Sharp GC, Kyriakos M, Bickel JT, Braley-Mullen H. Induction of granulomatous experimental autoimmune thyroiditis in mice with in vitro activated effector T cells and anti-IFN-gamma antibody. J Immunol 1992;149:2219–2226.
69. Sugihara S, Fujiwara H, Niimi H, Shearer GM. Self-thyroid epithelial cell (TEC)-reactive CD8+ T cell lines/clones derived from autoimmune thyroiditis lesions. J Immunol 1995;155:1619–1628.
70. Tang H, Mignon-Godefroy K, Meroni PL, Garotta G, Charreire J, Nicoletti F. The effects of a monoclonal antibody to interferon-gamma on experimental autoimmune thyroiditis (EAT): prevention of disease and decrease of EAT-specific T cells. Eur J Immunol 1993;23:275–278.
71. Nabozny GH, Kong YM. Circumvention of the induction of resistance in murine experimental autoimmune thyroiditis by recombinant IL-1β. J Immunol 1992;149:1086–1092.
72. Zhang W, Kong YM. IL-12 interferes with tolerance induction to experimental autoimmune thyroiditis. FASEB J 1998;12:A1096.

73. Fuller BE, Giraldo AA, Waldmann H, Cobbold SP, Kong YM. Depletion of CD4+ and CD8+ cells eliminates immunologic memory of thyroiditogenicity in murine experimental autoimmune thyroiditis. Autoimmunity 1994;19:161–168.
74. Carayanniotis G, Masters SR, Noelle RJ. Suppression of murine thyroiditis via blockade of the CD40-CD40L interaction. Immunology 1997;90:421–426.
75. Metcalfe RA, Tandon N, Tamatani T, Miyasaka M, Weetman AP. Adhesion molecule monoclonal antibodies inhibit experimental autoimmune thyroiditis. Immunology 1993;80:493–497.
76. Tamura K, Woo J, Murase N, Carrieri, G Nalesnik MA, Thomson AW. Suppression of autoimmune thyroid disease by FK 506: influence on thyroid-infiltrating cells, adhesion molecule expression and anti-thyroglobulin antibody production. Clin Exp Immunol 1993;91:368–375.
77. McMurray RW, Tang H, Braley-Mullen H. The role of α4 integrin and intercellular adhesion molecule-1 (ICAM-1) in murine experimental autoimmune thyroiditis. Autoimmunity 1996;23:9–23.
78. Mignon-Godefroy K, Rott O, Brazillet M-P, Charreire J. Curative and protective effects of IL-10 in experimental autoimmune thyroiditis (EAT): evidence for IL-10-enhanced cell death in EAT. J Immunol 1995;154:6634–6643.
79. Lewis M, Fuller BE, Giraldo AA, Kong YM. Resistance to experimental autoimmune thyroiditis is correlated with the duration of raised thyroglobulin levels. Clin Immunol Immunopathol 1992;64:197–204.
80. Bagchi N, Sundick RS, Hu LH, Cummings GD, Brown TR. Distinct regions of thyroglobulin control the proliferation and suppression of thyroid-specific lymphocytes in obese strain chickens. Endocrinology 1996;137:3286–3290.
81. Kong YM, Okayasu I, Giraldo AA, Beisel KW, Sundick RS, Rose NR, et al. Tolerance to thyroglobulin by activating suppressor mechanisms. Ann NY Acad Sci 1982;392:191–209.
82. Fuller BE, Okayasu I, Simon LL, Giraldo AA, Kong YM. Characterization of resistance to murine experimental autoimmune thyroiditis: duration and afferent action of thyroglobulin- and TSH-induced suppression. Clin Immunol Immunopathol 1993;69:60–68.
83. Parish NM, Rayner D, Cooke A, Roitt IM. An investigation of the nature of induced suppression to experimental autoimmune thyroiditis. Immunology 1988;63:199–203.
84. Kong YM, Giraldo AA, Waldmann H, Cobbold SP, Fuller BE. Resistance to experimental autoimmune thyroiditis: L3T4+ cells as mediators of both thyroglobulin-activated and TSH-induced suppression. Clin Immunol Immunopathol 1989;51:38–54.
85. Guimaraes VC, Quintans J, Fisfalen M-E, Straus FH, Fields PE, Medeiros-Neto G, et al. Immunosuppression of thyroiditis. Endocrinology 1996;137:2199–2207.
86. Peterson KE, Braley-Mullen H. Suppression of murine experimental autoimmune thyroiditis by oral administration of porcine thyroglobulin. Cell Immunol 1995;166:123–130.
87. Nabozny GH, Simon LL, Kong YM. Suppression in experimental autoimmune thyroiditis: the role of unique and shared determinants on mouse thyroglobulin in self-tolerance. Cell Immunol 1990;131:140–149.
88. Nabozny GH. Functional characteristics and autoantigenic requirements of CD4+ suppressor T cells in murine experimental autoimmune thyroiditis. PhD Dissertation, Wayne State University, 1991.
89. Flynn JC, Kong YM. In vivo evidence for CD4+ and CD8+ suppressor T cells in vaccination-induced suppression of murine experimental autoimmune thyroiditis. Clin Immunol Immunopathol 1991;60:484–494.
90. Maron R, Zerubavel R, Friedman A, Cohen IR. T lymphocyte line specific for thyroglobulin produces or vaccinates against autoimmune thyroiditis in mice. J Immunol 1983;131:2316–2322.
91. Remy J-J, Texier B, Chiocchia G, Charreire J. Characteristics of cytotoxic thyroglobulin-specific T cell hybridomas. J Immunol 1989;142:1129–1133.
92. Nabozny GH, Cobbold SP, Waldmann H, Kong YM. Suppression in murine experimental autoimmune thyroiditis: in vivo inhibition of CD4+ T cell-mediated resistance by a nondepleting rat CD4 monoclonal antibody. Cell Immunol 1991;138:185–196.
93. Hutchings PR, Cooke A, Dawe K, Waldmann H, Roitt IM. Active suppression induced by anti-CD4. Eur J Immunol 1993;23:965–968.
94. Tang H, Braley-Mullen H. Intravenous administration of deaggregated mouse thyroglobulin suppresses induction of experimental autoimmune thyroiditis and expression of both Th1 and Th2 cytokines. Int Immunol 1997;9:679–687.
95. Roubaty C, Bedin C, Charreire J. Prevention of experimental autoimmune thyroiditis through the anti-idiotypic network. J Immunol 1990;144:2167–2172.
96. Nabozny GH, Flynn JC, Kong YM. Synergism between mouse thyroglobulin- and vaccination-induced suppressor mechanisms in murine experimental autoimmune thyroiditis. Cell Immunol 1991;136:340–348.

5 Animal Models for Insulin-Dependent Diabetes Mellitus

Sabine Bieg, PhD, *and Åke Lernmark,* MD

CONTENTS

INTRODUCTION
ANIMAL MODELS
LESSONS FROM ANIMAL MODELS
CONCLUSIONS AND FUTURE OUTLOOK
REFERENCES

INTRODUCTION

Insulin-dependent diabetes mellitus (IDDM) in humans is a complex disease. Environmental and genetic factors contribute in variable proportions to the etiopathogenesis. In order to develop effective strategies to predict, prevent, and treat diabetes, it is important to identify and characterize the individual factors involved in the disease process and to study synergistic effects that may control progression toward the clinical onset of diabetes. In human diabetes, this goal has proven cumbersome and complicated to pursue, owing to the lack of knowledge of the development of human autoimmune diseases, lack of human pancreatic islet tissue to study the target organ, as well as complex inheritance patterns (*see also* Chapter 12). Thus, the use of animals to study IDDM has contributed fundamentally to the current knowledge and to hypotheses aimed at clarifying the nature of the disease. The reader is referred to recent excellent reviews on animals with IDDM, including the nonobese diabetic (NOD) mouse *(1–3)* and the BioBreeding (BB) rat *(4,5)*. This chapter will describe important animal models for IDDM and some of the implications of the research data that have been obtained by studying diabetes in these animals.

ANIMAL MODELS

Diabetes in animals occurs spontaneously, such as in the NOD mouse and the BB rat, or can be induced experimentally by genetic manipulation, virus infections, or chemicals. There are also animal models available for acute and chronic diabetes complications *(6)*. Diabetes may develop in larger mammals, such as primates and canines, but for practical reasons, rodent diabetes models are the most commonly used to study the disease. Consequently, the rodent type of diabetes has been characterized more exten-

From: *Contemporary Endocrinology: Autoimmune Endocrinopathies*
Edited by: R. Volpe © Humana Press Inc., Totowa, NJ

sively and will therefore be discussed in greater detail. In contrast to experimentally induced diabetes, the BB rat, the Long-Evans Tokushima Lean (LETL) rat, the NOD mouse, and the Chinese hamster develop spontaneous diabetes. Diabetes in these animals resemble that of human IDDM in some, but not in all features. These animals are nonetheless useful, and are being used to study potential etiologic and pathogenic pathways with the objective that understanding rodent IDDM may help to identify mechanisms that are relevant for IDDM in humans.

The BB Rat

The BB rat was discovered at the BioBreeding Laboratory in Ottawa, Canada, after spontaneously diabetic rats had been found in a colony of outbred Wistar rats *(4,7)*. Selective inbreeding of diabetic rats in different laboratories resulted in several lines of diabetes-prone (DP) BB rats *(5)*. Diabetes in DP-BB rats is gender independent and becomes clinically overt at 60–90 d of age. The symptoms, which are similar to human IDDM, include weight loss, polyuria, polydipsia, and ketoacidosis. The pathology of the pancreatic islet lesions reveals infiltration by mononuclear cells and β-cell destruction. Several independent morphometric analyses demonstrate a major reduction in the β-cell mass at the time of clinical onset. Without insulin treatment, the condition is terminal. The cumulative incidence of diabetes in DP BB reaches 100% if the animals are kept under specific pathogen-free (SPF) conditions. In the major histocompatibility complex- (MHC) identical diabetes-resistant (DR) line, BB-DR, diabetes has been reported at a cumulative incidence of <1% in some colonies *(8)* or does not occur at all *(5,9)*.

The genetics of the BB rat diabetes has provided important new information on the inheritance of complex diseases. The mechanisms of diabetes development may be explained by the identification of the individual genes, which seem to interact with the environment to initiate the disease pathogenesis. Dissection of the BB rat diabetes demonstrates linkage to at least three genes *(10)*. The first genetic factor *(iddm1)* is the lymphopenia *(11)* on chromosome 4, and it was mapped in a cross between inbred DP and DR rats *(10)*. The second gene *(iddm2)* is the MHC on chromosome 20. It was mapped in a cross between DP and Lewis rats *(10)* confirming previous studies in crosses between rats with different MHC types *(12)*. The diabetes phenotype in BB rats is accompanied by the autosomal-recessive peripheral T-cell deficiency (lymphopenia) *(13)* and polyendocrine phenomena, such as autoimmune thyroiditis *(14,15)*. The immunopathogenesis of BB rat diabetes has been studied in adoptive transfer experiments demonstrating the importance of T cells in the disease process *(16,17)* as well as different ways to manipulate the immune system to prevent diabetes *(4,18)*. The defined genetics and the autoimmune diabetes phenotype of the BB rat makes this rat an important animal to study with regard to mechanisms of diabetes development.

The LETL Rat

Kawano and coworkers reported the LETL rat 1989 as a model for Type 1 diabetes *(19)*. The animals develop diabetes at around 90–120 d of age. Depending on the mating constellation, the incidence varies between about 65% (both parents diabetic) and 23% (diabetic mother and nondiabetic father). There does not seem to be a gender bias in the development of diabetes in the offspring. LETL rats develop clinical and subclinical symptoms similar to humans and BB rats. However, in contrast to BB rats, the LETL rats have normal lymphocyte numbers. Breeding studies have indicated that diabetes segregates with at least two recessive genes *(19)*. Similar to what has been observed in the NOD mouse, LETL rats develop a Sjögren's-like syndrome, but no thyroiditis. The congenic Long-Evans Tokushima Otsuka (LETO) rat, which does not develop insulitis or diabetes, is used as a control strain for LETL. The absence of lymphopenia would make the LETL rat of great interest for IDDM investigations.

The NOD Mouse

Spontaneously diabetic mice were first discovered in Japan during the development of a cataract-prone subline (CTS) from noninbred ICR mice in Japan *(20)*. Selective inbreeding of the diabetic offspring resulted in the establishment of the NOD mouse, along with a congenic nonobese, nondiabetic (NON) mouse strain *(1,21)*. In animals kept in standard facilities, diabetes affects primarily female NOD mice with a cumulative incidence of about 60–90% at around 30 wk of age, in contrast to about 30% in male mice. In mice kept under SPF conditions, the cumulative incidence is reported to be nearly 100%, irrespective of gender. Insulitis starts at around 6 wk of age as a focal lymphocyte aggregation close to the islets (peri-insulitis) and progresses as a massive infiltration of mononuclear cells toward clinical onset. However, not every affected animal progresses to diabetes, and there are numerous reports on NOD mice with peri-insulitis as a sign of subclinical disease *(3)*. As in DP BB rats, the clinical symptoms in diabetic NOD mice closely resemble the Type 1 diabetes syndrome in humans, but also include the infiltration of the salivary and lacrimal glands (in 21.4 and 30% of the animals, respectively). The animals are insulin-dependent after clinical onset *(2)*. More than 16 genetic loci, including the MHC, have to date been linked to insulitis and diabetes in the NOD mouse *(22)*. Taken together, the overall view of the NOD mouse IDDM is that the etiology is dysregulation of the immune system, perhaps the lack of T-cell regulatory cells and cytokines.

The Chinese Hamster

Chinese hamsters develop a mild form of spontaneous diabetes. About 2% of a population develops severe ketoacidosis, whereas glycosuria can be detected at 4 wk of age already. It is not altogether clear whether diabetes in the Chinese hamster is autoimmune, since the incidence of insulitis is very low. Islet lesions are marked by the degranulation of β cells. The inheritance mode of diabetes in this model seems to be autosomal-recessive *(23)*. Recent views are that the Chinese hamster diabetes represents a Type 2 diabetes process with an early loss of glucose transporter expression *(24)* and replicative ability of β cells *(25)*. Further studies are needed to determine the genetic difference between the normal M and diabetic L sublines to identify potential markers for the diabetes etiology.

Diabetes Induced by Genetic Manipulation

IDDM develops after complete or partial loss of insulin production in the pancreas *(26)*. The destruction of the insulin-producing cells is associated with numerous autoimmune phenomena *(3,27)*, which may be the results of an activation of autoreactive effector T-cells causing β-cell damage. The presentation of tissue-specific autoantigens by antigen-presenting cells on high-risk alleles of the MHC and signaling factors, such as cytokines and costimulatory molecules, may have synergistic effects in this activation. Insulitis may occur in rodents, in particular, the peri-insulitis observed in the NOD mouse without subsequent development of diabetes. It is unknown to what extent this takes place in humans as well, and additional studies of children dying from infectious diseases are needed *(28)*. The presence of inflammatory cells in the islets of Langerhans implies that many factors are involved in the insulitis process. These factors need to be tested individually for their ability to cause islet inflammation and β-cell damage. Transgenic technology has made it possible to generate animals, particularly mice, in which the pancreas has artificially been made a target for an immune reaction *(29–32)*. In these highly controlled disease models, individual factors can be tested for their immunogenicity on a diabetes-resistant background. The following is a short summary of recent transgenic mice developing diabetes.

In one of the first transgenic models for diabetes, β cells in an otherwise diabetes resistant mouse strain were made to express MHC class I *(33)* or class II *(29,34,35)* molecules that are associated with rodent diabetes. In either case, diabetes, but not necessarily insulitis, was induced. The diabetes was most likely owing to a decrease in insulin production resulting from protein synthesis competition between proinsulin and the MHC molecules, all expressed under the control of the insulin gene promoter. Taken together, the transgenic mouse experiments failed to support the popularized view that β-cell autoimmunity was owing to an aberrant expression of MHC class II molecules *(36)*.

According to subsequent studies, coexpression of MHC molecules and proinflammatory cytokines, such as tumor necrosis factor (TNF-α), interferon (IFN)α, IFN-γ, and interleukin (IL-2), can induce islet inflammation by macrophages, CD4$^+$, and CD8$^+$ T cells. This has also been found in MHC-transgenic mice expressing immune costimulatory signals, such as B7, or the CD80/CD86 complex in the islets. Except for IL-2 *(37)*, expression of these factors individually can induce insulitis, but not diabetes *(38–40)*. In mice that express H-2^{g7}, the NOD mouse-specific diabetes susceptibility MHC haplotype, and that have been made transgenic for the T-cell receptor (TCR) variable region Vβ of a diabetogenic T-cell clone, insulitis develops very early and proceeds later to diabetes *(29,41)*. This model is considered useful for studying the progression of diabetes insulitis under the influence of individual genetic factors in the mouse *(41)*.

Another approach to investigating the cause of insulitis and subsequent diabetes is to generate transgenic mice that express specific antigens on their β cells and analyze the nature and degree of islet inflammation. Antigens, such as heat-shock proteins (hsp), or proteins from viruses, such as the glycoprotein (GP) from lymphocytic choriomeningitis virus (LCMV), have been expressed as transgenes under the control of the rat insulin promoter (RIP) *(32,42,43)*. In the RIP-LCMV model, self-reactive CD8$^+$ T cells are activated after infection with the respective virus, and as a consequence of tissue-specific antigen expression, autoimmune diabetes develops after destruction of the β cells, mediated by MHC class I-restricted CD8$^+$ T cells, using perforin and cytokines, such as IFN-γ and TNF-α *(44,45)*. When influenza hemagglutinin (HA) is expressed on the β cells of mice transgenic for HA-reactive T cells, insulitis and diabetes develop *(46)*. The manifestations and severity of disease were, however dependent on the genetic background of the respective transgenic mouse *(46,47)*. Since these transgenic mice display an inducible and highly controlled form of autoimmunity, the nature and number of activation factors necessary for the induction of self-reactive T cells can be studied. It will also be possible to dissect further the mechanisms that promote the pathogenesis to proceed from peri-insulitis to insulitis associated with β-cell killing and development of diabetes. It remains to be clarified to what extent intraislet inflammation occurs without β-cell destruction. It needs to be noted that every transgene under the control of the rat insulin promoter *(32)* may reduce β-cell function owing to competition with the endogenous mouse insulin promoter *(35)*.

Experimentally Induced Diabetes

Drugs or chemicals can induce diabetes in previously nondiabetic subjects or worsen hyperglycemia in already-known patients *(48)*. Certain drugs may induce insulin resistance or β-cell damage, resulting in impaired insulin release and finally diabetes. Administration of these chemicals to animals has similar effects, and these chemicals are often used to study not only the induction of IDDM, but also metabolic and symptomatic effects as well as possible treatments *(49–53)*.

Streptozotocin (STZ) is a broad-spectrum antibiotic. It is transported into the β cell through its glucose transporters *(54)*, and interferes with the cellular metabolism. It may generate free radicals, ultimately leading to DNA breaks and finally β-cell destruction *(55)*. STZ is used widely to induce diabetes in rats *(43,56)*, mice *(53,57,58)*, hamsters *(59)*, dogs *(60)*, lambs *(61)*, and monkeys *(60,62)*. Its antitumor capacities are used to treat malignant β-cell tumors clinically in human patients. It is noted that the β cytotoxic effect of STZ is much less in humans than in rodents, and diabetes seldom ensues after treatment of islet cell tumors *(63)*. The use of STZ to induce an IDDM-like disease process emanates from studies in different strains of mice.

STZ can be administered in a single high dose, causing β-cell death within 24 h. Multiple low doses of STZ induce pancreatic insulitis and slow-onset diabetes *(52)*. Diabetes may be induced by adoptive transfer *(64,65)*. The effect of STZ to induce insulitis is MHC-dependent *(66)*, and the progression to diabetes after the initial sub-diabetogenic five low-dose injections *(51)* may be inhibited by antibodies against MHC class II molecules *(66)* or with different T-lymphocyte antibodies *(67,68)*. More recently, the mechanisms of β-cell-mediated killing has been shown to be dependent on CD28/B7 costimulation *(69)*. The β-cell-specific effect of TSZ in the mouse and the association between an initial β-cell destruction followed by progression to chronic diabetes in association with insulitis make the multiple low-dose diabetes a useful model for autoimmune diabetes. This model seems, however, unique to the mouse, and numerous attempts to replicate this STZ regimen, for example, in rats have failed so far *(70)*.

Administration of alloxan, chlorotozin, Vacor *(71)*, or cyproheptadine *(72)* also causes chronic diabetes through β-cell destruction *(48,70,73)*. The utility in animals varies, since these drugs may have only minor effects or they are too toxic.

Polyinosinic polycytidylic acid (poly[I: C]) is an immune activator. It induces the expression of interferons and enhances the activity of natural killer (NK) cells. Poly(I: C) has been shown to prevent diabetes in NOD mice, possibly by inducing regulatory T cells *(74)*. In BB rats, however, administration of poly(I: C) accelerates (in BB DP) or induces (BB DR) diabetes, but has no effect on Wistar rats *(75)*. There are divergent reports on whether the additional depletion of RT6+ cells is necessary to induce diabetes after poly(I: C) administration in BB DR rats *(75,76)*. High-serum IFN-α levels have been associated with early onset of diabetes in BB rats. However, serum IFN-α is also increased in diabetes-resistant Wistar rats after poly(I: C) administration *(75,77)*. Since serum IFN levels are increased after virus infection as well, the poly(I: C) model is generally regarded as an experimental model for viral infection and diabetes development. The number of natural killer (NK) cell is increased in poly(I: C)-treated BB rats. Depletion of NK cells, however, did not prevent diabetes after poly(I: C) treatment *(78)*. Based on macrophage

Table 1
MHC Genes in Humans, Rats, and Mice

	Human leukocyte antigens, HLA	Rat RT 1	Mouse H-2
Class I	A	A	I
	B	E	K
	C	C	D
Class II	DQ	B	I-A
	DR	D	I-E
	DP	—	—

depletion experiments in Kilham rat virus (KRV) and poly(I: C)-treated BB DR rats, it has recently been suggested that macrophages and macrophage-derived cytokines, such as IL-1β, Il-12, and TNF-α, are activated by poly(I: C) and might be critically involved in poly(I: C)-mediated diabetes (79). These studies underline the possible importance of antigen-presenting cells in the disease process whether initiated by virus or treatment that would mimic virus exposure.

It has long been questioned whether autoimmunity associated with IDDM may be induced by failure of tolerance induction. Thymectomy at about 5 wk of age, followed by multiple low-dose irradiation induced chronic insulin-dependent diabetes in about 30% of nondiabetogenic PVG/c rats (80,81). The onset of diabetes was accompanied by elevated plasma glucose levels, ketosis, and lipidemia. Lymphocytic insulitis was found in both overtly diabetic and nondiabetic rats. Adoptive transfer of activated lymphocytes into syngeneic recipients induced diabetes, whereas reconstitution of thymectomized and irradiated rats with lymphocytes from untreated syngeneic donors prevented diabetes (81). It was also observed that the MHC type of responder rats was RT1^u, identical to that of the BB rat. Other MHC types were more resistant. These models of IDDM in the rat have yet to gain wider use and understanding.

Genetics

As in human IDDM, insulin-dependent diabetes in animal models has a strong genetic background. In both the NOD mouse and the BB rat, there is a strong linkage to certain MHC alleles conferring susceptibility or resistance (see Table 1). However, there seem to be differences between the number and impact of other genes and loci that have been linked to the phenotype diabetes in the different models. It is also noted that the genetic background is important to IDDM induced in mice by multiple low-dose STZ (50,66) or by virus-inducing β-cell destruction and IDDM (82). Novel techniques in gene mapping and the development of genetic maps of both rats and mice have made it possible to map genetic factors in IDDM in these animals. The presence of chromosomal regions that are syntenic between the rodents and the human genome makes it possible to carry out homology mapping. This approach implies the identification of a gene in the animal that allows the human counterpart to be identified and used to test the possible importance of a gene in human diseases.

GENETIC BACKGROUND OF DIABETES

The BB Rat. The genetic predisposition for diabetes in the DP BB rat is limited to at least three genes on the BB rat background. The autosomal-recessive lymphopenia gene

(*Lyp*) on rat chromosome 4 in BB rats (*Iddm1*) *(10)* induces the almost complete absence of peripheral T cells mainly of the CD8+ and RT6+ subtype. This phenotype is present from birth *(83,84)*. In a cross between BB DP and Lewis rats, it was demonstrated that the RT1 locus (*Iddm2*) on chromosome 20 was linked to diabetes *(10)*. Both DP and DR BB rats express the RT1^u haplotype *(85)*. Interestingly, the class II haplotype of LETL rats is RT1.B^u D^u *(19)*, indicating that RT1B^u alleles originally derived from the Wistar rat are a susceptibility factor for insulitis and diabetes also in other strains of rats.

DR BB rats are wild-type (+) for the lymphopenia locus and have normal lymphocyte levels *(13)*. Depletion of RT6+ peripheral lymphocytes resulted in a rapid induction of the disease in DR BB rats *(86)*. These data indicate that the missing RT6+ T-cell subset has immunoregulatory functions, most likely in conjunction with other lymphocyte subsets *(17,87)*. Diabetes in the BB rat might be the result of a poised equilibrium of immune effector cells *(88)*. Since lymphopenia is associated with a deletion of a major regulatory T-cell subset, the identification of the lymphopenia gene, *lyp*, might offer new insights into not only the lymphocyte differentiation pathway, but also to the ontogeny of autoreactivity. A newly developed BB-DR rat line congenic for *Lyp* might may help to identify the gene *(9)* and to determine its function. In backcrosses between BB (RT1^u, *Lyp/Lyp*) and Fischer (RT1^{lv}, +/+) rats, only about 50% of RT1^u *Lyp/Lyp* F2 offspring develop diabetes, indicating the presence of a third gene conferring resistance to diabetes *(10)*. This third genetic factor, *iddm3*, is located outside the MHC region. The inbred BB rat and its newly developed congenic lines should allow a final dissection of the gene controlling diabetes in this particular model. In summary, crosses between inbred DP BB rats and other inbred strains of rats have made it possible to map three genes that have the most significant impact on diabetes development. The use of defined crosses and marker-assisted breeding should make it possible to clone *iddm1-3* positionally and identify the mechanisms by which these genes are associated with disease development.

The NOD Mouse. Diabetes in the NOD mouse has a marked polygenic background. The autoimmune origin of the disease implies that candidate genes maintain central immunological functions. Exclusion mapping in order to identify possible candidate disease genes resulted in the linkage of NOD mouse diabetes to more than 17 loci on at least 5 different chromosomes in the mouse genome *(89–91)*. The genome scan also revealed the MHC locus (*Idd-1*) on mouse chromosome 17 as a major genetic factor. The NOD mouse has a recombinant H-2 class I locus (K^d, D^b) and a unique MHC class II locus, H-2 I-A^{g7} *(92)*. Owing to a deletion in the promoter region of the gene for the α-chain of the H-2 molecule, I-E is not expressed. This might be directly related to the development of diabetes, since transgenic expression of I-E$_\alpha$ prevents disease *(3)*. Similar to the human HLA-DQ susceptibility alleles, the amino acid on position 57 in the I-A β-chain may be critical for diabetes development *(22)*. This issue is yet to be resolved since transgenic mice with a substitution at position 56 are also protected from developing diabetes *(93)*. A single amino acid residue may therefore not suffice to control susceptibility or resistance to diabetes. Except for *Idd-1*, which shows different degrees of penetrance *(22)*, it is only *Idd-3* on chromosome 3 that shows linkage to both insulitis and diabetes *(94)*. *Idd-3* is located near the interleukin-2 gene (*IL-2*) on chromosome 3. Other polymorphisms have been located at *Thy-1* on chromosome 9 (*Idd-2*) and *bcl-2* on chromosome 1 *(95)*, which might correlate to the presence of apoptosis-resistant T cells in NOD mice. Interestingly, the CTLA-4 (cytotoxic T-lymphocyte-associated antigen 4) and the CD28 costimulatory molecules are defectively expressed in NOD mice *(96)*. Both these molecules are coded for at the *idd-5* locus, suggesting that one or both of these molecules may be involved in NOD mouse apoptosis resistance and diabetes susceptibility. The dissection of the NOD mouse IDDM genes should make it possible to identify allelic variants of several genes that interact to initiate insulitis and subsequent diabetes.

Currently Available Rodent Strains with a Genetic Background for Diabetes

Among the number of rodent subcolonies available for the study of Type 1 diabetes, a few are well established and may serve as the founders of newly developed strains. By international convention, a line is considered inbred only after at least 24 generations of sister/brother breeding. Table 2 gives an overview of the most commonly used inbred diabetic and nondiabetic strains. For NOD mice, Table 2 also lists some of the most recently developed congenic lines generated on the diabetes-prone NOD genetic background. In addition to those listed here, new lines and strains that develop diabetes on the basis of genetic manipulation are developed constantly *(9,97,98,98a,98b)*.

Autoimmunity

ISLET PATHOLOGY

In all animal models, insulitis precedes the clinical onset of diabetes. Insulitis is a gradual process, and the degree of inflammation can vary among individual islets from the same animal. It also differs histologically between the different models. In the BB rat and the LETL rat, inflammatory cell infiltration of the pancreatic islets starts shortly before clinical onset *(7,99)*. The infiltration proceeds rapidly into the islets, gradually dissolving the architecture of the islet. At the time of clinical onset, the islets have undergone severe atrophy. The β cells have been destroyed, and islet neogenesis is blocked. Analyses of phenotypes and local cytokine production indicated that in early stages of prediabetic insulitis, mostly macrophages were present *(100,101)*. The macrophage infiltration is followed by the progressive infiltration of $CD4^+$ and $CD8^+$ T cells, $CD4^-CD8^-$ NK cells, and B lymphocytes *(102–104)*. Insulitis in nondiabetic BB rats consists of a scattered infiltration of mostly macrophages in the exocrine and endocrine tissue.

NOD mouse insulitis starts at around 6 wk of age as a focal lymphocyte aggregation outside the islet (peri-insulitis) and in the islet capsule. It then progresses with age as a massive infiltration of mononuclear cells toward clinical onset, which is often restricted to one part of the islet. Again, not every affected animal progresses to diabetes. Islet lesions from diabetic and late prediabetic NOD mice contain all major mononuclear cell subsets. The development of insulitis and diabetes requires $CD4^+$ T cells and $CD8^+$ T cells as shown in adoptive transfer experiments *(105)*, and particularly, IFN-γ and IL-2-secreting $CD4^+$ T-cell subsets seem to have initiating functions. Macrophages seem to be present first, followed by T and B lymphocytes and NK cells.

THE IMMUNE RESPONSE

B-Cell Reactivity. Serum antibodies to β-cell proteins are used to predict the onset of diabetes and identify potential T-cell antigens. Islet cell antibodies (ICA) have been found in about 80% of NOD mice, whereas the occurrence of islet cell surface antigens (ICSA) *(106,107)* is common among both NOD mice and BB rats *(106–111)*. Depending on the fixation of the pancreatic tissue used for immunodetection of the antibodies, ICA

Chapter 5 / Animal Models for IDDM

Table 2
Colonies and Lines of BB Rats and NOD Mice

Colonies	Maintenance	Incidence of diabetes [%]	Age of onset [d of age]	Incidence of insulitis [%]	Specific features	References
BB rat						
BB/Wistar (BB/W)	SPF	>80	80–150	85–100 at >56 d of age	Thyroiditis in 50%	(98a)
BB/Worcester (BB/Wor)	VAF (virus antibody-free)	60–90	60–120	100		(14)
BB/Ottawa-Karlsburg (BB/OK)	SPF	50	60–120	96	Diabetes depends on mating	(98b)
BB/E	SPF	50–60	96 ± 18		DR subline also lymphopenic	(100)
BB/Mol	SPF	96	56–130		Commercial	
NOD mouse						
NOD/Lt (Leiter)	SPF	90 in female 83 in male	80–200	95% at >35 d		(75,170)
NOD/Shi (Shionogi)	SPF	70–80 in female <20 in male				(21)
NOD/Wehi (Walter and Eliza Hall Institute)	SPF	<10 in female <1 in male	150		Possible suppressor-cell population	(81)

Control strains	Incidence of diabetes and insulitis	Genetic features	Immune features	References
BB rats				
BB-DR	<1%	Same MHC as BB-DP	No lymphopenia	(13,14)
BB/E-DR			Lymphopenia	(100)
NOD-derived strains				
NOD/scid	0	H-2^{g7}	Block in T- and B-lymphocyte development	(56,75)
NOD/nu/nu	0		Athymic	(3)
NOR/Lt	0	Integrated retroviral genome, H-2^{g7}	Sialitis	(139)
NON/Lt	0	Diabetes-resistant MHC		(220)

in the NOD mouse seem to bind to different antigens in the cytoplasm, and one of them might be a glycolipid *(112)*. Up to 80% of NOD mice have autoantibodies to insulin, which have also been reported in BB rats. Autoantibodies to the 65-kDa isoform of the enzyme glutamic acid decarboxylase (GAD) have been found in both models *(113–115)*, although the presence of GAD antibodies is possibly restricted to some subcolonies, and reports are therefore controversial *(116,117)*. When present at diabetes onset, GAD antibodies in both models disappear within weeks. NOD mice also develop antibodies against a protein that is crossreactive with a bacterial heat-shock protein (hsp65) preceded by the presence of specific T cells. One report describes serum antibodies recognizing peripherin, a 58-kDa islet protein crossreacting with the NOD specific I-A class II *(118)*. Antibodies directed against proteins of other endocrine organs, such as thyroid peroxidase and gastric parietal cells, are also present *(83)*.

T-Cell Reactivity. Islet cell antigen-specific T-cell lines or clones have yet to be reported for the DP BB rat, although autoreactive T-cell lines could be established from infiltrated islets and the spleen *(119)*. Autoreactive T cells seem to be present in early lymphoid tissue, such as the thymus *(88,120)*. T-cell lines activated with islet cell extracts have been found to transfer diabetes into diabetes-resistant recipient rats *(121)* or to protect DP BB rats from diabetes *(122)*. We and others have found autoreactive thymocytes in diabetes-resistant strains that have been characterized by either their ability to secrete inflammatory cytokines or that are able to transfer diabetes *(120)*. Owing to their overrepresentation within the lymphocyte population and their presence in islet infiltrates in BB rats, particular interest has been assigned to NK cells as diabetes effector cells.

There are extensive data available on T-cell reactivity in the NOD mouse. For more information on this area of research, the reader may consult more detailed reviews *(123)*. In summary, it has been found that autoreactive T cells in the NOD mouse recognize several antigens that are present on β cells *(124–127)*. This reactivity has been used to identify antigenic epitopes on the respective molecules and to characterize the respective T cells, both of which are used as the basis for therapeutic interventions. The T-cell reactivity against GAD65 has been characterized extensively and has led to the identification of a number of epitopes on the GAD molecule that might also be recognized by human T cells. Some data have indicated clonal T-cell preference in islets from very young NOD mice, but their common antigen is unknown *(128)*. Although one would expect this to be reflected in the preference of certain T-cell receptor (TCR) β chains, it has been found that T-cell clones recognizing the insulin B-chain epitope between amino acid (AA) positions 9–23 rather seem to have a restricted TCR α-chain usage *(129)*. However, NOD mice transgenic for the TCR Vβ of a T-cell clone isolated from inflamed NOD islets show accelerated onset of the disease *(29,124)*. The p277 peptide of the human heat shock protein (hsp) 60 molecule is also recognized by autoreactive T cells in the NOD mouse *(130)*. Depending on the administration mode, p277 seems to address distinct T-cell populations, either inhibiting or accelerating the disease *(131,132)*. Many of the T-cell clones recognizing any of these antigens are able to transfer diabetes, and the administration of these antigens has been shown to influence disease development *(125–127)*. In transgenic NOD mice, such as Fas-deficient NOD-lpr/lpr or athymic NOD-nu/nu mice, the ontogeny or the costimulatory requirements for autoreactive T cells to attack β cells can be tested tested.

Environmental Influences

Although most of the common rodent models for spontaneous diabetes have a genetically determined predisposition, the incidence of diabetes is dramatically dependent on the surrounding conditions. Virus antibody-free (VAF) or SPF conditions are necessary to maintain a high incidence. Consequently, a number of factors that are part of the environment have been found to alter the disease process. It is generally assumed that environmental factors may deviate the immune response from being autoaggressive. Current studies are focused on understanding the role of T cells producing IFN-γ or IL-2 (Th1 response) to mediate and IL-4 or IL-10 (Th2 response) possibly to reduce self-reactivity.

INFECTIOUS AGENTS

Viruses. There are viruses that can either induce or prevent diabetes. In genetically susceptible hosts, viruses, such as the encephalomyocarditis virus variant D (EMCV-D) *(133)*, reoviruses *(134)*, mengoviruses *(135)*, or rubella *(136)*, can induce diabetes by specifically infecting and destroying the β cells *(137)*. Although this type of β-cell damage is not autoimmune and often reversible, the expression of LCMV antigens on the β-cell surface of transgenic animals leads to the autoimmune destruction by CD8$^+$ cytotoxic T cells *(138)*. Retroviral and rubella virus genome sequences have been found to be already integrated in NOD mouse and Golden Syrian genome, respectively *(136,139)*. The presence of retroviral particles in β cells was positively associated with insulitis lesions in these animals, suggesting that the activation of these endogenous viruses leads either to an alteration of the β cell into an autoimmune target or to the expression of novel autoantigen-attracting autoreactive cells. Rather than T cells, macrophages seem to be important mediators of this process *(140)*. PC-2 is a Coxsackie B4 virus antigenic epitope homologous to a sequence in the GAD65 molecule, so autoreactive T cells could be cross primed by the viral epitope *(141)*. In diabetes-resistant BB rat strains, Kilham rat virus (KLV) infection can also induce diabetes *(8)*.

Viruses can also prevent diabetes. Another EMCV variant (EMCV-B) is nondiabetogenic and can be used in mice as a vaccine against an infection with the diabetogenic EMCV-D variant. LCMV infection seems to prevent diabetes in NOD mice and BB-DP rats, possibly by downregulation of a particular CD4$^+$ cell subset *(142–144)*. Mouse hepatitis virus (MHV), lactate dehydrogenase virus (LDHV), pichinde, vaccinia, and Sendai virus have also been shown to be preventive *(143,145–147)*.

Other Pathogens. Bacteria and fungi may contribute to the pathogenesis of IDDM as well. Both in NOD mice and BB rats, vaccination with Bacillus Calmette Guerin (BCG) or complete Freund's adjuvants containing *Mycobacterium tuberculosis* protects from developing diabetes provided the treatment is initiated during the first 2 wk of life *(4,27)*. *Staphylococcal* enterotoxins have been shown to prevent diabetes in NOD mice *(148)*. It has been suggested that the protection is mediated by superantigen-induced expansion of β-chain-variable, region-specific T cells releasing anti-inflammatory cytokines, such as IL-10 and IL-4 *(149,150)*.

DIET

Standard rodent chow contains wheat, soybeans, and alfalfa, which may all trigger diabetes in the BB rat and in the NOD mouse. Biochemical analysis has suggested that proteins or peptides might be the triggering factors. Protein- and peptide-free diets prevent the development of diabetes in the BB rat as well as diets with restricted amounts of essential fatty acids *(151,152)*. The addition of 1% skim milk or 1% gliadin to a protein-free diet partially abrogates its protective effect. A diet containing hydrolyzed casein as a protein source (AIP-76), also prevents diabetes in NOD mice and BB rats. Recently, an alteration of the intraislet cytokine profile has been found in AIP-76-fed BB rats, suggesting that diet-induced disease protection is the result of the activation of immune cells with suppressor function *(153,154)*. Ingestion of cows' milk or bovine serum albumin (BSA) during infanthood has been suggested to be an important trigger for human Type 1 diabetes *(155)*. However, animal studies are inconclusive in this respect. In NOD mice neither cows' milk nor BSA seems to have any effect on diabetes incidence *(156)*, whereas the induction of tolerance to BSA early in life prevented the disease in BB rats *(157)*.

Toxic Agents

As already discussed, several drugs are β-cell toxic and can induce insulitis and diabetes. In rats and mice, STZ, alloxan and Vacor induce diabetes in animal models by interfering with the cellular metabolism resulting in β-cell destruction. In diabetes-prone animal models, such as the NOD mouse or the BB rat, they might therefore amplify the autoimmune response toward the β cells and by that accelerate the onset of the disease.

Chronic Stress

BB rats exposed to daily stress, such as rotation, vibration, or restraint, develop diabetes with a higher incidence than unaffected control animals *(158)*. In NOD mice, chronic stress between the 6th and 8th week of age as well as the long-time repeated injection of 0.9% saline decreased the incidence of diabetes in both sexes. Prenatal stress accelerated the onset of diabetes *(159–161)*. It is suspected that the stressors modulate the development of diabetes by neuroendocrine–immune interactions involving glucocorticoids and cytokines.

Sex Hormones

The incidence of diabetes is about fourfold higher in NOD females than in males. However, diabetes onset can be accelerated in males by castration, and androgen treatment inhibits diabetes development in female NOD mice *(37)*, suggesting an immunosuppressive effect mediated by androgens.

LESSONS FROM ANIMAL MODELS

Where human studies are difficult or even impossible to perform, studies using animal models are used to address the basic questions about the development of diabetes. How does β-cell directed autoimmunity develop? Is there a single agent triggering diabetes, or does the disease develop after the synergic impact of a multitude of genetical and environmental factors, and finally, can a preventive strategy be developed on the basis of this knowledge?

Paradigms for Diabetes Immunopathology

The Principle of Causality vs the Chaotic Model

It is evident from both human and animal data that genetic predisposition alone does not always lead to the development of diabetes. As described in the previous paragraphs, a multitude of physiological and environmental factors seem to contribute to the development of the diabetic syndrome. However, there are divergent opinions on the significance of these factors, both to trigger the disease and to establish and maintain its chronicity. According to the causal models, there is an acute impact that triggers the destruction of the β cells. This might be owing to the display of a β-cell-specific antigen to the immune system as a result of a β-cell tropic virus lysing the infected cells. Alternatively, viral antigenic epitopes may be homologous to β-cell-specific protein determinants and activate crossreacting T cells. In both cases, CD8+ T cells would be induced to attack and destroy β cells specifically, causing insulitis and diabetes. The presence of CD4+ T cells in insulitis lesions or the development of autoantibodies would therefore be a secondary phenomena. This hypothesis is supported by the frequent finding of CD8+ cells in islet lesions *(162,163)* as well as by data on NODβ$_{2m}$^{null} mice, which do not develop diabetes owing to a defect in MHC class I expression *(164,165)*. On the other hand, it has been repeatedly shown that CD4+ cells are a requirement for initiating diabetes.

A more holistic approach to explaining disease etiology offers the chaotic model responding to the variety of genetic, physiological, and environmental factors that have been associated with diabetes in human populations and animals. The chaotic model postulates the existence of harmful and not harmful forms of autoimmunity, reflected in the frequent occurrence of insulitis without diabetes in both the BB rat and the NOD mouse, disregarding their disease-prone genotype. Whether destructive autoimmunity develops or not may be owing to the occurrence and combination of various physiological and environmental impacts. These would add to the genetic predisposition and the momentary state of the immune system at a given time, so that the initial impact may not be the decisive one. The various impacts combine and accumulate until a phenotype, such as β-cell-reactive T cells or autoantibodies, becomes measurable. The model proposes that the development of the diabetic phenotype is therefore a chaotic process along which the immune system is offered multiple pathways to respond to triggering factors *(166)*. Prediction of diabetes will only be possible if these options of the immune system themselves become understandable and predictable. Recently, the transgression from nondestructive to destructive insulitis has been linked to the amount of the chemokines MIP 1β and MIP 1α, which are expressed in the pancreas and might affect local inflammatory T cells *(167,168)*, suggesting that genetic susceptibility is at least partially accountable for either form of autoimmunity.

TOLERANCE AND AUTOIMMUNITY

Autoimmunity is defined as a breakdown in the immune system's ability to tolerate self. This might involve failures in the establishment of central as well as peripheral tolerance. As early as during thymic T-cell maturation, the expression of diabetogenic MHC class II molecules with a low affinity for self-peptides by the thymus epithelium might allow self-reactive T cells to escape into the periphery instead of being negatively selected *(169–171)*. This might occur in the BB rat, where a block in intrathymic T-cell maturation might allow positive, but not negative selection *(172)*. Intrinsic thymic defects or aberrant intrathymic cytokine expression could contribute to the expansion of an autoreactive T-cell population *(88,173,174)*. Accordingly, some groups have been able to show a restriction of the peripheral TCR-Vβ or TCR-Vα repertoire *(175–177)*, although these results contradict the findings of others *(124,178,179)*. Along with abnormalities in bone marrow precursor cells and thymocytes, there is also evidence for functional defects in mature T cells. NOD mouse and BB rat T cells are hyporesponsive to proliferative signals. For the NOD mouse, this phenotype has been linked to the diminished production of T-cells cytokines, such as IL-2 and IL-4, and a defect in intracellular signaling, possibly controlled by *idd4 (168)*.

Intrathymic injection or transplantation with islet cells *(69,180–182)* as well as neonatal tolerization with GAD65 *(125,126)* or insulin *(178)* prevented diabetes *(183)*. It has therefore been suggested that β-cell specific self-antigens may not be expressed or presented in sufficient amount in the thymus *(184,185)*. T cells may therefore not be exposed to these self determinants during intrathymic selection. Assuming that this scenario is a common feature also in nonautoimmunity-prone individuals, it is likely that these autoreactive T cells are controlled in the periphery. If peripheral regulation fails, autoimmunity develops. It has been implied that the amount of self-antigen present in the target tissue is important to initiate immunoregulatory responses *(186)*. Cytokines, such as IFN-γ and TNF, can upregulate MHC class II expression and may therefore lead to the presentation of self-peptides on the β cell and to the activation of T cells *(50)*. Inflammatory cytokines can also suppress antagonistic T-cell subsets, mainly of the Th2 subset, contributing to a dysfunctional immune regulation. In BB-DP rats, the *Lyp*-dependent, missing RT6$^+$ T-cell subset seems to regulate autoreactive T cells *(187,188)*, indicating that the identification of *Lyp* may help to understand why suppression of autoreactivity fails to develop.

Aberrant or missing expression of T-cell costimulatory signals can inhibit or induce the activation of a self-reactive cell population. In CD28-deficient or CTLA-4-Ig transgenic NOD mice, diabetes is accelerated *(189)*. CTLA-4 and CD28 regulate T-cell apoptosis, and their expression has been shown to be defective in the NOD mouse. *Idd5* in the NOD mouse is located on mouse chromosome 1, a locus that includes the genes for CTLA-4 and CD28. On the other hand, neonatal blockage of CD28-mediated costimulation prevents NOD mice from developing diabetes *(190)*. The coexpression of B7-1 together with LCMV-GP *(42)* or TNF-α *(191)* on β cells also induced diabetes.

THE TH1/TH2 MODEL AND THE "FAILURE OF IMMUNOREGULATION" THEORY

The Th1/Th2 paradigm has been extended in favor of the more recent hypothesis that a failure in immunosuppression or immunodysregulation leads to destructive autoimmunity. This theory is opposed to the previously discussed notion of the causal relationship between a failure in the establishment of central tolerance and autoimmunity. Under normal circumstances, inflammatory Th1 cells and the antagonistic Th2-cell subset maintain a steady-state equilibrium with the help of cytokines, such as paracrine and autocrine regulators. Several findings support the idea of Th1 cells mediating diabetes, including the presence of IFN-γ and IL-2 in islet lesions *(192,193)*, the induction of diabetes by transgenic expression of IFN-γ in the islets *(194)*, and the prevention of the disease by administration of anti IFN-γ antibodies *(195)*. IL-12, an activation factor for Th1 cells, accelerates diabetes *(196)*. It is much less clear whether Th2 cells serve to regulate/suppress a pending Th1 response. There are still controversial findings about the beneficial effect of Th2 cells or Th2-associated cytokines, such as Il-4 and IL-10, in the NOD mouse on diabetes development *(197–201)*. Essentially, the questions is whether Th2 cells are downregulated by an overgrown Th1 population because of selective stimulation of the latter by a specific antigen *(202,203)* shifting the cytokine profile to an increased IFN-γ/IL-4 *(179)* or IFN-γ/IL-10 ratio *(88)*, or whether an intrinsic defect prevents

Th2 cells from compensating the Th1 response. NOD mice show reduced secretion of IL-4 and IL-2 and have defective suppressor T-cell function *(197,204)*. NK-like thymocytes and peripheral NK cells are an important source for IL-4, which is required to initiate and stimulate Th2 development. Consequently, the absence or functional defects of NK cells have also been associated with diabetes in the NOD mouse *(205; see also* Chapters 1 and 2*)*.

There is also evidence for an age-related onset of immunodysregulation in NOD mice, which might account for the age-related onset of diabetes *(206)*. TNF-α *(207)* and lymphotoxin α/β *(208)* might both be critical for the development of diabetes owing to their ability to shape the autoreactive T-cell repertoire. TNF-α is a pleiotropic cytokine. It is involved in T- and B-cell development, and can maintain expression of tissue-specific homing receptors, such as MadCAM-1 and ICAM-1. In adult NOD mice, TNF-α administration prevents diabetes, whereas neonatal administration critically enhances autoimmunity (for a review, *see 208a*) pointing toward TNF as a critical factor for immune regulation. The level of endogenous TNF-α during the ontogeny might therefore be important for the regulation of autoimmunity.

Molecular Mimicry

Molecular mimicry has been defined as the three-dimensional structural homology between a nontolerized exogenous antigen and a tolerized antigen, by which T cells become activated and tolerance to the latter is broken. Predisposition can happen as early as in the thymus, where thymocytes might not be exposed to certain antigens owing to cryptic epitopes or to insufficient expression. Therefore, central tolerance cannot be established and the T-cells become activated in the periphery, for example, after an infection. Several stretches of amino acid sequences in GAD65 and insulin show sequence homology with virus antigens. The best example of homology is the Coxsackie virus antigen P2-C *(141)*. The exact sequence homology extend to six amino acids (PEVKEK). Human polyclonal antibodies against the homologous sequence react with both proteins *(209)*; thus, it is most likely that there are HLA class II restricted T-helper cell epitopes that contain the PEVKEK sequence *(210,211)*. Autoantibodies in IDDM, however, do not specifically react with both the P2-C-protein and with GAD65 *(212)*. The alternative approach to molecular mimicry is to compare sequences of peptides that are eluted from MHC class II molecules associated with IDDM. Preliminary data suggest that new types of proteins or antigens in viruses and bacteria may be identified. These approaches to study the role of autoantigens in IDDM are very important, since they may result in a targeted drug design to reduce immunological β-cell autoreactivity.

Allergy and Diet

Food can play an important role in the development of autoimmune diseases. This is most classically shown in enteropathic celiac disease, induced by the ingestion of wheat, rye, and barley *(213)*. The strong impact of diet on the development of diabetes in the animal models, especially the BB rat, has given rise to the notion that Type 1 diabetes is also induced by an allergy against food components. Wheat gluten *(214)* and soy protein *(215)* can trigger diabetes in the BB rat and in the NOD mouse. It is possible that presumably protein components are recognized as foreign by the immune system and trigger an immune response. A crossreactivity between food-derived and self-peptides has also been suggested. Regardless of the type of developing hypersensitivity reaction, the allergic reaction includes the activation of T cells and the release of inflammatory mediators, such as IgE and cytokines, such as IL-4, which act on body tissue and cause the clinical condition. Recent data have indicated that proinflammatory cells are reduced in BB rats that have been fed a nondiabetogenic diet on the bases of hydrolyzed casein *(153)*. Although the study of immunological consequences of diabetogenic food components needs to be extended, the American Academy of Pediatrics infant-feeding guidelines have already been reformulated since soybean extracts have proven as diabetogenic factors in animal diabetes models.

Prediction and Prevention of Diabetes

Owing to its high predictability in disease-prone animal models, diabetes development can be manipulated in the presymptomatic, preclinical, or postclinical phase. Some of these approaches are rather systemic and may describe the significance of a specific factor for the development of autoimmunity rather than offer a therapeutic strategy to treat human diabetes. NOD mice with transgenic MHC alleles *(216–220)*, transgenic immune receptors *(221)*, or cytokines that are expressed in the islets *(222,223)* do not develop diabetes and might fall into this category.

Immunotherapy and immunotargeting administered in the presymptomatic and preclinical phase might be more suitable for human application. However, it is difficult to define the preclinical phase in human diabetes, which is still an obstacle for the development of an effective prophylaxis, especially since there seems to be a time window in the prediabetic phase during which treatments, such as the administration of anti-TNF-α antibodies or CFA, are most protective. Both in the NOD mouse and in the BB rat, antibodies against MHC class II, CD4, or CD8 as well as the IL-2 receptor *(224–227)* or the chronic administration of cytokines, such as TNF-α *(228, 229)* and IL-2 *(230,231)*, can prevent diabetes. This was also achieved by administrating immunosuppressive agents, such as cyclosporin A *(232,233)* and FK 506, or immunostimulating substances, such as BCG and Complete Freund's Adjuvant (CFA) *(234–236)*. Chronic β-cell tolerance can be induced by injecting islet antigens into the thymus *(126)* or administration intranasally or orally to young diabetes-prone mice. Insulin and GAD have been studied particularly extensive and are primary candidates for immunotargeting in the preclinical state. Nicotinamide is being tried in randomized studies, based also on studies in BB rats and NOD mice.

Treatment of clinically overt diabetes can be achieved in NOD mice by the administration of monoclonal antibodies (MAbs) to T-cell-surface receptors, such as the TCR, CD4, or CD8. MAbs against CD4 or against intercellular adhesion molecule (ICAM) 1 and LFA-1 as well as antagonists for the IL-1 receptor inhibited the recurrence of diabetes after pancreas transplantation into diabetic animals *(237,238)*. Also, new substances, such as Linomide, are developed *(239)*, which may help to improve the success rate after transplantation of allo- or xenografts *(240,241)*. Finally, by transgenic expression of insulin in non-β cells, such as the proopiomelanocortin (POMC) expressing cells in the intermediate lobe of the pituitary, the serum insulin level could be restored *(242)*.

CONCLUSION AND FUTURE OUTLOOK

Using animal models for the study of human diseases ultimately has two major reasons: to identify immunopathogenic pathways and to develop therapeutic strategies to treat patients or high-risk individuals. Considering that each species differs in its genetic pool, environmental habitat, and behavior, it is still remarkable that there seem to be many similarities in the disease pathogenesis and its genetic background.

Both the BB rat and the NOD mouse have been very valuable in studying different pathogenic pathways of IDDM, although there are obvious differences between the two models. The restricted genetic background of diabetes in the BB rat facilitates the investigation of immunogenetic linkages, whereas research in the NOD mouse takes advantage of a vast array of well-established mouse immunogenetic techniques. Many questions about the pathogenesis of diabetes and ways to treat it are yet to be answered, but it has become clear that early therapy affecting or targeted to the immune system has the better chance to protect from developing diabetes. Successful cyclosporin therapy of BB rat diabetes *(243)* and prophylactic treatment of NOD mice with insulin or nicotinamide *(27)* have already provided the basis for ongoing human trials. Treatment with immunosuppressive agents, such as glucocorticoids *(244)*, cyclosporin A *(245–247)*, or plasmapheresis *(248)*, combined with iv γ-globulin has had some effect in preserving residual β-cell function in new-onset patients. Most immunosuppressive agents have been analyzed in numerous small, often open clinical trials conducted on newly diagnosed diabetic patients *(27,249)*. Recent efforts to modify the diabetogenic lymphocyte pool in young BB rats and NOD mice using a variety of immunization and tolerization protocols have produced promising results *(4,27)*. Classic procedures of plasmapheresis and cytopheresis, and a variety of other immunological approaches, such as T-cell receptor antibodies, soluble HLA class II molecules loaded with GAD peptides, GAD peptides competing with antigen presentation, oral vaccination, GAD65 vaccination, and many more are being considered. Although none of the currently available and tested therapeutic agents represent a prevention or cure for IDDM, animal research and the development of new technology may eventually open new ways for successful preventive strategies for human patients *(249; see also* Chapter 17*)*.

REFERENCES

1. Leiter E. The genetics of diabetes susceptibility in mice. FASEB J 1989;3:2231–2241.
2. Berggren P-O. (1993) New concepts in the pathogenesis of NIDDM, 2nd ed. In: Östenson C-G, ed. Toronto-Stockholm on Perspective in Diabetes Research: Adv Exp Med Biol. Plenum, New York, 1993, pp. 24–45.
3. Makino S, Kunimoto K, Muraoka Y, Mizushima Y, Katagiri K, Tochino Y. Breeding of a non-obese, diabetic strain of mice. Jikken Dobutsu 1980;29:1–13.
4. Crisá L, Mordes JP, Rossini, AA. Autoimmune diabetes mellitus in the BB rat. Diabetes Metab Rev 1992;8:9–37.
5. Pettersson A, Jacob H, Lernmark Å. Lessons from the animal models: the BB rat. In: Palmer JP, ed. Diabetes Prediction, Prevention and Genetic Counseling in IDDM. John Wiley, New York, 1996, pp. 182–200.
6. Velasquez MT, Kimmel PL, Michaelis OET. Animal models of spontaneous diabetic kidney disease. FASEB J 1990;4:2850–2859.
7. Nakhooda AF, Like AA, Chappel CI, Murray FT, Marliss EB. The spontaneously diabetic Wistar rat. Metabolic and morphologic studies. Diabetes 1977;26:100–112.
8. Guberski DL, Thomas VA, Shek WR, Like AA, Handler ES, Rossini AA, et al. Induction of type 1 diabetes by Kilham's rat virus in diabetes-resistant BB wor rats. Science 1991;254:1010–1013.
9. Field CJ. A diet producing a low diabetes incidence modifies immune abnormalities in diabetes-prone BB rats. J Nutr 1995;125:2595–2603.
10. Jacob H, Pettersson A, Wilson D, Lernmark Å, Lander ES. Genetic dissection of autoimmune type 1 diabetes in the BB rat. Nature Genet 1992;2:56–60.

11. Jackson R, Rassi N, Crump T, Haynes B, Eisenbarth GS. The BB diabetic rat. Profound T-cell lymphocytopenia. Diabetes 1981;30:887–889.
12. Colle E, Ono S, Fuks A, Guttman RD, Seemayer TA. Association of susceptibility to spontaneous diabetes in rat with genes of major histocompatibility complex. Diabetes 1988;37:1483–1486.
13. Markholst H, Andreasen B, Eastman S, Lernmark Å. Diabetes segregates as a single locus in crosses between inbred BB rats prone or resistant to diabetes. J Exp Med 1991;174:297–300.
14. Awata T, Guberski DL, Like AA. Genetics of the BB rat: Association of autoimmune disorders (diabetes, insulitis, and thyroiditis) with lymphopenia and major histocompatibility complex class II. Endocrinology 1995;136:5731–5735.
15. Pettersson A, Wilson D, Daniels T, Tobin S, Jacob JJ, Lander ES, et al. Thyroiditis in the BB rat is associated with lymphopenia but occurs independently of diabetes. J Autoimmunity 1995;8:493–505.
16. Like AA, Weringer EJ, Holdash A, McGill P, Atkinson D, Rossini AA. Adoptive transfer of autoimmune diabetes mellitus in Biobreeding/Worcester (BB/W) inbred and hybrid rats. J Immunol 1985;34: 1583–1586.
17. Whalen BJ, Griner DL, Mordes JP, Rossini AA. Adoptive transfer of autoimmune diabetes mellitus to athymic rats: synergy of CD4+ and CD8+ T cells and prevention of RT6+ T cells. J. Autoimmunity 1994;7:819–831.
18. Nepom BS, Nepom GT, Coleman M, Kwok WW. Critical contribution of beta chain residue 57 in peptide binding ability of both HLA-DR and -DQ molecules. Proc Natl Acad Sci USA 1996;33:7 202–7206.
19. Kawano K, Hirashima T, Mori S, Saitoh Y, Kurosumi M, Natori T. New inbred strain of Long-Evans Tokushima lean rats with IDDM without lymphopenia. Diabetes 1991;40:1375–1381.
20. Makino S, Kunimoto K, Muraoka Y, Mizushima Y, Katagiri K, Tochima Y. Breeding of non-obese diabetic strain of mice. Exp Anim 1980;29:1–13.
21. Tochino Y. The NOD mouse as a model of type 1 diabetes. Crit Rev Immunol 1987;1:49–81.
22. Bodansky HJ, Staines A, Stephenson C, Haigh D, Cartwright R. Evidence for an environmental effect in the aetiology of insulin dependent diabetes in a transmigratory population. Brit Med J 1992; 304:1020–1022.
23. Tochino Y. The NOD mouse as a model of type I diabetes. Crit Rev Immunol 1987;8:49–81.
24. Lo D, Burkly LC, Widera G, Cowing C, Flavell RA, Palmiter RD, et al. Diabetes and tolerance in transgenic mice expressing class II MHC molecules in pancreatic beta cells. Cell 1988;53:159–168.
25. Frankel BJ, Korsgren O, Andersson A. DNA replication in pancreatic islets and adrenals in diabetic Chinese hamsters. Horm Res 1993;39:67–72.
26. Palmer JP, Lernmark Å. Pathophysiology of type 1 (Insulin-Dependent) diabetes. In: Daniel Porte J, Sherwin RS, eds. Ellenberg and Rifkin's Diabetes Mellitus: Theory and Practice. Elsevier, Stamford, CT, 1996, pp. 455–486.
27. Bach JF. Insulin-dependent diabetes mellitus as an autoimmune disease. Endocrine Rev 1994;15: 516–542.
28. Jenson AB, Rosenberg HS, Notkins AL. Pancreatic islet-cell damage in children with fatal viral infections. Lancet 1980;ii:354–358.
29. Katz JD, Wang B, Haskins K, Benoist C, Mathis D. Following a diabetogenic T cell from genesis through pathogenesis. Cell 1993;74:1089–1100.
30. Shizuru JA, Sarvetnick N. Transgenic mice for the study of diabetes mellitus. Trends Endocrinol Metab 1991;2:97–104.
31. Lipes MA, Eisenbarth GS. Transgenic mouse models of type I diabetes. Diabetes 1990;39:879–884.
32. Hanahan D. Transgenic mouse models of self-tolerance and autoreactivity by the immune system. Annu Rev Cell Biol 1990;6:493–537.
33. Allison J, Campbell IL, Morahan G, Mandel TE, Harrison LC, Miller JFAP. Diabetes in transgenic mice resulting from over-expression of class I histocompatibility molecules in pancreatic β cells. Nature 1988;333:529–533.
34. Lo D, Burkly LC, Widera G. Diabetes and tolerance in transgenic mice expressing class II MHC molecules in pancreatic beta cells. Cell 1988;53:159–168.
35. Markmann J, Lo D, Naji A, Palmiter RD, Brinster RL, Heber-Katz E. Antigen presenting function of class II MHC expressing pancreatic beta cells. Nature 1988;336:476–479.
36. Bottazzo GF, Dean BM, McNally JM, MacKay EH, Swift PGF, Gamble DR. *In situ* characterization of autoimmune phenomena and expression of HLA molecules in the pancreas in diabetic insulitis. N Engl J Med 1985;313:353–360.

37. Homo-Delarche F, Fitzpatrick F, Christeff N, Nunez EA, Bach JF, Dardenne M. Sex steroids, glucocorticoids, stress and autoimmunity. J Steroid Biochem Mol Biol 1991;40:619–637.
38. Garchon HJ, Bedossa P, Eloy L, Bach JF. Identification and mapping to chromosome 1 of a susceptibility locus for periinsulitis in non-obese diabetic mice. Nature 1991;353:260–262.
39. Cand'eias S, Katz J, Benoist C, Mathis D, Haskins K. Islet-specific T-cell clones from nonobese diabetic mice express heterogeneous T-cell receptors. Proc Natl Acad Sci USA 1991;88:6167–6170.
40. Sarvetnick N, Liggitt D, Pitts SL, Hansen SE, Stewart TA. Insulin-dependent diabetes mellitus induced in transgenic mice by ectopic expression of class II MHC and interferon-gamma. Cell 1988;52:773–782.
41. Gonzalez A, Katz JD, Mattei MG, Kikutani H, Benoist C, Mathis D. Genetic control of diabetes progression. Immunity 1997;7:873–883.
42. von Herrath MG, Guerder S, Lewicki H, Flavell RA, Oldstone MB. Coexpression of B7-1 and viral ("self") transgenes in pancreatic beta cells can break peripheral ignorance and lead to spontaneous autoimmune diabetes. Immunity 1995;3:727–738.
43. Ohashi PS, Oehen S, Aichele P, Pircher H, Odermatt B, Herrera P, et al. Induction of diabetes is influenced by the infectious virus and local expression of MHC class I and tumor necrosis factor-alpha. J Immunol 1993;150:5185–5194.
44. Grodsky GM, Ma YH, Cullen B, Sarvetnick N. Effect on insulin production sorting and secretion by major histocompatibility complex class II gene expression in the pancreatic beta-cell of transgenic mice. Endocrinology 1992;131:933–938.
45. Elliott EA, Flavell RA. Transgenic mice expressing constitutive levels of IL-2 in islet beta cells develop diabetes. Int Immunol 1994;6:1629–1637.
46. Ehl S, Hombach J, Aichele P, Hengartner H, Zinkernagel RM. Bystander activation of cytotoxic T cells: studies on the mechanism and evaluation of in vivo significance in a transgenic mouse model. J Exp Med 1997;185:1241–1251.
47. Higuchi Y, Herrera P, Muniesa P, Huarte J, Belin D, Ohashi P, et al. Expression of a tumor necrosis factor alpha transgene in murine pancreatic beta cells results in severe and permanent insulitis without evolution towards diabetes. J Exp Med 1992;176:1719–1731.
48. von Herrath M, Holz A. Pathological changes in the islet milieu precede infiltration of islets and destruction of beta-cells by autoreactive lymphocytes in a transgenic model of virus-induced IDDM. J Autoimmunity 1997;10:231–238.
49. von Herrath MG, Homann D, Gairin JE, Oldstone MB. Pathogenesis and treatment of virus-induced autoimmune diabetes: novel insights gained from the RIP-LCMV transgenic mouse model. Biochem Soc Trans 1997;25:630–635.
50. von Herrath MG, Oldstone MB. Interferon-gamma is essential for destruction of beta cells and development of insulin-dependent diabetes mellitus. J Exp Med 1997;185:531–539.
51. Bonnevie-Nielsen V, Steffes MW, Lernmark Å. A major loss in islet mass and ß-cell function precedes hyperglycemia in mice given multiple low doses of streptozotocin. Diabetes 1981;30:424–429.
52. Like AA, Rossini AA. Streptozotocin-induced pancreatic insulitis: new model of diabetes mellitus. Science 1976;93:415–417.
53. Groot PC, Moen CJ, Dietrich W, Stoye JP, Lander ES, Demant P. The recombinant congenic strains for analysis of multigenic traits: genetic composition. FASEB J 1992;6:2826–2835.
54. Pipeleers D, Van De Winkel M. Pancreatic B cells possess defense mechanisms against cell-specific toxicity. Proc Natl Acad Sci USA 1986;83:5267–5271.
55. Uchigata Y, Yamamoto H, Nagai H, Okamoto H. Effect of poly(ADP-ribose) synthetase inhibitor administration to rats before and after injection of alloxan and streptozotocin on islet proinsulin synthesis. Diabetes 1983;32(4):316–318.
56. McAleer MA, Reifsnyder P, Palmer SM, Prochazka M, Love JM, Copeman JB, et al. Crosses of NOD mice with the related NON strain. A polygenic model for IDDM. Diabetes 1995;44:1186–1195.
57. Oehen S, Ohashi PS, Aichele P, Burki K, Hengartner H, Zinkernagel RM. Vaccination or tolerance to prevent diabetes. Eur J Immunol 1992;22:3149–3153.
58. Kagi D, Odermatt B, Ohashi PS, Zinkernagel RM, Hengartner H. Development of insulitis without diabetes in transgenic mice lacking perforin-dependent cytotoxicity. J Exp Med 1996;183:2143–152.
59. Degermann S, Reilly C, Scott B, Ogata L, von B-H, Lo D. On the various manifestations of spontaneous autoimmune diabetes in rodent models. Eur J Immunol 1994;24:3155–3160.
60. Herold KC, Baumann E, Vezys V, Buckingham F. Expression and immune response to islet antigens following treatment with low doses of streptozotocin in H-2d mice. J Autoimmunity 1997;10:17–25.

61. Herold KG, Lenschow DJ, Bluestone JA. CD28/B7 regulation of autoimmune diabetes. Immunol Res 1997;16:71–84.
62. Herold KC, Vezys V, Koons A, Lenschow D, Thompson C, Bluestone JA. CD28/B7 costimulation regulates autoimmune diabetes induced with multiple low doses of streptozotocin. J Immunol 1997; 58:984–991.
63. Grama D, Eriksson B, Martensson H, Cedermark B, Ahr'en B, Kristoffersson A, et al. Clinical characteristics, treatment and survival in patients with pancreatic tumors causing hormonal syndromes. World J Surg 1992;16:632–639.
64. Kiesel U, Freytag G, Biener J, Kolb H. Transfer of experimental autoimmune insulitis by spleen cells in mice. Diabetologia 1980;19:516–520.
65. Buschard K, Rygaard J. Passive transfer of streptozotocin induced diabetes mellitus with spleen cells. Acta Pathol Microbiol Scand 1977;85(C):469–472.
66. Mustafa MI, Diener P, Hojeberg B, Van der-Meide P, Olsson T. T cell immunity and interferon-gamma secretion during experimental allergic encephalomyelitis in Lewis rats. J Neuroimmunol 1991;31: 165–177.
67. Kendall MD. Functional anatomy of the thymic microenvironment. J Anat 1991;177:1–29.
68. Herold KC, Vezys V, Sun Q, Viktora D, Seung E, Reiner S, et al. Regulation of cytokine production during development of autoimmune diabetes induced with multiple low doses of streptozotocin. J Immunol 1996;156:3521–3527.
69. Baumann EE, Buckingham F, Herold KC. Intrathymic transplantation of islet antigen affects CD8+ diabetogenic T-cells resulting in tolerance to autoimmune IDDM. Diabetes 1995;44:871–877.
70. Herold KC, Bloch TN, Vezys V, Sun Q. Diabetes induced with low doses of streptozotocin is mediated by V beta 8.2+ T-cells. Diabetes 1995;44:354–359.
71. Pont A, Rubino JM, Bishop D, Peal R. Diabetes mellitus and neuropathy following Vacor ingestion in man. Arch Intern Med 1979;39:185–187.
72. Herold KC, Vezys V, Gage A, Montag AG. Prevention of autoimmune diabetes by treatment with anti-LFA-1 and anti-ICAM-1 monoclonal antibodies. Cell Immunol 1994;57:489–500.
73. Yoon J-W, Austin M, Onodera T, Notkins AL. Isolation of a virus from the pancreas of a child with diabetic ketoacidosis. N Engl J Med 1975;300:1174–1179.
74. Ferner RE, Antsiferov ML, Kelman AW, Alberti KG, Rawlins MD. The relationships between dose and concentration of tolbutamide and insulin and glucose responses in patients with non-insulin-dependent diabetes. Eur J Clin Pharmacol 1991;40:163–168.
75. Serreze DV, Prochazka M, Reifsnyder PC, Bridgett MM, Leiter EH. Use of recombinant congenic and congenic strains of NOD mice to identify a new insulin-dependent diabetes resistance gene. J Exp Med 1994;180:1553–1558.
76. Wilander E. Streptozotocin-diabetes in the Chinese hamster. Long-term effects on the light microscopic structure of the pancreatic islet tissue, liver and kidney. Acta Pathol Microbiol Scand A 1974; 82:767–776.
77. Mauer SM, Sutherland DE, Steffes MW, Lee CS, Najarian JS, Brown DM. Effects of kidney and pancreas transplantation on streptozotocin-induced malignant kidney tumors in rats. Cancer Res 1974; 34:1643–1645.
78. Pitkin RM, Van Orden DE. Fetal effects of maternal streptozotocin-diabetes. Endocrinology 1974;94:1247–1253.
79. Hoftiezer V, Carpenter AM. Comparison of streptozotocin and alloxan-induced diabetes in the rat, including volumetric quantitation of the pancreatic islets. Diabetologia 1973;9:178–184.
80. Schein PS, Rakieten N, Cooney DA, Davis R, Vernon ML. Streptozotocin diabetes in monkeys and dogs, and its prevention by nicotinamide. Proc Soc Exp Biol Med 1973;143:514–518.
81. McClive PJ, Baxter AG, Morahan G. Genetic polymorphisms of the non-obese diabetic (NOD) mouse. Immunol Cell Biol 1994;72:137–142.
82. Zouali H, Vaxillaire M, Lesage S, Sun F, Velho G, Vionnet N, et al. Linkage analysis and molecular scanning of glucokinase gene in NIDDM families. Diabetes 1993;42:1238–1245.
83. Aanstot HJ, Kang SM, Kim J, Lindsay LA, Roll U, Knip M, et al. Identification and characterization of glima 38, a glycosylated islet cell membrane antigen, which together with GAD(65) and IA2 marks the early phases of autoimmune response in type 1 diabetes. J Clin Invest 1996;97:2772–2783.
84. Adamus G, Aptsiauri N, Guy J, Heckenlively J, Flannery J, Hargrave PA. The occurrence of serum autoantibodies against enolase in cancer-associated retinopathy. Clin Immunol Immunopathol 1996; 78:120–129.

85. Colle E, Guttmann RD, Seemayer TA, Michel F. Spontaneous diabetes mellitus syndrome in the rat. IV. Immunogenetic interactions of MHC and non-MHC components of the syndrome. Metabolism 1983;32:54–61.
86. Agardh D, Gaur LK, Agardh E, Landin-Olsson M, Agardh C-D, Lernmark Å. HLA-DQB1*0201/0302 is associated with severe retinopathy in patients with insulin-dependent diabetes mellitus. Diabetologia 1996;39:1313–1317.
87. Bellgrau D, Lagarde C. Cytotoxic T-cell precursors with low-level CD8 in the diabetes-prone biobreeding rat: Implications for generation of an autoimmune T-cell repertoire. Proc Natl Acad Sci USA 1990;87:313–317.
88. Bieg S, Moller C, Olsson T, Lernmark A. The lymphopenia (lyp) gene controls the intrathymic cytokine ratio in congenic BioBreeding rats. Diabetologia 1997;40:786–792.
89. Podolin PL, Denny P, Lord CJ, Hill NJ, Todd JA, Peterson LB, et al. Congenic mapping of the insulin-dependent diabetes (Idd) gene, Idd10, localizes two genes mediating the Idd10 effect and eliminates the candidate Fcgr1. J Immunol 1997;159:1835–1843.
90. Wicker LS, Todd JA, Peterson LB. Genetic control of autoimmune diabetes in the NOD mouse. Annu Rev Immunol 1995;13:179–200.
91. Todd JA. Genetic analysis of susceptibility to type 1 diabetes. Springer Semin Immunopathol 1992;14:33–58.
92. Hattori M, Buse JB, Jackson RA, Glimcher L, Dorf ME, Minami M, et al. The NOD mouse: recessive gene in the major histocompatibility complex. Science 1986;231:733–735.
93. Alexander DP, Britton HG, Cohen NM, Mashiter K, Nixon DA, Smith FG, Jr. Streptozotocin induced diabetes in the newborn lamb. Biol Neonate 1971;17:381–393.
94. Ghosh S, Palmer SM, Rodrigues NR, Cordell HJ, Hearne CM, Cornall RJ, et al. Polygenic control of autoimmune diabetes in nonobese diabetic mice. Nature Genet 1993;4:404–409.
95. Brashear HR, Caccamo DV, Heck A, Keeney PM. Localization of antibody in the central nervous system of a patient with paraneoplastic encephalomyeloneuritis. Neurology 1991;41:1583–1587.
96. Pitkin RM, Reynolds WA. Diabetogenic effects of streptozotocin in rhesus monkeys. Diabetes 1970;19:85–90.
97. Golob EK, Rishi S, Becker KL, Moore C, Shah N. Effect of streptozotocin-induced diabetes on pancreatic insulin content of the fetus. Diabetes 1970;19:610–613.
98. Junod A, Lambert AE, Stauffacher W, Renold AE. Diabetogenic action of streptozotocin: relationship of dose to metabolic response. J Clin Invest 1969;48:2129–2139.
98a. Scott FW. Food-induced type 1 diabetes in the BB rat. Diabetes/Metabolism Rev 1996;12:341–359.
98b. Kloting I, Voigt B, Kov'acs P. Metabolic features of newly established congenic diabetes-prone BB.SHR rat strains. Life Sci 1998;62:973–979.
99. Logothetopoulos J, Valiquette N, Madura E, Cvet D. The onset of the progression of pancreatic insulitis in the overt, spontaneously diabetic, young adult BB rat studied by pancreatic biopsy. Diabetes 1984;33:33–36.
100. Walker R, Bone A, Cooke A, Baird J. Distinct macrophage subpopulations in pancreas of prediabetic BB/E rats. Diabetes 1988;37:1301–1304.
101. Huang X, Hultgren B, Dybdal N, Stewart TA. Islet expression of interferon-alpha precedes diabetes in both the BB rat and streptozotocin-treated mice. Immunity 1994;1:469–478.
102. Bass J, Kurose T, Pashmforoush M, Steiner DF. Fusion of insulin receptor ectodomains to immunoglobulin constant domains reproduces high-affinity insulin binding in vitro. J Biol Chem 1996;271:19,367–19,375.
103. Rabinovitch A. Immunoregulatory and cytokine imbalances in the pathogenesis of IDDM. Therapeutic intervention by immunostimulation? Diabetes 1994;43:613–621.
104. Bazan NG, Rodriguez-de-Turco EB. Platelet-activating factor is a synapse messenger and a modulator of gene expression in the nervous system. Neurochem Int 1995;26:435–441.
105. Björk E, Kämpe O, Karlsson FA, Pipeleers DG, Andersson A, Hellerström C, et al. Glucose regulation of the autoantigen GAD_{65} in human pancreatic islets. J. Clin Endocrinol Metab 1992;75:1574–1576.
106. Dyrberg T. Humoral autoimmunity in the pathogenesis of insulin-dependent diabetes mellitus. Studies in the spontaneously diabetic BB rat. Acta Endocrinol Suppl Copenh 1986;280:1–29.
107. Pipeleers D, Van de Winkel M, Dyrberg T, Lernmark A. Spontaneously diabetic BB rats have age-dependent islet beta-cell-specific surface antibodies at clinical onset. Diabetes 1987;36:1111–1115.
108. Pipeleers DG, In't Veld PA, Pipeleers-Marichal MA, Gepts W, van de Winkel M. Presence of pancreatic hormones in islet cells with MHC-class II antigen expression. Diabetes 1987;36:872–876.

109. Pipeleers D. The biosociology of pancreatic B cells. Diabetologia 1987;30:277–291.
110. Reddy S, Bibby N, Elliott RB. Longitudinal study of islet cell antibodies and insulin autoantibodies and development of diabetes in non-obese diabetic (NOD) mice. Clin Exp Immunol 1990;81:400–405.
111. Martignat L, Elmansour A, Audrain M, Julien JF, Charbonnel B, Sai P. Pancreatic expression of antigens for islet cell antibodies in non-obese diabetic mice. J Autoimmunity 1995;8:465–482.
112. Nayak RC, Omar MAK, Rabizadeh A, Srikanta S, Eisenbarth GS. "Cytoplasmic" islet cell antibodies. Evidence that the target antigen is a sialoglycoconjugate. Diabetes 1985;34:617–619.
113. Bain SC, Bennett AH, Todd JA. The British Diabetic Association Warren Repository. Autoimmunity 1990;7:83–85.
114. Bain SC, Rowe BR, Barnett AH, Todd JA. Parental origin of diabetes-associated HLA types in sibling pairs with type I diabetes. Diabetes 1994;43:1462–1468.
115. Baekkeskov S, Dyrberg T, Lernmark Å. Autoantibodies to a 64-kilodalton islet cell protein precede the onset of spontaneous diabetes in the BB rat. Science 1984;224:1348–1350.
116. Bingley PJ. Interactions of age, islet cell antibodies, insulin autoantibodies, and first-phase insulin response in predicting risk of progression to IDDM in ICA(+) relatives: The ICARUS data set. Diabetes 1996;45:1720–1728.
117. Björk E, Kampe O, Andersson A, Karlsson FA. Expression of the 64 kDa/glutamic acid decarboxylase rat islet cell autoantigen is influenced by the rate of insulin secretion. Diabetologia 1992;35:490–493.
118. Brosky G, Logothetopoulos J. Streptozotocin diabetes in the mouse and guinea pig. Diabetes 1969;18:606–611.
119. Bell GI, Pilkis SJ, Weber IT, Polonsky KS. Glucokinase mutations, insulin secretion, and diabetes mellitus. Annu Rev Physiol 1996;58:171–186.
120. Whalen BJ, Rossini AA, Mordes JP, Greiner DL. DR-BB rat thymus contains thymocyte populations predisposed to autoreactivity. Diabetes 1995;44:963–967.
121. Ellerman KE, Richards CA, Guberski DL, Shek WR, Like AA. Kilham rat triggers T-cell-dependent autoimmune diabetes in multiple strains of rat. Diabetes 1996;45:557–562.
122. Bellgrau D, Redd JM, Sellins KS. Peculiar T-cell signaling does not preclude positive selection in the diabetes-prone BB rat. Diabetes 1994;43:47–52.
123. Like AA, Rossini AA. Streptozotocin-induced pancreatic insulitis: new model of diabetes mellitus. Science 1976;193:415–417.
124. Haskins K, Portas M, Bergman B, Lafferty K, Bradley B. Pancreatic islet-specific T-cell clones from nonobese diabetic mice. Proc Natl Acac Sci USA 1989;86:8000–8004.
125. Kaufman DL, Clare-Salzler M, Tian J, Forsthuber T, Ting GSP, Robinson P, et al. Spontaneous loss of T-cell tolerance to glutamic acid decarboxylase in murine insulin-dependent diabetes. Nature 1993;366:69–72.
126. Tisch R, Yang X-D, Singer SM, Liblau RS, Fugger L, McDevitt HO. Immune response to glutamic acid decarboxylase correlates with insulitis in non-obese diabetic mice. Nature 1993;366:72–75.
127. Wegmann DR, Gill RG, Daniel D. The role of insulin-specific T cells in IDDM in NOD mice. 13th Immunology and Diabetes Workshop. Montvillargenne, France, 1994, p. 12.
128. Blue ML, Shin SI. Diabetes induction by subdiabetogenic doses of streptozotocin in BALB/cBOM mice. Noninvolvement of host B-lymphocyte functions. Diabetes 1984;33:105–110.
129. Nakhoda A, Wong HA. The induction of diabetes in rats by intramuscular administration of streptozotocin. Experientia 1979;35:1679–1680.
130. Lee DS, Tian J, Phan T, Kaufman DL. Cloning and sequence analysis of a murine cDNA encoding glutamate decarboxylase (GAD65). Biochim. Biophys. Acta 1993;1216:157–160.
131. Ferner RE. Drug-induced diabetes. Baillieres Clin Endocrinol Metab 1992;6:849–866.
132. Wilson GL, Leiter EH. Streptozotocin interactions with pancreatic beta cells and the induction of insulin-dependent diabetes. Curr Top Microbiol Immunol 1990;156:27–54.
133. Bae YS, Eun HM, Yoon JW. Genomic differences between the diabetogenic and nondiabetogenic variants of encephalomyocarditis virus. Virology 1989;170:282–287.
134. Onodera T, Ray UR, Melez KA, Suzuki H, Toniolo A, Notkins AL. Virus-induced diabetes mellitus. Autoimmunity and polyendocrine disease prevented by immunosuppression. Nature 1982;297:66–68.
135. Yoon JW, Morishima T, McClintock PR, Austin M, Notkins AL. Virus-induced diabetes mellitus: mengovirus infects pancreatic beta cells in strains of mice resistant to the diabetogenic effect of encephalomyocarditis virus. J Virol 1984;50:684–690.
136. Rayfield EJ, Kelly KJ, Yoon J.-W. Rubella virus-induced diabetes in the hamster. Diabetes 1986;35:1278–1281.

137. Hermitte L, Vialettes B, Naquet P, Atlan C, Payan MJ, Vague P. Paradoxical lessening of autoimmune processes in non-obese diabetic mice after infection with the diabetogenic variant of encephalomyocarditis virus. Eur J Immunol 1990;20:1297–1303.
138. von Herrath MG, Evans CF, Horwitz MS, Oldstone MB. Using transgenic mouse models to dissect the pathogenesis of virus-induced autoimmune disorders of the islets of Langerhans and the central nervous system. Immunol Rev 1996;152:111–143.
139. Gaskins HR, Prochazka M, Hamaguchi K, Serreze DV, Leiter EH. Beta cell expression of endogenous xenotropic retrovirus distinguishes diabetes-susceptible NOD/Lt from resistant NON/Lt mice. J Clin Invest 1992;90:2220–2227.
140. Yoon JW. Induction and prevention of type 1 diabetes mellitus by viruses. Diabetes Metab 1992;18: 378–386.
141. Kaufman DJ, Erlander MG, Clare-Salzler M, Atkinson MA, Maclaren NK, Tobin AJ. Autoimmunity to two forms of glutamate decarboxylase in Insulin-dependent diabetes mellitus. J Clin Invest 1992; 89:283–292.
142. Oldstone MB, Ahmed R, Salvato M. Viruses as therapeutic agents. II. Viral reassortants map prevention of insulin-dependent diabetes mellitus to the small RNA of lymphocytic choriomeningitis virus. J Exp Med 1990;171:2091–2100.
143. Oldstone MB. Viruses as therapeutic agents. I. Treatment of nonobese insulin-dependent diabetes mice with virus prevents insulin-dependent diabetes mellitus while maintaining general immune competence. J Exp Med 1990;171:2077–2089.
144. Dyrberg T, Schwimmbeck PL, Oldstone MBA. Inhibition of diabetes in BB rats by virus infection. J Clin Invest 1988;81:928–931.
145. Wilberz S, Partke HJ, Dagnaes H-F, Herberg L. Persistent MHV (mouse hepatitis virus) infection reduces the incidence of diabetes mellitus in non-obese diabetic mice. Diabetologia 1991;34:2–5.
146. Takei I, Asaba Y, Kasatani T, Maruyama T, Watanabe K, Yanagawa T, et al. Suppression of development of diabetes in NOD mice by lactate dehydrogenase virus infection. J Autoimmunity 1992;5:665–673.
147. Like AA, Guberski DL, Butler L. Influence of environmental viral agents on frequency and tempo of diabetes mellitus in BB/wor rats. Diabetes 1991;40:259–262.
148. Kawamura T, Nagata M, Utsugi T, Yoon JW. Prevention of autoimmune type I diabetes by CD4+ suppressor T cells in superantigen-treated non-obese diabetic mice. J Immunol 1993;151:4362–4370.
149. McDuffie M, Ostrowska A. Superantigen-like effects and incidence of diabetes in NOD mice. Diabetes 1993;42:1094–1098.
150. Radons J, Burkart V, Kolb H. MHC class II-dependent abnormal reactivity toward bacterial superantigens in immune cells of NOD mice. Diabetes 1997;46:379–385.
151. Elliott RB, Martin JM. Dietary protein: a trigger of insulin dependent diabetes in the BB rat? Diabetologia 1984;26:297–299.
152. Lefkowith J, Schreiner G, Cormier J, Handler ES, Driscoll HK, Greiner D, et al. Prevention of diabetes in the BB rat by essential fatty acid deficiency. Relationship between physiological and biochemical changes. J Exp Med 1990;171:729–743.
153. Scott FW, Cloutier HE, Kleemann R, Woerz P-U, Rowsell P, Modler HW, et al. Potential mechanisms by which certain foods promote or inhibit the development of spontaneous diabetes in BB rats: dose, timing, early effect on islet area, and switch in infiltrate from Th1 to Th2 cells. Diabetes 1997;46: 589–598.
154. Li XB, Scott FW, Park YH, Yoon JW. Low incidence of autoimmune type I diabetes in BB rats fed a hydrolysed casein-based diet associated with early inhibition of non-macrophage-dependent hyperexpression of MHC class I molecules on beta cells [see comments]. Diabetologia 1995;38:1138–1147.
155. Karjalainen J, Martin JM, Knip M, Ilonen J, Robinson BH, Savilathi E, et al. A bovine albumin peptide as a possible trigger of insulin-dependent diabetes mellitus. N Engl J Med 1992;327:302–307.
156. Paxson JA, Weber JG, Kulczyck, A Jr. Cow's milk-free diet does not prevent diabetes in NOD mice. Diabetes 1997;46:1711–1717.
157. Malkani S, Nompleggi D, Hansen JW, Greiner DL, Mordes JP, Rossini AA. Dietary cow's milk protein does not alter the frequency of diabetes in the BB rat. Diabetes 1997;46:1133–1140.
158. Lehman CD, Rodin J, McEwen B, Brinton R. Impact of environmental stress on the expression of insulin-dependent diabetes mellitus. Behav Neurosci 1991;105:241–245.
159. Saravia-Fernandez F, Durant S, el Hasnaoui A, Dardenne M, Homo-Delarche F. Environmental and experimental procedures leading to variations in the incidence of diabetes in the nonobese diabetic (NOD) mouse. Autoimmunity 1996;24:113–121.

160. Amrani A, Chaouloff F, Mormede P, Dardenne M, Homo-Delarche F. Glucose, insulin, and open field responses to immobilization in nonobese diabetic (NOD) mice. Physiol Behav 1994;56:241–246.
161. Durant S, Coulaud J, Amrani A, el-Hasnaoui A, Dardenne M, Homo-Delarche F. Effects of various environmental stress paradigms and adrenalectomy on the expression of autoimmune type 1 diabetes in the non-obese diabetic (NOD) mouse. J Autoimmunity 1993;6:735–751.
162. Utsugi T, Yoon JW, Park BJ, Imamura M, Averill N, Kawazu S, et al. Major histocompatibility complex class I-restricted infiltration and destruction of pancreatic islets by NOD mouse-derived beta-cell cytotoxic CD8+ T-cell clones in vivo. Diabetes 1996;45:1121–1131.
163. Nagata M, Santamaria P, Kawamura T, Utsugi T, Yoon JW. Evidence for the role of CD8+ cytotoxic T cells in the destruction of pancreatic beta-cells in nonobese diabetic mice. J Immunol 1994;152:2042–2050.
164. Wicker LS, Leiter EH, Todd JA, Renjilian RJ, Peterson E, Fischer PA, et al. Beta 2-microglobulin-deficient NOD mice do not develop insulitis or diabetes. Diabetes 1994;43:500–504.
165. Markmann JF, Bassiri H, Desai NM, Odorico JS, Kim JI, Koller BH, et al. Indefinite survival of MHC class I-deficient murine pancreatic islet allografts. Transplantation 1992;54:1085–1089.
166. Gazda LS, Gilchrist KA, Lafferty KJ. Autoimmune diabetes: caught in the causality trap? Immunol Cell Biol 1995;73:549–551.
167. Cameron MJ, Arreaza GA, Delovitch TL. Cytokine- and costimulation-mediated therapy of IDDM. Crit Rev Immunol 1997;17:537–544.
168. Gill BM, Jaramillo A, Ma L, Laupland KB, Delovitch TL. Genetic linkage of thymic T-cell proliferative unresponsiveness to mouse chromosome 11 in NOD mice. A possible role for chemokine genes. Diabetes 1995;44:614–619.
169. Serreze DV. Autoimmune diabetes results from genetic defects manifest by antigen presenting cells. FASEB J 1993;7:1092–1096.
170. Serreze DV, Gaskins HR, Leiter EH. Defects in the differentiation and function of antigen presenting cells in NOD/Lt mice. J Immunol 1993;150:2534–2543.
171. Carrasco M-E, Shimizu J, Kanagawa O, Unanue ER. The class II MHC I-Ag7 molecules from non-obese diabetic mice are poor peptide binders. J Immunol 1996;156:450–458.
172. Bellgrau D, Stenger D, Richards C, Bao F. The diabetic BB rat. Neither Th1 nor Th2? Horm Metab Res 1996;28:299–301.
173. Savino W, Boitard C, Bach JF, Dardenne M. Studies on the thymus in nonobese diabetic mouse. I. Changes in the microenvironmental compartments. Lab Invest 1991;64:405–417.
174. Tullin S, Farris P, Petersen JS, Hornum L, Jackerott M, Markholst H. A pronounced thymic B cell deficiency in the spontaneously diabetic BB rat. J Immunol 1997;158:5554–5559.
175. Gold D, Bellgrau D. Identification of a limited T-cell receptor b chain variable region repertoire associated with diabetes in the BB rat. Proc Natl Acad Sci USA 1991;88:9888–9891.
176. Simone EA, Yu L, Wegmann DR, Eisenbarth GS. T cell receptor gene polymorphisms associated with anti-insulin, autoimmune T cells in diabetes-prone NOD mice. J Autoimmunity 1997;10:317–321.
177. Komagata Y, Masuko K, Tashiro F, Kato T, Ikuta K, Nishioka K, et al. Clonal prevalence of T cells infiltrating into the pancreas of prediabetic non-obese diabetic mice. Int Immunol 1996;8:807–814.
178. Daniel D, Wegmann DR. Protection of nonobese diabetic mice from diabetes by intranasal or subcutaneous administration of insulin peptide B-(9-23). Proc Natl Acad Sci USA 1996;93:956–960.
179. Fox CJ, Danska JS. IL-4 expression at the onset of islet inflammation predicts nondestructive insulitis in nonobese diabetic mice. J Immunol 1997;158:2414–2424.
180. Gerling IC, Atkinson MA, Leiter EH. The thymus as a site for evaluating the potency of candidate beta cell autoantigens in NOD mice. J Autoimmunity 1994;7:851–858.
181. Posselt AM, Barker CF, Friedman AL, Naji A. Prevention of autoimmune diabetes in the BB rat by intrathymic islet transplantation at birth. Science 1992;256:1321–1324.
182. Herold KC, Montag AG, Buckingham F. Induction of tolerance to autoimmune diabetes with islet antigens. J Exp Med 1992;176:1107–1114.
183. Cetkovic C-M, Gerling IC, Muir A, Atkinson MA, Elliot JF, Leiter EH. Retardation or acceleration of diabetes in NOD/Lt mice mediated by intrathymic administration of candidate beta-cell antigens. Diabetes 1997;46:1975–1982.
184. Charlton B, Taylor E-C, Tisch R, Fathman CG. Prevention of diabetes and insulitis by neonatal intrathymic islet administration in NOD mice. J Autoimmunity 1994;7:549–560.
185. Egwuagu CE, Charukamnoetkanok P, Gery I. Thymic expression of autoantigens correlates with resistance to autoimmune disease. J Immunol 1997;159:3109–3112.

186. Akkaraju S, Ho WY, Leong D, Canaan K, Davis MM, Goodnow CC. A range of CD4 T cell tolerance: partial inactivation to organ-specific antigen allows nondestructive thyroiditis or insulitis. Immunity 1997;7:255–271.
187. Greiner DL, Mordes JP, Handler ES, Angelillo M, Nakamura N, Rossini AA. Depletion of RT6.1+ T lymphocytes induces diabetes in resistant BioBreeding/Worcester (BB/W) rats. J Exp Med 1987; 166:461–475.
188. Rossini AA, Faustman D, Woda BA, Like AA, Szymanski I, Mordes JP. Lymphocyte transfusions prevent diabetes in the Bio-Breeding/Worcester rat. J Clin Invest 1984;74:39–46.
189. Lenschow DJ, Herold K. C, Rhee L, Patel B, Koons A, Qin HY, et al. CD28/B7 regulation of Th1 and Th2 subsets in the development of autoimmune diabetes. Immunity 1996;5:285–293.
190. Arreaza GA, Cameron MJ, Jaramillo A, Gill BM, Hardy D, Laupland KB, et al. Neonatal activation of CD28 signaling overcomes T cell anergy and preve:nts autoimmune diabetes by an IL-4-dependent mechanism. J Clin Invest 1997;100:2243–2253.
191. Guerder S, Picarella DE, Linsley PS, Flavell RA. Costimulator B7-1 confers antigen-presenting-cell function to parenchymal tissue and in conjunction with tumor necrosis factor alpha leads to auto-immunity in transgenic mice. Proc Natl Acad Sci USA 1994;91:5138–5142.
192. Kolb H, Worz P-U, Kleemann R, Rothe H, Rowsell P, Scott FW. Cytokine gene expression in the BB rat pancreas: natural course and impact of bacterial vaccines. Diabetologia 1996;39:1448–1454.
193. Faulkner J-BE, Dempsey C-M, Mandel TE, Harrison LC. Both TH1 and TH2 cytokine mRNAs are expressed in the NOD mouse pancreas in vivo. Autoimmunity 1996;23:99–110.
194. Sarvetnick N, Shizuru J, Liggitt D, Martin L, McIntyre B, Gregory A, et al. Loss of pancreatic islet tolerance induced by β-cell expression of interferon-gamma. Nature 1990;346:844–847.
195. Debray S-M, Carnaud C, Boitard C, Cohen H, Gresser I, Bedossa P, et al. Prevention of diabetes in NOD mice treated with antibody to murine IFN gamma. J Autoimmunity 1991;4:237–248.
196. Trembleau S, Germann T, Gately MK, Adorini L. The role of IL-12 in the induction of organ-specific autoimmune diseases. Immunol Today 1995;16:383–386.
197. Rapoport MJ, Jaramillo A, Zipris D, Lazarus AH, Serreze DV, Leiter EH, et al. Interleukin 4 reverses T cell proliferative unresponsiveness and prevents the onset of diabetes in nonobese diabetic mice. J Exp Med 1993;178:87–99.
198. Mueller R, Krahl T, Sarvetnick N. Pancreatic expression of interleukin-4 abrogates insulitis and autoimmune diabetes in nonobese diabetic (NOD) mice. J Exp Med 1996;184:1093–1099.
199. Hancock WW, Polanski M, Zhang J, Blogg N, Weiner HL. Suppression of insulitis in non-obese diabetic (NOD) mice by oral insulin administration is associated with selective expression of interleukin-4 and -10, transforming growth factor-beta, and prostaglandin-E. Am J Pathol 1995;147:1193–1199.
200. Wogensen L, Lee MS, Sarvetnick N. Production of interleukin 10 by islet cells accelerates immune-mediated destruction of beta cells in nonobese diabetic mice. J Exp Med 1994;94:1379–1384.
201. Pakala SV, Kurrer MO, Katz JD. T helper 2 (Th2) T cells induce acute pancreatitis and diabetes in immune-compromised nonobese diabetic (NOD) mice. J Exp Med 1997;186:299–306.
202. Wegmann DR, Gill RG, Norbury G-M, Schloot N, Daniel D. Analysis of the spontaneous T cell response to insulin in NOD mice. J Autoimmunity 1994;7:833–843.
203. Haskins K, Wegmann D. Diabetogenic T-cell clones. Diabetes 1996;45, 1299–1305.
204. Bergerot I, Arreaza G, Cameron M, Chou H, Delovitch TL. Role of T-cell anergy and suppression in susceptibility to IDDM. Res Immunol 148:348–358.
205. Bach, JF, Mathis, D. (1997) The NOD mouse. Res Immunol 1997;148:285,286.
206. Delovitch TL, Singh B. The nonobese diabetic mouse as a model of autoimmune diabetes: immune dysregulation gets the NOD. Immunity 1997;7:727–738.
207. Pasparakis M, Alexopoulou L, Douni E, Kollias G. Tumour necrosis factors in immune regulation: everything that's interesting is...new! Cytokine Growth Factor Rev 1996;7:223–229.
208. Matsumoto M, Mariathasan S, Nahm MH, Baranyay F, Peschon JJ, Chaplin DD. Role of lymphotoxin and the type 1 TNF receptor in the formation of germinal centers. Science 1996;271:1289–1291.
208a. Cope A, Ettinger R, McDevitt H. The role of TNF alpha and related cytokines in the development and function of the autoreactive T-cell repertoire. Res Immunol 1997;148:307–312.
209. Hou J, Said C, Franchi D, Dockstader P, Chatterjee NK. Antibodies to glutamic acid decarboxylase and P2-C peptides in sera from Coxsackie virus B4-infected mice and IDDM patients. Diabetes 1994; 43:1260–1266.
210. Orchard TJ. From diagnosis and classification to complications and therapy. DCCT. Part II? Diabetes control and complications trial. Diabetes Care 1994;17:326–338.

211. Landgraf-Leurs MM, Drummer C, Froschl H, Steinhuber R, Von Schacky C, Landgraf R. Pilot study on omega-3 fatty acids in type I diabetes mellitus. Diabetes 1990;39:369–75.
212. Richter W, Mertens T, Schoel B, Muir P, Ritzkowsky A, Scherbaum WA, et al. Sequence homology of the disease-associated autoantigen glutamate decarboxylase with Coxsackie B4-2C protein and heat shock protein 60 mediates no molecular mimicry of autoantibodies. J Exp Med 1994;180:721–726.
213. Sturgess R, Day P, Ellis HJ, Lundin K. E, Gjertsen HA, Kontakou M, et al. Wheat peptide challenge in coeliac disease. Lancet 1994;343:758–761.
214. Scott B, Liblau R, Degermann S, Marconi LA, Ogata L, Caton AJ, et al. A role for non-MHC genetic polymorphism in susceptibility to spontaneous autoimmunity. Immunity 1994;1:73–83.
215. Hoorfar J, Scott FW, Cloutier HE. Dietary plant materials and development of diabetes in the BB rat. J Nutr 1991;121:908–916.
216. Hutchings P, Tonks P, Cooke A. Effect of MHC transgene expression on spontaneous insulin autoantibody class switch in nonobese diabetic mice. Diabetes 1997;46:779–784.
217. Hanson MS, Cetkovic C-M, Ramiya VK, Atkinson MA, Maclaren NK, Singh B, et al. Quantitative thresholds of MHC class II I-E expressed on hemopoietically derived antigen-presenting cells in transgenic NOD/Lt mice determine level of diabetes resistance and indicate mechanism of protection. J Immunol 1996;157:1279–1287.
218. Quartey-Papafio R, Lund T, Chandler P, Picard J, Ozegbe P, Day S, et al. Aspartate at position 57 of nonobese diabetic I-Ag7 beta-chain diminishes the spontaneous incidence of insulin-dependent diabetes mellitus. J Immunol 1995;154:5567–5575.
219. Serjeantson S, Theophilus J, Zimmet P, Court J, Crossley JR, Elliott RB. Lymphocytotoxic antibodies and histocompatibility antigens in juvenile-onset diabetes mellitus. Diabetes 1981;30:26–29.
220. Serreze DV, Leiter EH, Christianson GJ, Greiner D, Roopenian DC. Major histocompatibility complex class I-deficient NOD-B2mnull mice are diabetes and insulitis resistant. Diabetes 1994;43:505–509.
221. Chervonsky AV, Wang Y, Wong FS, Visintin I, Flavell RA, Janeway CA Jr, et al. The role of Fas in autoimmune diabetes. Cell 1997;89:17–24.
222. Grewal IS, Grewal KD, Wong FS, Picarella DE, Janeway CA Jr, Flavell RA. Local expression of transgene encoded TNF alpha in islets prevents autoimmune diabetes in nonobese diabetic (NOD) mice by preventing the development of auto-reactive islet-specific T cells. J Exp Med 1996;184:1963–1974.
223. Sarvetnick N. Mechanisms of cytokine-mediated localized immunoprotection. J Exp Med 1996;184:1597–1600.
224. Harada M, Makino S. Suppression of overt diabetes in NOD mice by anti-thymocyte serum or anti-Thy 1, 2 antibody. Jikken Dobutsu 1986;35:501–504.
225. Boitard C, Michie S, Serrurier P, Butcher GW, Larkins AP, McDevitt HO. In vitro prevention of thyroid and pancreatic autoimmunity in the BB rat by antibody to class II major histocompatibility complex gene products. Proc Natl Acad Sci USA 1985;82:6627–6631.
226. Boitard C, Bendelac A, Richard MF, Carnaud C, Bach JF. Prevention of diabetes in nonobese diabetic mice by anti-I-A monoclonal antibodies: transfer of protection by splenic T cells. Proc Natl Acad Sci USA 1988;85:9719–9723.
227. Hahn HJ, Lucke S, Kloting I, Volk HD, Baehr RV, Diamantstein T. Curing BB rats of freshly manifested diabetes by short-term treatment with a combination of a monoclonal anti-interleukin 2 receptor antibody and a subtherapeutic dose of cyclosporin A. Eur J Immunol 1987;17:1075–1078.
228. Satoh J, Seino H, Shintani S, Tanaka S-I, Ohteki T, Masuda T, et al. Inhibition of type 1 diabetes in BB rats with recombinant human tumor necrosis factor-α. J Immunol 1990;145:1395–1399.
229. Satoh J, Seino H, Abo T, Tanaka S, Shintani S, Ohta S, et al. Recombinant human tumor necrosis factor alpha suppresses autoimmune diabetes in nonobese diabetic mice. J Clin Invest 1989;84:1345–1348.
230. Zielasek J, Burkart V, Naylor P, Goldstein A, Kiesel U, Kolb H. Interleukin-2-dependent control of disease development in spontaneously diabetic BB rats. Immunology 1990;69:209–214.
231. Burstein D, Handler ES, Schindler J, Seals J, Mordes JP, Rossini AA. Effect of interleukin-2 on diabetes in the BB/Wor rat. Diabetes Res 1987;5:163–167.
232. Like AA, Dirodi V, Thomas S, Guberski DL, Rossini AA. Prevention of diabetes mellitus in the BB/W rat with Cyclosporin-A. Am J Pathol 1984;117:92–97.
233. Mori Y, Suko M, Okudaira H, Matsuba I, Tsuruoka A, Sasaki A, et al. Preventive effects of cyclosporin on diabetes in NOD mice. Diabetologia 1986;29:244–247.
234. Qin HY, Sadelain MW, Hitchon C, Lauzon J, Singh B. Complete Freund's adjuvant-induced T cells prevent the development and adoptive transfer of diabetes in nonobese diabetic mice. J Immunol 1993;150:2072–2080.
235. Qin HY, Singh B. BCG vaccination prevents insulin-dependent diabetes mellitus (IDDM) in NOD mice after disease acceleration with cyclophosphamide. J Autoimmunity 1997;10:271–278.

236. Lakey JR, Singh B, Warnock GL, Rajotte RV. BCG immunotherapy prevents recurrence of diabetes in islet grafts transplanted into spontaneously diabetic NOD mice. Transplantation 1994;57:1213–1217.
237. Kuttler B, Rosing K, Hahn HJ. Anti-CD4/CyA therapy causes prevention of autoimmune but not allogeneic destruction of grafted islets in BB rats. Transplant Proc 1997;29:2163–2165.
238. Uchikoshi F, Ito T, Kamiike W, Moriguchi A, Nozaki S, Ito A, et al. Anti-ICAM-1/LFA-1 monoclonal antibody therapy prevents graft rejection and IDDM recurrence in BB rat pancreas transplantation. Transplant Proc 1995;27:1527–1528.
239. Slavin S, Weiss L, Xia W, Gross DJ. Successful treatment of diabetes in NOD mice with advanced disease by islet isografts following immunoregulation with Linomide (quinoline-3-carboxamide). Cell Transplant 1996;5:627–630.
240. Rivereau AS, Darquy S, Chaillous L, Maugendre S, Gouin E, Reach G, et al. Reversal of diabetes in non-obese diabetic mice by xenografts of porcine islets entrapped in hollow fibres composed of polyacrylonitrile-sodium methallylsulphonate copolymer. Diabetes Metab 1997;23:205–212.
241. Mital D, Guo Z, Chong AS, Fu Z, Tian Y, Foster PF, et al. Successful xenotransplantation of adult porcine islets in NOD and BALB/c mice with leflunomide and cyclosporine. Transplant Proc 1997; 29:2166–2167.
242. Lipes MA, Davalli AM, Cooper EM. Genetic engineering of insulin expression in nonislet cells: implications for beta-cell replacement therapy for insulin-dependent diabetes mellitus. Acta Diabetol 1997;34:2–5.
243. Jaworski MA, Honore L, Jewell LD. Cyclosporin prophylaxis induces long-term prevention of diabetes, and inhibits lymphocytic infiltration in multiple target tissues in the high-risk BB rat. Diabetes Res 1986;3:1–6.
244. Elliott RB, Crossley JR, Berryman CC, James AG. Partial preservation of pancreatic β cell function in children with diabetes. Lancet 1981;ii:119–123.
245. Feutren G, Papoz L, Assan R, Vialettes B, Karsenty G, Vexiau P, et al. Cyclosporin increases the rate and length of remission in insulin-dependent diabetes of recent onset. Results of a multicenter double-blind trial. Lancet 1986;ii:119–123.
246. Bach JF. Cyclosporine in insulin-dependent diabetes mellitus. J Pediatr 1987;111:1073–1074.
247. Feutren G, Mihatsch MJ. Risk factors for cyclosporine-induced nephropathy in patients with autoimmune diseases. N Engl J Med 1992;326:1654–1660.
248. Sundkvist G, Hagopian WA, Landin-Olsson M, Lernmark Å, Ohlsson L, Ericsson C. et al. Islet cell antibodies (ICA) but not glutamic acid decarboxylase antibodies (GAD65-Ab) are decreased by plasmapheresis in patients with newly diagnosed insulin-dependent diabetes mellitus (IDDM). J Clin Endocrinol Metab 1994;78:1159–1165.
249. Skyler JS, Marks JB. Immune intervention in type 1 diabetes mellitus. Diabetes Rev 1993;1:15–42.

6 The Epidemiology of Autoimmune Thyroid Disease

Mark P. J. Vanderpump, MD, MRCP, and W. Michael G. Tunbridge, MD, FRCP

CONTENTS

    INTRODUCTION
    HYPERTHYROIDISM
    ASYMPTOMATIC AUTOIMMUNE THYROIDITIS
    HYPOTHYROIDISM
    POSTPARTUM THYROIDITIS (PPT)
    SCREENING FOR THYROID DYSFUNCTION
    REFERENCES

INTRODUCTION

Epidemiology is the study of the frequency of disease within the community, and requires analysis and interpretation of distribution patterns of disease in terms of possible causal factors. Proof of causal association between a factor and a disease, is however, seldom provided by an epidemiological study. Thyroid dysfunction can be classified according to the severity of clinical findings, serum hormone levels, the presence or absence of thyroid antibodies, or the biochemical or physiological effect in the target tissues. The problems encountered in epidemiological studies of thyroid disorders are those of definition, e.g., overt hypothyroidism and subclinical hypothyroidism, the selection criteria used, the influence of age, sex, environmental factors, and the different techniques used for the measurement of thyroid function (*see also* Chapter 9). The most commonly used initial tests in epidemiological surveys are measurements of serum total or free thyroxine (T_4) and sensitive (second-generation) thyroid-stimulating hormone (TSH).

Hospital records have limitations as an index of thyroid disease within a community, because referral may be highly selective and incomplete. Cross-sectional studies have determined the prevalence of hyperthyroidism and hypothyroidism, and the frequency and distribution of thyroid autoantibodies in different, mainly Caucasian, communities. Most have concentrated on middle-aged women and elderly people in the community, healthy persons undergoing routine medical examinations, or hospital inpatients, and only a few have documented the prevalence of thyroid disorders in a cross-section of the

From: *Contemporary Endocrinology: Autoimmune Endocrinopathies*
Edited by: R. Volpe © Humana Press Inc., Totowa, NJ

adult population in the community. The limitations of epidemiological studies of thyroid disorders should therefore be borne in mind when considering the purported frequency of thyroid diseases in different communities.

In iodine-replete areas, most persons with thyroid disorders have autoimmune disease, ranging from hyperthyroidism to hypothyroidism *(1)*. A cross-sectional study performed between 1972 and 1974 in Whickham, a mixed urban and rural area in northeastern England, has documented the prevalence of thyroid disorders in the community *(2)*. The 2779 subjects examined in the survey (82% of the available sample) represented a one in six sample of the adult population aged over 18 yr, and closely resembled the British population as a whole in terms of age, sex, and social class. Other cross-sectional studies from Europe, the US, and Japan have corroborated the findings of the Whickham survey, and therefore, its findings have a broad application to iodine-replete communities.

Until recently, relatively little data existed on the incidence of autoimmune thyroid diseases. Incidence rates provide a direct measure of the rate at which individuals in a given population develop a disease, and thus, provide a basis for statements about probability or risk of disease. By comparing incidence rates of a disease among population groups varying in one or more identified factors, analytic studies can detect whether a factor affects the risk of acquiring a disease and provide an estimate of the magnitude of the effect. Longitudinal studies are necessary to determine incidence rates, etiological risk factors, and the natural history of the disease process. The logistic and administrative difficulties of such studies explain their relative paucity. A recent 20-yr follow-up of the Whickham cohort determined outcomes in terms of thyroid disease in 87% of the total original survey population *(3)*. The cohort was, as in the first study, shown to be representative of the British population in terms of age and sex distribution and mortality over 20 yr. A total of 825 subjects had died and, in addition to death certificates, two-thirds had information from medical records or postmortem reports to document morbidity prior to death. Of the 1877 known survivors, 91% were examined for clinical, biochemical, and immunological evidence of thyroid dysfunction. This 20-yr follow-up study has therefore provided longitudinal data for autoimmune thyroid disease in a representative sample of a community. Following a review of this study and other available epidemiological data, the value of screening populations for autoimmune thyroid disease will be considered.

HYPERTHYROIDISM

In epidemiological studies, the clinical diagnosis of hyperthyroidism should be supported by measurements of serum T_4 (or triiodothyronine [T_3]) and TSH concentrations. Biochemical tests of thyroid function may reveal the diagnosis before it is clinically apparent. A rise in serum T_3 and fall in serum TSH are the earliest measures of thyroid overactivity, followed by a rise in serum T_4. The most common causes of hyperthyroidism are Graves' disease, followed by toxic multinodular goiter, whereas rarer causes include an autonomously functioning thyroid adenoma or thyroiditis. In epidemiological studies, however, the etiology is rarely ascertained.

Prevalence of Hyperthyroidism

Hoffenberg *(4)* quoted a UK survey of 106 general practices between May 1955 and April 1956 suggesting a prevalence of 25–30 cases/10,000 women and a hospital inpatient inquiry in 1967, which calculated 3 cases of hyperthyroidism/10,000 hospital discharges. In neither series, however, were diagnostic criteria specified. In the Whickham survey, the prevalence of undiagnosed hyperthyroidism, based on clinical features and elevated serum T_4 and free thyroxine index (FTI) values, was 4.7/1000 women *(2)*. Hyperthyroidism had been previously diagnosed and treated in 20/1000 women, rising to 27/1000 women when possible, but unproven cases were included, as compared with 1.6–2.3/1000 men, in whom no new cases were found at the survey. The mean age at diagnosis was 48 yr. In the few other cross-sectional studies of the adult population, the results were comparable to the Whickham data (Table 1). In a study at a primary care center in a rural area of Sweden, 2000 consecutive adult patients were tested with a serum TSH assay with a low detection limit (0.05 mU/L) *(5)*. Three women aged over 60 yr were identified with clinically unsuspected hyperthyroidism. An epidemiological study screened 2421 subjects aged over 40 yr (77% of the adult population) in a Japanese town with serum TSH and measured FT_4 in addition if the serum TSH was abnormal *(6)*. Three women (2/1000) and no men were found to be biochemically hyperthyroid. In a study by Kågedal et al. *(7)*, FTI and serum TSH were measured in 3885 women aged 39–60 yr who attended for cervical carcinoma screening in Sweden. Previously undiagnosed hyperthyroidism was found in 5/1000 with the etiology in most cases being toxic nodular goiter.

Several studies have assessed healthy volunteers. The data available from these highly selected populations of presumably well-motivated individuals must be treated with caution before being applied to the general population. Baldwin and Rowett *(8)* assessed 1544 patients volunteering for an annual physical examination at a general internal medicine clinic. Graves' disease was diagnosed in 15 patients (10/1000), 6 of whom were new cases. In Oakland, CA, FTI was measured in a health screening program in 2704 asymptomatic adult volunteers. The prevalence of overt hyperthyroidism was 5/1000 women of all ages and 9/1000 women aged over 40 *(9)*. In a study of a working population in Germany (6539 men, 345 women) the prevalence of overt hyperthyroidism was 0.3/1000 based on TSH, T3, T4, and thyrotrophin-releasing hormone (TRH) test *(10)*. A sample of 4110 subjects (2931 men, 1179 women; age 45.6 ± 10.3 yr [mean ± SD]) attending a health insurance medical were recruited at an annual examination in Sapporo, Japan *(11)*. In a documented iodine-sufficient area, hyperthyroidism, as defined by suppressed serum TSH and elevated FT_4 values, was found in 3/1000 men and 5/1000 women of whom two thirds had Graves' disease based on positive thyrotrophin receptor antibody results.

The prevalence data in elderly persons are conflicting. In a survey of 1210 persons aged over 60 yr in a single general practice in Birmingham, UK, only one woman was found to be hyperthyroid *(12)*. Among 1442 women aged over 60 yr in a Swedish rural district, 28 (20/1000) were found to be hyperthyroid on the basis of biochemical screening *(13)*. The prevalence of hyperthyroidism in 968 healthy volunteers aged over 55 yr from a healthy urban population in the US was 0.7% following assessment with a sensitive TSH assay and TRH stimulation test *(14)*. An investigation in a rural community in Norway of 1 in 4 subjects aged over 70 yr (86 men, 114 women) found previously diagnosed hyperthyroidism in 9/1000 women and in no men, and undiagnosed hyperthyroidism in no women, but in 1 man *(15)*. Campbell et al. *(16)* measured FTI followed by a TRH stimulation test in 427 subjects living in a community, residential care, and in a hospital aged 80 yr or over in New Zealand. Two subjects (sex not identified) were identified clinically at the examination with hyperthyroidism, and the prevalence was therefore 4.7/1000. A population study in Gothenburg of 601 women and 285 men aged

Table 1
Prevalence of Previously Undiagnosed Hyperthyroidism and Hypothyroidism at Testing in Epidemiological Surveys of Thyroid Dysfunction

Study name	Ref.	Sample number	Gender, M = men, W = women	Age, yr	Test of thyroid function	Hyperthyroidism N/1000 Men	Hyperthyroidism N/1000 Women	Hypothyroidism N/1000 Men	Hypothyroidism N/1000 Women
Whickham, UK	2	2779	M + W	18+	TSH + FTI	0	4.7	0	3.3
Mölnlycke, Sweden	5	2000	M + W	18+	TSH	0	2.5	1.3	12.0
Hisayama, Japan	6	2421	M + W	40+	TSH	0	2.0	4.0	7.0
Kisa, Sweden	7	3885	W	39–60	TSH + FTI	—	5.1	—	0
Connecticut, US	8	1544	M + W	18+	FTI	0	7.8	2.6	5.2
Oakland, US	9	2704	M + W	18+	TSH + TT3/4	0	5.4	3.5	6.1
Ludwigshafen, FRG	10	6884	M + W	18+?	TSH	0.3			0.2
Sapporo, Japan	11	4110	M + W	25+	TSH + THY AB	2.7	5.1	2.4	8.5
Birmingham, UK	12	1210	M + W	60+	TSH	0.9		7.8	20.5
Kisa, Sweden	13	1442	W	60+	TSH + FTI	—	19.4	—	5.5
Nærøy, Norway	15	200	M + W	70+	TSH + TT4	11.6	0	11.6	17.5
Gisborne, NZ	16	427	M + W	80+	FTI	4.7		9.4	
Göteborg, Sweden	31,32	1283	W	44–66	TSH	—	6.0		6.4
Barry, Wales	45	414	M + W	70+	THY AB+	—	—	4.8	
Southern Finland	52	3000	M + W	18+	TSH	—	—	2.0	

over 85 yr found previously undetected hyperthyroidism in two women, with an additional three cases suspected, but not confirmed in two women and one man *(17)*.

In studies of patients in the hospital, the point prevalence rates for previously undiagnosed hyperthyroidism are consistent with the rate in the Whickham survey. A selective study measured extensive thyroid function tests in 98 patients hospitalized with acute medical illnesses and identified only one patient with hyperthyroidism. Accurate diagnosis could be achieved by determination of FT_4 and serum TSH, and a drug history *(18)*. Gow et al. *(19)* assessed 299 hospital inpatients in Scotland for previously undiagnosed hyperthyroidism initially using a sensitive TSH assay and found that only one patient had biochemical evidence of hyperthyroidism after discharge. In an audit of thyroid-function testing, also in Scotland, of 630 medical admissions in 4 mo, 4 cases of hyperthyroidism (all women) were found and treated, only 2 of whom were suspected clinically *(20)*. Only one subject was found to be hyperthyroid when samples from 364 consecutive admissions to a large, acute care teaching hospital were assayed for serum TSH and FTI *(21)*. A survey of 190 elderly hospitalized patients found two patients with hyperthyroidism, but both had strong clinical indications (history of weight loss and new-onset atrial fibrillation) for measuring thyroid function *(22)*.

Subclinical Hyperthyroidism

The introduction of assays for serum TSH over 10 yr ago that were sensitive enough to distinguish between normal and low concentrations allowed subjects with subclinical hyperthyroidism to be identified. This is defined as a low-serum TSH concentration in the presence of normal-serum T_4 concentrations, and the absence of hypothalamic or pituitary disease, nonthyroidal illness, or ingestion of drugs that inhibit TSH secretion. The available studies differ in the definition of a low-serum TSH concentration and whether the subjects included were receiving T_4. The recently available third-generation assays have rarely been used in epidemiological studies.

In a study of 2000 consecutive adults attending a primary care center, 65 (3%), who were not receiving T_4 and were not new cases of overt hyperthyroidism, had a serum TSH concentration of 0.2 mU/L or less (normal range 0.2–4.0 mU/L) *(5)*. In 57% of the subjects who had a low but detectable serum TSH (≥0.05 <0.2 mU/L), the value was normal two to three weeks later. Two Japanese studies provide conflicting data with a prevalence of 5% in one community study of 2421 subjects aged over 40 *(6)* and 0.6% in 4110 healthy volunteers *(11)*. At the 20-yr follow-up of the Whickham survey cohort, 4% of 1704 survivors (now aged over 38 yr) had a serum TSH <0.5 mU/L (second-generation assay with detection limit of 0.05 mU/L, a coefficient of variation [CV] of 9% at 0.6 mU/L, and a normal range of 0.5–5.2 mU/L), decreasing to 3% if those subjects taking T_4 and those with newly diagnosed overt hyperthyroidism were excluded *(3)*. Use of a more sensitive third-generation TSH assay (detection limit of 0.01 mU/L, a CV of 10% at 0.08 mU/L and a normal range of 0.17–2.89 mU/L) in these 73 subjects found that 21 (29%) had a normal serum TSH level, 31 (42%) had a low, but detectable serum TSH (≥0.01 and <0.17 mU/L) including one subject with undiagnosed hyperthyroidism, and 21 (29%) had an undetectable serum TSH (<0.01 mU/L), including four subjects with undiagnosed hyperthyroidism. Thus, approx 2% of the population studied had a subnormal serum TSH and 1% had an undetectable serum TSH.

The prevalence of subclinical hyperthyroidism has been investigated in older populations. In 2575 survivors of the Framingham Heart Study aged over 60 yr, 4% had a low-serum TSH concentration (<0.1 mU/L) of whom half were taking T_4 *(23)*. In the community survey in Birmingham, UK, 6% had low-serum TSH concentrations, and 2% of women and 1% of men had undetectable values (<0.05 mU/L) *(12)*. Only 5% of these subjects with a below-normal serum TSH were taking T_4.

Incidence of Hyperthyroidism

The incidence data available for overt hyperthyroidism in men and women from large population studies are comparable (Table 2). In the US, an annual incidence of 0.3 cases/1000 was estimated in a survey of Olmsted County hospital referrals over 32 yr *(24)*, but the data were complicated by change in diagnostic procedures over 30 yr. A study based on a review of all thyroid function tests in Denmark performed over a 3-yr period in the Funen region, a demographically representative sample of the Danish population, found an annual incidence rate of 0.5/1000 in women and 0.1/1000 in men *(25)*. A nationwide survey of the incidence of thyrotoxicosis in Iceland, a country with a high iodine intake, identified by a questionnaire to all family and hospital doctors an annual incidence rate of 0.4/1000 women and 0.1/1000 men. Graves' disease was defined as a toxic diffuse goitre and accounted for over 80% of all causes *(26)*. A study of all hospital referrals between 1970 and 1974 in Malmö, a demographically well-defined population, found a mean annual incidence of 0.4/1000 women and 0.1/1000 men *(27)*. In these population studies, the age-specific incidence of Graves' disease varies considerably. The peak age-specific incidence was between 20 and 49 yr in two studies *(24,25)*, but increased with age in Iceland *(26)* and peaked at 60–69 yr in Malmö, Sweden *(27)*. The only available data in a black population from Johannesburg suggest a much lower annual incidence of hyperthyroidism in black Africans than in European whites of 0.09/1000 women and 0.007/1000 men *(28)*.

In a prospective study of 12 towns in England and Wales, the annual incidence of hyperthyroidism varied from 0.1 to 0.5/1,000 and was strongly correlated with the prevalence of endemic goiter among schoolchildren 60 yr earlier *(29)*. Subsequent to this survey, serum samples from 216 of the 290 cases identified were assayed for TSH-receptor antibodies. The incidence of antibody-negative hyperthyroidism correlated closely with the previous prevalence of endemic goiter, indicating a high current incidence of toxic nodular goiter in towns in which the incidence of goiter had been high many yr ago. The frequency of antibody-positive thyrotoxicosis, an indicator of Graves' disease, did not correlate with goiter in the past *(30)*.

Cohort studies provide higher incidence rates, which suggests that many cases of hyperthyroidism remain undiagnosed in the community, since routine testing is not undertaken. In the survivors of the Whickham survey cohort, 11 women had been diagnosed and treated for hyperthyroidism after the first survey and 5 women were diagnosed at the second survey *(3)*. The etiology in these 16 new cases was Graves' disease in 10 subjects, multinodular goiter in 3 subjects, an autonomously functioning thyroid adenoma in 1, chronic autoimmune thyroiditis in 1, and unknown in 1. The mean annual incidence of hyperthyroidism in women was 0.8/1000 survivors (95% confidence interval 0.5–1.4). The incidence rate was similar in the deceased women. No new cases were detected in men. An estimate of the probability of the development of hyperthyroidism

Chapter 6 / Epidemiology of Autoimmune Thyroid Disease

Table 2
Incidence of Hyperthyroidism and Hypothyroidism in Epidemiological Surveys of Thyroid Dysfunction

Study name	Ref.	Sample number	Gender, M = men, W = women	Age, yr	Length of follow-up	Hyperthyroidism N/1000/yr Men	Hyperthyroidism N/1000/yr Women	Hypothyroidism N/1000/yr Men	Hypothyroidism N/1000/yr Women
Whickham, UK	3	2779	M + W	18+	20 yr	<0.1	0.8	0.6	3.5
Oakland, US	9	2704	M + W	18+	1 yr	0.2	0.8	8.0	
Birmingham, UK	12	1210	M + W	60+	1 yr		0.9		11.1
Gothenburg, Sweden	17	1148	M + W	70+	10 yr	—	1.0	—	2
Olmsted, US	24	?	M + W	0+	32 yr	0.1	0.3	—	—
Funen, Denmark	25	450,000	M + W	0+	3 yr	0.1	0.5	—	—
Iceland	26	230,000	M + W	0+	3 yr	0.1	0.4	—	—
Malmö, Sweden	27	257,764	M + W	0+	5 yr	0.1	0.4	—	—
12 Towns in UK	29	1,641,949	M + W	0+	1 yr	0.1	0.4	—	—
Göteborg, Sweden	31,32	1283	W	44–66	4 yr	—	1.3	—	—
West Australia	42	1587	M + W	18+	6 yr	—	—	3	—
Barry, Wales	45	414	M + W	70+	5 yr	—	—	4	1–2

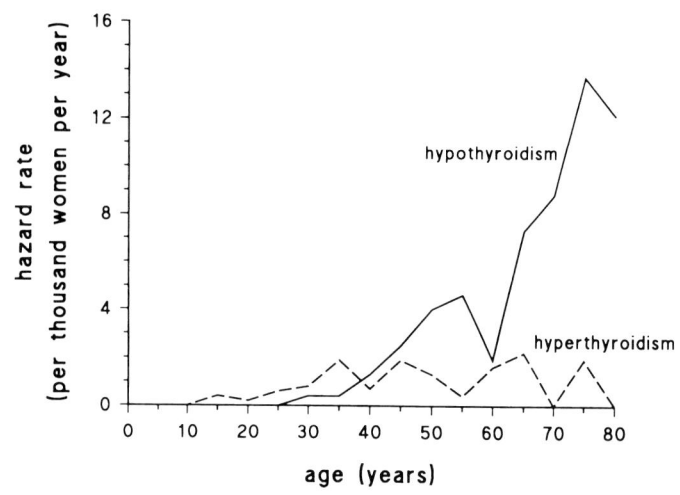

Fig. 1. Age-specific hazard rates for the development of overt hyperthyroidism and hypothyroidism in women at 20-yr follow-up of the Whickham survey *(3)*. Reproduced with permission.

in women at a particular time, i.e., the hazard rate, averaged 1.4/1000 between the ages of 35 and 60 yr (Fig. 1). Neither thyroid antibody status nor the presence of a goiter during the first survey was associated with he development of hyperthyroidism at follow-up.

Other cohort studies provide comparable incidence data. In the health screening program of 2704 asymptomatic volunteers, an annual incidence of symptomatic hyperthyroidism was estimated at 0.5/1000 *(9)*. A 6-yr follow-up of a representative sample of women aged 44–66 yr in Sweden investigated 1138 women using a serum T_3 assay followed by TRH stimulation test both in 1974–1975 and 1980–1981. Twenty-eight women gave a history of hyperthyroidism in the 1980–1981 questionnaire, eight of whom had developed hyperthyroidism during the 6 yr between the two investigations, and in addition, one woman was identified with overt hyperthyroidism in 1980–1981. Thus, the incidence was 1.3 cases/1000 women/year in this population *(31,32)*.

At the 1-yr follow-up of the 66 subjects aged over 60 yr in Birmingham who initially had serum TSH values below normal, only one man developed hyperthyroidism, 88% with undetectable serum TSH values (<0.05 mU/L) continued to have a subnormal value, and 76% with a value of between 0.05 and 0.5 mU/L had normal values at follow-up *(12)*. The lack of any association between subnormal serum TSH levels and thyroid antibody status and the absence of a clear relationship with FT_4 values suggested that significant thyroid pathology was not present in this group. In a follow-up investigation of 15 elderly in- and outpatients with a low-serum TSH and normal free T_4 and T_3 concentrations, two required antithyroid treatment and almost 50% had normal serum TSH concentrations when restudied during a mean follow-up of 8 mo *(33)*. Only six subjects initially found to have a below-normal serum TSH developed hyperthyroidism during 4 yr of follow-up of the Framingham sample *(34)*. The Gothenburg study of elderly women over 70 yr estimated an annual incidence of hyperthyroidism of 1/1000 *(17)*.

ASYMPTOMATIC AUTOIMMUNE THYROIDITIS

A substantial proportion of the population, particularly elderly women who live in iodine-replete areas, have circulating thyroid antibodies (antithyroid peroxidase [microsomal] and antithyroglobulin antibodies) and normal thyroid function. The presence of these antibodies correlates with the presence of focal thyroiditis in biopsy and in postmortem material of patients with no evidence of hypothyroidism during life *(35,36)*. In an analysis from several hundred necropsies, histological evidence of chronic autoimmune thyroiditis was found in 27% of adult women, with a rise in frequency over 50 yr, and 7% of adult men, and diffuse changes in 5% of women and 1% of men *(37)*.

Patients with hypothyroidism caused by either atrophic or goitrous autoimmune thyroiditis usually have high serum titers of those same antibodies. These antibodies also are often detected in serum of patients with Graves' disease and other thyroid diseases, but the titers are usually lower. There is considerable variation in the frequency and distribution of thyroid antibodies because of variations in techniques of detection, definition of abnormal titers, and inherent differences in the populations tested. Most of the available data are based on studies using hemagglutination and complement fixation tests for thyroglobulin and antithyroid microsomal antibody tests, respectively, and not the newer radioimmunoassays for either thyroglobulin or thyroid peroxidase.

In all the early studies, regardless of the methodology, a progressive increase in prevalence of thyroid antibodies was revealed with age in women, as compared with a uniformly low prevalence with no age trend in men. A random sample of the population of a single practice in northeastern England found antibodies to thyroglobulin (thyroglobulin antibodies; TGA) by the tanned red cell test in a titer of 1:25 or more in 16% of women and 4% of men *(38)*. High antibody titers were found in 5% of women and 1% of men, which is similar to the prevalence of diffuse thyroiditis found in the necropsy study by Williams and Doniach *(37)*. A population study in Carterton, New Zealand, defined the age and sex prevalence of TGA and antithyroid cytoplasmic antibodies. TGA was found in 2% of women aged 25 yr, rising to 15% at 75 yr, but in men, there was a low prevalence with no age trend. Cytoplasmic antibodies occurred in 4% of women aged 35 yr, rising to 20% at age 75, and infrequently in men *(39)*. Another population study in Australia of various autoantibodies, including epithelial cells of human thyroid gland detected by indirect immunofluorescence, confirmed this trend of a progressive increase in prevalence with age and a uniformly higher prevalence in women *(40)*. Those trends were confirmed in the original Whickham survey, but the frequency of positive tests was lower *(2)*. Specifically, 2% of the subjects surveyed had positive tests for anti-TGA antibodies, and only 0.7% had these antibodies and no antithyroid microsomal antibodies. Microsomal antibodies, measured by an immunofluorescent technique with serum diluted 1:10, were found in 7% (women 10%, men 3%). The mean serum TSH concentrations were significantly higher in both men and women with positive antibody tests, and 3% of the sample (5% of women, 1% of men) had both positive antibody tests and a serum TSH value >6 mU/L. Fifty percent of those subjects who were thyroid antibody-positive had serum TSH >6 mU/L. Conversely, 60% of those with serum TSH >6 mU/L were thyroid antibody-positive, and 80% of those with serum TSH >10 mU/L were thyroid antibody-positive.

In a random sample of 507 adults in southern Finland, the prevalence of asymptomatic chronic autoimmune thyroiditis was between 2 and 5%, based on elevated serum TSH values and high titers of either anti-TGA or antithyroid microsomal antibodies *(41)*. The prevalence of antithyroid microsomal antibodies was 7% (women 10%, men 3%) in an Australian survey *(42)*, and the prevalence of chronic autoimmune thyroiditis as defined by an elevated TSH and positive antibody test was 5% if the serum TSH was even minimally elevated, and 3% if it was >10 mU/L. The prevalence in women in the sixth decade was 15%, with a subsequent fall, suggesting selective mortality in more elderly women. A lower prevalence of thyroid antibodies in the very elderly was also found in an Italian study *(43)*, which speculated that the appearance of organ-specific antibodies at an older age might therefore be a risk factor for a shorter life expectancy. In the Framingham cohort of subjects aged over 60 yr, two-thirds of those with serum TSH concentrations >10 mU/L had positive tests for antithyroid microsomal antibodies *(44)*, and in 414 asymptomatic elderly people aged over 70 yr in the UK, 15 and 13% had elevated titers of antithyroid microsomal and anti-TGA antibodies, respectively; 9% had elevated titers of both antibodies *(45)*. In summary, a significant proportion of subjects in the community have asymptomatic chronic autoimmune thyroiditis of whom a substantial proportion have subclinical hypothyroidism.

In recent studies in which antithyroid peroxidase antibodies were measured by radioimmunoassay, the results were similar. For example, antibodies were found in 18% of 698 female blood donors from seven towns in England and Wales *(46)*, with a rise in prevalence from 15% at age 18–24 yr to 24% at age 55–64 yr. In contrast to many of the earlier studies, the prevalence of antithyroid peroxidase antibodies and anti-TGA antibodies was similar. Geographical differences in the prevalence of thyroid antibodies were not significant, and did not correlate with either the goiter prevalence or with current differences in iodine intake. In another study of 342 elderly subjects in Italy (mean age 80 yr), antithyroid peroxidase antibodies measured by radioimmunoassay occurred in 10% of women and 2% of men *(47)*.

At the 20-yr follow-up of the Whickham survey *(3)*, 1704 survivors had tests for antithyroid peroxidase or TGA antibodies, 19% had positive tests for the former antibodies, and 5% had positive tests for the latter. Seventeen percent of women and 7% of men who initially had negative tests now had positive tests, 9% of women and 2% of men had positive tests on both occasions, and 2% of women and 0.5% of men no longer had positive tests. The thyroid antibodies were most often detected in women aged 55–65 yr at follow-up (and who were therefore aged 35–45 yr at the time of the first survey). There was no evidence that a positive thyroid antibody test at the original survey was a risk factor for premature death in this cohort *(48)*. Over half of the women in whom the tests changed from positive to negative were receiving T_4 treatment for hypothyroidism, a change noted in some patients by others *(49,50)*. In other shorter longitudinal studies, one-third of 160 subjects who were initially antibody-positive in a population survey no longer had detectable antibodies 6 yr later *(42)*, whereas in another study of 51 elderly subjects, all remained thyroid antibody-positive at a 5-yr follow-up *(45)*.

HYPOTHYROIDISM

The earliest biochemical abnormality in hypothyroidism is a rise in serum TSH associated with normal serum T_4 and T_3 concentrations (subclinical hypothyroidism), followed by a fall in serum T_4, at which stage most patients have symptoms and benefit from treatment (overt hypothyroidism). In persons living in iodine-replete areas, the cause is either chronic autoimmune disease (atrophic autoimmune thyroiditis or goitrous autoimmune thyroiditis [Hashimoto's thyroiditis]) or destructive treatment for thyrotoxicosis, but this is rarely discussed in the available studies.

Prevalence of Hypothyroidism

In 1959, Lowrey and Starr determined protein-bound iodine (PBI) levels in a selected group of 5755 physicians, blood donors, and hospital employees *(51)*. Despite the limitations in methodology and selection bias, 10/1000 men and 20/1000 women were estimated as definitely hypothyroid after further tests, which included serum cholesterol, basal metabolic rate, radioiodine uptake, and thyroxine binding globulin. In the Whickham survey, the prevalence of newly diagnosed overt hypothyroidism was 3/1000 women *(2)*. The prevalence of previously diagnosed and treated hypothyroidism was 14/1000 women, rising to 19/1000 women when possible, but unproven cases were included. The overall prevalence in men was <1/1000. The mean age at diagnosis was 57 yr. One-third had been previously treated by surgery or radioiodine for hyperthyroidism. Excluding iatrogenic causes, the prevalence of hypothyroidism was 10/1000 women, rising to 15/1000 when possible, but unproven cases were included. The diagnosis was based on clinical features and high serum TSH and low FTI values in the new cases, and from the original records in the previously diagnosed and treated cases.

The figure of 3 new cases/1000 women in the Whickham survey is comparable to other studies (Table 1). The prevalence of hypothyroidism was investigated in 3000 subjects who comprised more than 65% of all subjects over 20 yr in the population registers of two Finnish towns *(52)*. Six subjects had frank hypothyroidism, and therefore, the prevalence of previously unrecognized hypothyroidism was 2/1000. In a study of 2000 consecutive patients by Eggertsen et al. *(5)*, 16 spontaneous cases (15 women) were found, and in addition, 71 subjects were already receiving thyroid hormone therapy (52 for spontaneous hypothyroidism). A survey of 2421 residents aged 40 or over in a Japanese town discovered overt hypothyroidism in 4/1000 men and 7/1000 women *(6)*. Two studies have examined prevalence of hypothyroidism in middle-aged women. Serum TSH was determined in 1283 women aged 44–66 yr representative of the general population *(31)*. No women with previously unknown hypothyroidism were found at the clinical examination, 4% were on T_4 (0.7% because of spontaneous hypothyroidism), and 1% had markedly elevated serum TSH concentrations of whom the majority required T_4 within 4 yr. A thyroid panel using serum FTI and TSH as the initial test in 3885 middle-aged women found 6/1000 with previously undiagnosed hypothyroidism *(7)*. Following an assessment of 1544 patients volunteering for an annual physical examination at a general internal medicine clinic, six subjects (four women, two men) had clinical and biochemical evidence of hypothyroidism *(8)*. A similar prevalence of newly diagnosed hypothyroidism of 6/1000 women was found in a screening program in 2704 asymptomatic adult volunteers using the FTI in an Oakland hospital clinic *(9)*. A study of a working population in Germany (6539 men, 345 women) found only one case of unsuspected overt hypothyroidism *(10)*, but in a similar study of healthy volunteers in Japan (2931 men, 1179 women), the prevalence was 2/1000 men and 9/1000 women *(11)*.

The prevalence was higher in surveys of the elderly in the community. A random sample of 114 apparently well elderly over 65 yr living in an English community found two subjects with unsuspected hypothyroidism *(53)*. The overall prevalence of hypothyroidism, including those already taking T_4, in Birmingham of 1210 subjects aged 60 and over was 4% of women and 0.8% of men aged over 60 yr *(12)*. In a survey of 1442 women aged 60 yr or over by Falkenberg et al. *(13)*, 8 women (6/1000) were detected on the basis of symptoms and signs of hypothyroidism, elevated serum TSH >13 mU/L, and a therapeutic response to T_4. In addition, 9 women were already on T_4, but only two because of primary hypothyroidism. In subjects aged 60 yr or more in Framingham, 4% had serum TSH concentration >10 mU/L, of whom one-third had low-serum T_4 concentrations (54). Of the 968 healthy volunteers aged over 55 yr from an urban population in the US, elevated serum TSH levels (>6 mU/L) were found in 7%, but low TT_4 levels were found in only 0.6% of total sample (14). A study of 200 elderly men and women aged 70 yr and over in a Norwegian rural community found 4% of women and no men with known hypothyroidism, and newly diagnosed hypothyroidism (raised serum TSH >6 mU/L, low TT_4 <70 nmol/L) in 2% of women and 1% of men (15). The prevalence of newly discovered hypothyroidism was 10/1000 in a sample of elderly subjects aged over 80 yr in New Zealand (16).

The testing of hospital inpatients, predominantly elderly women, might be expected to reveal a higher proportion of unsuspected hypothyroidism (55), but this is not supported by recent studies. Overt hypothyroidism, very rarely suspected clinically, was found in approx 2% of patients admitted for treatment of an acute illness in studies of 98, 299, and 630 admissions (18–20). In another similar study, however, 6% of 364 patients admitted consecutively to an acute care teaching hospital had unrecognized or untreated thyroid failure (low-serum FTI and elevated TSH values) (21). These subjects tended to be older and have more severe illnesses, but limiting testing to women over 50 yr in this study would have missed 40% of those with significant hypothyroidism.

Subclinical Hypothyroidism

The term subclinical hypothyroidism is used to describe the finding of a raised serum TSH, but a normal FT_4 in an asymptomatic patient (56). It represents a compensated state in which increased TSH output is required to maintain normal circulating thyroid hormone levels. An elevated serum TSH is a sensitive indicator of some degree of thyroid failure and, in contrast to below normal serum TSH levels, a clear inverse relationship is found with FT_4 levels. Serum TSH concentrations do not change as a function of age among adult men, but in women over 40 yr the concentrations increase markedly. If, however, women with thyroid antibodies are excluded, there is no age-related increase (2). Nearly all of the older women with elevated serum TSH values have subclinical hypothyroidism. With respect to epidemiological studies, the definition of subclinical hypothyroidism varies from any increase in serum TSH to values >10 mU/L or more stringently, a serum TSH value >10 mU/L and a positive test for circulating thyroid antibodies in serum. It is commonly found either postradioiodine therapy (57) or postsurgery (58) in up to 50% of apparently euthyroid patients. It may be evident for only a few months, but more often it represents a stage in the progression toward overt thyroid failure. Less frequent causes include external beam irradiation of malignant tumours of the head and neck, and drugs. In the community, the most common etiology is chronic autoimmune thyroiditis.

In the Whickham survey, 8% of women (10% of women aged over 55 yr) and 3% of men had subclinical hypothyroidism (2). The results were similar in a study of a Japanese population aged 40 yr and over where the prevalence of subclinical hypothyroidism was 6% in women and 3% in men (6). Community studies of elderly persons have confirmed the high prevalence in this age group, approx 10% of subjects over 60 yr having serum TSH values above the normal range (12,13,44). In surveys of hospital inpatients, the point prevalence rates were similar, being between 3 and 6% (19–21).

Incidence of Hypothyroidism

After destructive treatment of hyperthyroidism, the incidence of overt hypothyroidism is greatest in the first year after either radioiodine or surgery. If the serum TSH remains raised, then the rate of progression toward overt hypothyroidism is between 2 and 6%/yr after either treatment *(57–59)*. In a long-term follow-up study conducted in a Birmingham, UK clinic of 1918 patients with hyperthyroidism treated with either radioiodine at a dose calculated from thyroid size and radioiodine uptake scan, an empirical dose of radioiodine (3, 5, or 10 mC [110, 185, or 370 mBq]), or partial thyroidectomy *(60)*, all treatments resulted in a similar control of hyperthyroidism (more than 90%). After the calculated dose of radioiodine, 18% were hypothyroid at 5 yr and 42% at 20 yr, equivalent to a constant annual incidence of 2%. The results in the patients treated with an empirical dose of radioiodine were only available for 5 years, at which time just <40% were hypothyroid (8%/yr). After partial thyroidectomy, only 2% were hypothyroid at 5 yr, but 28% were hypothyroid at 20 yr; annual incidence was 0.4% for the first decade and almost 3%/yr for the second decade. A 9-yr follow-up in Malmö found a cumulative incidence of 32% for surgery and 78% for radioiodine treatment for Graves' disease *(61)*. Treatment of Graves' disease with antithyroid drugs alone is also associated with the eventual development of hypothyroidism in 5–20% of cases from either autoimmune thyroiditis or the presence of TSH-blocking antibodies *(62,63)*.

The 20-yr follow-up of the Whickham cohort has provided incidence data and allowed the determination of risk factors for hypothyroidism in this period *(3)*. The mean incidence of spontaneous hypothyroidism in the surviving women over the 20-yr follow-up was 3.5/1000/yr (95% confidence interval [CI] 2.8–4.5) rising to 4.1/1000/yr (95% CI 3.3–5.0) if all cases including those who had received destructive treatment for thyrotoxicosis are included. Only 9% of cases of spontaneous hypothyroidism in surviving women were diagnosed when they were less than age 45 yr, and 51% were diagnosed between the ages of 45–64 yr. The hazard rate, that is, the estimate of the probability of a woman developing hypothyroidism at a particular time, increased with age to 13.7/1000 in women aged between 75 and 80 yr (Fig. 1). The mean incidence during the 20-yr follow-up period in men (all spontaneous except for one case of lithium-induced hypothyroidism) was 0.6/1000/yr (95% CI 0.3–1.2). The incidence rates for the deceased women and men were similar.

The risk of having developed hypothyroidism by the time of follow-up was examined with respect to risk factors identified in the first survey. The odds ratios (with 95% CI) of developing spontaneous hypothyroidism in surviving women is shown in Table 3. Either raised serum TSH or positive thyroid antibodies alone or in combination are associated with a significantly increased risk of hypothyroidism. The odds are greatly increased when both risk factors are present and each had a similar effect. In men, the odds ratio (with 95% CI) of developing hypothyroidism with:

1. Raised serum TSH was 44 (19–104).
2. Positive thyroid antibodies alone was 25 (10–63).
3. Both raised serum TSH and positive thyroid antibodies was 173 (81–370).

The smaller number of observed cases in men resulted in wide, but highly significant confidence limits, but also did not allow the independent effects of these risk factors to be calculated. In the surviving women, the annual risk of developing spontaneous hypothyroidism was 4%/yr, in those who both had raised serum TSH values and were thyroid

Table 3
Development of Spontaneous Hypothyroidism
in Surviving Women at 20-Yr Follow-up of Whickham Survey:
Odds Ratios (with 95% CI)

TSH raised, regardless of THY AB status	14 (9–24)
THY AB+, regardless of TSH status	13 (8–19)
If THY AB-, effect of raised TSH alone	8 (3–20)
If THY AB+, additional effect of raised TSH	5 (2–11)
If TSH normal, effect of THY AB+ alone	8 (5–15)
If TSH raised, additional effect of THY AB+	5 (1–15)
TSH raised and THY AB+ combined	38 (22–65)

antibody-positive, 3%/yr if only serum TSH was raised, and 2%/yr if only thyroid antibodies were positive; at the time of follow-up, the respective rates of hypothyroidism were 55, 33, and 27%. The probability of developing hypothyroidism in women was plotted against log serum TSH as measured at first survey (Fig. 2). The graph indicates that a rise in serum TSH above 2 mU/L is associated with an increased probability of hypothyroidism, and this is further increased if antithyroid antibody-positive and decreased if antithyroid antibody-negative. The development of hypothyroidism also correlated with the strength of titer of antithyroid microsomal antibodies at first survey. Neither a positive family history of any form of thyroid disease, the presence of a goiter at either the first or the follow-up survey, nor parity at first survey was associated with an increased risk of hypothyroidism. These results confirm those from a 4-yr follow-up of a subgroup of women in the Whickham survey cohort in whom overt hypothyroidism had developed at a rate of 5%/yr in those who initially had a raised serum TSH and a positive test for thyroid antibodies *(64)*. Either alone, however, was not associated with an increased risk of hypothyroidism at 4 yr.

The other incidence data for hypothyroidism are from short (and often small) follow-up studies (Table 2). The longitudinal population study in Australia of 1587 individuals screened initially for antithyroid microsomal antibodies *(41)* reported 31 subjects with positive antithyroid microsomal antibodies developing elevated serum TSH (≥3.6 mU/L) over 6 yr, resulting in an annual incidence of approx 3/1000. However, since thyroid hormone levels were not measured, it is not clear how many of these subjects were overtly hypothyroid. Among 22 women with asymptomatic chronic autoimmune thyroiditis, overt hypothyroidism developed at a rate of 7%/yr, increasing to 10%/yr in those who initially had serum TSH values >19 mU/L *(65,66)*. A population sample in Sweden of 1283 women aged between 44 and 66 yr followed for 4 yr estimated an annual incidence of between 1 and 2 cases/1000. However, it was acknowledged that this may be falsely low, since only the 16 women with initially high-serum TSH concentrations were followed up, and four of these were begun on T_4 when clinically euthyroid because of the presence of a goiter and abnormal laboratory test results *(31)*. In a recent follow-up study of 437 healthy women aged 40–60 yr in the Netherlands, 24% of those who initially had a positive test for antithyroid microsomal antibodies and normal serum TSH concentrations had an elevated serum TSH concentration (>4.2 mU/L) 10 yr later, as compared with 3% in the antibody-negative group *(67)*. As in the 20-yr follow-up of the Whickham cohort, serum TSH concentrations in the upper part of the normal range in this study also appeared to have a predictive value.

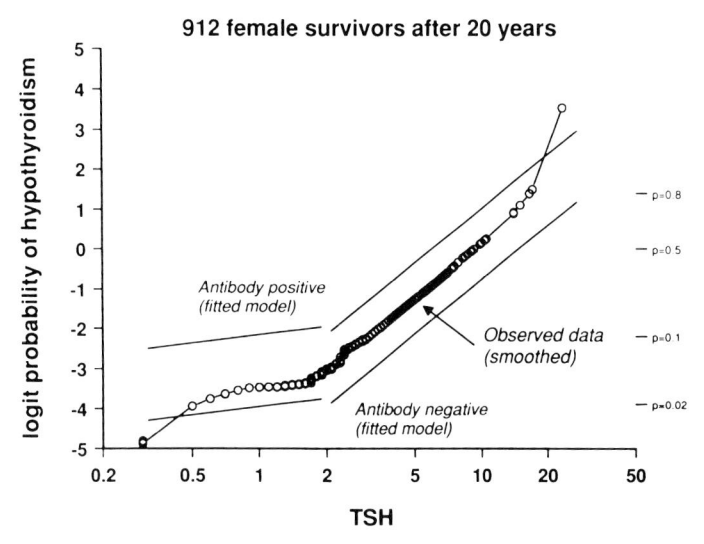

Fig. 2. Logit probability (log odds) for development within 20 yr of hypothyroidism with increasing values of serum TSH at first survey in 912 survivors *(3)*. Reproduced with permission.

There are conflicting incidence data on hypothyroidism in elderly subjects. In a 4-yr follow-up of 258 healthy elderly men and women, hypothyroidism developed at a rate of 7%/annum if thyroid antibodies were positive and serum TSH values were >10 mU/L *(68)*, whereas Lazarus et al. *(45)* had found that the prognostic significance of raised thyroid antibodies in a sample of 414 healthy elderly subjects was less than that seen in middle-aged or younger subjects. At 5-yr follow-up, the annual rate of developing hypothyroidism was approx 0.4% for the whole group and 2.2% for those with both elevated serum TSH and thyroid antibodies. A longitudinal population study of elderly women in Gothenburg estimated the incidence of hypothyroidism to be 2/1000/yr between ages 70 and 79 *(17)*. In a survey of a Birmingham practice of 1210 subjects aged over 60 yr, 18% of those with high serum TSH on initial testing had proceeded to overt hypothyroidism by 1 yr. Over half of these subjects with elevated serum TSH values were antithyroid microsomal antibody-positive initially and they were the more likely to progress *(12)*.

POSTPARTUM THYROIDITIS (PPT)

Approx 10% of women booking into antenatal clinics at 16 wk gestation are antithyroid peroxidase antibody- (antithyroid microsomal antibody) positive, which is compatible with the prevalence of thyroid antibodies in community surveys. PPT is a transient, destructive autoimmune thyroiditis that occurs between the 12th and 16th wk postpartum in 40–50% of such women *(69; see also* Chapter 11). The presence of antithyroid microsomal antibodies early in pregnancy increases the risk of developing PPT, and lymphocytic infiltration of the thyroid has been observed. It usually presents as a temporary, usually painless episode of hypothyroidism, occasionally preceded by a short episode of hyperthyroidism *(70)*. An association with symptoms of depression exists *(71)*, but these symptoms are more common among thyroid antibody-positive than antibody-negative women, and this association is independent of thyroid status *(72)*.

A proportion of women progress to permanent hypothyroidism following an episode of PPT, particularly those with high antibody titers. In one study, 17% of Japanese patients developed hypothyroidism during a 5–16 yr follow-up period (mean 9 yr) *(73)*, whereas in Wales, about a quarter of women with PPT became hypothyroid within the next 5 yr after delivery *(74)*. It is not clear whether pregnancy actually alters the final incidence of autoimmune thyroid disease or merely brings forward the time that thyroid disease develops. These studies suggest that if PPT occurs in 5% of all pregnancies and 20% develop permanent hypothyroidism, 1% of all parous women will be hypothyroid within a fairly short time after pregnancy. As already discussed, about 1% of Caucasian women have hypothyroidism, and therefore, PPT would be expected to occur before the majority of these cases of hypothyroidism. This would seem unlikely, since the Whickham follow-up study showed that the annual risk of spontaneous hypothyroidism increases dramatically with age from 1.4/1000 at ages 20–25 yr to 14/1000 at ages 75–80 yr (Fig. 1) and parity was not a risk factor. If over 20% of patients with Hashimoto's thyroiditis spontaneously recover satisfactory thyroid function *(75)*, it is possible that intensive follow-up of PPT patients will lead to the initiation of thyroxine treatment when the hypothyroidism is fluctuating, but will ultimately recover to normal.

SCREENING FOR THYROID DYSFUNCTION

It is desirable to detect any disease in its early stage, particularly when treatment is available that will benefit the affected person and forestall or improve the natural history of the condition. Thyroid disorders secondary to autoimmune thyroid disease are among the most prevalent of medical conditions, their symptoms and signs may be subtle and nonspecific, and they can be mistakenly attributed to other illnesses, particularly in the elderly. On the basis of the epidemiological studies of autoimmune thyroid disorders in iodine-replete communities reviewed in this chapter, who should be tested for thyroid dysfunction, when, and with what? The evidence from the community studies is that general testing of the apparently healthy population will detect only a few cases of overt thyroid disease and is unjustified.

Among postmenopausal women, however, up to 10% have subclinical hypothyroidism. Does this condition warrant detection? It may not have any ill effects, and treatment is not without risk. However, hypothyroidism is an insidious condition and can be readily overlooked. Questionnaires that aim to identify at-risk subjects in the community do not differentiate between those with and those without elevated serum TSH values *(76)*. There is some evidence that nonspecific symptoms and psychometric scores can be improved by T_4 with a retrospective awareness of disability *(77,78)*, and that T_4 may have beneficial effects on cardiovascular function and lipoprotein metabolism in subjects with subclinical hypothyroidism *(79–81)*. The adverse effects of subclinical hypothyroidism on cholesterol concentrations have long been associated with a theoretical increased risk of cardiovascular disease in cross-sectional studies *(82)*. A recent study found an association between subclinical hypothyroidism and raised low-density lipoprotein cholesterol, low high-density lipoprotein cholesterol, and raised lipoprotein(a) *(83)*. A reanalysis of intervention studies between 1976 and 1995 showed that subclinical hypothyroidism is up to three times more common in subjects with increased plasma cholesterol concentrations, but that total cholesterol is only slightly raised (up to 30%) in subclinical hypothyroidism *(84)*. A cost-utility analysis using a computer decision model to assess the consequences and costs of including serum TSH screening with cholesterol screening concluded that testing 35-yr-old men and women with repeat estimates every

5 yr for 50 yr would be beneficial and was as favorable as screening for hypertension *(85)*. The cost of detecting subclinical hypothyroidism was $9223 for women and $22,595 for men/quality-adjusted life year, but this cost was heavily dependent on the cost of the TSH assay kit ($10–50). Over half of the benefit in quality adjusted life years was accounted for by preventing progression to overt hypothyroidism, 30% by improving associated mild symptoms, and 2% estimated owing to prevention of cardiovascular disease. However, recent data from the 20-yr follow-up of the Whickham survey cohort found, in a multiple logistic regression analysis, no association between evidence of autoimmune thyroid disease (defined as either treated hypothyroidism, positive thyroid antibodies, or raised serum TSH) documented at the first survey with mortality or the development of ischemic heart disease *(48)*.

Most clinicians treat those subjects who have both raised serum TSH concentrations and positive thyroid antibody tests, even if symptoms are absent, provided that no contraindication is present, in view of the annual risk of developing hypothyroidism of approx 5%. If serum TSH alone is raised the annual risk of developing hypothyroidism is approx 3%/yr. The higher the serum TSH level, the greater the prognostic significance for the development of overt hypothyroidism. The risks of lifelong T_4, such as precipitating symptoms of ischemic heart disease *(86)* or the theoretical risks of osteoporosis *(87)*, can be balanced against the need for regular long-term follow-up in the expectation that one-third of these women will become hypothyroid within 20 yr. If thyroid antibodies alone are found, serum TSH should be measured approx every 3–5 yr.

The case for detection of subclinical hyperthyroidism, which will be an inevitable consequence of screening with serum TSH determinations, is even less clear. Approx 4% of men and women in the community have serum TSH levels below the normal range, with the prevalence being only slightly higher in women (cf. subclinical hypothyroidism). Subjects with slightly low, but detectable serum TSH values form a large proportion of this group. They have no evidence of thyroid disease clinically and are difficult to classify, but only rarely will they have undiagnosed hyperthyroidism. Some may have transient decreases in TSH, whereas others may be taking medication that suppresses TSH or have a nonthyroidal illness. The prevalence of clinically euthyroid subjects with undetectable TSH values and normal levels of FT_4 and FT_3 is approx 1%. In addition to the risk of subsequent development of overt hyperthyroidism, atrial fibrillation *(88,89)* and osteoporosis *(90)* are other possible long-term complications. The annual incidence of overt hyperthyroidism, which is usually more clinically obvious than hypothyroidism, is as little as 1/1000/yr in women and negligible in men *(3)*. The benefits of detection and treatment of hyperthyroidism were not included in the cost-utility analysis of TSH screening *(85)*.

Certain groups do have a high risk of developing autoimmune thyroid disease and require at least annual surveillance of thyroid function. This can be part of a computerized testing program of serum TSH measurements in primary care, with a recall system and follow-up serum-free T_4 measurements if the TSH is found to be abnormal. Those who would benefit most from this review are patients who have been treated for hyperthyroidism, and who are therefore at risk for either recurrent hyperthyroidism or hypothyroidism. Other patients who should have an assessment of thyroid function once include those with atrial fibrillation or hyperlipidemia *(91,92)*. Periodic assessment is indicated in those receiving amiodarone and lithium *(93)*. There is a high frequency of asymptomatic thyroid dysfunction in unselected patients with diabetes, and it was recently calculated that including an annual test of thyroid function in the annual review of diabetic complications was cost-effective *(94)*. The threefold increase in the prevalence of thyroid antibodies in patients with breast cancer suggests that it may be worth screening this group for thyroid dysfunction *(95)*. The evidence from the studies of patients hospitalized for acute illness is that the occurrence of autoimmune thyroid disease is no more common than in the general population. Therefore, testing should be limited, but with a high index of clinical suspicion, particularly in elderly women, and with an awareness of the difficulties in interpreting thyroid function tests in the presence of acute illness. An exception is possibly screening patients with psychiatric disorders, such as bipolar affective disorder with rapid cycling *(96)* and refractory depression *(97)*, for hypothyroidism, although the effect of T_4 treatment in such patients is uncertain and delaying testing for 3 wk avoids transient disturbances of thyroid function *(98)*. Symptoms of depression, as in PPT, are associated with positive thyroid antibodies rather than raised serum TSH concentrations, which suggests an immunological rather than an endocrinological basis for these symptoms. There is no consensus on whether healthy women should be screened for PPT *(99)*, although since women with Type 1 diabetes are three times more likely to develop postpartum thyroid dysfunction *(100)*, it is recommended that all such women should be screened in the first trimester. Any women with a past history of PPT should be offered annual surveillance of thyroid function in view of the long-term risk of permanent hypothyroidism. For most purposes, a determination of serum TSH, done by a sensitive immunoradiometric assay is the single most useful test for screening thyroid function in a selected population at risk (101).

REFERENCES

1. Vanderpump MPJ, Tunbridge WMG. The epidemiology of thyroid diseases. In: Braverman LE, Utiger RD, eds. The Thyroid: A Fundamental and Clinical Text, 7th ed. JB Lippincott-Raven, Philadelphia, 1996, pp. 474–482.
2. Tunbridge WMG, Evered DC, Hall R, Appleton D, Brewis M, Clark F, et al. The spectrum of thyroid disease in the community: The Whickham Survey. Clin Endocrinol 1977;7:481–493.
3. Vanderpump MPJ, Tunbridge WMG, French JM, Appleton D, Bates D, Clark F, et al. The incidence of thyroid disorders in the community—a twenty-year follow-up of the Whickham survey. Clin Endocrinol 1995;43:55–69.
4. Hoffenberg R. Aetiology of hyperthyroidism—part I. Br Med J 1974;3:452–456.
5. Eggertsen R, Petersen K, Lundberg P-A, Nyström E, Lindstedt G. Screening for thyroid disease in a primary care unit with a thyroid stimulating hormone assay with a low detection limit. Br Med J 1988; 297:1586–1591.
6. Okamura K, Ueda K, Sone H, Ikenoue H, Hasuo Y, Sato K, et al. A sensitive thyroid stimulating hormone assay for screening of thyroid functional disorder in elderly Japanese. J Am Geriatr Soc 1989; 37:317–322.
7. Kågedal B, Månson JC, Norr A, Sörbo B, Tegler L. Screening for thyroid disorders in middle-aged women by computer-assisted evaluation of a thyroid hormone panel. Scand J Clin Lab Invest 1981;41: 403–408.
8. Baldwin DB, Rowett D. Incidence of thyroid disorders in Connecticut. JAMA 1978;239:742–744.
9. dos Remedios LV, Weber PM, Feldman R, Schurr DA, Tsoi TG. Detecting unsuspected thyroid dysfunction by the free thyroxine index. Arch Intern Med 1980;140:1045–1049.
10. Schaaf L, Pohl T, Schmidt R, Vardali I, Teuber J, Schlote-Sauter B, et al. Screening for thyroid disorders in a working population. Clin Invest 1993;71:126–131.
11. Konno N, Yuri K, Taguchi H, Miura K, Taguchi S, Hagiwara K, et al. Screening for thyroid diseases in an iodine sufficient area with sensitive thyrotrophin assays, and serum thyroid autoantibody and urinary iodide determinations. Clin Endocrinol 1993;38:273–281.
12. Parle JV, Franklyn JA, Cross KW, Jones SC, Sheppard MC. Prevalence and follow-up of abnormal thyrotrophin (TSH) concentrations in the elderly in the United Kingdom. Clin Endocrinol 1991;34: 77–83.

13. Falkenberg M, Kågedal B, Norr A. Screening of an elderly female population for hypo- and hyperthyroidism by use of a thyroid hormone panel. Acta Med Scand 1983;214:361–365.
14. Bagchi N, Brown TR, Parish RF. Thyroid dysfunction in adults over age 55 years. A study in an urban US community. Arch Intern Med 1990;150:785–787.
15. Brochmann H, Bjøro T, Gaarder PI, Hanson F, Frey HM. Prevalence of thyroid dysfunction in elderly subjects. A randomized study in a Norwegian rural community (Nærøy). Acta Endocrinol 1988;117:7–12.
16. Campbell AJ, Reinken J, Allan BC. Thyroid disease in the elderly in the community. Age Ageing 1981;10:47–52.
17. Sundbeck G, Lundberg P-A, Lindstedt G, Jagenburg R, Edén S. Incidence and prevalence of thyroid disease in elderly women: results from the longitudinal population study of elderly people in Gothenburg, Sweden. Age Ageing 1991;20:291–298.
18. Kaplan MM, Reed Larsen P, Cranzt FR, Dzau VJ, Rossing TH. Prevalence of abnormal thyroid function test results in patients with acute medical illnesses. Am J Med 1982;72:9–16.
19. Gow SM, Elder A, Caldwell G, Bell G, Seth J, Sweeting VM, et al. An improved approach to thyroid function testing in patients with non-thyroidal illness. Clin Chim Acta 1986;158:49–58.
20. Small M, Buchanan L, Evans R. Value of screening thyroid function in acute medical admissions to hospital. Clin Endocrinol 1990;32:185–191.
21. DeGroot LJ, Mayor G. Admission screening by thyroid function tests in an acute general care teaching hospital. Am J Med 1992;93:558–564.
22. Simons RJ, Simon JM, Demers LM, Santen RJ. Thyroid dysfunction in elderly hospitalized patients. Effect of age and severity of illness. Arch Intern Med 1990;150:1249–1253.
23. Sawin CT, Geller A, Kaplan MM, Bacharach P, Wilson PWF, Hershman JM. Low serum thyrotropin (thyroid-stimulating hormone) in older persons without hyperthyroidism. Arch Intern Med 1991;151:165–168.
24. Furszyfer J, Kurland LT, McConahey WM, Elveback LR. Graves' disease in Olmsted County, Minnesota, 1935 through 1967. Mayo Clin Proc 1970;45:636–644.
25. Mogensen EF, Green A. The epidemiology of thyrotoxicosis in Denmark. Incidence and geographical variation in the Funen region 1972–1974. Acta Med Scand 1980;208:183–186.
26. Haraldsson A, Gudmundsson ST, Larusson G, Sigurdsson G. Thyrotoxicosis in Iceland 1980–1982. An epidemiological survey. Acta Med Scand 1985;217:253–258.
27. Berglund J, Christensen SB, Hallengren B. Total and age-specific incidence of Graves' thyrotoxicosis, toxic nodular goitre and solitary toxic adenoma in Malmö 1970–1974. J Intern Med 1990;227:137–141.
28. Kalk WJ, Kalk J. Incidence and causes of hyperthyroidism in blacks. S Afr Med J 1989;75:114–116.
29. Barker DJB, Phillips DIW. Current incidence of thyrotoxicosis and past prevalence of goitre in 12 British towns. Lancet 1984;ii:567–570.
30. Phillips DIW, Barker DJ, Rees Smith B, Didcote S, Morgan D. The geographical distribution of thyrotoxicosis in England according to the presence or absence of TSH-receptor antibodies. Clin Endocrinol 1985;23:283–287.
31. Nyström E, Bengtsson C, Lindquist O, Noppa H, Lindstedt G, Lundberg P-A. Thyroid disease and high concentration of serum thyrotrophin in a population sample of women. Acta Med Scand 1981;210:39–46.
32. Nyström E, Bengtsson C, Lindquist O, Lindberg S, Lindstedt G, Lundberg P-A. Serum triiodothyronine and hyperthyroidism in a population sample of women. Clin Endocrinol 1984;20:31–42.
33. Stott DJ, McLellan AR, Finlayson J, Chu P, Alexander WD. Elderly patients with suppressed serum TSH but normal free thyroid levels usually have mild thyroid overactivity and are at increased risk of developing overt hyperthyroidism. Q J Med 1991;78:77–84.
34. Sawin CT, Geller A, Kaplan MM, Bacharach P, Wilson PWF, Hershman JM. Low serum thyrotropin (thyroid-stimulating hormone) in older persons without hyperthyroidism. Arch Intern Med 1991;151:165–168.
35. Goudie RB, Anderson JR, Gray KG. Complement fixing thyroid antibodies in hospital patients with asymptomatic thyroid lesions. J Pathol Bacteriol 1959;90:389–400.
36. Bastenie PA, Neve P, Bonnyns M, Vanhaelst L, Chailly M. Clinical and pathological significance of asymptomatic atrophic thyroiditis. Lancet 1967;i:915–919.
37. Williams ED, Doniach I. The post mortem incidence of focal thyroiditis. J Pathol Bacteriol 1962;83:255–264.
38. Dingle PR, Ferguson A, Horn DB, Tubmen J, Hall R. The incidence of thyroglobulin antibodies and thyroid enlargement in a general practice in North East England. Clin Exp Immunol 1966;1:277–284.

39. Couchman KG, Wigley RD, Prior IAM. Autoantibodies in the Carterton Population Survey. J Chronic Dis 1970;23:45–53.
40. Hooper B, Whittingham S, Matthews JD, Mackay IR, Curnow DH. Autoimmunity in a rural community. Clin Exp Immunol 1972;12:79–87.
41. Gordin A, Maatela J, Miettinen A, Helenius T, Lamberg B-A. Serum thyrotrophin and circulating thyroglobulin and thyroid microsomal antibodies in a Finnish population. Acta Endocrinol 1979;90:33–42.
42. Hawkins BR, Cheah PS, Dawkins RL, Whittingham S, Burger HG, Patel Y, Mackay IR, et al. Diagnostic significance of thyroid microsomal antibodies in randomly selected population. Lancet 1980;ii:1057–1059.
43. Mariotti S, Sansoni P, Barbesino G, Caturegli P, Monti D, Cossarizza A, et al. Thyroid and other organ-specific autoantibodies in healthy centenarians. Lancet 1992;339:1506–1508.
44. Sawin CT, Castelli WP, Hershman JM, McNamara P, Bacharach P. The aging thyroid. Thyroid deficiency in the Framingham Study. Arch Intern Med 1985;145:1386–1388.
45. Lazarus JH, Burr ML, McGregor AM, Weetman AP, Ludgate M, Woodhead JS, et al. The prevalence and progression of autoimmune thyroid disease in the elderly. Acta Endocrinol 1984;106:199–202.
46. Prentice LM, Phillips DIW, Sarsero D, Beever K, McLachlan SM, Rees Smith B. Geographical distribution of subclinical autoimmune thyroid disease in Britain: A study using highly sensitive direct assays for autoantibodies to thyroglobulin and thyroid peroxidase. Acta Endocrinol 1990;123:493–498.
47. Roti E, Gardini E, Minelli R, Bianconi L, Braverman LE. Prevalence of anti-thyroid peroxidase antibodies in serum in the elderly: comparison with other tests for anti-thyroid antibodies. Clin Chem 1992;38:88–92.
48. Vanderpump MPJ, Tunbridge WMG, French JM, Appleton D, Bates D, Clark F, et al. The development of ischemic heart disease in relation to autoimmune thyroid disease in a 20-year follow-up study of an English community. Thyroid 1996;6:155–160.
49. Jansson R, Karlsson A, Dahlberg PA. Thyroxine, methimazole, and thyroid microsomal autoantibody titres in hypothyroid Hashimoto's thyroiditis. Br Med J 1985;290:11,12.
50. Takusu N, Yamada T, Takusu M, Komiya I, Nagasawa Y, Asawa T, et al. Disappearance of thyrotropin-blocking antibodies and spontaneous recovery from hypothyroidism in autoimmune thyroiditis. N Engl J Med 1992;326:513–518.
51. Lowrey R, Starr P. Chemical evidence of incidence of hypothyroidism. JAMA 1959;171:2045–2048.
52. Gordin A, Heinonen OP, Saarinen P, Lamberg B-A. Serum-thyrotrophin in symptomless autoimmune thyroiditis. Lancet 1972;i:551–554.
53. Hodkinson HM, Denham MJ Thyroid function tests in the elderly in the community. Age Ageing 1977;6:67–70.
54. Sawin CT, Bigos ST, Land S, Bacharach P. The aging thyroid. Relationship between elevated serum thyrotropin level and thyroid antibodies in elderly patients. Am J Med 1985;79:591–595.
55. Bahemuka M, Hodkinson HM. Screening for hypothyroidism in elderly inpatients. Br Med J 1975;2:601–603.
56. Franklyn JA. "Subclinical hypothyroidism": to treat or not to treat, that is the question. Clin Endocrinol 1995;43:443–444.
57. Toft AD, Irvine WJ, Seth J, Hunter WM, Cameron EHD. Thyroid function in the long-term follow-up of patients treated with iodine-131 for thyrotoxicosis. Lancet 1975;ii:576–578.
58. Evered DC, Young ET, Tunbridge WMG, Ormston BJ, Green E, Petersen VB, et al. Thyroid function after subtotal thyroidectomy for hyperthyroidism. Br Med J 1975;1:25–27.
59. Lundström B, Gillquist J The importance of elevated TSH in serum after subtotal thyroidectomy for hyperthyroidism. Acta Chir Scand 1981;147:645–647.
60. Franklyn JA, Daykin J, Droic Z, Farmer M, Sheppard MC. Long term follow-up of treatment of thyrotoxicosis by three different methods. Clin Endocrinol 1991;34:71–76.
61. Berglund J, Christensen SB, Dymling JF, Hallengren B. The incidence of recurrence and hypothyroidism following treatment with antithyroid drugs, surgery or radioiodine in all patients with thyrotoxicosis in Malmö during the period 1970–1974. J Intern Med 1991;229:435–442.
62. Tamai H, Kasagi K, Takaichi Y, Takamatsu J, Komaki G, Matsubayashi S, et al. Development of spontaneous hypothyroidism in patients with Graves' Disease treated with antithyroidal drugs: clinical, immunological, and histological findings in 26 patients. Metabolism 1989;69:49–53.
63. Shigemasa C, Mitani Y, Taniguchi S, Adachi T, Ueta Y, Urabe K, et al. Three patients who spontaneously developed persistent hypothyroidism during or following treatment with antithyroid drugs for Graves' hyperthyroidism. Arch Intern Med 1990;150:1150–1159.

64. Tunbridge WMG, Brewis M, French JM, Appleton D, Bird T, Clark F, et al. Natural history of autoimmune thyroiditis. Br Med J 1981;282:258–262.
65. Gordin A, and Lamberg B-A. Natural course of symptomless autoimmune thyroiditis. Lancet 1975;ii: 1234–1238.
66. Gordin A, Lamberg B-A. Spontaneous hypothyroidism in symptomless autoimmune thyroiditis. A long-term follow-up study. Clin Endocrinol 1981;15:537–543.
67. Geul KW, van Sluisveld ILL, Grobbee DE, Docter R, de Bruyn AM, Hooykaas H, et al. The importance of thyroid microsomal antibodies in the development of elevated serum TSH in middle-aged women: associations with serum lipids. Clin Endocrinol 1993;39:275–280.
68. Rosenthal KJ, Hunt WC, Garry PJ, Goodwin JS. Thyroid failure in the elderly. Microsomal antibodies as discriminant for therapy. JAMA 1987;258:209–213.
69. Hall R. Pregnancy and autoimmune endocrine disease. Balliere's Clin Endocrinol Metab 1995;9: 137–155.
70. Gerstein HC. How common is post-partum thyroiditis? A methodologic overview of the literature. Arch Intern Med 1990;150:1397–1399.
71. Harris B, Othman S, Davies JA, Weppner GJ, Richards CJ, Newcombe RG, et al. Association between post-partum thyroid dysfunction and thyroid antibodies and depression. Br Med J 1992;305:152–156.
72. Tachi J, Amino N, Tamaki H, Aozasa M, Iwatani Y, Miyai K. Long term follow-up and HLA association in patients with post-partum hypothyroidism. J Clin Endocrinol Metab 1988;66:480–484.
73. Lazarus JH, Hall R, Othman S, Parkes AB, Richards CJ, McCulloch B, et al. The clinical spectrum of postpartum thyroid disease. Q J Med 1996;89:429–435.
74. Othman S, Phillips DIW, Parkes AB, Richards CJ, Harris B, Fung H, et al. A long term follow-up of postpartum thyroiditis. Clin Endocrinol 1990;32:559–564.
75. Takasu N, Komiya I, Asawa T, Nagasawa Y, Yamada T. Test for recovery from hypothyroidism during thyroxine therapy in Hashimoto's thyroiditis. Lancet 1990;336:1084–1086.
76. Parle JV, Franklyn JA, Cross KW, Jones SC, Sheppard MC. Assessment of a screening process to detect patients aged 60 years and over at high risk of hypothyroidism. Br J Gen Pract 1991;41:414–416.
77. Cooper DS, Halpern R, Wood LC, Levin AA, Ridgeway ED. L-thyroxine therapy in subclinical hypothyroidism: a double-blind, placebo-controlled trial. Ann Intern Med 1984;101:18–24.
78. Monzani F, Del Guerra P, Caraccio N, Pruneti CA, Pucci CA, Luisi M, et al. Subclinical hypothyroidism: neurobehavioral features and beneficial effects of L-thyroxine treatment. Clin Invest 1993;71: 367–371.
79. Bell GM, Todd WTA, Forfar JC, Martyn C, Wathen CG, Gow S, et al. End-organ responses to thyroxine therapy in subclinical hypothyroidism. Clin Endocrinol 1985;22:83–89.
80. Nyström E, Caidahl K, Fager G, Wikkelsö C, Lundberg P-A, Lindstedt G. A double-blind cross-over 12-month study of L-thyroxine treatment of women with "subclinical" hypothyroidism. Clin Endocrinol 1988;29:63–76.
81. Franklyn JA, Daykin J, Betteridge J, Hughes E.A, Holder R, Jones SR, et al. Thyroxine replacement therapy and circulating lipid concentrations. Clin Endocrinol 1993;38:453–459.
82. Bastenie PA. Hypothyroidism and coronary heart disease. Acta Cardiol 1982;37:365–373.
83. Kung AWC, Pang RWC, Janus ED. Elevated serum lipoprotein(a) in subclinical hypothyroidism. Clin Endocrinol 1995;43:445–449.
84. Tanis BC, Westendorp RGJ, Smelt AHM. Effect of thyroid substitution on hypercholesterolaemia in patients with subclinical hypothyroidism: a re-analysis of intervention studies. Clin Endocrinol 1996; 44:643–649.
85. Danese MD, Powe NR, Sawin CT, Ladenson PW. Screening for mild thyroid failure at the periodic health examination: a decision and cost-effectiveness analysis. JAMA 1996;276:285–292.
86. Gammage M, Franklyn J. Hypothyroidism, thyroxine treatment and the heart. Heart 1997;77:189–190.
87. Faber J, Galloe AM. Changes in bone mass during prolonged subclinical hyperthyroidism due to L-thyroxine treatment: a meta-analysis. Eur J Endocrinol 1994;130:631–642.
88. Tenerz A, Forberg R, Jansson R. Is a more active attitude warranted in patients with subclinical thyrotoxicosis? J Intern Med 1990;228:229–233.
89. Sawin CT, Geller A, Wolf PA, Belanger AJ, Baker E, Bacharach P, et al. Low serum thyrotropin concentrations as a risk factor for atrial fibrillation in older persons. N Engl J Med 1994;331:1249–1252.
90. Földes J, Tarján G, Szathmari M, Varga F, Krasznai I, Horvath Cs. Bone mineral density in patients with endogenous subclinical hyperthyroidism: is this thyroid status a risk factor for osteoporosis. Clin Endocrinol 1993;39:521–527.

91. Glueck CJ, Lang J, Tracy T, Speirs J. The common finding of covert hypothyroidism at initial clinical evaluation for hyperlipoproteinaemia. Clin Chim Acta 1991;201:113–122.
92. O'Kane MJ, Neely RDG, Trimble ER, Nicholls DP. The incidence of asymptomatic hypothyroidism in new referrals to a hospital lipid clinic. Ann Clin Biochem 1991;28:509–511.
93. Vanderpump MPJ, Tunbridge WMG. The effects of drugs on endocrine function. Clin Endocrinol 1993;39:389–397.
94. Perros P, McCrimmon RJ, Shaw G, Frier BM. Frequency of thyroid dysfunction in diabetic patients: value of annual screening. Diabetic Med 1996;12:622–627.
95. Giani C, Fierabracci P, Bonacci R, Giglotti A, Campani D, De Negri F, et al. Relationship between breast cancer and thyroid disease: relevance of autoimmune thyroid disorders in breast malignancy. J Clin Endocrinol Metab 1996;81:990–994.
96. Oomen HAPC, Schipperijn AMJ, Drexhage HA. The prevalence of affective disorder and in particular of a rapid cycling of bipolar disorder in patients with abnormal thyroid function tests. Clin Endocrinol 1996;45:215–223.
97. Howland RH. Thyroid dysfunction in refractory depression: implications for pathophysiology and treatment. J Clin Psychiatry 1993;54:47–54.
98. White AJ, Barraclough B. Thyroid disease and mental illness; a study of thyroid disease in psychiatric admissions. J Pychomatic Res 1988;32:99–106.
99. Vanderpump MPJ, Ahlquist JAO, Franklyn JA, Clayton RN. Development of consensus for good practice and audit measures in the management of hypothyroidism and hyperthyroidism. Br Med J 1996;313:539–544.
100. Alvarez-Marfany M, Roman SH, Drexler AJ, Robertson C, Stagnaro-Green A. Long-term prospective study of post-partum thyroid dysfunction in women with insulin dependent diabetes mellitus. J Clin Endocrinol Metab 1994;79:10–16.
101. Ross DS, Daniels GH, Gouveia D. The use and limitations of a chemiluminescent thyrotrophin assay as a single thyroid function test in an out-patient endocrine clinic. J Clin Endocrinol Metab 1990;71:764–769.

7   Sex Hormones and Immune Responses

William J. Kovacs, MD, and Nancy J. Olsen, MD

CONTENTS

> INTRODUCTION
> INNATE IMMUNITY IS MODULATED BY HORMONAL STATUS
> IMMUNE RESPONSES TO PARASITIC INFECTIONS MAY BE MODULATED BY HORMONAL STATUS
> AUTOIMMUNE DISEASES ARE MODULATED BY HORMONAL STATUS
> CELLULAR TARGETS OF HORMONE ACTION IN THE IMMUNE SYSTEM: HORMONE RECEPTORS
> CELLULAR AND MOLECULAR EFFECTS OF GONADAL STEROIDS ON INNATE IMMUNITY
> MECHANISMS OF ACTIONS OF HORMONES IN THE ADAPTIVE ARM OF THE IMMUNE SYSTEM
> CONCLUSIONS
> ACKNOWLEDGMENTS
> REFERENCES

INTRODUCTION

The immune system is an interacting network of cells and mediators that serves to defend the host against invasion by either infectious agents or malignant cells. The system discerns self from nonself; when this recognition breaks down, pathologic inflammatory states or autoimmune disease may develop. In considering the role of hormones in modulating immune function in health and disease, it is useful to consider two main functional arms of the immune system (Table 1). The first might be described as innate immunity, and probably represents, from the evolutionary perspective, the most primitive components of the system *(1)*. Innate or natural immunity is not dependent on prior recognition of a foreign antigen and generally serves as an early line of defense against invasion. Innate responses lack high degrees of specificity, but are rapidly deployed. When such innate immune responses are mobilized in error or in excess, inflammatory damage may result. Components of innate or natural immune reactions include the complement proteins and macrophages along with their secreted products, such as interleukin 1 (IL-1) and tumor necrosis factor α (TNF-α). Innate or natural immune responses may be activated during sepsis and shock or when a malignancy is

From: *Contemporary Endocrinology: Autoimmune Endocrinopathies*
Edited by: R. Volpe © Humana Press Inc., Totowa, NJ

Table 1
Cellular and Soluble Mediators of Innate and Acquired Immunity

Immune system components	Cellular mediators	Soluble mediators
Innate immunity	Macrophages	IL-1, IL-6, IL-12, TNF-α
	NK cells	—
Adaptive immunity	T lymphocytes	IL-2, IL-4, IL-10, other
	B lymphocytes	Antibodies

present. The second major functional arm of the immune system is more specific, and may be referred to as "adaptive" because previous exposure to an antigen has taken place. Major components of this aspect of immune function include T and B lymphocytes, along with their respective secreted products, cytokines and antibodies. Chronic infectious diseases usually activate adaptive immune responses. Overresponsiveness or inappropriate triggering of the various components of the immune system may result in autoimmune diseases, such as rheumatoid arthritis, thyroiditis, or systemic lupus erythematosus. In some clinical situations, both innate and specific responses contribute to pathogenesis of autoimmune disorders. For example, rheumatoid arthritis is an autoimmune process that is most dependent on antigen-specific T cells. However, innate immune mediators such as IL-1 and TNF-α also contribute to ongoing tissue damage.

Clinical and experimental evidence suggests that gonadal steroid hormones modulate both innate and adaptive immune responses. The well-described sexual dimorphisms of diseases involving the immune system, including chronic infections and autoimmune syndromes, might thus be owing in part to actions of these hormones to modulate immune functions of the host. Human diseases and animal models of these diseases are complex, and undoubtedly multifactorial. Direct proof of a role for hormones in directing the host's response to immune system challenge is sometimes difficult to establish. However, an increasing number of experimental systems provide substantial evidence for direct and important interactions between gonadal steroids and cellular targets within the immune system. Some of these data are derived from animal models that allow assessment of the effects of altered hormonal status. Other data derive from clinical experiences with the alterations in hormonal status that occur in humans during pregnancy or with pharmacologic administration of these agents. Understanding the mechanisms of gonadal steroid hormone action within the immune system is likely to provide insight into aspects of the pathogenesis of disorders as diverse as septic shock, helminthic infections, and autoimmune syndromes.

INNATE IMMUNITY IS MODULATED BY HORMONAL STATUS

Innate immune responses are principally mediated by nonlymphoid mononuclear cells (macrophages and monocytes) that circulate in the peripheral blood or reside fixed in organs, such as the liver or synovium. These cells and their products, chiefly IL-1, IL-6, and TNF-α, are important components of the early host response to infection, shock, or wounding. Activation of these proinflammatory mediators (for example, by bacterial lipopolysacharride [LPS] during Gram-negative bacteremia) elicits a host response that may include fever and an altered pattern of hepatic protein production, called the acute-phase response. A common consequence of such innate immune activation is the injury of normal tissues.

Clinical observations in humans and experimental work on animal models have indicated that androgens may exacerbate the adverse aspects of the innate immune response elicited by shock. Males usually predominate in clinical series of patients suffering septic shock (2). Whether this male predominance is due to hormonal differences or to other risk factors incurred by males is not known. In animal models, however, the evidence strongly suggests that testosterone adversely affects the outcome of septic shock. Only 10% of C3H/HeN male mice survive induction of polymicrobial sepsis (accomplished by cecal ligation and puncture), whereas 60% of females are alive 10 d after such a septic insult (3). Androgen receptor blockade by flutamide treatment reduces the mortality rate among male mice subjected to combined hemorrhagic and septic shock by 30% (4). Antiandrogen treatment is associated with normalization of rates of in vitro splenocyte proliferation and of secretion of the mediators IL-1, IL-6, and IL-2 (5). Whether these cytokines actually contribute to differences in morbidity and mortality, however, remains undetermined. The observed differences in survival and in immunologic parameters are not attributable to alterations in glucocorticoids, since plasma levels of corticosterone are not altered by flutamide treatment.

IMMUNE RESPONSES TO PARASITIC INFECTIONS MAY BE MODULATED BY HORMONAL STATUS

Host responses to parasitic infections are complex, and although a variety of data exist that suggest hormonal modulation of some aspects of antiparasitic immunity, the overall picture is far from clear. Innate immune mechanisms are involved in combating infection by intracellular organisms, such as protozoa. Most parasites infecting vertebrates are resistant to lysis by complement; some protozoa can be phagocytosed by macrophages, but are able to evade phagocytic killing. Specific immune responses are therefore required for defense against many parasites, and every conceivable type of immune response has been observed against these organisms. Helper (CD4$^+$) T lymphocytes, which recognize parasite antigens, are mobilized to contain tissue spread of some parasites within granulomas. Antigen-specific cytotoxic T lymphocytes may attack some parasitic organisms directly. T cells also produce soluble mediators, notably IL-4, which can activate components of the innate immune system, such as macrophages, to amplify granuloma formation. B cells may be stimulated by IL-4 to produce high levels of IgE. Antibody- (IgE) directed cytotoxic attack is involved in the response to some parasites, notably helminths. Despite these various immune responses, parasitic diseases are characterized by chronicity owing to the inability of the host to eliminate the parasite, which utilizes many evasive mechanisms to escape detection and eradication. As a result of the long-term immunostimulation that develops, initially protective responses may evolve into destructive processes and may contribute significantly to morbidity and mortality of these diseases. An example is the severe liver fibrosis resulting from delayed-type hypersensitivity reaction to hepatic egg deposition in chronic *Schistosoma mansoni* infection, leading to portal hypertension.

Reports of sexual dimorphism of parasitic diseases include observations of increased prevalence or severity in males for some infections and in females for others (Table 2). Such sexual dimorphism could be the consequence of direct hormonal effects on the parasites themselves (6), or hormonal modulation of host immune responses or the resultant chronic inflammatory reaction. Alternatively, gender differences for human

Table 2
Sexually Dimorphic Disease Expression in Parasitic Infections[a]

Infections with greater severity in females
    Schistosomiasis (mouse)
    T. Crassiceps (mouse)
Infections with greater severity in males
    Malaria (mouse)
    Leishmania (mouse)
    Chagas disease (human)
    Lymphatic filariasis (human)
    Onchoceriasis (human)

[a]Host species reported indicated in parentheses.

disorders and animal models may be the result of behavioral differences that subject males and females to different environmental risks. The issue of hormonal status has been examined in only a few models.

Infections with the helminths *Schistosoma mansoni* and *Taenia crassiceps* elicit largely adaptive immune responses in the host. Both of these infections show evidence of greater severity in females *(7,8)*. Female CBA/J mice have higher rates of mortality from experimental *S. mansoni* infection than males, despite infection of both sexes with equal numbers of the immature cercariae *(7)*. Spleen and liver weights are significantly higher in the females, but hematocrits are lower, consistent with more severe disease *(7)*. Females have higher burdens of mature worms, suggesting that conditions for maturation of the parasite are more favorable in females than in males. Castration of normal males results in a pattern of infection that is indistinguishable from that seen in females. The mortality rate after 16 wk of infection is 80% in females and castrate males, compared to only 40% in intact males or testosterone-treated females *(9)*. The influence of hormonal status appears to be exerted during early stages of infection; if manipulations are carried out 5 wk after *S. mansoni* infection, rather than prior to parasite exposure, no differences are observed. The results are not specific for a given strain of mice: two inbred strains (C57 Bl/6 and CBA/J) and one outbred strain (CF1) showed similar results. These results indicate that the hormonally mediated effects target early life forms of the parasite, with the presence of testosterone providing a generally less favorable environment for worm development.

Infection of female BALB/c mice with *T. crassiceps* results in parasite levels that are four to five times higher than in males *(8)*. Gonadectomy in males leads to higher levels of disease intensity in this infection, but in females, removal of the ovaries results in lower parasite burdens. Direct addition of estradiol, testosterone, or progesterone to parasites in vitro does not have any effect on growth of the organisms. The data therefore suggest that sexual dimorphism in this parasitic infection is modulated by effects of gonadal steroid hormones on the immune system of the host. As in the case of *S. mansoni*, the mechanism of hormonal modulation of the adaptive immune response is not known.

A number of parasitic infections (Table 2) show greater prevalence or severity in males. Three of these are protozoan organisms (Leishmania, Chagas' disease, and malaria). Innate immune responses, especially macrophage activation, are important for host defense against these organisms, which usually reside in an intracellular location. In experimental leishmaniasis, castration of males results in a decrease in the parasite load, whereas treatment of females with testosterone results in a higher number of parasites

(10). The stronger innate immunity that is postulated to be relatively protective of the female in septic shock, as discussed above, may also provide more protection of females against these disorders. Adaptive immunity may also be modulated; androgens suppress Th1-type responses that are known to be protective in leishmaniasis *(11)*. In experimental models of malaria, male gender (or testosterone administration) is associated with an accelerated or nonhealing form of the disease *(12,13)*. The responsible mechanism in this disorder may involve diminished numbers of B cells and correspondingly lower levels of antibodies to the parasite *(14)*.

Two parasitic infections with observed male predominance (lymphatic filariasis and onchoceriasis) are due to helminths. It is not readily apparent why these infections appear to have the opposite gender bias from other helminthic infections (schistosomiasis, cistercercosis). One potential difference is in the pattern of T-cell responses and cytokine profiles specific to the host response to these organisms. Cytokines derived from the Th1 subset (IL-2; interferon-gamma [IFN-γ]) may be relatively protective against filariasis, but as noted above, androgens may suppress the Th1 response *(15,16)*, whereas estrogen is stimulatory *(17)*.

AUTOIMMUNE DISEASES ARE MODULATED BY HORMONAL STATUS

As the site of T-cell development and maturation, the thymus gland has a pivotal role in the development of specific immune responses. It is here that immature T cells learn to distinguish self from nonself. Failure of appropriate deletion mechanisms may lead to escape of cells with potentially autoreactive specificities to enter the peripheral T-cell repertoire. Precise mechanisms of T-cell selection are incompletely understood. However, interactions between the thymocyte and epithelial cell components based on expression of major histocompatibility complex (MHC) molecules are critical to selecting which thymocytes mature and which die by apoptosis within the thymus gland *(18)*.

Development of B cells takes place in the bone marrow. Uncommitted or undefined lymphoid progenitor cells follow a well-defined sequence of cellular transitions to produce a virgin B cell *(19)*. The sequence of B-cell maturation is mediated by cytokines and growth factors, at least some of which are derived from underlying stromal cells. Processes of cellular selection and generation of the peripheral B-cell repertoire probably take place in the bone marrow. These are not yet as well defined as in the thymus.

Peripheral T lymphocytes possess surface antigen receptors, and B lymphocytes display surface immunoglobulins that define cellular specificity for antigen. Under appropriate conditions of antigen engagement, these receptors trigger activation of the cell to produce soluble products, either cytokines or antibodies. Abnormal autoimmune responses in the peripheral lymphoid compartment may be owing to defects in the central selection mechanisms, resulting in escape of cells with autoimmune specificities or to intrinsic abnormalities in the lymphocytes themselves. An example of the latter is the generalized hyperresponsiveness of B cells in patients with systemic lupus erythematosus, which may produce inappropriately high levels of antibodies in response to exogenous antigens *(20)*. Whether such lymphocyte abnormalities are genetic or acquired is currently unknown.

Human autoimmune diseases show a female predominance (Table 3). These include multisystem autoimmune syndromes such as rheumatoid arthritis *(21)*, systemic lupus erythematosus (SLE) *(22)*, scleroderma (systemic sclerosis) *(23)* and Sjögren's Syndrome *(24)*, as well as organ-specific disorders, such as Graves' disease *(25)* and Addison's disease

Table 3
Sexual Dimorphism of Autoimmune Disease

Autoimmune disease or syndrome	Prevalence ratios female:male
Rheumatoid arthritis	2.5:1
SLE	9:1
Scleroderma	5:1
Sjögren's syndrome	9:1
Graves' disease	5:1
Addison's disease	2.5:1
Multiple sclerosis	1.8:1

(26; see also Chapters 9 and 13). Neurologic syndromes with autoimmune features, including multiple sclerosis (27), also occur with greater frequency in females.

Examination of age-specific incidence rates in males and females provides further evidence for the importance of hormonal influences in the onset of these disorders. Systemic lupus erythematosus in children does not show a marked predilection for females. However, with the onset of puberty in teen years, the proportion of new cases in females shows a dramatic increase, and this trend continues in succeeding years (22) (Fig. 1). Rheumatoid arthritis is unusual in persons <20 yr of age, but subsequently shows a higher incidence in females, especially in the third and fourth decades of life (21) (Fig. 1).

Studies in lupus patients suggest that hormonal status may be related to disease susceptibility or disease exacerbations. Female patients with SLE have serum levels of androgens that are lower than those in control subjects (28,29). Although differences between the groups were not statistically significant, lower levels of androgens were observed in the patients with more active disease (28,29). These findings suggest that hormonal background may be involved in the development of SLE. Other evidence implicating a role for hormones in the development of SLE is derived from reports of autoimmune disease in hypogonadal males such as those with Klinefelter's syndrome (30). Although such reports are suggestive of an association, systematic studies to determine either the prevalence of hypogonadism in male lupus patients or the prevalence of autoimmunity in hypogonadal patients have not been done.

Pregnancy provides an opportunity to assess possible effects of an altered hormonal milieu on the expression of autoimmune diseases. A relationship between disease activity and pregnancy is most obvious for patients with rheumatoid arthritis, who commonly show amelioration of disease during the second and third trimesters. The disease generally flares again several months after delivery. A very similar pattern of pregnancy-induced remission and postpartum exacerbation is seen in multiple sclerosis patients (31). Hench (32) first postulated a hormonal basis for changes in disease manifestations associated with pregnancy. However, pregnancy is associated with changes in levels of many hormones, and nonhormonal mechanisms also require consideration. Recent studies suggest that the extent of disparity between maternal and fetal histocompatibility (HLA) haplotypes may be correlated with the degree of modulation of disease activity observed in patients with rheumatoid arthritis (33). Patients with SLE may experience exacerbations of disease activity during pregnancy (34). However, other studies suggest that the frequency of lupus flares is not more frequent during pregnancy (35). Reasons for these reported differences are not clear.

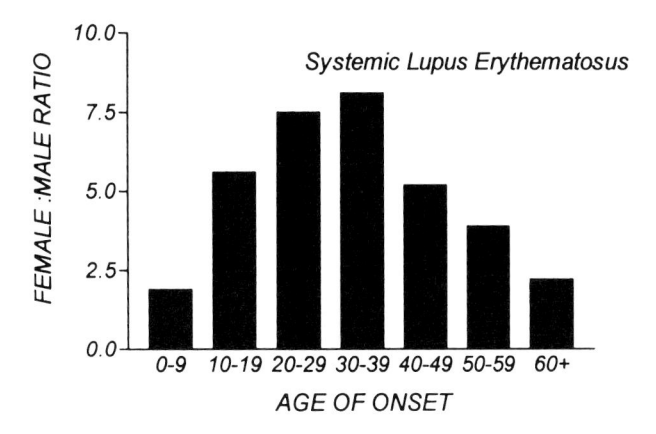

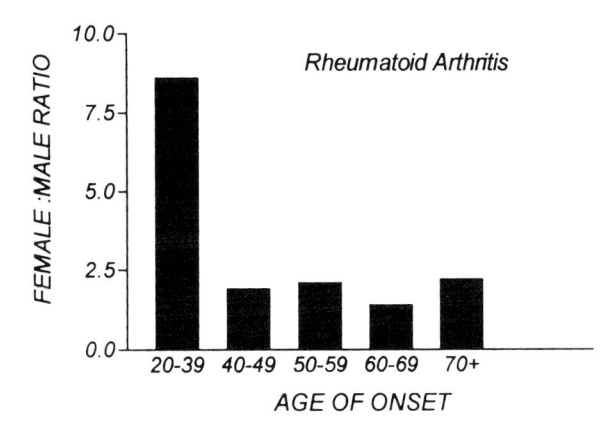

Fig. 1. Ratios of females to males at various ages of onset for SLE (top) and rheumatoid arthritis (bottom). For both diseases, the highest female:male ratio is seen in the 20–39 age group, corresponding with the peak childbearing years in females (adapted from Wallace et al. [22] and Linos et al. [21]).

Administration of exogenous estrogen or stimulation of endogenous estrogen production may alter the course of autoimmune processes. A recent report documents the onset of classical SLE occurring in three women within 3 mo of ovulation induction therapy for treatment of infertility (36). All three patients had completed at least six cycles of treatment, resulting in very high serum levels of estradiol. Cases such as these have led to concern about the potential for estrogen to exacerbate disease activity in lupus. An ongoing, multicenter, double-blind trial comparing estrogen to placebo has been designed to determine whether hormone-replacement therapy in postmenopausal lupus patients poses significant risks (37).

Interest in the use of androgens for treatment of SLE was triggered by studies suggesting that danazol (Danocrine) had efficacy in some patients (38,39). Furthermore, hypogonadal male patients who are treated to normalize serum levels of testosterone also have been reported to show symptomatic and serologic improvement (40,41). These results have suggested that treatment of female lupus patients with androgens might also be beneficial. Unfortunately, virilizing side effects limit tolerability of therapy in females. A weaker androgen with less potential for masculinization is 19-nortestosterone, but this agent had no significant efficacy in female patients in one study, and male patients in the same study actually showed worsening of disease activity *(42)*. In vivo conversion of the hormone to a metabolite with estrogenic activity was postulated, but not demonstrated. An alternative hormone treatment that has been investigated for treatment of SLE is the adrenal androgen dehydroepiandrosterone (DHEA) *(43)*. Preliminary analyses from a double-blind trial of DHEA in female patients with lupus suggest that use of this agent allows reduction in the dose of prednisone required to control disease activity in a subset of patients *(44)*. Serum levels of testosterone were not reported with the other preliminary findings. Whether DHEA exerts a steroid-sparing effect by acting at a known steroid hormone receptor, through an unidentified member of this receptor family, or whether this is an immunomodulatory effect owing to metabolic conversion to more active androgens remains to be determined. Further trials with this agent in the treatment of SLE are in progress.

Most models of autoimmune disease in animals occur preferentially or with greater severity in females than in males. The classic description of this phenomenon was made in the NZB/W murine lupus model. Disease prevalence and the rate of progression to mortality are greater in females than males of this F1 hybrid strain. Female mice of the MRL/lpr and SWRxSJL strains also show autoimmune manifestations at a rate that is significantly greater than that of corresponding males *(45,46)*. Autoimmune diabetes in the nonobese diabetic (NOD) mouse shows higher levels in females than in males, a pattern that has been reported in all NOD colonies *(47)*. Autoimmune insulitis occurs in both sexes, but onset of overt disease occurs significantly sooner in females *(47)*. Variability of diabetes prevalence in males appears to be related to differences in environmental factors, possibly related to viral infection. These external factors appear to be of greater importance to disease penetrance in the male than in the female *(48)*. Only the BXSB mouse, which develops a lupus-like disease, shows higher levels of autoimmune manifestations in the male; the disease-susceptibility gene in this particular strain maps to the Y chromosome *(49)*.

The autoimmune disease of both NZB/W and NOD mice is significantly altered by changes in androgenic hormonal status. Castration of NZB/W male mice results in a mortality curve that is equivalent to intact females. Treatment of females with androgens results in almost complete abolition of disease manifestations *(50–52)*. Conversely, estradiol administration to castrate females enhances disease progression *(51)*. Removal of the thymus prevents the ameliorating actions of androgens in these mice, suggesting that the pathway of interaction between male hormones and the immune manifestations includes the thymus *(53)*. Diabetes in the NOD mouse strain is also affected by hormonal status. Disease manifestations are accelerated by castration and reversed by androgen replacement *(54,55)*.

CELLULAR TARGETS OF HORMONE ACTION IN THE IMMUNE SYSTEM: HORMONE RECEPTORS

Gonadal steroid hormones exert most of their known effects by interaction with specific intracellular receptor proteins. These receptors are ligand-activated transcription factors that regulate the expression of specific gene products by target cells. Receptors for gonadal steroid hormones have been identified in a variety of cells of the immune system *(56)* (Table 4).

Table 4
Receptors for Gondadal Steroid Hormones in Cells of the Immune System

Steroid hormone	Localization of receptors in the immune system		
	Thymus	Spleen/blood	Bone marrow
Androgen	Thymocytes	Macrophages	B cells
	Thymic epithelium		Stromal cells
Estrogen	Thymocytes	CD8+ T cells	Stromal cells
	Thymic epithelium		
Progesterone	Thymic epithelium	?	?

Androgen receptors (ARs) are expressed in both lymphoid and stromal cell components of the thymus. Although AR is present in all major thymocyte subclasses, increased levels of expression have been demonstrated in the more immature components of the gland, including the CD4$^-$CD8$^-$ and CD4$^-$CD8$^+$ subpopulations *(57)*. Ligand binding assays have also demonstrated expression of AR in murine thymic epithelial cell lines of both cortical and medullary origin *(58)*. Lymphoid and stromal cell components of bone marrow have also been shown to contain AR *(59)*. However, numerous studies have failed to demonstrate AR in peripheral lymphoid tissues, including spleen *(60–62)* and peripheral blood or thoracic duct *(63,64)*. Expression of AR by lymphoid cells appears to be limited to immature forms in thymus and bone marrow. Peripheral leukocytes of the monocyte/macrophage lineage have been shown to express AR. For example, macrophage-like cells within synovial tissues have been shown to be AR-positive by immunohistochemistry *(65)*.

Estrogen receptors (ERs) have been demonstrated in the thymus by a variety of techniques including ligand binding assays *(66,67)*, immunohistochemistry *(68)*, and Northern blot analysis *(69)*. Subcellular localization within the thymus is less well defined, but may include both lymphoid and epithelial cells *(56)*. In the bone marrow compartment, the presence of ER in stromal cells has been demonstrated using reverse transcription-polymerase chain reaction (RT-PCR) amplification *(70)*. Unlike AR, ER also appears to be expressed in peripheral lymphoid cells, especially the CD8$^+$ subset of T cells *(64,71,72)*.

Receptors for progesterone have been demonstrated in the thymus by hormone binding and immunohistochemical techniques *(56,68,73)*. Although specific cell types expressing the receptor have not been definitively identified, the data are consistent with localization to nonlymphoid thymus cells, which are most likely epithelial in origin.

CELLULAR AND MOLECULAR EFFECTS OF GONADAL STEROIDS ON INNATE IMMUNITY

Estrogens have been found to downregulate the activation of macrophages in most experimental systems. Talc-induced peritoneal adhesion formation in mice can be quantitatively assessed by measurement of the thickness of the peritoneal membrane. In vivo treatment with 17β estradiol (E2) results in decreased membrane thickening by 65% compared to vehicle-treated controls ($p < 0.01$) *(74)*. Estrogen treatment does not reduce the number of macrophages in the lesions. However, the activation state of the lesional cells is diminished as shown by a decrease in mRNA for the murine monocyte chemoattractant protein designated JE/MCP-1. Similar effects on JE/MCP-1 expression are observed in macrophage-like cell lines *(74)*. Molecular mechanisms underlying the interaction between estrogens and JE/MCP-1 expression have not as yet been defined, but may be mediated through estrogen response elements in the JE/MCP-1 promoter.

Macrophages and monocytes produce IL-1, a soluble mediator of the pyrogenic and acute-phase protein responses. The available data concerning effects of estrogen on levels of IL-1 are somewhat contradictory, with some studies finding that estrogen elevates and others indicating that it decreases levels of this cytokine. Isolated peritoneal macrophages from female mice produce more IL-1 than cells from males after LPS treatment in vivo *(75)* or in vitro *(76)*. The difference appears to be estrogen-dependent, since the highest level of IL-1 is produced by cells isolated during the proestrus phase of the female reproductive cycle *(75)*, is diminished after ovariectomy, and is restored by estrogen replacement *(77)*. Some investigators have reported similar findings in humans —women's peripheral blood mononuclear cells produce greater amounts of IL-1 than cells from men under LPS stimulation, and women excrete greater amounts of IL-1 in the urine than men *(78)*. In contrast to these studies, other investigators have found that spontaneous IL-1 from cultured human monocytes increases after ovariectomy and is suppressed by estrogen replacement therapy *(79)*. Furthermore, bone marrow cells isolated from rats after ovariectomy also produce more IL-1 than cells isolated from sham-operated control rats *(80)*. The reasons for these conflicting findings are not apparent. Some differences might be expected between IL-1 expression or regulation between specialized tissue macrophages (bone) and isolated peripheral blood mononuclear cells, and some methodological differences exist (LPS stimulation vs nonstimulatory conditions; isolated adherent cells vs unseparated blood mononuclear cells). For the present, however, the discrepancies are unexplained.

Expression of other monocyte products also has been reported to be modulated by gonadal steroids, but only limited data are available and, again, some are apparently contradictory. Estrogens have been reported both to stimulate and to inhibit IL-6 production *(81–83)*. In some studies, levels of the monokine TNF-α have not shown gender-related differences *(76)*, but other investigators have demonstrated a suppressive effect of estrogen on TNF-α release *(79)*. Suppression of IL-6 production by peripheral blood monocytes may contribute to the downregulatory effects of androgens on immunoglobulin production *(84)*. Hormone doses as low as 10^{-11} M have been found to have a significant inhibitory effect *(85)*. In vitro addition of progesterone to human peripheral blood monocytes results in suppression of IL-1 activity as measured by bioassay *(86)*. However, concentrations of 10^{-6} M or greater were required, suggesting that this effect is unlikely to occur under physiologic conditions.

MECHANISMS OF ACTIONS OF HORMONES IN THE ADAPTIVE ARM OF THE IMMUNE SYSTEM

Gonadal steroid hormones have long been recognized to exert effects on the thymus. Thymic enlargement in castrate cattle was reported by Henderson in 1904 *(87)*. In 1941, Selye found that injection of testosterone into male rats resulted in dose-related thymic atrophy, whereas other organs, such as the seminal vesicles and prostate, showed remarkable enlargement *(88)* (Fig. 2). Thymic atrophy in response to androgens has also been observed in vertebrate animals as different as turtles *(89)*, fish *(90)*, and rodents *(91)*. Conversely, when androgen levels are lowered by castration, thymic enlargement occurs

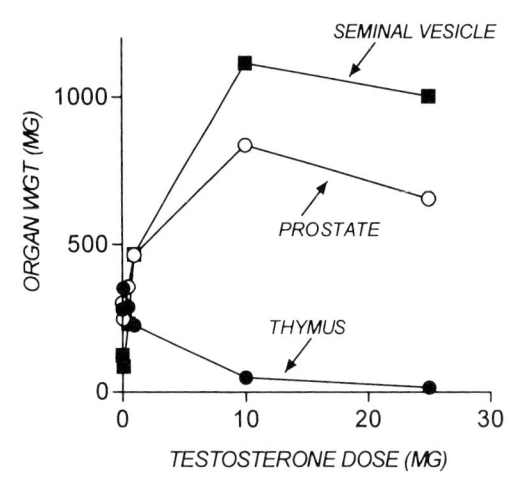

Fig. 2. Average values for the weight of seminal vesicle (closed square), prostate (open circle), and thymus in male rats treated with various doses of testosterone. Only the thymus shows a dose-related decrease in weight. (Adapted from Selye *[88]*).

owing largely to accelerated rates of thymocyte proliferation *(92)*. Castration-induced thymic enlargement is accompanied by phenotypic alterations in thymocyte subpopulations, with a small but significant decrease in the relative number of CD4$^-$CD8$^+$ thymocytes *(93)*. Subsequent androgen replacement leads to a relative loss of cortical thymocytes of the CD4$^+$CD8$^+$ subset *(93)*. Mechanisms of androgen-induced thymic involution may include enhanced production of TGF-β *(94)* and accelerated apoptosis.

The remarkable sensitivity of thymus size to levels of androgens is well recognized, but the rapidity with which such changes can occur has been recognized only recently *(95)*. A single dose of testosterone (1 mg) administered to castrate male mice results in a 50% reduction in thymic size 4 h later. This amount of decrease is comparable to that seen after administration of dexamethasone, a recognized inducer of thymocyte apoptosis. Since such a rapid change is unlikely to be owing to egress of cells from the thymus or to arrest of cellular proliferation, the third possibility, acceleration of thymocyte apoptosis, was investigated in detail. Detection of DNA fragmentation was utilized as the hallmark of apoptosis or programmed cell death. Since this is the normal pathway for negative selection of the vast majority of thymoctes, sensitive methods were required to detect levels of apoptosis exceeding the usual background rate. Furthermore, since apoptotic cells are rapidly removed from the gland, an in vitro organ culture procedure was required. Detection of soluble DNA fragments by ELISA, immunodetection of fragmented DNA *in situ*, and electrophoretic analysis of thymocyte DNA all indicated that at least one mechanism responsible for androgen-induced thymic atrophy is acceleration of thymocyte apoptosis. It seems likely that such changes impact on thymocyte selection processes, which in turn may lead to generation of an altered peripheral T cell repertoire.

Injection of estrogen also induces thymic atrophy *(96–98)*. A single dose of estradiol (1 mg) in a mouse induces a remarkable reduction in thymocyte numbers that persists for at least 20 d following the injection *(99)*. Similar results are obtained by adding estrogen to fetal thymic lobes in organ culture *(100)*. Most of the decrease in cellularity following estrogen administration is accounted for by loss of cortical cells with the "double-positive" CD4$^+$CD8$^+$ phenotype *(98)*. Cells with intermediate levels of the T-cell receptor CD3 are relatively increased, consistent with the observed preservation of the medullary zone of thymus tissue *(99)*. The CD4+CD8− subset shows a greater increase than the CD4−CD8+ subset *(97)* (opposite to the effect of androgens) *(93)*. Mechanisms responsible for the thymic changes induced by estrogens have not been established. Acceleration of apoptosis has been postulated as one explanation for the relatively rapid effects, but direct demonstration of estrogen-mediated thymocyte apoptosis has not been reported. It is possible that effects on cell trafficking, which appear to be more prominent for estrogens than for androgens, may contribute to the observed thymic changes.

Pregnancy is associated with a significant decrease in thymic size *(101–103)*. Whether the high levels of progesterone observed during pregnancy mediate this effect is not known *(56)*. Progesterone alone has no effect on thymic size or on the distribution of thymocyte subsets in mice *(98)*.

Peripheral T Lymphocytes

Although receptors for androgens have not been demonstrable in peripheral T lymphocytes, effects on peripheral T-cell functions have been described. Manipulation of androgen levels in vivo generally appears to alter responses of the CD8+ cytotoxic/suppressor subset of peripheral T cells with increased androgen levels mediating enhanced suppressor effects *(93,104)*. Removal of androgens by castration results in increased production of the cytokines IL-2 and IFN-γ *(15)*. Both of these molecules are produced by the Th1 subset of helper T cells, suggesting that androgens act to keep this component of T-cell-mediated functions in negative regulatory balance. Androgen-induced modulations of T-cell function generally require in vivo treatments rather than direct in vitro addition of the hormone to mature T cells. This is consistent with the hypothesis that effects of androgens on peripheral T-cell function are most likely due to changes in generation of the T-cell repertoire, which take place at the level of the thymus.

Estrogens enhance activity of the helper/inducer subset of T cells identified by CD4 and reduce the activity of the CD8+ suppressor/cytotoxic T-cell subset. These effects are exerted at least in part at the level of the mature T cell. Both in vivo and in vitro estrogen administration results in increased cytolytic activity of CD4+ T cells *(105)* and suppression of the classic delayed-type hypersensitivity (DTH) response *(106)*. Direct addition of estrogen to cultured human blood peripheral blood mononuclear cells reduces the activity of suppressor T cells as measured by effects on immunoglobulin production *(107)*. In vitro effects of estrogen measured in cell cultures are consistent with the reported expression of the ER in peripheral blood T cells *(64,71)*.

Emerging data from diverse systems indicate that estrogens have effects on the trafficking of T cells in vivo. Administration of estrogen results in increased numbers of T cells in some locations, notably the liver *(96,108)*, whereas other sites, including intestinal lymphoid tissues, show decreased T-cell numbers *(109)*. Activation of liver T-cell maturation can result in generation of potentially autoreactive specificities, since normal selection mechanisms used in the thymus are not operative *(96)*. Altered T-cell trafficking is seen in a model of drug-induced lupus using cloned pathogenic T-cells designated D10 *(110)*. Normal female AKR mice that are injected with D10 cells produce higher autoantibody levels than males. Although pathologic changes in renal and pulmonary tissues are observed in both males and females, liver abnormalities are limited to females and are responsive to hormonal modulation. Splenic homing of injected T cells is significantly greater in females than in males; this response was reduced by oophorectomy.

Mechanisms responsible for this action of estrogens may involve alterations in the expression of endothelial adhesion molecules *(111)*.

Estrogens directly regulate at least one product of mature T cells. Female mice produce higher levels of the Th1 cytokine interferon gamma (IFN-γ) than do males *(112,113)*. In vitro treatment of mitogen-stimulated spleen cells results in an increase in mRNA for IFN-γ, an effect mediated by transcriptional regulation at the level of the IFN-γ promoter *(17)*.

Bone Marrow

During pregnancy in normal mice, total numbers of bone marrow B cells are reduced *(114)*. These changes can be recapitulated in nonpregnant female mice by implantation of estradiol-containing pellets to produce levels of the hormone similar to those achieved during pregnancy *(115)*. All developing B-cell subpopulations following the earliest pro-B-cell stage show decreases. The major effects of estrogens on B cells occur at the pre-B-cell stage of development, with reduced numbers of IL-7-responsive pre-B cells available for further maturation *(114)*. In vitro cultures containing bone marrow cells and stromal cells show that direct cell-to-cell contact between these populations is not required in order to mediate the effects of estrogen. These data have been interpreted as suggesting a role for stromal-derived soluble molecules, the precise nature of which has not as yet been determined *(116)*.

Progesterone alone has no significant effect on developing B cells. However, progesterone does have a synergistic effect with estrogen on the number of bone marrow B cells, resulting in a highly significant decrease in the number of bone marrow B cells *(117)*. These results suggest that the two hormones together may be involved in mediating the effects observed during pregnancy, when levels of both are significantly increased.

Androgens also influence B-cell development. Castration of male mice leads to expansion of B-cell populations in the bone marrow *(118)*. An increased number of bone marrow B cells is observed as soon as 9 d following castration surgery and increases of approx 50% are maintained for at least 2–3 mo *(59)*. The changes are reversed by androgen replacement with either testosterone or dihydrotestosterone, and are not altered by thymectomy *(59)*. Whether the androgen effect is directly mediated by lymphoid or stromal cells of the bone marrow is unclear. Ligand binding and immunoblot techniques demonstrate AR positivity in both immature B cells and stromal components of murine bone marrow *(59)*. These findings suggest that either compartment is a potential target for androgen action.

Peripheral B Cells

Immunoglobulin production by mature B lymphocytes is enhanced by estrogens, whereas the number of B cells is not increased *(56)*. Levels of potentially pathogenic autoantibodies are increased in normal mice treated in vivo with estrogens *(119–121)*. In one study, castrated normal male mice treated in vivo with estrogen implants produced anticardiolipin antibodies at levels similar to those observed in normal females *(121)*. Most of the autoantibodies produced were of the IgG class, especially the IgG2b subclass, along with some increase for IgM. However, IgA antibodies to cardiolipin were not detected. Treatment of ovariectomized female MRL+/+ mice with estradiol results in higher levels of serum immunoglobulins, especially of the IgM class and of the IgG2a subclass *(106)*. Antigen-specific antibody responses were tested in these animals after cutaneous sensitization with oxazolone (OXA). Increased levels of anti-OXA antibodies were apparent for the IgG, but not IgM class *(106)*. Other data suggest that T cells mediate effects of estrogens on B cells *(107)*. This model would be consistent with the observation that estrogen receptors are present in peripheral blood T cells, but have not been reported in normal B cells *(56)*.

Androgens appear to exert suppressive effects on peripheral B-cell numbers. Castration of normal male mice results in expansion of the number of B cells in the spleen *(15,54)*. Since spleen cells do not express the AR *(60,60–62)*, it seems likely that this is an indirect effect. Experiments in thymectomized mice have indicated that the thymus (known to express AR in both lymphoid and nonlymphoid cells) is not required for androgen effect on splenic B-cell numbers *(59)*. The bone marrow (where AR is known to be expressed) thus seems likely to be the locus of androgen action that results in changes in B-cell populations in the periphery.

Androgens may also influence the functional status of peripheral B cells. Testosterone has been reported to suppress immunoglobulin production from cultured human peripheral blood mononuclear cells *(84,85)*. The cultures used in most of these studies contained cells of the monocyte lineage as well as mature B cells. In partially purified B-cell populations, the effect of androgens on immunoglobulin production is less marked. Testosterone was also found to inhibit monocyte production of IL-6, a known B-cell modulator *(85)*. Thus, effects of androgens on immunoglobulin synthesis may be indirect and mediated by blood monocytes.

CONCLUSIONS

Gonadal steroid hormones are important modulators of the immune response. Specific cellular components of the immune system express receptors for these hormones, permitting direct communication between the endocrine and immune systems. Sexually dimorphic patterns of immunologic diseases suggest that immuno–endocrine interactions make a significant contribution to disease susceptibility or expression. The female predominance of autoimmune disease has often been cited in support of such an hypothesis. A variety of data also indicate that gonadal steroid hormones may modulate disorders ranging from the septic shock syndrome to chronic infections. Advances have been made in elucidating the impact of gonadal steroid hormones on immune cell functions, in particular, their modulation of the production of soluble mediators by these cells. However, most of the cellular and molecular mechanisms underlying the effects of gonadal steroids on immunity remain unexplored. Understanding how sex hormones modulate immune function could open new avenues for therapeutic interventions in immune system disorders.

ACKNOWLEDGMENTS

This work was supported by grants from the National Institutes of Health (DK 41053 and AI 41575), the Lupus Foundation of America, and the Department of Veterans Affairs.

REFERENCES

1. Abbas AK, Lichtman AH, Pober JS. Cellular and Molecular Immunology. W.B. Saunders, Philadelphia, 1994.
2. Bone RC. Toward an epidemiology and natural history of SIRS (systemic inflammatory response syndrome). JAMA 1992;268:3452–3455.

3. Zellweger R, Wichmann MW, Ayala A, Stein S, DeMaso CM, Chaudry IH. Females in proestrus state maintain splenic immune functions and tolerate sepsis better than males. Crit Care Med 1997;25:106–110.
4. Angele MK, Wichmann MW, Ayala A, Cioffi WG, Chaudry IH. Testosterone receptor blockade after hemorrhage in males. Restoration of the depressed immune functions and improved survival following subsequent sepsis. Arch Surg 1997;132:1207–1214.
5. Wichmann MW, Angele MK, Ayala A, Cioffi WG, Chaudry IH. Flutamide: a novel agent for restoring the depressed cell-mediated immunity following soft-tissue trauma and hemorrhagic shock. Shock 1997;8:242–248.
6. Barrabes A, Goma-Mouanda J, Reynouard F, Combescot C. [17 beta-estradiol receptors in Schistosoma mansoni. Contribution to the explanation of the protective power of this hormone in Schistosoma mansoni bilharziasis in the mouse. Preliminary study] [French]. Annales de Parasitologie Humaine et Comparee 1986;;61:637–641.
7. Eloi-Santos S, Olsen NJ, Correa-Oliveira R, Colley DG. Schistosoma mansoni: mortality, pathophysiology, and susceptibility differences in male and female mice. Exp Parasitol 1992;75:168–175.
8. Huerta L, Terrazas LI, Sciutto E, Larralde C. Immunological mediation of gonadal effects on experimental murine cysticercosis caused by *Taenia crassiceps* metacestodes. J Parasitol 1992;78:471–476.
9. Nakazawa M, Fantappie MR, Freeman GL Jr, Eloi-Santos S, Olsen NJ, Kovacs WJ, et al. Schistosoma mansoni: susceptibility differences between male and female mice can be mediated by testosterone during early infection. Exp Parasitol 1997;85:233–240.
10. Mock BA, Nacy CA. Hormonal modulation of sex differences in resistance to Leishmania major systemic infections. Infect Immun 1988;56:3316–3319.
11. Launois P, Maillard I, Pingel S, Swihart KG, Xenarios I, Acha-Orbea H, et al. IL-4 rapidly produced by V beta 4 V alpha 8 CD4+ T cells instructs Th2 development and susceptibility to Leishmania major in BALB/c mice. Immunity 1997;6:541–549.
12. Krucken J, Schmitt-Wrede HP, Markmann-Mulisch U, Wunderlich F. Novel gene expressed in spleen cells mediating acquired testosterone-resistant immunity to *Plasmodium chabaudi* malaria. Biochem Biophys Res Commun 1997;230:167–170.
13. Mossmann H, Benten WP, Galanos C, Freudenberg M, Kuhn-Velten WN, Reinauer H, et al. Dietary testosterone suppresses protective responsiveness to *Plasmodium chabaudi* malaria. Life Sci 1997; 60:839–848.
14. Benten WP, Ulrich P, Kuhn-Velten WN, Vohr HW, Wunderlich F. Testosterone-induced susceptibility to *Plasmodium chabaudi* malaria: persistence after withdrawal of testosterone. J Endocrinol 1997; 153:275–281.
15. Viselli SM, Stanziale S, Shults K, Kovacs WJ, Olsen NJ. Castration alters peripheral immune function in normal male mice. Immunology 1995;84:337–342.
16. Fox CJ, Danska JS. IL-4 expression at the onset of islet inflammation predicts nondestructive insulitis in nonobese diabetic mice. J Immunol 1997;158:2414–2424.
17. Fox HS, Bond BL, Parslow TG. Estrogen regulates the IFN-gamma promoter. J Immunol 1991;146: 4362–4367.
18. Sprent J, Gao EK, Webb SR. T cell reactivity to MHC molecules: immunity versus tolerance. Science 1990;248:1357–1363.
19. Tarlinton D. B-cell differentiation in the bone marrow and the periphery. Immunol Rev 1994;137: 203–229.
20. Liossis SN, Kovacs B, Dennis G, Kammer GM, Tsokos GC. B cells from patients with systemic lupus erythematosus display abnormal antigen receptor-mediated early signal transduction events. J Clin Invest 1996;98:2549–2557.
21. Linos A, Worthington JW, O'Fallon WM, Kurland LT. The epidemiology of rheumatoid arthritis in Rochester, Minnesota: a study of incidence, prevalence, and mortality. Am J Epidemiol 1980;111:87–98.
22. Wallace DJ, Metzger AL. Systemic lupus erythematosus: clinical aspects and treatment. In: Koopman WJ, ed. Arthritis and Allied Conditions. Williams and Wilkins, Baltimore, 1997, pp. 1319–1345.
23. Mayes MD. Scleroderma epidemiology. Rheum Dis Clin North Am 1996;22:751–764.
24. Manthorpe R, Frost-Larsen K, Isager H, Prause JU. Sjogren's Syndrome: A review with emphasis on immunological features. Allergy 1981;36:139–153.
25. Furszyfer J, Kurland LT, McConahey WM, Woolner LB, Elveback LR. Epidemiologic aspects of Hashimoto's thyroiditis and Graves' disease in Rochester, Minnesota (1935–1967), with special reference to temporal trends. Metabolism: Clin Exp 1972;21:197–204.
26. Weetman AP. Autoimmunity to steroid-producing cells and familial polyendocrine autoimmunity. Baillieres Clin Endocrinol Metab 1995;9:157–174.

27. Duquette P, Pleines J, Girard M, Charest L, Senecal-Quevillon M, Masse C. The increased susceptibility of women to multiple sclerosis. Can J Neurol Sci 1992;19:466–471.
28. Jungers P, Nahoul K, Pelissier C, Dougados M, Tron F, Bach JF. Low plasma androgens in women with active or quiescent systemic lupus erythematosus. Arthritis Rheum 1982;25:454–457.
29. Lahita RG, Bradlow HL, Ginzler E, Pang S, New M. Low plasma androgens in women with systemic lupus erythematosus. Arthritis Rheum 1987;30:241–248.
30. French MA, Hughes P. Systemic lupus erythematosus and Klinefelter's syndrome. Ann Rheum Dis 1983;42:471–473.
31. Abramsky O. Pregnancy and multiple sclerosis. Ann Neurol 1994;36 Suppl:S38–S41.
32. Hench PS. The Ameliorating effect of pregnancy on chronic atrophic (infectious rheumatoid) arthritis, fibrositis, and intermittent hydrarthrosis. Mayo Clin Proc 1938;13:161–167.
33. Nelson JL, Hughes KA, Smith AG, Nisperos BB, Branchaud AM, Hansen JA. Maternal–fetal disparity in HLA class II alloantigens and the pregnancy-induced amelioration of rheumatoid arthritis. N Engl J Med 1993;329:466–471.
34. Petri M, Howard D, Repke J. Frequency of lupus flare in pregnancy. The Hopkins Lupus Pregnancy Center experience. Arthritis Rheum 1991;34:1538–1545.
35. Gladman DD, Urowitz MB. Rheumatic disease in pregnancy. In: Burrow JN, Ferris TF, eds. Medical Complications During Pregnancy. W.B. Saunders, Philadelphia, 1995, pp. 501–529.
36. Ben-Chetrit A, Ben-Chetrit E. Systemic lupus erythematosus induced by ovulation induction treatment. Arthritis Rheum 1994;37:1614–1617.
37. Petri M, Buyon J, Skovron ML, Kim M. Disease activity and health status (SF-36) in post-menopausal systemic lupus erythematosus: the SELENA trial. Arthritis Rheum 1998;40:S208.
38. Morley KD, Parke A, Hughes GR. Systemic lupus erythematosus: two patients treated with danazol. Br Med J Clin Res Ed 1982;284:1431–1432.
39. Agnello V, Pariser K, Gell J, Gelfand J, Turksoy RN. Preliminary observations on danazol therapy of systemic lupus erythematosus: effects on DNA antibodies, thrombocytopenia and complement. J Rheumatol 1983;10:682–687.
40. Bizzaro A, Valentini G, Di Martino G, Daponte A, De Bellis A, Iacono G. Influence of testosterone therapy on clinical and immunological features of autoimmune diseases associated with Klinefelter's syndrome. J Clin Endocrinol Metab 1987;64:32–36.
41. Olsen NJ, Kovacs WJ. Case Report: testosterone treatment of systemic lupus erythematosus in a patient with Klinefelter's syndrome. Am J Med Sci 1995;310:158–160.
42. Lahita RG, Cheng CY, Monder C, Bardin CW. Experience with 19-nortestosterone in the therapy of systemic lupus erythematosus: worsened disease after treatment with 19- nortestosterone in men and lack of improvement in women. J Rheumatol 1992;19:547–555.
43. Van Vollenhoven RF, Engleman EG, McGuire JL. An open study of dehydroepiandrosterone in systemic lupus erythematosus. Arthritis Rheum 1994;37:1305–1310.
44. Petri M, Lahita RG, McGuire JL, Van Vollenhoven RF, Strand V, Kunz A, et al. Results of the GL701 (DHEA) multicenter steroid-sparing SLE study. Arthritis Rheum 1998;40:S327.
45. Steinberg AD, Roths JB, Murphy ED, Steinberg RT, Raveche ES. Effects of thymectomy or androgen administration upon the autoimmune disease of MRL/Mp-lpr/lpr mice. J Immunol 1980;125: 871–873.
46. Vidal S, Gelpi C, Rodriguez-Sanchez JL. (SWR x SJL)F1 mice: a new model of lupus-like disease. J Exp Med 1994;179:1429–1435.
47. Pozzilli P, Signore A, Williams AJ, Beales PE. NOD mouse colonies around the world—recent facts and figures [Review]. Immunol Today 1993;14:193–196.
48. Bowman MA, Leiter EH, Atkinson MA. Prevention of diabetes in the NOD mouse: implications for therapeutic intervention in human disease. Immunol Today 1994;15:115–120.
49. Merino R, Iwamoto M, Fossati L, Muniesa P, Araki K, Takahashi S, et al. Prevention of systemic lupus erythematosus in autoimmune BXSB mice by a transgene encoding I-E alpha chain. J Exp Med 1993; 178:1189–1197.
50. Roubinian JR, Papoian R, Talal N. Androgenic hormones modulate autoantibody responses and improve survival in murine lupus. J Clin Invest 1977;59:1066–1070.
51. Roubinian JR, Talal N, Greenspan JS, Goodman JR, Siiteri PK. Effect of castration and sex hormone treatment on survival, anti- nucleic acid antibodies, and glomerulonephritis in NZB/NZW F1 mice. J Exp Med 1978;147:1568–1583.
52. Roubinian JR, Talal N, Greenspan JS, Goodman JR, Siiteri PK. Delayed androgen treatment prolongs survival in murine lupus. J Clin Invest 1979;63:902–911.

53. Roubinian JR, Papoian R, Talal N. Effects of neonatal thymectomy and splenectomy on survival and regulation of autoantibody formation in NZB/NZW F1 mice. J Immunol 1977;118:1524–1529.
54. Fitzpatrick F, Lepault F, Homo-Delarche F, Bach JF, Dardenne M. Influence of castration, alone or combined with thymectomy, on the development of diabetes in the nonobese diabetic mouse. Endocrinology 1991;129:1382–1390.
55. Fox HS. Androgen treatment prevents diabetes in nonobese diabetic mice. J Exp Med 1992;175:1409–1412.
56. Olsen NJ, Kovacs WJ. Gonadal steroids and immunity. Endocr Rev 1996;17:369–384.
57. Viselli SM, Olsen NJ, Shults K, Steizer G, Kovacs WJ. Immunochemical and flow cytometric analysis of androgen receptor expression in thymocytes. Mol Cell Endocrinol 1995;109:19–26.
58. Kovacs WJ, Olsen NJ. Unpublished work, 1997.
59. Viselli SM, Reese KR, Fan J, Kovacs WJ, Olsen NJ. Androgens alter B cell development in normal male mice. Cell Immunol 1997;82:99–104.
60. Takeda H, Chodak G, Mutchnik S, Nakamoto T, Chang C. Immunohistochemical localization of androgen receptors with monoclonal and polyclonal antibodies to androgen receptor. J Endocrinol 1990;126:17–23.
61. Kumar N, Shan L-X, Hardy MP, Bardin CW. Mechanism of androgen-induced thymolysis. Endocrinology 1995;136:4887–4893.
62. Rife SU, Marquez MG, Escalante A, Velich T. The effect of testosterone on the immune response. 1. Mechanism of action on antibody-forming cells. Immunol Invest 1990;19:259–270.
63. Kovacs WJ, Olsen NJ. Androgen receptors in human thymocytes. J Immunol 1987;139:490–493.
64. Cohen JH, Danel L, Cordier G, Saez S, Revillard JP. Sex steroid receptors in peripheral T cells: absence of androgen receptors and restriction of estrogen receptors to OKT8-positive cells. J Immunol 1983;131:2767–2771.
65. Cutolo M, Silvano A, Villaggio B, Clerico P, Indiveri F, Carruba G, et al. Evidence for the presence of androgen receptors in the synovial tissue of rheumatoid arthritis patients and healthy controls. Arthritis Rheum 1992;35:1007–1013.
66. Grossman CJ, Sholiton LJ, Nathan P. Rat thymic estrogen receptor—I. Preparation, location and physiochemical properties. J Steroid Biochem 1979;11:1233–1240.
67. Gulino A, Screpanti I, Torrisi MR, Frati L. Estrogen receptors and estrogen sensitivity of fetal thymocytes are restricted to blast lymphoid cells. Endocrinology 1985;117:47–54.
68. Kawashima I, Sakabe K, Seiki K, Fujii-Hanamoto H, Akatsuka A, Tsukamoto H. Localization of sex steroid receptor cells, with special reference to thymulin (FTS)-producing cells in female rat thymus. Thymus 1991;18:79–93.
69. Kawashima I, Seiki K, Sakabe K, Ihara S, Akatsuka A, Katsumata Y. Localization of estrogen receptors and estrogen receptor-mRNA in female mouse thymus. Thymus 1992;20:115–121.
70. Smithson G, Medina K, Ponting I, Kincade PW. Estrogen suppresses stromal cell-dependent lymphopoiesis in culture. J Immunol 1995;155:3409–3417.
71. Cutolo M, Accardo S, Villaggio B, Clerico P, Bagnasco M, Coviello DA, et al. Presence of estrogen-binding sites on macrophage-like synoviocytes and CD8+, CD29+, CD45RO+ T lymphocytes in normal and rheumatoid synovium. Arthritis Rheum 1993;36:1087–1097.
72. Larsson P, Goldschmidt TJ, Klareskog L, Holmdahl R. Oestrogen-mediated suppression of collagen-induced arthritis in rats. Studies on the role of the thymus and of peripheral CD8+ T lymphocytes. Scand J Immunol 1989;30:741–747.
73. Sakabe K, Seiki K, Fujii-Hanamoto H. Histochemical localization of progestin receptor cells in the rat thymus. Thymus 1986;8:97–107.
74. Frazier-Jessen MR, Mott FJ, Witte PL, Kovacs EJ. Estrogen suppression of connective tissue deposition in a murine model of peritoneal adhesion formation. J Immunol 1996;156:3036–3042.
75. Wichmann MW, Zellweger R, DeMaso CM, Ayala A, Chaudry IH. Enhanced immune responses in females, as opposed to decreased responses in males following haemorrhagic shock and resuscitation. Cytokine 1996;8:853–863.
76. Li P, Allen H, Banerjee S, Franklin S, Herzog L, Johnston C, et al. Mice deficient in IL-1 beta-converting enzyme are defective in production of mature IL-1 beta and resistant to endotoxic shock. Cell 1995;80:401–411.
77. Hu SK, Mitcho YL, Rath NC. Effect of estradiol on interleukin 1 synthesis by macrophages. Int J Immunopharmacol 1988;10:247–252.
78. Lynch EA, Dinarello CA, Cannon JG. Gender differences in IL-1 alpha, IL-1 beta, and IL-1 receptor antagonist secretion from mononuclear cells and urinary excretion. J Immunol 1994;153:300–306.

79. Pacifici R, Brown C, Puscheck E, Friedrich E, Slatopolsky E, Maggio D, et al. Effect of surgical menopause and estrogen replacement on cytokine release from human blood mononuclear cells. Proc Natl Acad Sci USA 1991;88:5134–5138.
80. Kimble RB, Matayoshi AB, Vannice JL, Kung VT, Williams C, Pacifici R. Simultaneous block of interleukin-1 and tumor necrosis factor is required to completely prevent bone loss in the early post-ovariectomy period. Endocrinology 1995;136:3054–3061.
81. Li ZG, Danis VA, Brooks PM. Effect of gonadal steroids on the production of IL-1 and IL-6 by blood mononuclear cells in vitro. Clin Exp Rheumatol 1993;11:157–162.
82. Jilka RL, Hangoc G, Girasole G, Passeri G, Williams DC, Abrams JS, et al. Increased osteoclast development after estrogen loss: mediation by interleukin-6. Science 1992;257:88–91.
83. Girasole G, Jilka RL, Passeri G, Boswell S, Boder G, Williams DC, et al. 17 beta-estradiol inhibits interleukin-6 production by bone marrow-derived stromal cells and osteoblasts in vitro: a potential mechanism for the antiosteoporotic effect of estrogens. J Clin Invest 1992;89:883–891.
84. Kanda N, Tsuchida T, Tamaki K. Testosterone inhibits immunoglobulin production by human peripheral blood mononuclear cells. Clin Exp Immunol 1996;106:410–415.
85. Kanda N, Tsuchida T, Tamaki K. Testosterone suppresses anti-DNA antibody production in peripheral blood mononuclear cells from patients with systemic lupus erythematosus. Arthritis Rheum 1997;40: 1703–1711.
86. Polan ML, Daniele A, Kuo A. Gonadal steroids modulate human monocyte interleukin-1 (IL-1) activity. Fertil Steril 1988;49:964–968.
87. Henderson J. On the relationship of the thymus to the sexual organs. I. The influence of castration on the thymus. J Physiol 1904;31:222–229.
88. Selye H. Effect of dosage on the morphogenetic actions of testosterone. Proc Soc Exp Biol Med 1941;46:142–146.
89. Leceta J, Zapata A. Seasonal changes in the thymus and spleen of the turtle, Mauremys caspica. A morphometrical, light microscopical study. Dev Comp Immunol 1985;9:653–668.
90. Slater CH, Fitzpatrick MS, Schreck CB. Characterization of an androgen receptor in salmonid lymphocytes: possible link to androgen-induced immunosuppression. Gen Comp Endocrinol 1995;100: 218–225.
91. Greenstein BD, Fitzpatrick FT, Adcock IM, Kendall MD, Wheeler MJ. Reappearance of the thymus in old rats after orchidectomy: inhibition of regeneration by testosterone. J Endocrinol 1986;110:417–422.
92. Olsen NJ, Viselli SM, Shults K, Stelzer G, Kovacs WJ. Induction of immature thymocyte proliferation after castration of normal male mice. Endocrinology 1994;134:107–113.
93. Olsen NJ, Watson MB, Henderson GS, Kovacs WJ. Androgen deprivation induces phenotypic and functional changes in the thymus of adult male mice. Endocrinology 1991;129:2471–2476.
94. Olsen NJ, Zhou P, Ong H, Kovacs WJ. Testosterone induces expression of transforming growth factor-beta 1 in the murine thymus. J Steroid Biochem Mol Biol 1993;45:327–332.
95. Olsen NJ, Viselli SM, Fan J, Kovacs WJ. Androgens accelerate thymocyte apoptosis. Endocrinology 1998;139:748–752.
96. Okuyama R, Abo T, Seki S, Ohteki T, Sugiura K, Kusumi A, et al. Estrogen administration activates extrathymic T cell differentiation in the liver. J Exp Med 1992;175:661–669.
97. Screpanti I, Morrone S, Meco D, Santoni A, Gulino A, Paolini R, et al. Steroid sensitivity of thymocyte subpopulations during intrathymic differentiation. Effects of 17 beta-estradiol and dexamethasone on subsets expressing T cell antigen receptor or IL- 2 receptor. J Immunol 1989;142:3378–3383.
98. Rijhsinghani AG, Thompson K, Bhatia SK, Waldschmidt TJ. Estrogen blocks early T cell development in the thymus. Am J Reprod Immunol 1996;36:269–277.
99. Nakayama M, Otsuka K, Sato K, Hasegawa K, Osman Y, Kawamura T, et al. Activation by estrogen of the number and function of forbidden T-cell clones in intermediate T-cell receptor cells. Cell Immunol 1996;172:163–171.
100. Rijhsinghani A, Bhatia SK, Kantamneni L, Schlueter A, Waldschmidt TJ. Estrogen inhibits fetal thymocyte development in vitro. Am J Reprod Immunol 1997;37:384–390.
101. Phuc LH, Papiernik M, Berrih S, Duval D. Thymic involution in pregnant mice. I. Characterization of the remaining thymocyte subpopulations. Clin Exp Immunol 1981;44:247–252.
102. Phuc LH, Papiernik M, Dardenne M. Thymic involution in pregnant mice. II. Functional aspects of the remaining thymocytes. Clin Exp Immunol 1981;44:253–261.
103. Rijhsinghani AG, Bhatia SK, Tygrett LT, Waldschmidt TJ. Effect of pregnancy on thymic T cell development. Am J Reprod Immunol 1996;35:523–528.

104. Weinstein Y, Berkovich Z. Testosterone effect on bone marrow, thymus, and suppressor T cells in the (NZB X NZW)F1 mice: its relevance to autoimmunity. J Immunol 1981;126:998–1002.
105. Muller D, Chen M, Vikingsson A, Hildeman D, Pederson K. Oestrogen influences CD4+ T-lymphocyte activity *in vivo* and *in vitro* in β_2-microglobulin-deficient mice. Immunology 1995;86:162–167.
106. Carlsten H, Verdrengh M, Taube M. Additive effects of suboptimal doses of estrogen and cortisone on the suppression of T lymphocyte dependent inflammatory responses in mice. Inflamm Res 1996;45:26–30.
107. Paavonen T, Andersson LC, Adlercreutz H. Sex hormone regulation of in vitro immune response. Estradiol enhances human B cell maturation via inhibition of suppressor T cells in pokeweed mitogen-stimulated cultures. J Exp Med 1981;154:1935–1945.
108. Kimura M, Tomita Y, Watanabe H, Sato S, Abo T. Androgen regulation of intra-and extra-thymic T cells and its effect on sex differences in the immune system. Int J Androl 1995;18:127–136.
109. Boll G, Reimann J. Oestrogen treatment depletes extrathymic T cells from intestinal lymphoid tissues. Scand J Immunol 1996;43:345–350.
110. Yung R, Chang S, Hemati N, Johnson K, Richardson B. Mechanisms of drug-induced lupus. IV. Comparison of procainamide and hydralazine with analogs in vitro and in vivo. Arthritis Rheum 1997;40:1436–1443.
111. Cid MC, Kleinman HK, Grant DS, Schnaper HW, Fauci AS, Hoffman GS. Estradiol enhances leukocyte binding to tumor necrosis factor (TNF)-stimulated endothelial cells via an increase in TNF-induced adhesion molecules E-selectin, intercellular adhesion molecule type 1, and vascular cell adhesion molecule type 1. J Clin Invest 1994;93:17–25.
112. Huygen K, Palfliet K. Strain variation in interferon gamma production of BCG- sensitized mice challenged with PPD II. Importance of one major autosomal locus and additional sexual influences. Cell Immunol 1984;85:75–81.
113. McFarland HI, Bigley NJ. Sex-dependent, early cytokine production by NK-like spleen cells following infection with the D variant of encephalomyocarditis virus (EMCV-D). Viral Immunol 1989;2:205–214.
114. Medina KL, Smithson G, Kincade PW. Suppression of B lymphopoiesis during normal pregnancy. J Exp Med 1993;178:1507–1515.
115. Kincade PW, Medina KL, Smithson G. Sex hormones as negative regulators of lymphopoiesis. Immunol Rev 1994;137:119–134.
116. Kincade PW, Medina KL, Smithson G, Scott DC. Pregnancy: a clue to normal regulation of B lymphopoiesis. Immunol Today 1994;15:539–544.
117. Medina KL, Kincade PW. Pregnancy-related steroids are potential negative regulators of B lymphopoiesis. Proc Natl Acad Sci USA 1994;91:5382–5386.
118. Wilson CA, Mrosa SA, Thomas DW. Enhanced production of B lymphocytes after castration. Blood 1995;85:1535–1539.
119. Verthelyi D, Ahmed SA. 17 beta-estradiol, but not 5 alpha-dihydrotestosterone, augments antibodies to double-stranded deoxyribonucleic acid in nonautoimmune C57BL/6J mice. Endocrinology 1994;135:2615–2622.
120. Ahmed SA, Verthelyi D. Antibodies to cardiolipin in normal C57BL/6J mice: induction by estrogen but not dihydrotestosterone. J Autoimmunity 1993;6:265–279.
121. Verthelyi D, Ansar AS. Characterization of estrogen-induced autoantibodies to cardiolipin in non-autoimmune mice. J Autoimmunity 1997;10:115–125.

8 Autoantigens in the Autoimmune Endocrinopathies

Jadwiga Furmaniak, MD, PhD,
Jane Sanders, BSc, PhD,
and Bernard Rees Smith, BSc, PhD, DSc

CONTENTS

    INTRODUCTION
    AUTOANTIGENS IN THE PITUITARY GLAND
    THYROID AUTOANTIGENS
    PARATHYROID AUTOANTIGENS
    ISLET CELL AUTOANTIGENS
    ADRENAL AND GONADAL AUTOANTIGENS
    CONCLUDING REMARKS
    REFERENCES

INTRODUCTION

Identification and characterization of specific autoantigens are integral parts of research into the understanding of the pathogenesis of autoimmune diseases. In the case of endocrine autoimmunity, the pituitary, thyroid, parathyroids, pancreatic islet cells, adrenals, and gonads can be subject to autoimmune attack, and many of the autoantigens involved have been identified and studied in detail (Table 1).

Identification of specific autoantigens in autoimmune diseases appears to be important for several reasons:

1. To confirm the autoimmune nature of the disease *(1)*.
2. To study B- and T-cell responses.
3. To characterize autoantibodies.
4. To develop methods to measure autoantibodies.
5. To study genetic, population, environmental, and evolutionary aspects of autoimmunity.

In the majority of cases, organ-specific autoantigens are proteins of well-defined functions and activities, such as enzymes or receptors, but the expression of these antigens in the affected organs is often not as specific as believed until recently. For example, thyroglobulin (Tg) and thyroid peroxidase (TPO) are truly organ-specific antigens and

From: *Contemporary Endocrinology: Autoimmune Endocrinopathies*
Edited by: R. Volpe © Humana Press Inc., Totowa, NJ

Table 1
Autoantigens in Endocrine Autoimmunity

Pituitary gland	Not yet identified unequivocally
Thyroid gland	Tg, TPO, TSHR
Parathyroid glands	Calcium-sensing receptor (Ca-SR)
Islet cells	GAD
	IA-2 (ICA512) protein(s) from the protein tyrosine phosphatase family
	Insulin
Adrenal glands	21-OH
	17α-OH
	Cytochrome P450 side-chain cleavage enzyme (P450scc)
Gonads	17α-OH, P450scc in association with adrenal autoimmunity; in isolated autoimmune gonadal failure—autoantigens not yet identified unequivocally

are not expressed in other organs. In contrast, glutamic acid decarboxylase (GAD), IA-2, or the calcium-sensing receptor (Ca-SR) are expressed and functional in other tissues in addition to those affected by autoimmunity.

Different approaches can be used to identify autoantigens. For example, proteins reactive with specific autoantibodies may be purified from their respective native human tissue and their properties and functional activity characterized. With this approach, amino acid sequencing may be particularly useful in identifying antigens homologous to known human proteins. Alternatively, oligonucleotide sequences of autoantigen genes can be determined by using autoantibodies to screen cDNA expression libraries prepared from RNA isolated from the organs involved in autoimmunity. Expression of the recombinant proteins in different systems can be very useful in studies to confirm autoantigen specificity. Furthermore, the availibility of recombinant autoantigen preparations not contaminated with other proteins from the target organ are invaluable in a number of studies, for example, in investigating the properties of autoantigens, developing new assays to measure autoantibodies, and studies of T-cell responses.

Here, we review recent progress in the identification and characterization of autoantigens in the autoimmune endocrinopathies.

AUTOANTIGENS IN THE PITUITARY GLAND

Lymphocytic hypophysitis thought to be related to autoimmune responses in the pituitary was reported for the first time in 1962 *(2)*, but this condition is seen rarely, most probably owing to a relatively low prevalence and/or the absence of definite criteria for diagnosis *(3)*. However, the association of clinically suspected and histologically confirmed cases of lymphocytic hypophysitis with other autoimmune diseases (insulin-dependent diabetes mellitus [IDDM], autoimmune thyroid disease [AITD], Addison's disease, atrophic gastritis, or autoimmune hypoparathyroidism) argues in favor of an autoimmune origin *(3–7; see also* Chapter 14).

Autoantibodies to pituitary antigens are difficult to detect using standard immunofluorescence techniques. This is owing mainly to the presence of the immunoglobulin Fc receptors on adrenocorticotropic hormone (ACTH)-secreting cells, and these receptors are responsible for nonspecific staining when unfractionated sera or intact IgG preparations are used *(6)*. Consequently, only when special techniques, such as use of autoantibody (Fab)$_2$ preparations, are employed, is it possible to assess the presence of pituitary autoantibodies by immunofluorescence. Consequently, reports that sera from patients suspected of hypophysitis contain autoantibodies to different cells in the pituitary or hypothalamus need to be confirmed and studied in detail *(6)*.

Reports based on Western blotting analyses of human, porcine or rat pituitaries have suggested that sera from patients with various autoimmune diseases contain autoantibodies to a range of pituitary proteins (from 14 to 98 kDa) *(8–10)*. In one study *(10)*, antibodies to a protein of mol wt 22 kDa was reported to be present in 57% of patients with IDDM and less frequently in patients with noninsulin-dependent diabetes mellitus (NIDDM) (24%) or healthy control subjects (6%). The apparent reactivity of patient and control sera with multiple protein bands in Western blotting suggests that these early observations should be considered with caution.

A number of different proteins have been postulated as candidate pituitary autoantigens; a particular association of lymphocytic hypophysitis with IDDM suggests that by analogy with glutamic acid decarboxylase or IA-2 *(3,5,7,10,11)*, the antigen(s) involved might be expressed in both islet cells and the brain. However, as lymphocytic infiltration of the pituitary gland has been reported to be associated with a number of other conditions, such as pregnancy, hyperprolactinemia, pituitary hormone deficiencies, autoimmune thyroiditis, or other autoimmune diseases *(3–7)*, the possibility of finding a "common" autoantigen is perhaps less likely. In order to elucidate the nature of autoimmune responses to hypophysis, future studies should follow similar approaches at molecular, genetic, and environmental levels to studies of other autoimmune diseases.

THYROID AUTOANTIGENS

Clinical descriptions of AITD date back to the early and mid-1780s when Parry, Graves, and Basedow independently reported cases of what is today known as Graves' disease *(12; see also* Chapter 9). In 1912, Hashimoto described patients with goiter and diffuse lymphocytic infiltration of the thyroid, thyroid cell atrophy, and fibrosis *(13)*, and then in the 1950s, the presence of autoantibodies to thyroid antigens was demonstrated. Autoantibodies to Tg were reported in serum from patients with Hashimoto's disease in 1956 *(14)* and autoantibodies to a thyroid microsomal antigen distinct from thyroglobulin by Belyavin and Trotter in 1959 *(15)*. Long-acting thyroid stimulator (not related to thyroid stimulating hormone [TSH]) in sera from patients with Graves' disease was described for the first time in 1956 *(16)* and subsequently shown to be an autoantibody to the TSH receptor (TSHR) in 1974 *(17)*. The evidence of a second thyroid colloid autoantigen distinct from Tg has been reported *(18)*, but it has not been characterized. More recently, there have been suggestions that the Na^+/I^- symporter (NIS) may also be an autoantigen in AITD *(19)*, but more comprehensive investigations are necessary before this can be accepted.

Thyroglobulin

Tg is a large water-soluble thyroid glycoprotein synthesized by thyrocytes and secreted into the thyroid lumen. It consists of two identical subunits with molecular weight of about 330 kDa and has a key role as a precursor of thyroid hormones *(20)*.

The gene coding for human Tg is located on the long arm of chromosome 8, spans at least 300 kbp, and contains at least 37 exons with up to 64 large introns *(21)*. The differences in the exon/intron organization of the Tg gene in its 5' and 3'-ends suggests that Tg is derived from two evolutionary different gene components *(21–23)*.

The mature human Tg monomer consists of 2748 amino acids and is characterized by the presence of three types of repetitive motifs at the N-terminus and a highly homologous sequence to acetylcholinesterase at the C-terminus *(24)*. The four hormonogenic domains are situated at both ends of the Tg molecule, one site at the N-terminus (Tyr 5) where most of the T_4 is formed and the other three at the C-terminus (Tyr 2553, 2567, 2746), which are involved in T_3 synthesis *(24–27)*. It appears that preferential iodination of these sites is dependent primarily on the native structure of Tg, since the same tyrosyl sites are involved in both chemical and enzymatic iodination *(28)*. There are 20 putative N-linked glycosylation sites on Tg, and carbohydrate residues contribute to about 10% of the Tg molecular weight. The presence of a limited number of O-linked sugars has also been reported *(24,29)*, and 16 out of the 20 N-linked glycosylation sites have been confirmed to bear sugars with the majority of these being associated with complex-type carbohydrates *(29)*. It has been shown that the sugar residues on Tg are important for its function related to hormone synthesis processes *(30)*. In addition, different types of sugars have been reported on Tg from thyroid carcinoma *(31–35)*.

The number of autoantibody epitopes on Tg appears limited (only two or three) despite the very large size of the molecule *(20,36)*. There is compelling evidence that the autoantibody binding sites on Tg are conformational, i.e., formed by three-dimensional folding of the protein *(20,36)*. In contrast, T-cell epitopes on Tg appear to be linear and present even on small fragments of the protein peptide chain *(20,36)*. Although sugar residues appear to be important for Tg processing and iodination, there is no evidence that they are important for autoantibody binding *(20,36)*.

High levels of Tg Ab are usually found in patients with AITD, and the antibody prevalences reported vary depending on the detection method used. Using highly sensitive assays, Tg Abs were found in up to 70% of patients with Graves' disease and 95–100% of patients with Hashimoto's thyroiditis *(36,37)*. In addition, Tg Abs are found in patients with other organ-specific or nonorgan-specific autoimmune diseases *(36)*. Studies based on sensitive direct radioimmunoassays have shown that 18% of female healthy blood donors without evidence of autoimmune disease had detectable Tg Ab. This prevalence increased with age, up to 30% for the age group of 55–64 yr old. The overall prevalence for Tg Ab in a group of male healthy blood donors was 12% *(36)*.

Autoantibodies that can bind both Tg and TPO have been reported to be present in sera from patients with AITD, and it is believed that these antibodies bind to Tg and TPO through different antigen-combining sites on the immunoglobulin variable (V) regions rather than through the shared epitope on the two molecules *(38,39)*.

Studies with human monoclonal antibodies (MAbs) to Tg have provided valuable insights into our understanding of the interaction between Tg Abs and Tg *(40,41)*. These studies confirmed earlier observations that there appear to be differences in the epitopes recognized by Tg Abs in sera from different patients compared to the epitopes recognized by Tg Abs in sera from apparently healthy blood donors *(40,42,43)*. In particular, the epitopes recognized predominantly by Tg Ab from healthy blood donors appear different from epitopes recognized predominantly by Tg Ab from patients with AITD *(40)*. Studies with human monoclonal Tg Ab also confirmed that there are only two major Ab epitopes on the Tg molecule and these epitopes are dependent on the protein conformation *(40,41)*. Analysis of Tg Ab V region sequences has shown that Tg Ab with similar epitope specificities can be derived from different germlines and can have different complementarity determining region sequences. This indicates that Tg Ab directed to the same or closely related epitope show considerable heterogeneity at the molecular level *(40)*. Furthermore, V region sequence analyses suggested a degree of somatic mutation within the IgG heavy chain and to a lesser extent within the light-chain gene sequences consistent with antigen-driven selection mechanisms *(40,41)*. However, to date, the amino acid sequences on Tg itself that are involved in forming the major autoantibody binding epitopes, have not been determined (*see also* Chapter 4).

Thyroid Peroxidase

More than 20 years after its first description, thyroid microsomal antigen was identified as TPO, a membrane-bound hemoprotein responsible for iodination of tyrosines on Tg. TPO is a glycosylated protein and consists of 933 amino acids with a peptide chain mol. wt. of approx 110 kDa *(20)*.

The gene coding for TPO is located on the short arm of chromosome 2 covering over 150 kbp, and comprising 17 exons and 16 introns. Evidence for two variants of the TPO protein synthesized through alternate gene splicing has been reported *(20,44)*. One variant is the full length protein of 933 amino acids, and the other, alternate spliced variant has 171 bp missing (between 1670 and 1840 bp) and codes for a protein of 876 amino acids *(20)*. It has been suggested that the two variants were responsible for the typical double-band appearance of TPO on the SDS-polyacrylamide gels. However, detailed studies have shown that these two TPO bands represent full-length TPO containing different sugar residues and do not appear to be related to the presence of differently sized TPO peptide chains *(45–48)*. Analysis of the TPO gene sequence indicates a 42% homology with the human myeloperoxidase gene, suggesting a common ancestral origin *(46)*. Homology of the TPO sequence to other peroxidases and to a segment of cytochrome-c oxidase has also been reported *(20,46)*.

A detailed structure of TPO has not been established as yet, but TPO is known to consist of a single peptide chain with a short hydrophobic domain at the C-terminal end, which anchors the protein to thyroid cell endoplasmic reticulum and apical membrane. Peroxidase activity and autoantibody binding sites are associated with the large hydrophilic part of TPO. Intrachain disulfide bridge(s) appears to be important for the correct folding of TPO, and the integrity of the disulfide bonds is critical for both TPO enzyme activity and TPO Ab binding *(20)*. Treatment with trypsin cleaves TPO at a site close to the transmembrane section and allows release of a water-soluble fragment of mol wt approx 100 kDa with the TPO enzyme activity and TPO Ab binding activity essentially intact *(20)*. The native, membrane-bound form of TPO is found in thyroid homogenates as a disulfide-linked dimer consisting of two polypeptide chains (approx 110 kDa each), which on reduction resolve into single 110-kDa chains *(49,50)*. Reports on the presence of detectable levels of TPO in sera from AITD patients have not been confirmed when using a sensitive TPO radioimmunoassay, and this is consistent with the membrane-bound nature of TPO and its relatively low abundance in the thyroid *(36,51)*.

Following molecular cloning of TPO, it has been possible to produce recombinant TPO in different expression systems. Recombinant TPO expressed in bacteria (in the majority of cases as a fusion protein) is unglycosylated and unlikely to fold correctly. Although the TPO fragments expressed in *Escherichia coli* have been used in studies to characterize TPO Ab epitopes, it seems likely that the linear epitopes identified in these studies are part of more complex conformational epitopes *(52–54)*.

With this argument in mind, it is also possible to analyze TPO Ab binding to fragments of TPO expressed in the in vitro transcription/translation (TnT) system *(55)*. In the TnT reactions, TPO is produced under relatively mild conditions, which should be considered an advantage in comparison with bacterial expression.

Yeast-expressed recombinant TPO (both full-length and the 100-kDa hydrophilic fragment) appears to be glycosylated and reactive with TPO antibodies; however, only low levels of expression have been found *(56)*. In contrast, full-length and the water-soluble fragment of TPO expressed in mammalian cells (for example CHO cells) show characteristics typical of native TPO, including their glycosylation patterns and TPO Ab binding *(52)*. However, the technical complexity and relatively high cost of large-scale mammalian cell culture reduce its attractiveness for use in the production of large amounts of recombinant TPO.

To date, the baculovirus-insect cell system appears to be the most suitable for expressing relatively high levels of recombinant human TPO *(48)*. *Tricoplusia ni* (High Five) cells have been found particularly useful, and recombinant TPO in amounts of up to 30 mg/L culture medium can be produced using these cells. Furthermore, recombinant TPO produced by appropriately infected High Five cells cultured in medium supplemented with a heme precursor is glycosylated (containing both high-mannose and complex-type sugar residues), reacts well with TPO autoantibodies, and shows TPO enzyme activity comparable with that of native TPO *(48)*.

Autoantibodies to TPO are characteristic of AITD, and using sensitive assays, the antibodies are found in over 90% of patients with Graves' disease and almost all patients with Hashimoto's thyroiditis *(36,37)*. Like Tg Ab, TPO Ab are also found in apparently healthy female blood donors at the overall prevalence of 18% *(36)*. This prevalence increases with age up to 30% for the age group of 55–64 yr old *(36)*. In contrast, about 10% of healthy male blood donors have detectable TPO Abs *(36)*. TPO Ab are frequently found in patients with nonthyroid autoimmune diseases, and this is consistent with the observation that more than one organ is often subject to autoimmune attack at either the disease and/or serological level *(36)*. Measurement of Tg Abs and TPO Abs in pregnant women appears particularly useful as a marker for risk of miscarriage and in prediction of thyroid dysfunction after pregnancy *(36,57–59)*.

Analysis of the interaction of human monoclonal and/or recombinant TPO autoantibodies with TPO has indicated that there are two major autoantibody binding domains on human TPO *(54,55,60)*. Both these domains are formed by three-dimensional folding of the TPO peptide chain *(36,45,55)*. Epitopes recognized by TPO Ab are distinctive for individual sera, do not change over time, and tend to be inherited in some families. To date, however, disease specific and nondisease-specific epitopes on human TPO have not been observed *(54)*.

As in the case of Tg Abs, TPO Ab V regions are not unique and are derived from germline genes used by other antibodies and autoantibodies. There is evidence of somatic mutation, which affects heavy-chain genes to a greater degree than the light-chain genes *(54)*.

Some laboratories have reported that TPO Abs can inhibit TPO enzyme activity in the guaiacol and/or iodide oxidation assays in vitro, but other studies have suggested that these effects are not evident either with TPO Abs from different patients' sera or with human monoclonal TPO Abs *(36)*. Recently, using a sensitive chemiluminescence method, the inhibiting effect of TPO F(ab')$_2$ fragments on porcine TPO enzyme activity in a guaiacol assay has been demonstrated *(61)*. However, TPO Abs are known to react poorly with porcine TPO (Nakajima and Rees Smith, unpublished observations), and the significance of this latest observation is not clear at present.

Recent developments in our understanding of TPO protein structure and function and the characteristics of TPO Abs have been in main part owing to progress in and application of recombinant DNA technology. However, in order to understand fully TPO structure and its relationship to peroxidase activity, as well as TPO Ab binding activity, crystallographic analysis of TPO and TPO/TPO Ab complexes is necessary. Thus far, crystallographic analysis of a recombinant human TPO Fab has been reported, but production of TPO crystals suitable for detailed structural analysis has not been achieved as yet *(62,63)*.

TSH Receptor

The TSHR is a key protein in the control of thyroid function and is a major thyroid autoantigen. The human receptor consists of a polypeptide chain of 764 amino acids with a calculated peptide chain mol wt of about 84 kDa. The receptor is encoded by 10 exons spread over 60 kbp located on chromosome 14; a single exon encodes the transmembrane segment, whereas 9 exons encode the extracellular domain *(64,65)*.

The TSHR is a member of the extensive G-protein-coupled receptor family, which shares a common structure of seven-transmembrane spanning regions linked by three sets of alternating intracellular and extracellular loops. All the receptors have an extracellular amino-terminus and an intracellular carboxy-terminus *(66)*. The TSHR together with the follicle-stimulating hormone (FSH) receptor and the lutinizing hormone (LH)/chorionic gonadotropin (CG) receptor belong to a subgroup of the G protein coupled receptors characterized by a large and heavily glycosylated extracellular domain. This domain is principally responsible for hormone binding *(67–72)*, but contributions from membrane spanning in terms of increasing binding affinity may be important. The TSHR is highly homologous between species, showing a high overall DNA sequence identity varying from 75 to 90% between the TSHRs cloned to date *(73)*.

Mutations in the TSHR gene that result in the change of only one amino acid residue can lead to either loss or gain of TSHR function, resulting in activation or inactivation of the receptor (for review, *see 74,75*). Activating mutations in the majority of cases involve amino acids within the transmembrane domain, mainly in the third intracellular loop and transmembrane sections VI and VII *(76)*. Activating mutations are principally associated with autonomously functioning thyroid adenomas, and these are somatic mutations *(77)*. However, in the case of congenital, nonautoimmune hyperthyroidism, the mutations are germline and are inherited in an autosomal, dominant fashion. Patients with congenital, nonautoimmune hyperthyroidism present with thyrotoxicosis and thyroid hyperplasia without opthalmopathy or thyroid autoantibodies. However, onset of the disease can be at birth or as late as adulthood, which suggests that other factors may be involved in the development of this type of thyrotoxicosis. In several cases, germline mutations affect the same amino acids as the somatic mutations found in autonomous adenomas *(77)*. Recently, activating mutations have been identified in differentiated thyroid carcinoma *(75,77)*. However, the same mutations have been described in nonmalignant toxic adenoma, and consequently, whether certain TSHR mutations are specific for thyroid carcinoma remains uncertain at present.

Loss-of-function mutations have been identified in congenital hypothyroidism, and these germline mutations have an autosomal-recessive inheritance pattern *(75,77)*. It has been shown that two alleles containing a mutation are needed for clinical disease to present, suggesting that a single normal TSHR allele may be sufficient for thyroid function *(78)*.

The extracellular domain of the TSHR is approx 415 amino acids long and contains six potential N-linked glycosylation sites *(67,70–72)*. The human TSHR expressed in CHO-K1 cells has been shown to be present as two full-length species of approx 100 and 120 kDa by Western blotting analysis with mouse MAbs to the TSHR *(79–81)*. Pulse-labeling experiments using L cells expressing the TSHR have suggested that the 100-kDa product is a precursor for the upper 120-kDa band *(80)*. More extensive studies, including the treatment of the TSHR with glycosidases, have shown that the upper 120-kDa TSHR band is resistant to digestion with endoglycosidase H (specific for high-mannose sugar residues), but sensitive to neuraminidase (which removes sialic acid residues). In contrast, the lower 100-kDa TSHR band is resistant to neuraminidase, but sensitive to endoglycosidase H digestion, and treatment with this enzyme results in the appearance of a band of approx 84-kDa (the expected molecular weight of the unglycosylated TSHR). Both the upper and lower TSHR bands are sensitive to PNGaseF digestion, which removes all sugar residues, and treatment with this enzyme produces a single 84-kDa band consisting of the deglycosylated TSHR polypeptide chain. These studies indicate that the upper 120-kDa band of the TSHR doublet contains predominantly complex-type carbohydrate, whereas the lower 100-kDa band contains mainly high-mannose-type sugar residues *(73,80,82,83)*. Confirmation of these conclusions has been obtained by analysis of the receptor using biotin-labeled lectins specific for different types of sugar residues. Lectins from *Canavalia ensiformis* and *Galanthus nivalis* (GNL) bound to the lower 100-kDa TSHR band indicating the presence of high-mannose sugar residues, whereas lectins from *Datura stramonium* (DSL) and *Maackia amurensis* (MALII), specific for complex-type sugars, bound specifically to the upper 120-kDa TSHR band, indicating the presence of complex carbohydrates. During the glycosylation process, high-mannose-type sugar residues are at first attached to the glycosylation sites on the peptide chain; these residues are then modified by forming complex-type structures, and this process gives rise to the mature glycosylated protein. Overall, therefore, current data indicate that the 120-kDa form of the TSHR is the mature fully glycosylated form, whereas the 100-kDa represents an immaturely glycosylated precursor.

Owing to the differences in glycosylation, the two full length TSHR bands can be separated using lectin-affinity chromatography *(73)* and the TSH binding activity of the unretarded column fractions measured. Using a GNL affinity column (specific for high mannose residues), the immature high-mannose-containing 100-kDa form of TSHR can be bound by the column. The unretarded column fractions contain the 120-kDa band (mature TSHR), and these fractions retain approx 80% of the TSH binding activity of the unfractionated load material. When a DSL affinity column (specific for b-1,4 linked *N*-acetylglucosamine characteristic for complex-type sugars) is used, the mature 120-kDa form of the receptor is bound to the column, and the 100-kDa, high-mannose precursor is present in the unretarded fractions. These unretarded fractions only contain 20% of the TSH binding activity loaded onto the column. Experiments such as these indicate that the presence of complex carbohydrates on the TSHR is important for high-affinity TSH binding. The importance of correct TSHR glycosylation in the ability of the receptor to bind TSH explains in part at least the difficulties in producing recombinant receptors (which can bind TSH or TSHR autoantibodies with high affinity) in expression systems other than those based on mammalian cells. In addition to the observations on the importance of TSHR glycosylation for binding of TSH to the receptor, it has been shown that the extracellular domain of the TSHR alone is insufficient for high-affinity TSH binding *(84–89)*. The role of the transmembrane segment in either direct binding of the ligand and/or stabilizing the TSHR/TSH complex after its formation is still not clear *(90)*. Overall, analysis of TSH binding to the receptor indicates that correct folding, glycosylation, and the presence of the transmembrane region, as well as the extracellular domain are all required for high-affinity TSH binding.

Early observations indicated that the TSHR is susceptible to proteolytic cleavage in the extracellular domain to form two subunits that are joined by an S—S bond *(20,36)*. The A subunit contains most of the extracellular domain, but the B subunit contains the seven-transmembrane spanning domain *(20,36)*. Recently, it has been suggested that the TSHR can undergo cleavage at two sites within the C-terminus of the extracellular domain, giving rise to two A subunits and releasing a small C-terminal peptide of approx 50 amino acids *(91)*. However, cleavage of the TSHR into the A and B subunits does not appear important for TSH binding *(92)*. Native human TSHR extracted from thyroid tissue obtained at operation is found to be present mostly in the cleaved subunit form in Western blotting analysis with only a small amount of the full-length receptor detected *(73,79)*. This is in contrast to the recombinant human TSHR expressed in CHO-K1 cells, which is present predominantly in the uncleaved form *(79)*. The differences in the amounts of cleaved and uncleaved receptors found between recombinant and native human TSHRs could be owing to practical difficulties in preventing rapid protease digestion of the receptor in thyroid tissue removed at operation, but it is relatively simple to add protease inhibitors to cultured cells expressing the receptor as soon as they are harvested. Experimental evidence from L cells expressing recombinant TSH receptor and cultured thyroid cells suggests that cleavage of the full-length receptor into the A and B subunits may be dependent on a matrix metalloprotease *(93,94)*. Cleavage of the receptor may lead to the release of the extracellular domain into the medium, and the same process could possibly be involved in shedding of the extracellular domain of the receptor into the bloodstream *(73,93,94)*. However, the presence of the soluble TSHR extracellular domain in serum has not been demonstrated conclusively as yet.

This reservation should be borne in mind when considering suggestions that splicing variants might be a source of the TSHR extracellular domain in the bloodstream that could act as a nonfunctional autoantigen. It has been proposed that such a variant may be involved in the pathogenesis of thyroid-associated ophthalmopathy, and the best characterized of these is a 1.3-kbp human TSHR transcript coding for the extracellular domain of the receptor *(95)*.

In order to increase our understanding of the pathogenesis of autoimmune thyroid disease, more information is needed on the sites of interaction between the TSHR and both TSH and TSHR autoantibodies (TRAb). Early observations of the inhibiting effect of TRAb on TSH binding suggested that the binding of TSH and TRAb to the receptor was mutually exclusive *(96)*. Consequently, after cloning of the TSHR, numerous studies were carried out to identify the regions involved in TSH and TRAb binding. Methods used included the expression of chimeras of the TSHR and the LH/CG receptor *(97–99)*, and TSHR constructs containing amino acid mutations, substitutions, or deletions *(100, 101)* expressed in Chinese hamster ovary (CHO) cells. These studies concluded that the sites of interaction between TSH and TRAb on the receptor were not identical, but appeared to overlap and cover most of the extracellular domain.

Another approach to identify the hormone and autoantibody binding sites for TRAb was to study the effects of synthetic peptides corresponding to various regions of the TSHR extracellular domain on the stimulation of cAMP production by TSH and TRAb. Some of these studies reported that the binding sites for TRAb with TSH antagonistic activity were located in the C-terminal segment of the extracellular domain, whereas TRAb with TSH agonist activity bound to the N-terminal part of the TSHR extracellular domain *(102)*. However, unlike binding of TSH to the receptor, which requires both the transmembrane and extracellular domains, the extracellular domain alone appears sufficient for autoantibody binding *(85,86,103)*. In addition, the first 261 *N*-terminal amino acids of the TSHR expressed in CHO-K1 cells have been reported to inhibit the binding of TRAb from Graves' sera to solubilized porcine TSHR *(104)*. This observation would suggest that an N-terminal fragment of the TSHR extracellular domain is involved in TRAb binding. However, whether this fragment alone has the ability to form a TRAb binding site is not clear at present. Overall, despite extensive studies, the nature of the binding site(s) for TSH and TRAb on the receptor is not yet clear.

Pure, stable TSHR preparations that can bind TRAb would be important reagents for developing improved methods of measuring TRAb in patient sera. Consequently, recombinant TSHR has been produced in different expression systems, and the interaction of these recombinant receptors with TRAb investigated. As discussed above, there is compelling evidence that binding of TRAb to the receptor is, in part at least, dependent on the correct glycosylation of the extracellular domain. For example, the TSHR extracellular domain expressed in *E. coli* is unglycosylated and in general does not bind TRAb *(87, 105)*, whereas the TSHR expressed in the baculovirus-insect cell system was reported to inhibit binding of patient autoantibodies to the receptor only in the glycosylated form (containing *N*-acetylglucosamine, galactose, and mannose), but not the unglycosylated form *(106)*. A similar observation has been made with the TSHR extracellular domain expressed in CHO-K1 cells in which the extracellular domain containing only high-mannose-type sugars was unable to bind TSHR autoantibodies, whereas the extracellular domain, which was fully glycosylated, was shown to be capable of autoantibody binding *(107)*. In our own studies *(83)*, Western blotting analysis of TSHR produced in CHO-K1 cells and affinity-purified showed that 7/18 Graves' sera with high levels of TRAb reacted with the 120-kDa TSHR band containing complex-type sugars. In addition to reactivity with the 120-kDa band, two of these sera also reacted with a 50-kDa specific band believed to represent the A subunit derived from the "mature" fully glycosylated TSHR. However, no reactivity was detected in any of the sera tested ($n = 18$) with the 100-kDa TSHR band containing high-mannose-type sugar residues *(83)*. TSHR produced by rabbit reticulocytes in an in vitro transcription/translation system is unglycosylated (mol wt approx 84 kDa), and although these preparations react well with both polyclonal and monoclonal TSHR antibodies, there are conflicting reports on their ability to bind TSHR autoantibodies *(108,109)*. In view of the important role of carbohydrate residues in the formation of the binding site(s) for TSH and TRAb, it seems highly unlikely that the TSHR produced in the TnT system could bind TSH or TRAb with high affinity *(109)*. Taken together, different studies strongly suggest that the fully glycosylated "mature" and correctly folded TSHR is important for both TSH and TRAb binding; however, the specific sites on the TSHR that bind TSH or TRAb have yet to be identified.

Other Thyroid Autoantigens

SECOND COLLOID ANTIGEN

Since it was first described by Balfour et al. in 1961, the nature of the "second colloid" thyroid autoantigen has not been studied extensively *(18)*. Autoantibodies to this antigen have been reported to be present in 40–50% of cases of Graves' disease, almost all cases of Hashimoto's thyroiditis, and 35–45% of cases of atrophic thyroiditis *(36)*. "Second colloid" autoantibodies were also detected in 12% of apparently healthy individuals. In addition, these antibodies appeared to be associated with congenital hypothyroidism and were also found in mothers of hypothyroid children *(36)*. However, the importance of these autoantibodies in the diagnosis and monitoring of AITD is not clear at present.

Na^+/I^- SYMPORTER

One of the main physiological functions of the thyroid gland is the uptake and accumulation of I^- ions, which are essential for thyroid hormone synthesis. This process is regulated by a thyroid plasma membrane-associated protein, which simultaneously transports two ions: Na^+ and I^- (Na^+/I^- symporter) *(19)*. Na^+/I^- symporter cDNAs (first from rat and subsequently from human thyroid cells) have been now cloned *(110,111)*. The human NIS cDNA (1929 bp) codes for an approx 70-kDa protein consisting of 643 amino acids. NIS proteins are characterized by 12 transmembrane domains and appear to be only expressed in the thyroid. Furthermore, NIS expression has not been found in thyroid cells that had lost their ability to concentrate iodine *(19,110,111)*.

Understanding the relationship between the structure and function of the NIS protein will clearly have an important impact on our understanding of thyroid physiology and pathophysiology.

There have been recent reports of autoantibodies to NIS, but overall the data currently available are unconvincing. Morris et al. *(112)* reported initially that synthetic peptides corresponding to rat NIS bound IgG preparations from Graves' and (to a lesser extent) from Hashimoto's sera. However, subsequent studies from the same laboratory *(113)* with peptides corresponding to human NIS were unable to confirm the results obtained with rat NIS. Endo et al. *(114)* have carried out Western blotting analysis of rat NIS and reported reactivity with Graves' and Hashimoto's sera, but more comprehensive studies, including those with additional control autoantigen preparations, are needed.

Although there is no definite evidence at the present time that NIS is a target for autoimmune attack, NIS does have some features in common with other well-established autoantigens. In particular, the protein is thyroid-specific and critical for thyroid function. Thus, it can be compared with TPO, Tg, and the TSHR, and with the major adrenal autoantigen steroid 21-hydroxylase *(36,115)*.

PARATHYROID AUTOANTIGENS

Idiopathic hypoparathyroidism (IHP) is one of the major components of autoimmune polyglandular syndrome (APS) Type 1 *(116; see also* Chapter 15). It may also present as a sporadic disease, sometimes associated with Hashimoto's thyroiditis in women *(6)*. The association of IHP with other autoimmune diseases and reports of the presence of autoantibodies reactive with parathyroid tissue in IHP suggest an autoimmune pathogenesis *(6,117)*. Parathyroid autoantibodies have been reported to show a complement-dependent cytotoxic effect on cultured bovine parathyroid cells *(6,116)*. However, reliable detection of parathyroid autoantibodies using the indirect immunofluorescence technique (IFT) on cryostat sections of parathyroid tissue is problematic because of the frequent presence of mitochondrial antibodies in sera from patients with IHP, which makes interpretation difficult *(6,116)*.

Recently, at least one major parathyroid autoantigen has been identified as the calcium-sensing receptor (Ca-SR) *(118)*. In this study, sera from patients with IHP of different disease durations reacted in Western blotting analysis with the 120–140 kDa Ca-SR doublet in membrane preparations of human parathyroid tissue and of HEK-293 cells expressing recombinant human Ca-SR. Similar protein bands were recognized in these preparations by a rabbit antibody to the Ca-SR. When overlaping extracellular and transmembrane sections of the Ca-SR were produced labeled with ^{35}S in an in vitro transcription/translation system, 14/25 (56%) IHP sera reacted with the extracellular domain of the Ca-SR. In contrast, none of 22 normal and 50 autoimmune control sera were positive. Furthermore, adsorption of positive sera with membranes prepared from HEK-293 cells expressing recombinant Ca-SR inhibited the ability of the sera to bind to ^{35}S-labeled Ca-SR.

The Ca-SR is of major importance in the regulation of parathyroid hormone secretion and renal tubular calcium reabsorption *(119)*. The receptor is a member of the G-protein-coupled receptor family with the characteristic seven-membrane spanning domains. However, at the amino acid level, the Ca-SR sequence differs markedly from the sequences of other receptors from the same family, except for the metabotropic glutamate receptors *(119)*. The Ca-SR consists of 1085 amino acids with the first 613 N-terminal amino acids forming the extracellular domain of the receptor. Sequence identity at the amino acid level between the Ca-SR cloned from different species is more than 90%, suggesting that the genes coding for this receptor are derived from a single common ancestral gene. Tissue expression of the Ca-SR is not limited to parathyroid or renal cortex and medulla cells, but is also found in thyroid C cells, pituitary, hypothalamus, and other regions of the brain *(119,120)*.

Overall, it appears that the Ca-SR is a major autoantigen in IHP, but the role of autoimmune attack on the receptor in disease pathogenesis is not clear at present. Preliminary studies have suggested that Ca-SR autoantibodies do not have an effect on Ca-SR activity in cell culture *(118)*. In terms of the prevalence of Ca-SR autoantibodies, Li et al. *(118)* studied a group of IHP patients with established disease and found 14/25 (56%) positive. More investigations are needed, particularly in patients before overt clinical symptoms or with short disease duration, since the prevalence of Ca-SR autoantibodies in these two groups may be higher. It is possible that measurement of Ca-SR autoantibodies could be helpful in the assessment and monitoring of IHP. Furthermore, their measurement may be of value in predicting IHP development in patients with autoimmune endocrinopathies who are at risk for the disease.

ISLET CELL AUTOANTIGENS

There is compelling evidence that IDDM is an autoimmune disease, in particular, the observation of lymphocytic infiltration of pancreatic islet cells, detection of islet cell-reactive autoantibodies and lymphocytes, and the association with certain human leukocyte antigen (HLA) alleles as well as the association of IDDM with other autoimmune diseases *(121)*. In addition, spontaneous and induced animal models of diabetes provide further support for the autoimmune origin of IDDM *(121; see also* Chapters 5 and 12).

Autoantibodies reactive with cytoplasmic components of islet cells were described in 1974 by Bottazzo et al. *(122)*, and the indirect IFT used in these studies is still the most common method for detecting islet cell autoantibodies (ICA) *(121)*. Differences in immunofluorescence staining patterns with different sera suggest that ICA are heterogenous in nature *(121)*. In recent years, there has been considerable progress in identifying the antigens reactive with autoantibodies in sera from patients with IDDM. These antigens include both well-characterized and poorly characterized proteins (for review, *see 121, 123,124*). However, current data indicate that GAD, two IA-2 proteins of the protein tyrosine phosphatase family, and insulin appear to be the three major islet cell autoantigens. Extensive studies have indicated that autoantibodies to GAD and to IA-2 proteins are the major components (but not the only components) of ICA, and autoantibodies to GAD, IA-2 and insulin are now considered the most relevant for IDDM prediction, diagnosis, and monitoring *(121,123,125)*.

Glutamic Acid Decarboxylase

Elegant studies over several years allowed Baekkeskov and her colleagues to show that sera from IDDM patients immunoprecipitate a 64-kDa islet cell protein and to identify this protein as the 65-kDa isoform of GAD *(126,127)*.

GAD is an enzyme responsible for the synthesis of γ-aminobutyric acid (GABA) from glutamic acid. GABA is a major inhibitory neurotransmitter of central and peripheral nervous systems *(128,129)*. In pancreatic islet cells, GABA is most probably involved in the paracrine signaling between β and α cells. There are two isoforms of GAD, 65 and 67 kDa *(128,129)*, and these are coded for by different genes; GAD_{65} is encoded by a gene on chromosome 10, and GAD_{67} by a gene on chromosome 2 *(130)*. Analysis of GAD-coding genes from different organisms indicates that GAD_{65} and GAD_{67} gene sequences are well conserved and are derived from a common ancestor *(129)*. The GAD_{65} molecule consists of 585 amino acids, whereas GAD_{67} consists of 594 amino acids *(128–131)*. There is about 65% overall amino acid homology between the two GAD isoforms with the greatest diversity at the N-terminus. The remaining parts of the sequence show about 78% homology. GAD_{65} is expressed mostly in the brain and in islet cells, although expression in other tissues (testes and ovary) has also been reported. GAD_{67} is expressed mostly in the brain, but some expression in islet cells and testes and ovary is also evident. There are differences in tissue expression between the two GAD isoforms in different species *(129)*. GAD_{65} is associated with synaptic vesicles in neurons and synaptic-like microvesicles in islet β cells. Both GAD isoforms are synthesized as hydrophilic, soluble molecules. GAD_{65}, but not GAD_{67}, undergoes posttranslational modification involving palmitoylation at the N-terminus, which was thought originally to be important for membrane anchoring of GAD_{65}. However, studies with recombinant GAD_{65} expressed in mammalian cells have indicated that palmitoylation is not essential for GAD_{65} anchoring into the membrane, and membrane targeting of GAD_{65} appears to be dependent on its hydrophobic N-terminal amino acids *(129)*. In the native form, both GAD_{65} and GAD_{67} are found as noncovalently linked homodimers *(129)*. GAD_{65} exists as two forms, an α form and a β form, which run as two distinct bands on SDS-polyacrylamide gels. Native GAD_{65} consists of one α form and one β form, noncovalently linked. Recently, it has been shown that only the α form of GAD_{65} undergoes phosphorylation following membrane anchoring, which may be related to the role of this GAD_{65} form within the membrane. However, phosphorylation itself does not appear to be related to the membrane-anchoring process *(132)*.

The availability of purified GAD preparations with characteristics similar to those of native GAD is important for research into the autoimmunity of diabetes, including studies of B- and T-cell responses to GAD. The complex relationship between the three-dimensional structure of the GAD molecule and the formation of autoantibody binding sites indicates that a correctly folded protein should be used for studies on GAD autoantibodies. This material can be obtained by careful purification of native GAD preparations (for example, from pig or rat brains) *(133,134)* or producing recombinant GAD in the appropriate expression system. Brain GAD preparations usually have their functional properties essentially preserved, but it is difficult to separate GAD_{65} completely from GAD_{67} *(129,133,134)*. Out of the currently available recombinant protein expression systems, prokariotic cells have been used for producing both GAD_{65} and GAD_{67} molecules *(135)* and some reactivity of autoantibodies in IDDM sera with bacterially expressed GAD_{65} demonstrated *(135)*. Recombinant GAD_{65} produced in an in vitro TnT system reacts with autoantibodies well, but it is difficult to purify and produce large amounts of GAD_{65} or GAD_{67} this way *(136,137)*. Immunoreactive recombinant GAD_{65} has been expressed successfully in larger amounts in insect cells and mammalian cells, including COS7 cells, hamster fibroblasts (BHK77.3), and myeloma cells *(138–142)*. In our experience, yeast provides a very useful and relatively inexpensive expression system for producing relatively large quantities of recombinant GAD_{65}, which shows excellent reactivity with autoantibodies *(143,144)*.

The conformational nature of autoantibody binding sites on the GAD_{65} molecule has been demonstrated in several studies using differently modified GAD proteins and IDDM sera or human monoclonal GAD_{65} autoantibodies (for review, *see 121,129*). Two major regions in the central and the C-terminal parts of the GAD_{65} molecule appear to be involved in forming the autoantibody binding sites *(121,129)*. The exact number and positions of amino acids reported to be involved varies with the different modifications introduced into the GAD_{65} molecule in different studies. There is, however, agreement that the C-terminal length of amino acids from about 451 to 570 is important as well as the amino acids in the middle of the sequence (amino acids from about 240 to 360). Autoantibody binding to GAD_{65} does not appear to be dependent on the region between amino acids 361 and 436, which contains the pirydoxal phosphate binding site related to GAD enzyme activity *(121,129,145)*. This observation can be considered consistent with reports that GAD_{65} Abs in patients with IDDM do not affect GAD enzyme activity *(121,129)*. A small proportion (20–30%) of IDDM sera contain antibodies reactive with GAD_{67}, and this is believed to be owing to crossreactivity of a population of GAD_{65} Abs with both GAD isoforms *(121,129)*. There is heterogeneity in epitope recognition by GAD_{65} Abs in sera from patients with IDDM, and in the majority of cases, Abs reactive with both central and C-terminal regions are found in the same individual *(121,129,145)*. Preliminary studies have indicated that there are no clear differences in epitope recognition by GAD_{65} Abs in sera from children who develop IDDM compared to GAD_{65} Ab in sera from apparently healthy children who have not progressed to IDDM *(129,145)*. However, the level of GAD_{65} Ab in apparently healthy children tends to be lower *(129,145)*. Studies with a number of GAD_{65}-specific human MAbs have contributed greatly to the analysis of the regions of GAD_{65} important for autoantibody binding and have allowed valuable insights into GAD_{65} Ab V region sequences. These analyses have indicated that there is no clear relationship between the epitope region recognized and the Ab V region sequence. Furthermore, the patterns of somatic mutations of the germline sequences have the characteristics of antigen-driven selection mechanisms *(146–148)*. GAD_{65} Abs in patients with IDDM are different from those found in patients with Stiff Man Syndrome (SMS). In particular, GAD_{65} Abs in SMS are usually present at high levels, tend to react with nonconformational epitopes, and have the ability to inhibit GAD enzyme activity *(129)*.

Although the epitopes recognized by GAD Abs in SMS are mostly distinct from those reactive with GAD Abs in IDDM sera and are contained within the N-terminal, central, and C-terminal parts of the sequence, some of SMS sera also contain GAD Abs, which bind to the same conformation-dependent epitopes that are targeted by GAD Abs in IDDM *(129,149)*. Furthermore, GAD_{65} Abs in sera from patients with APS Type 1 or 2 seem to show subtle differences in their characteristics compared to GAD_{65} Abs in isolated IDDM, and this may reflect some differences in the autoimmune mechanisms involved in the pathogenesis of these disorders *(129,150–152)*.

Evidence that different environmental factors, in particular, viral infections, may be involved in the etiology of IDDM has been reported in several studies *(153)*, and the finding of some amino acid sequence homology between human GAD_{65} and Coxsackie virus P2-C protein can be considered to support this concept. However, sequence homology between microbial agents and human proteins alone is not sufficient to establish a definite link between an infection and a disease *(153,154)*. Further studies on the association of Coxsackie virus infection and IDDM, including studies on T-cell responses, might be helpful in establishing if molecular mimicry is involved in the autoimmune responses in IDDM *(153)*.

IA-2 and IA-2β

Early immunoprecipitation experiments by Christie and his collegues indicated that sera from IDDM patients contained Abs reactive with 50-, 40-, and 37-kDa proteins released by trypsin treatment of islet cell proteins *(121,155)*. The 50-kDa protein was found to be related to GAD_{65} *(121,123,129)*, and the 40- and 37-kDa proteins were identified as fragments of IA-2 and IA-2β. IA-2 and IA-2β are proteins of the protein tyrosin phosphatase (PTP) family. The equivalent of IA-2β in rat islet cells is referred to as phogrin (phosphatase homolog in granules of insuloma). IA-2 and IA-2β are associated with the secretory granule membrane, and are expressed in the brain, islet cells (α, β, and δ cells), pituitary, and adrenal glands *(156)*.

IA-2 is a single-chain protein consisting of 979 amino acids with mol wt of about 106 kDa and a short transmembrane section almost in the middle of the seqeunce (amino acids 577–600). The N-terminal (extracellular) domain contains two N-linked glycosylation sites; the C-terminal (intracellular) domain contains a potential casein kinase II phosphorylation site, a potential tyrosine phosphorylation site, a potential protein kinase C phosphorylation site, and a PTP core sequence *(157)*. The IA-2 gene is located on chromosome 2 *(158)*. The sequence of the islet cell antigen known as ICA512 is contained within and is 100% homologous to the IA-2 sequence (between amino acids 389 and 914) *(121,155)*.

IA-2β has a mol wt of about 111 kDa, being larger than IA-2. The amino acid sequence is organised in a similar way to IA-2, with the transmembrane domain almost in the middle of the sequence, and the C-terminal domain containing potential phosphorylation

Table 2
GAD$_{65}$ Autoantibodies
and IA-2 Autoantibodies in 113 IDDM Patients
of Different Ages and with Different Disease Durations

	GAD$_{65}$ Ab(+)	GAD$_{65}$ AB(−)
IA-2Ab(+)	39	13
IA-2Ab(−)	34	27

sites and the PTP core sequence *(157)*. The N-terminal part of the protein contains one potential N-linked glycosylation site, and there is evidence that IA-2 and IA-2β are differently glycosylated *(155,159)*. There is about 74% amino acid sequence homology between IA-2 and IA-2β within the intracellular (C-terminal) domain, but only 27% homology between the N-terminal region amino acids. Although both IA-2 and IA-2β contain a PTP domain, PTP enzyme activity has not been detected in either protein as yet *(155)*.

Current data indicate that autoantibodies in sera from IDDM patients are directed exclusively to epitopes within the intracellular parts of IA-2 and IA-2β *(155,159)*, and IA-2 Abs are found more frequently than IA-2β Abs. Early studies indicated that IA-2 Abs cross-react with IA-2β and suggested that IA-2β Abs were not found in the absence of IA-2 Abs. This suggested that the autoimmune response to IA-2β was secondary to the response to IA-2 *(121,155,156)*. However, it has been reported recently that Abs directed to epitopes unique for IA-2β can be detected in some sera *(159,160)*. The exact binding sites for IA-2/IA-2β Abs on their respective antigens have not been well documented, but there is evidence that the autoantibodies are heterogenous and are directed to several different epitopes within the C-terminal domain. The epitopes appear to be predominantly conformational (although Abs to linear epitopes may be present) and do not tend to crossreact with other proteins of the PTP family *(155,159)*.

GAD$_{65}$ Abs and IA-2/IA-2β Abs appear to be the major components of ICA activity *(121,123,129,155,156)*. However, IA-2 Abs are more frequently detected in young patients (below 15 yr of age) with shorter disease duration *(121,155)*. The majority of studies on IA-2 Abs prevalence in different patient groups are based on assays employing ^{35}S-labeled IA-2 intracellular domain produced in an in vitro TnT system *(121,123, 155–157,159,160)*. An alternative and more convenient assay has been developed recently, and this is based on purified ^{125}I-labeled recombinant IA-2 intracellular domain expressed in *E. coli (161)*. The ^{125}I assay shows good agreement with the ^{35}S assay ($r = 0.84$) *(161)*, and in a group of 113 IDDM patients of different ages and with different disease durations, IA-2 Ab were detected using the ^{125}I-based assay in 52 (46%). In the same group of patients, GAD$_{65}$ Ab (by ^{125}I-labeled assay) were detected in 73 patients (65%) (Table 2) *(143,161)*.

It is of note that 13 patients in this group were positive for IA-2Abs in the absence of GAD$_{65}$ Abs. IA-2 Abs were found to have the highest prevalence (14/21, 67%) in the patients of/or below 15 yr of age and with recent-onset diabetes (2 wk or less from diagnosis) (Table 3). This was followed by a prevalence of 62% (16/26) in a group of patients of/or below the age of 15 with relatively short disease duration (2 wk to 2 yr) (Table 3). Older patients (above the age of 15 yr) had a IA-2 Ab prevalence of 45% 2 wk or less from diagnosis, and a IA-2 Ab prevalence of 25% from more than 2 wk to 2 yr from diagnosis (Table 3). In the group of patients with disease duration of longer than 2 yr,

Table 3
Relationship Among IA-2 and GAD Ab Positivity,
Disease Duration, and Age of Patients in 101 IDDM Sera

IDDM duration	Age of patients	n	IA-2 Ab positivity, %	GAD Ab positivity, %
Recent onset	≤15 yr	21	14/21 (67%)	15/21 (71%)
(2 wk)	>15 yr	11	5/11 (45%)	8/11 (73%)
2 wk to 2 yr	≤15 yr	26	16/26 (62%)	19/26 (73%)
	>15 yr	8	2/8 (25%)	5/8 (63%)
>2 yr	≤15 yr	32	10/32 (31%)	16/32 (50%)
	>15 yr	3	1/3 (33%)	2/3 (67%)

the prevalence of IA-2 Ab was about 30% (Table 3). The prevalence of GAD_{65} Abs in these different patient groups was far less dependent than IA-2 Ab on age, and the disease duration ranged from 63 to 73% in the three different groups (Table 3) *(143,161)*.

Overall, measurement of autoantibodies to IA-2 complement those of autoantibodies to GAD_{65}, and both measurements are valuable in the prediction, diagnosis, and monitoring of IDDM.

Insulin

Autoantibodies to insulin in children with IDDM before exogenous insulin treatment was commenced were first described in 1983 by Palmer et al. *(162)*. Insulin, the major secretory product of pancreatic β-islet cells, was successfully purified in the 1920s and is a very well-characterized protein *(163)*. It consists of a water-soluble, two-chain peptide (the 21 amino acids long A chain and the 30 amino acids long B chain) linked by disulfide bridges, and this is derived from a single-chain proinsulin peptide *(163–165)*. Insulin is the only truly islet cell-specific autoantigen described to date, since the insulin gene (on human chromosome 11) is not expressed in any other cell, except the pancreatic β cell *(163–165)*. This is in contrast to GAD or IA-2 proteins *(see above)*.

Insulin autoantibodies tend to be a characteristic feature of IDDM in very young children (below 5 yr of age), and their presence indicates a faster rate of progression to IDDM in first-degree relatives of IDDM patients *(156)*. Autoantibodies to water-soluble insulin are not detected by IFT, and the fluid-phase radioligand assay is currently most commonly used for measurement of insulin autoantibodies *(156,166)*. However, combined measurement of autoantibodies to the ICA components GAD_{65} and IA-2 together with insulin autoantibodies is currently believed to provide the best way of monitoring of individuals suspected of autoimmune diabetes *(121,125, 55,156)*.

Other Autoantigens

Extensive studies have been carried out to identify other autoantigens that might be involved in the pathogenesis of autoimmune diabetes mellitus. These studies were mostly based on screening of cDNA libraries with sera from prediabetic or diabetic patients, and several different candidate proteins have been isolated and characterized. Some of these (such as GAD or carboxypeptidase H) were known and had been cloned prior to the discovery of their relationship with diabetes. In addition to the major autoantigens considered in detail in previous sections, a number of other proteins have been reported to be related to autoimmune diabetes, for example, islet cell autoantigen 69 kDa (ICA69), carboxypeptidase H, ganglioside GM2-1, imogen 38, glima 38, peripherin, heat-shock protein 65, and very recently unidentified peptides selected from a phage display library *(121,124,156)*. However, none of these antigens seem to have as important a role as GAD_{65}, IA-2/IA-2β, and insulin in the autoimmunity of diabetes, at least in terms of humoral responses.

The relationship between diatary exposure of young children to cows' milk and diabetes has received a great deal of attention. In particular, sequence homologies between bovine serum albumin and one potential islet cell antigen (ICA69) have been used to support a "molecular mimicry" hypothesis for the development of islet autoimmunity *(121)*. Current extensive research at the molecular, humoral, cellular, genetic, and environmental levels should allow any relationship between exogenous factors and autoimmune diabetes to be established in due course.

ADRENAL AND GONADAL AUTOANTIGENS

Studies on diseases of adrenal cortex date back to the 1850s with the description of adrenocortical failure by Addison *(167)*. The existence of adrenal-specific autoantibodies was described for the first time by Anderson et al. *(168)*, and in 1963, an indirect immunofluorescence test for adrenal autoantibodies was described by Blizzard and Kyle *(169)*. Since then, IFT based on sections of human, bovine, or monkey adrenal tissues have been the most commonly used technique to detect the presence of adrenal cortex autoantibodies (ACA) in patients' sera *(6,170)*. Steroid-producing cell autoantibodies (StCA) reactive with different types of cells producing steroid hormones (in adrenals, testes, ovaries, and placenta) were first described by Anderson et al. in 1968 using IFT *(171)*. StCA are detected predominantly in ACA-positive patients with Addison's disease who have premature ovarian failure (POF) or in the context of APS Type 1 *(6,116,172)*.

In 1988, an adrenal-specific 55-kDa autoantigen was immunoprecipitated from ^{125}I-labeled human adrenal microsomes using Addison sera *(173)*, and in 1992, three steroidogenic enzymes were shown to be autoantigens in adrenal autoimmune disease. (*See also* Chapters 13, 15, and 16.)

Steroid 21-Hydroxylase (21-OH)

21-OH was identified as a major autoantigen in independent studies in two separate laboratories *(174,175)*. In our own investigations, identification of 21-OH was based on (1) purification of native 21-OH from human adrenals and Western blotting analysis using Addison sera and a rabbit antibody to 21-OH and (2) analysis of the reactivity of ACA-positive Addison sera with recombinant human 21-hydroxylase produced in yeast *(174,176)*. Winqvist et al. *(175)* also used Western blotting with patients' sera, and rabbit antisera, and a combination of immunoprecipitation and absorption studies to identify 21-OH as a major adrenal autoantigen.

The initial reports on identification of 21-OH as a major adrenal autoantigen were confirmed by studies in several laboratories using different expression and detection methods *(177–179)*.

21-OH is an adrenal-specific enzyme of the cytochrome p450 family with a key role in the synthesis of steroid hormones, such as cortisol and aldosterone *(180–182)*. There are two 21-OH genes (CYP21) with an overall 98% nucleotide sequence homology located in tandem on the short arm of chromosome 6 in the same region as HLA class III genes *(183,184)*. 21-OH is coded for by the CYP21B gene, whereas the CYP21A gene is inactive (pseudogene) *(183)*. Gene conversion and rearrangement episodes between CYP21B and CYP21A can result in 21-OH enzyme deficiency leading to adrenal hyperplasia *(180–182)*. In addition, some single amino acid mutations in the 21-OH sequence are associated with reduced 21-OH enzyme activity and classical or nonclassical adrenal hyperplasia *(180–182)*. Over 95% of cases of congenital adrenal hyperplasia are owing to deficiency of 21-hydroxylation. The three different clinical forms of congenital adrenal hyperplasia are salt wasting, simple virilizing, and nonclassical. These represent different levels of disease severity with the nonclassical form being the mildest *(180)*.

21-OH is a single chain 55-kDa (494 amino acids) protein, which is integrated into the membrane of the smooth endoplasmic reticulum *(183,185,186)*. It catalyzes the conversion of progesterone and 17-hydroxyprogesterone into deoxycorticosterone and 11-deoxycortisol. The 21-OH molecule is not soluble in water without detergents, and the hydrophobic domains responsible for targeting and anchoring of the protein into the membrane are situated at the N-terminal end *(183,185,186)*. The heme group and substrate binding sites associated with 21-OH enzyme activity are located in the C-terminal end of the molecule. There is good evidence that 21-OH enzyme activity is dependent on correct folding of the peptide chain, and even single amino acid substitutions can cause a marked reduction in enzyme activity, most probably through changes in protein conformation *(187–189)*.

The relationship between ACA measured by IFT and 21-OH autoantibodies (measured by several different techniques) has been investigated in detail *(177,190–195)* and these studies show that 21-OH is a major autoantigen in autoimmune adrenal disease, irrespective of whether it presents as isolated Addison's disease or APS Type 1 or Type 2 *(192,195)*.

Once 21-OH had been identified as a major adrenal autoantigen, studies on the location of its autoantibody binding site(s) were carried out. These included Western blotting analysis and/or immunoprecipitation assays with fragments of 21-OH and 21-OH containing amino acid muations prepared in an in vitro TnT system, yeast, or bacteria. Studies with 21-OH containing N-terminal, internal, and C-terminal amino acid sequence deletions expressed in the TnT system or in yeast indicated that the central and the C-terminal regions of the 21-OH sequence (amino acids 241–494) are important for autoantibody binding *(196,197)*. The importance of the C-terminal part of the 21-OH molecule was confirmed in studies of 21-OH fragments expressed in *E. coli (177)*. 21-OH-containing amino acid mutations within this region, for example, Pro453 to Ser, which occur naturally and are associated with impaired enzyme activity and nonclassical adrenal hyperplasia, showed markedly reduced ability to bind autoantibodies *(197)*. Mutations at Cys428, which do not occur naturally, but are likely to affect enzyme activity (as Cys428 is proposed to coordinate with heme), also result in a decrease in 21-OH autoantibody binding *(183,198,199)*. Naturally occurring mutations within the central part of the 21-OH molecule (at Ile172 to Asn and Arg339 to His) have a smaller effect on autoantibody binding *(197,199)*. In contrast, the naturally occurring mutation of Pro30 to Leu in the N-terminal region, which is associated with an approx 50% reduction in 21-OH enzyme activity *(180–182,200)*, has no effect on autoantibody binding *(199)*.

The observation of a relationship between 21-OH Ab binding and sites important for 21-OH enzyme activity prompted direct studies on the effect of 21-OH Abs on 21-OH enzyme activity. These investigations showed that IgGs from Addison sera positive for 21-OH Abs caused a marked, dose-dependent inhibition of 21-OH enzyme activity in vitro *(201)*. However, studies of adrenal steroid synthesis markers (in particular, the pattern of change in the 17-hydroxyprogesterone to cortisol ratio in response to ACTH stimulation) in patients with high levels of 21-OH Abs suggest that an inhibiting effect of 21-OH Abs on 21-OH enzyme activity is not usually evident in vivo *(202)*.

The involvement of long stretches of amino acids in the central and C-terminal regions of 21-OH in forming most of the autoantibody binding sites on 21-OH suggests that the binding sites depend on the three-dimensional folding of the 21-OH peptide chain (i.e., conformation-dependent) *(115,196–199)*. Furthermore, 21-OH Abs in different patient sera show different reactivities with 21-OH fragments and/or 21-OH-containing amino acid mutations, and this suggests that 21-OH Abs are heterogenous *(175,196–199)*. However, analyses of this type with 21-OH Abs in sera from patients with APS Type 1, Type 2, isolated Addison's disease or ACA-positive patients without overt Addison's disease (with impaired or unimpaired adrenal function) have not shown significant differences between the epitopes recognized by 21-OH Abs in different patient groups *(203)*.

Taken together, recent studies indicate that autoantibody epitopes on human steroid 21-OH are conformational, and are formed by both central and C-terminal parts of the molecule. A close relationship between the amino acid sequences important for 21-OH enzyme activity and the autoantibody binding site(s) is also apparent.

Autoantibodies to 21-OH can be detected by Western blotting using native or recombinant proteins *(174–176,204)*. The binding of 21-OH Ab to 21-OH in Western blotting analysis might be considered inconsistent with the conformational nature of autoantigenic epitopes on 21-OH. However, other autoantibodies reactive with the conformational epitopes can bind to autoantigens in Western blotting, for example, in the cases of glutamic acid decarboxylase and thyroid peroxidase *(55,205)*. The reasons for these reactivities are probably complex, but may be related, in part at least, to some renaturation, i.e., refolding of the protein after blotting. Another important factor in detection of antibodies and antigens by Western blotting is the purity of the antigen preparation loaded onto the gel; it can be difficult to detect small amounts of a particular antigen in a complex mixture of proteins because of high background limitations. However, when pure (or highly purified) preparations of antigen are used, much more of the material of interest can be loaded onto the gel, and this can allow detection of small amounts of renatured (or nondenaturated) antigen even in the presence of a considerable excess of denatured antigen. Although Western blotting analysis can be sensitive and specific, it is expensive and time-consuming, and the results are, at best, semiquantitative.

Consequently, a sensitive and convenient assay to measure 21-OH Abs has been developed based on ^{125}I-labeled recombinant 21-OH expressed in yeast *(195)*. In the assay, ^{125}I-labeled recombinant 21-OH is allowed to react with 21-OH Abs in test sera, and the immune complexes formed precipitate with solid-phase protein A. 21-OH Ab levels are calculated from a standard curve prepared using dilutions of a 21-OH Ab-positive serum. The precision of the ^{125}I assay is good, with inter- and intra-assay coefficients of variation of about 2% *(195)*.

Using this assay, 21-OH Abs could be detected in 43/60 (72%) of patients with isolated Addison's disease, 11/12 (92%) patients with APS Type 1, 27/27 (100%) patients with

APS Type 2, and 24/30 (80%) sera from patients who were positive for ACA by IFT, but had no overt Addison's disease. Low levels of 21-OH Abs were found using the ^{125}I assay in 2.5% of apparently healthy blood donors, 1.3% of Graves' sera, 2.7% of IDDM sera, and 1.5% of sera from patients with Hashimoto's thyroiditis *(195)*. 21-OH Abs were not detected in any of the myasthenia gravis, NIDDM, or POF sera studied *(195)*. These results can be compared with the observation that low levels of GAD_{65} Abs are found in a small proportion of healthy blood donors and in patients with autoimmune diseases other than IDDM *(55,136,137)*.

When ACAs were measured by IFT in 808 children with organ-specific autoimmune diseases without adrenal insufficiency, ACAs were detectable in 14 children (1.7%) *(206)*. Ten of these ACA-positive children (who were also 21-OH Ab-positive) and 12 ACA-negative children were followed up by evaluation of adrenocortical function and autoantibody status *(206)*. Overt Addison's disease developed in 9 (90%) ACA/21-OH Ab-positive children after 3–121 mo, and 1 remaining child had subclinical hypoadrenalism throughout the observation period of 24 mo. The calculated cumulative risk of developing Addison's disease (including subclinical) for ACA/21-OH Ab-positive children was 100% at 11 yr. The rate of progression to adrenal failure in children was not related to ACA titer, sex, adrenal function, type of pre-existing autoimmune disorder, or HLA status. This study shows that in children, ACA/21-OH Abs are important predictive markers for the development of Addison's disease with all its potentially life-threatening consequences *(206)*. In contrast, the cumulative risk for developing Addison's disease in ACA-positive adult patients with organ-specific autoimmune diseases (other than Addison's disease) was about 32%. Consequently, detection of ACA/21-OH Abs in adults is only a moderate marker of progression toward clinical Addison's disease *(207)*.

Overall, identification 21-OH as the major adrenal autoantigen and the development of new assays to measure 21-OH autoantibodies should provide improved diagnosis, monitoring, and prediction of autoimmune adrenal disease. In addition, availability of purified preparations of 21-OH should allow the crystallographic analysis of adrenal autoantigen–autoantibody complexes to be carried out, and this should be of further help in improving our understanding of the interaction between the adrenal and immune system at the molecular level.

Steroid 17α-Hydroxylase (17α-OH)

Screening of a human fetal adrenal cDNA expression library with sera from patients with APS Type 1 enabled 17α-OH to be identified as an adrenal autoantigen by Krohn et al. *(208)*. In this study, APS Type 1 sera, but not serum from one adult Addison patient reacted with a fragment of recombinant 17α-OH expressed in bacteria, and the authors suggested that 17α-OH might be an autoantigen associated with Addison's disease in children in the contex of APS Type 1.

17α-OH is a heme binding protein and, like 21-OH, is a member of the p450 cytochrome family. 17α-OH is coded for by a single gene on human chromosome 10, and it is expressed in adrenals and gonads, but not placenta *(179,209)*. There is about 30% homology at the amino acid level between the 21-OH and 17α-OH sequences. Furthermore, hydropathy profiles, predicted α- and β-structures, and computer modeling of protein conformation, including the substrate binding pocket, suggest that the overall structures of 17α-OH and 21-OH are rather similar *(188,189)*.

Table 4
Adrenal Autoantibodies in Different Patient Groups[a]

Group	ACA	21-OH	StCA	17α-OH	P450scc
APS 1	8/11 (73)	7/11 (64)	5/11 (45)	6/11 (55)	5/11 (45)
APS II[b]	21/24 (87)	23/24 (96)	8/22 (36)	8/24 (33)	10/24 (42)
ACA(+)[c]	56/56 (100)	48/56 (86)	12/56 (21)	11/56 (20)	11/56 (20)
Addison[d]	14/17 (82)	41/64 (64)	1/17 (6)	3/64 (5)	6/64 (9)
Isolated POF	0/17	0/17	0/17	1/17 (6)	0.17

[a]Percentages are given in parentheses.
[b]StCA data were only available for 22 of 24 APS II sera.
[c]ACA–positive patients without Addison's disease.
[d]Immunofluorescence data (ACA and StCA) were only available for 17 out of the 64 Addison sera studied. Of the 17 sera, 13 (76%) were positive for 21-OH autoantibodies.

The initial report on identification of 17α-OH as an adrenal autoantigen was followed by a number of studies on the reactivity of sera from patients with different forms of Addison's disease with 17α-OH *(177–179,194)*. A detailed study based on immunoprecipitation of ^{35}S-labeled autoantigens produced in an in vitro TnT system provided comprehensive information on the prevalence of autoantibodies to 21-OH and 17α-OH (Table 4) *(192)*. 17α-OH Abs were found in 55% of patients with APS Type 1, 33% of patients with APS Type 2, 5% of patients with isolated Addison's disease, and 20% of patients who were ACA-positive by IFT, but who did not have overt Addison's disease *(192)*. Prevalence of 17α-OH Abs was clearly lower than that of 21-OH Abs (Table 4). Studies on the autoantibody binding sites on 17α-OH have suggested the presence of four distinct regions reactive with Abs in sera from patients with APS Type 1 *(210)*. Although only a limited number of sera ($n = 6$) were tested in this study, there was evidence of heterogeneity in terms of different sera recognizing different epitopes *(210)*. To date, studies on the effect of 17α-OH Abs on 17α-OH enzyme activity have not yet been reported.

Cytochrome P450 Side-Chain Cleavage Enzyme

The reactivity of sera from APS Type 1 patients with cytochrome P450scc was demonstrated by immunoblotting and immunoprecipitation studies with native and recombinant P450scc *(178,204)*. In addition, an inhibiting effect of P450scc Abs in APS Type 1 serum on P450scc enzyme activity in vitro has been reported *(204)*.

The gene coding for P450scc has been assigned to human chromosome 15, and expression of P450scc protein has been reported in the adrenals, gonads, and placenta *(179,211)*. There is about 20% overall amino acid homology between P450scc and 21-OH sequences, and the predicted structure of P450scc appears to differ more extensively from that of 17α-OH and 21-OH *(183,188,211)*.

Studies from different laboratories have indicated some discrepancies in the observed prevalence of P450scc Ab in various patient groups *(175,178,204)*. However, as in the case of 17α-OH Abs, a study based on immunoprecipitation of ^{35}S-labeled autoantigens produced in an in vitro TnT system allowed clarification of some of these discrepancies as shown in Table 4 *(192)*. In the group of patients with APS Type 1, 45% of sera were positive for P450scc Abs, compared to 36% of sera in the APS Type 2 group, 9% of sera in isolated Addison's disease, and 20% in a group of patients who were ACA-positive by IFT, but did not have overt Addison's disease (Table 4) *(192)*. The prevalence of P450scc Abs in these patient groups was always lower than that of 21-OH Abs, but similar to that of 17α-OH Abs. Furthermore, all sera that were positive for 17α-OH and/or P450scc Abs were also positive for 21-OH Abs, except for one sample. In addition, a comparison of StCA (measured by IFT) with 17α-OH and P450scc Ab measurements suggested that 17α-OH and P450scc are the major components of the StCA antigen *(192)*.

Other Autoantigens

In addition to autoantibodies to 21-OH, 17α-OH, and P450scc, autoantibodies to aromatic L-amino acid decarboxylase (AADC) have been reported in patients with APS Type 1 *(212–214)*. Among patients with APS Type 1, AADC Abs were found more often in those with hepatitis, vitiligo, or IDDM *(214)*. AADC is involved in generation of serotonin and dopamine, and is expressed in monoaminergic neurons of the peripheral and central nervous system, pancreatic islet β cells and other cells capable of amine precursor uptake and decarboxylation, including the liver and the kidney *(214)*.

A 51-kDa protein of unknown function, present in granulosa cells and placenta, has also been reported to be an autoantigen in patients with adrenal insufficiency associated with gonadal failure *(215)*. However, the significance of autoantibodies to these autoantigens in adrenal autoimmunity and their diagnostic value remain to be demonstrated *(214,216)*.

In one recent study, the existence of autoantibodies to 3β-hydroxysteroid dehydrogenase has been suggested, and reported to be associated with premature ovarian failure and the presence of StCA *(217)*. However, two separate laboratories were unable to show reactivity to this enzyme in patients with APS Type 1 (with or without gonadal failure) or Addison's disease *(177,194)*.

One of the disease components of APS Type 1 is chronic mucocutaneous candidiasis, and this is believed to be related to selective T-cell deficiency *(6)*. Antibodies to the candidal antigens enolase, heat-shock protein 90, pyruvate kinase, and alcohol dehydrogenase have been reported to be present in sera from patients with APS Type 1, and detection of these antibodies could be helpful in the diagnosis of infections with *Candida albicans (218)*. An observation that candidal infections usually precede the onset of Addison's disease in patients with APS Type 1 has led to a suggestion that molecular mimicry between candidal and adrenal proteins could be involved in the pathogenesis of Addison's disease *(218)*. However, to date there is no evidence for such mechanisms being responsible for the development of adrenal autoimmunity.

Overall, therefore, autoimmune responses in autoimmune adrenal disease may involve antigens other than 21-OH, 17α-OH, and P450scc, but reactivity to these three steroidogenic enzymes, particularly to 21-OH, appears to predominate.

Autoantigens Involved in Gonadal Failure

Premature ovarian failure is associated most commonly with APS Type 1 and to a much lesser extent with APS Type 2 *(116,219,220)*. StCA are detectable in most of these cases *(6,116,172,219,220)*. Furthermore, in female patients with evidence of adrenal autoimmunity, but without overt gonadal failure, the presence of StCA can be considered a serological marker of potential ovarian failure *(221; see also* Chapter 14). Recent studies on the relationship between the ACA, StCA, and autoantibodies to the three steroidogenic enzymes (21-OH, 17α-OH, and P450scc) have indicated that 17α-OH and P450scc Abs are the major components of StCA measured by IFT *(178,192)*. Consequently, these two enzymes appear to be key gonadal autoantigens in patients with ovarian failure associated with autoimmune adrenal disease.

The significance of autoantibodies to the (so far unidentified) 51-kDa antigen present in granulosa cells and placenta *(215)* has yet to be demonstrated.

Whether autoantibodies to specific gonadal autoantigens exist in cases of gonadal failure not associated with adrenal autoimmunity is not clear as yet. In a study of 17 patients with idiopathic POF, autoantibodies to 17α-OH and P450scc were not detectable by immunoprecipitation assay based on ^{35}S-labeled antigens produced in an in vitro TnT, except for one patient who had very low levels of 17α-OH Abs *(192)*. Reports from other laboratories have also indicated a lack of reactivity to 17α-OH, P450scc, 3β-hydroxy-steroid dehydrogenese, or aromatase in sera from patients with POF *(220,222)*. Studies of the interaction of sera from POF patients with different preparations of ovarian antigens using different systems have failed to demonstrate convincingly the presence of specific gonadal autoantibodies *(220,223)*. Furthermore, these studies suggested that any reactivity to ovarian proteins may be secondary and related to ovarian damage rather than to autoimmune reaction *(223)*. LH and FSH receptors have been reported to be autoantigens involved in POF. However, this observation has not been confirmed in other independent studies, including a recent report on the lack of an inhibitory effect of POF sera on hormone binding to recombinant LH and FSH receptors expressed in mammalian cells in culture *(223–225)*.

Although autoimmunity to specific gonadal autoantigens is now clearly established to be present in patients with ovarian failure associated with adrenal autoimmune disease, currently available data do not provide convincing evidence of an autoimmune origin for isolated POF *(223)*.

CONCLUDING REMARKS

Many autoantigens involved in the pathogenesis of autoimmune endocrinopathies have been identified and characterized in the last few decades. Some of these antigens do not fulfill strictly the criteria of organ specificity, which were believed in the 1950s and 1960s to be features of autoimmune responses in organ-specific autoimmune diseases, including autoimmune endocrinopathies *(1,226)*. This is consistent with the current appreciation that complex molecular, genetic, evolutionary, and environmental factors are involved in autoimmune responses.

General improvement in health care, life expectancy, and in the treatment available for patients affected by autoimmune diseases in particular may lead to an increase in the prevalence and incidence of autoimmune disease in the world population. A recent survey of epidemiological reports suggested that about 1 in 30 people resident in the US (more than 8,500,000 people) are currently affected by autoimmune disease *(227)*. Graves' disease/hyperthyroidism, IDDM, pernicious anemia, rheumatoid arthritis, thyroiditis/hypothyroidism, and vitiligo are the most prevalent, and 93% of affected individuals have one of these conditions *(227)*. Overall the impact of autoimmune diseases on health care services and the quality of life of affected individuals and their families in all parts of the world is likely to be greater than generally realized *(227)*, thus emphasizing the importance of autoimmunity research.

REFERENCES

1. Rose NR, Bona C. Defining criteria for autoimmune diseases (Witebsky's postulates revisited). Immunol Today 1993;14:426–430.
2. Goudie RB, Pinkerton PH. Anterior hypophysitis and Hashimoto's disease in a young woman. J Pathol Bacteriol 1962;83:584–585.
3. Ezzat S, Josse RG. Autoimmune hypophysitis. Trends Endocrinol Metab 1997;8:74–80.
4. Bottazzo GF, Pouplard A, Florin-Christensen A, Doniach D. Autoantibodies to prolactin-secreting cells of human pituitary. Lancet 1975;2:97–101.
5. Mirakian R, Cudworth AG, Bottazzo GF, Richardson CA, Doniach D. Autoimmunity to anterior pituitary cells and the pathogenesis of insulin-dependent diabetes mellitus. Lancet 1982:April 3:755–759.
6. Muir A, Maclaren NK. Autoimmune diseases of the adrenal glands, parathyroid glands, gonads and hypothalamic-pituitary axis. Endocrinol Metab Clin North Am 1991;20:619–644.
7. Thodou E, Asa SL, Kontogeorgos G, Kovacs K, Horvath E, Ezzat S. Clinical case seminar: lymphocytic hypophysitis: clinicopathological findings. J Clin Endocrinol Metab 1995;80:2302–2311.
8. Crock P, Salvi M, Miller A, Wall J, Guyda H. Detection of anti-pituitary autoantibodies by immunoblotting. J Immunol Methods 1993;162:31–40.
9. Yabe S, Murakami M, Maruyama K, Miwa H, Fukumura Y, Ishii S, et al. Western blot analysis of rat pituitary antigens recognized by human antipituitary antibodies. Endocr J 1995;42:115–119.
10. Kobayashi T, Yabe S, Kikuchi T, Kanda T, KobayashiI. Presence of anti-pituitary antibodies and GAD antibodies in NIDDM and IDDM. Diabetes Care 1997;20:864–866.
11. Song Y-H, Li Y, Maclaren NK. The nature of autoantigens targeted in autoimmune endocrine diseases. Immunol Today 1996;17:232–238.
12. Volpé R. Hypothesis: the immunoregulatory disturbance in autoimmune thyroid disease. Autoimmunity 1988;2:55–72.
13. Hashimoto H. Zur Kenntnis der lymphomatosen veranderung der schildruse (strume lymphomatosa). Arch Klin Chir 1912;97:219–248.
14. Roitt IM, Doniach D, Campbell PN, Hudson RV. Autoantibodies in Hashimoto's disease. Lancet 1956;2:820–821.
15. Belyavin G, Trotter WR. Investigations of thyroid antigens reacting with Hashimoto sera. Lancet 1959;March 28:648–652.
16. Adams DD, Purves HD. Abnormal responses in the assay of thyrotropin. Proc Univ Otago Med Sch 1956;34:11-12.
17. Rees Smith B, Hall R. Thyroid-stimulating immunoglobulins in Graves' disease. Lancet 1974;August 24:427–431.
18. Balfour BM, Doniach D, Roitt IM, Couchman KG. Fluorescent antibody studies in human thyroiditis: autoantibodies to an antigen of the thyroid colloid distinct from thyroglobulin. Br J Exp Pathol 1961; 42:307–316.
19. Spitzweg C, Heufelder AE. Update on the thyroid sodium iodide symporter: a novel thyroid antigen emerging on the horizon. Eur J Endocrinol 1997;137:22–23.
20. Furmaniak J, Rees Smith B. Review: The structure of thyroid autoantigens. Autoimmunity 1990; 7:63–80.
21. Baas F, van Ommen G-JB, Bikker H, Arnberg AC, de Vijlder JJM. The human thyroglobulin gene is over 300 kb long and contains introns of up to 64 kb. Nucleic Acids Res 1986;14:5171–5186.
22. Mori N, Itoh N, Salvaterra PM. Evolutionary origin of cholinergic macromolecules and thyroglobulin. Proc Natl Acad Sci USA 1987;84:2813–2817.
23. Takagi Y, Omura T, Go M. Evolutionary origin of thyroglobulin by duplication of esterase gene. FEBS 1991;282:17–22.
24. Malthiery Y, Lissitzky S. Primary structure of human thyroglobulin deduced from the sequence of its 8448-base complementary DNA. Eur J Biochem 1987;165:491–498.
25. Edelhoch H. The structure of thyroglobulin and its role in iodination. Rec Prog Horm Res 1965;21:1–24.
26. Kondo, Y Inoue K, Kotani T, Ohtaki S. Immunoelectron microscopy of the hormonogenic sites of the thyroglobulin molecule. Mol Cell Endocrinol 1988;57:261–267.
27. Palumbo G, Gentile F, Condorelli GL, Salvatore G. The earliest site of iodination in thyroglobulin is residue number 5. J Biol Chem 1990;265:8887–8892.
28. Xiao S, Dorris ML, Rawitch AB, Taurog A. Selectivity in tyrosyl iodination sites in human thyroglobulin. Arch Biochem Biophys 1996;334:284–294.

29. Yang S-Y, Pollock HG, Rawitch AB. Glycosylation in human thyroglobulin: location of the N-linked oligosaccharide units and comparison with bovine thyroglobulin. Arch Biochem Biophys 1996;327: 61–70.
30. Malle B, Lejeune P-J, Baudry N, Niccole P, Carayon P, Franc J-L. N-glycans modulate *in vivo* and *in vitro* thyroid hormone synthesis. J Biol Chem 1995;270:29,881–29,888.
31. Yamamoto K, Tsuji T, Tarutani O, Osawa T. Structural changes of carbohydrate chains of human thyroglobulin accompanying malignant transformations of thyroid glands. Eur J Biochem 1984;143: 133–144.
32. Hotta T, Ishii I, Ishihara H, Tejima S, Tarutani O, Takahashi N. Comparative study of the oligosaccharides of human thyroglobulins obtained from normal subjects and patients with various diseases. J Appl Biochem 1985;7:98–103.
33. Tarutani O, Ui N. Properties of thyroglobulins from normal thyroid and thyroid tumor on a concanavalin A-Sepharose column. J Biochem 1985;98:851–857.
34. Yamamoto K, Tsuji T, Tarutani O, Osawa T. Phosphorylated high mannose-type and hybrid-type oligosaccharide chains of human thyroglobulin isolated from malignant thyroid tissue. Biochim Biophys Acta 1985;838:84–91.
35. Sinadović J, Cvejić D, Savin S, Jančić-Zuguricas M, Mićić JV. Altered terminal glycosylation of thyroglobulin in papillary thyroid carcinoma. Exp Clin Endocrinol 1992;100:124–128.
36. Furmaniak J, Rees Smith B. Thyroid antibodies. In: Wheeler MH, Lazarus JH, eds. Diseases of the Thyroid. Chapman & Hall, London, 1994, pp. 117–130.
37. Winter WE. Review: The Immunoendocrinopathies. Part 2: autoimmune thyroid disease, autoimmune Addison disease and related disorders. Am Assoc Clin Chem 1996;14:45–52.
38. Ruf J, Feldt-Rasmussen U, Hegedüs L, Ferrand M, Carayon P. Bispecific thyroglobulin and thyroperoxidase autoantibodies in patients with various thyroid and autoimmune diseases. J Clin Endocrinol Metab 1994;79:1404–1409.
39. Ruf J, Ferrand M, Durand-Gorde J-M, Carayon P. Autoantibodies and monoclonal antibodies directed to an immunodominant antigenic region of thyroglobulin interact with thyroperoxidase through an interspecies idiotype. Autoimmunity 1994;19:55–62.
40. Prentice L, Kiso Y, Fukuma K, Horimoto M, Petersen V, Grennan F, et al. Monoclonal thyroglobulin autoantibodies: variable region analysis and epitope recognition. J Clin Endocrinol Metab 1995;80: 977–986.
41. McIntosh RS, Asghar MS, Watson PF, Kemp EH, Weetman AP. Cloning and analysis of IgGκ and IgGλ anti-thyroglobulin autoantibodies from a patient with Hashimoto's thyroiditis. J Immunol 1996; 157:927–935.
42. Caturegli P, Mariotti S, Kuppers RC, Burek CL, Pinchera A, Rose NR. Epitopes on thyroglobulin: a study of patients with thyroid disease. Autoimmunity 1994;18:41–49.
43. Saboori AM, Caturegli P, Rose NR, Mariotti S, Pinchera A, Burek CL. Tryptic peptides of human thyroglobulin: II. Immunoreactivity with sera from patients with thyroid diseases. Clin Exp Immunol 1994;98:459–463.
44. Kimura S, Hong YS, Kotani T, Ohtaki S, Kikkawa F. Structure of the human thyroid peroxidase gene: comparison and relationship to the human myeloperoxidase gene. Biochemistry 1989;28:4481–4489.
45. Kiso Y, Furmaniak J, Morteo C, Rees Smith B. Analysis of carbohydrate residues on human thyroid peroxidase (TPO) and thyroglobulin (Tg) and effects of deglycosylation, reduction and unfolding on autoantibody binding. Autoimmunity 1992;12:259–269.
46. McLachlan SM, Rapoport B. Review: The molecular biology of thyroid peroxidase: cloning, expression and role as autoantigen in autoimmune thyroid disease. Endocr Rev 1992;13:192–206.
47. Cetani F, Costagliola S, Tonacchera M, Panneels V, Vassart G, Ludgate M. The thyroperoxidase doublet is not produced by alternative splicing. Mol Cell Endocrinol 1995;115:125–132.
48. Grennan Jones F, Wolstenholme A, Fowler S, Smith S, Ziemnicka K, Bradbury J, et al. High-level expression of recombinant immunoreactive thyroid peroxidase in the High Five insect cell line. J Mol Endocrinol 1996;17:165–174.
49. Berman M, Magee M, Koenig RJ, Kaplan MM, Arscott P, Maastricht J, et al. Differential autoantibody responses to thyroid peroxidase in patients with Graves' disease and Hashimoto's thryoiditis. J Clin Endocrinol Metab 1993;77:1098–1101.
50. Baker JR, Arscott P, Johnson J. An analysis of the structure and antigenicity of different forms of human thyroid peroxidase. Thyroid 1994;4:173–178.

51. Premawardhana LDKE, Kiso Y, Phillips DI, Morteo C, Furmaniak J, Rees Smith B. Is TPO detectable in the circulation? Thyroid 1993;3:225–228.
52. McLachlan SM, Rapoport BR. Autoimmune endocrinopathies 2. Recombinant thyroid autoantigens: the keys to the pathogenesis of thyroid disease. J Int Med 1993;234:347–359.
53. Nagayama Y. Continuous versus discontinuous B-cell epitopes on thyroid-specific autoantigens—thyrotropin receptor and thyroid peroxidase. Eur J Endocrinol 1995;132:9–11.
54. McLachlan SM, Rapoport B. Genetic and epitopic analysis of thyroid peroxidase (TPO) autoantibodies: markers of the human thyroid autoimmune response. Clin Exp Immunol 1995;101:200–206.
55. Grennan F, Sanders J, Wolstenholme A, Furmaniak J, Rees Smith B. Analysis of TPO autoantibody epitopes using immunoprecipitation assay based on ^{35}S-labelled intact and modified TPO. J Endocrinol 1996;148 suppl:OC31.
56. Wedlock N, Furmaniak J, Fowler S, Kiso Y, Bednarek J, Baumann-Antczak A, et al. Expression of human thyroid peroxidase in the yeasts *Saccharomyces cerevisiae* and *Hensenula polymorpha*. J Mol Endocrinol 1993;10:325–336.
57. Weetman AP. Editorial: Insulin-dependent diabetes mellitus and postpartum thyroiditis: an important association. J Clin Endocrinol Metab 1994;79:7–9.
58. Hall R. Pregnancy and autoimmune endocrine disease. Baillière's Clin Endocrinol Metab 1995;9:137–155.
59. Roberts J, Jenkins C, Wilson R, Pearson C, Franklin IA, Maclean MA, et al. Recurrent miscarriage is associated with increased numbers of CD5/20 positive lymphocytes and an increased incidence of thyroid antibodies. Eur J Endocrinol 1996;134:84–86.
60. Horimoto M, Petersen VS, Pegg CAS, Fukuma N, Wakabayashi N, Kiso Y, et al. Production and characterisation of a human monoclonal thyroid peroxidase autoantibody. Autoimmunity 1992;14:1–7.
61. Kaczur V, Vereb Gy, Molnár I, Krajczár G, Kiss E, Farid NR, et al. Effect of anti-thyroid peroxidase (TPO) antibodies on TPO activity measured by chemiluminescence assay. Clin Chem 1997;43:1392–1396.
62. Chacko S, Padlan EA. Structural studies of human autoantibodies. Crystal structure of a thyroid peroxidase autoantibody Fab. J Biol Chem 1996;271:12,191–12,198.
63. Gardas A, Sohi MK, Sutton BJ, McGregor AM, Banga JP. Purification and crystallisation of the autoantigen thyroid peroxidase from human Graves' thyroid tissue. Biochem Biophys Res Commun 1997;234:366–370.
64. Libert F, Passage E, Lefort A, Vassart G, Mattei M-G. Localisation of human thyrotropin receptor gene to chromosome region 14q31 by in situ hybridisation. Cytogen Cell Genet 1990;54:82–83.
65. Gross B, Misrahi M, Sar S, Milgrom E. Composite structure of the human thryotropin receptor gene. Biochem Biophys Res Commun 1991;177:679–687.
66. Lefkowitz RJ, Coron MG. Adrenergic Receptors. J Biol Chem 1988;263:4993–4996.
67. Nagayama Y, Kaufman KD, Seto P, Rapoport B. Molecular cloning, sequence and functional expression of the cDNA for the human thyrotropin receptor. Biochem Biophys Res Commun 1989;165:1184–1190.
68. Akamizu T, Ikuyama S, Saji M, Kosugi S, Cozak C, McBridge OW, et al. Cloning, chromosomal assignment and regulation of the rat thyrotropin receptor: expression of the gene is regulated by thyrotropin, agents that increase cAMP levels and thyroid autoantibodies. Proc Natl Acad Sci USA 1990;87:5677–5681.
69. Parmentier M, Libert F, Maenhaut C, Lefort A, Gérard C, Perret J, et al. Molecular cloning of the thyrotropin receptor. Science 1989;246:1620–1622.
70. Libert F, Lefort A, Gerard C. Parmentier M, Perret J, Ludgate M, et al. Cloning, sequencing and expression of the human thyrotropin (TSH) receptor: evidence for binding of autoantibodies. Biochem Biophys Res Commun 1989;165:1250–1255.
71. Frazier AL, Robbins LS, Stork PJ. Sprengel R, Segaloff DL, Cone RD. Isolation of TSH and LH/CG receptor cDNAs from human thyroid: regulation of tissue specific splicing. Mol Endocrinol 1990;4:1264–1276.
72. Misrahi M, Loosfelt H, Atger M, Sar S, Guiochon-Mantel A, Milgrom E. Cloning, sequencing and expression of the human TSH receptor. Biochem Biophys Res Commun 1990;166:394–403.
73. Sanders, J, Oda, Y, Roberts, S-A, Maruyama, M, Furmaniak, J, Rees Smith, B. Understanding the TSH receptor function/structure relationship. In: Newer Aspects of Graves' Disease—Basic and Clinical Aspects. Baillière's Clin Endocrinol Metab 1997;11:451–479.
74. Shenker A. G protein-coupled receptor structure and function: the impact of disease-causing mutations. Baillière's Clin Endocrinol Metab 1995;9:427–451.

75. Spiegel AM. Mutations in G proteins and G protein coupled receptors in endocrine disease. J Clin Endocrinol Metab 1996;81:2434–2442.
76. Van Sande J, Parma J, Tonacchera M. Swillens S, Dumont J, Vassart G. Somatic and germline mutations of the TSH receptor gene in thyroid diseases. J Clin Endocrinol Metab 1995;80:2577–2585.
77. Russo D, Arturi F, Chiefari E, Filetti S. Molecular insights into TSH receptor abnormality and thyroid disease. J Endocrinol Invest 1997;20:36–47.
78. Clifton-Bligh RJ, Gregory JW, Ludgate M. John R, Persani L, Asteria C, et al. Two novel mutations in the thyrotropin (TSH) receptor gene in a child with resistance to TSH. J Clin Endocrinol Metab 1997; 82:1094–1100.
79. Oda Y, Sanders J, Roberts S, Maruyama M, Kato R, Perez M, et al. Binding characteristics of antibodies to the TSH receptor. J Mol Endocrinol 1998;20:233–244.
80. Misrahi M. Ghinea N, Sar S, Saunier B, Jolivet A, Loosfelt H, et al. Processing of the precursors of the human thyroid stimulating hormone receptor in various eukaryotic cells (human thyrocytes, transfected L cells and baculovirus infected insect cells). Eur J Biochem 1994;222:711–719.
81. Chazenbalk GD, Kakinuma A, Jaume JC, McLachlan SM, Rapoport B. Evidence for negative cooperativity among human thyrotropin receptors over expressed in mammalian cells. Endocrinology 1996;137:4586–4591.
82. Loosfelt H, Pichon C, Jolivet A, Misrahi M, Caillou B, Jamous M, et al. Two-subunit structure of the human thyrotropin receptor. Proc Natl Acad Sci USA 1992;89:3765–3769.
83. Sanders JF, Roberts S, Oda Y, Maruyama M, Furmaniak J, Rees Smith B. Analysis of carbohydrate residues on human recombinant TSH receptor. J Endocrinol Invest 1997;20(Suppl):26.
84. Davies Jones E, Rees Smith B. A water soluble fragment of the thyroid stimulating hormone receptor which binds both thyroid stimulating hormone and thyroid stimulating hormone receptor antibodies. J Endocrinol 1984;100:113–118.
85. Davies Jones E, Hashim FA, Kajita Y, Creagh FM, Buckland PR, Petersen VB, et al. Interaction of autoantibodies to thyrotropin receptor with a hydrophilic subunit of the thyrotropin receptor. Biochem J 1985;228:111–117.
86. Harfst E, Nussey SS, Johnstone AP. Interaction of thyrotropin and thyroid stimulating antibodies with recombinant extracellular region of human TSH receptor. Lancet 1992;339:193–194.
87. Harfst E, Johnstone AP, Nussey SS. Characterisation of the extracellular region of the human thyrotrophin receptor expressed as a recombinant protein. J Mol Endocrinol 1992;9:227–236.
88. Huang GC, Page MJ, Nicholson LB, Collison KS, McGregor AM, Banga JP. The thyrotrophin hormone receptor of Graves' disease: overexpression of the extracellular domain in insect cells using recombinant baculovirus, immunoaffinity purification and analysis of autoantibody binding. J Mol Endocrinol 1993;10:127–142.
89. Vlase H, Matsuoka N, Graves PN, Magnusson RP, Davies TF. Folding dependent binding of thyrotropin (TSH) and TSH receptor autoantibodies to the murine TSH receptor ectodomain. Endocrinology 1997;138:1658–1666.
90. Brennan A, Petersen VB, Petersen MM, Rees Smith B, Hall R. Time-dependent stabilisation of the TSH–TSH receptor complex. FEBS 1980;111:35–38.
91. Chazenbalk GD, Tanaka K, Nagayama Y, Kakinuma A, Jaume JC, McLachlan SM, et al. Evidence that the thyrotropin receptor ectodomain contains not one, but two, cleavage sites. Endocrinology 1997; 138:2893–2899.
92. Chazenbalk GD, McLachlan SM, Nagayama Y, Rapoport B. Is receptor cleavage into two subunits necessary for thyrotropin action? Biochem Biophys Res Commun 1996;225:479–484.
93. Couet J, Sar S, Jolivet A, Hai M-TV, Milgrom E, Misrahi M. Shedding of human thyrotropin receptor ectodomain. J Biol Chem 1996;271:4545–4552
94. Couet J, de Bernard S, Loosfelt H, Saunier B, Milgrom E, Misrahi M. Cell surface protein disulfide isomerase is involved in the shedding of human thyrotropin receptor ectodomain. Biochemisty 1996;35: 14,800–14,805.
95. Paschke R, Metcalfe A, Alcalde L, Vassart G, Weetman A, Ludgate M. Presence of nonfunctional thyrotropin receptor transcripts in retroocular and other tissues. J Clin Endocrinol Metab 1994;79: 1234–1238.
96. Furmaniak J, Rees Smith B. Immunity to the thyroid-stimulating hormone receptor. Springer Semin Immunopathol 1993;14:309–321.
97. Nagayama Y, Russo D, Chazenbalk GD, Wadsworth HL, Rapoport B. Extracellular domain chimeras of the TSH and LH/CG receptors reveal the mid-region (amino acids 171-260) to play a vital role in high affinity TSH binding. Biochem Biophys Res Commun 1990;173:1150–1156.

98. Nagayama Y, Wadsworth HL, Russo D, Chazenbalk GD, Rapoport B. Binding domains of stimulatory and inhibitory thyrotropin (TSH) receptor autoantibodies determined with chimeric TSH-lutropin/chorionic gonadotropin receptors. J Clin Invest 1991;88:336–340.
99. Watanabe Y, Tahara K, Hirai A, Tada H, Kohn LD, Amino N. Subtypes of anti-TSH receptor antibodies classified by various assays using CHO cells expressing wild type or chimeric human TSH receptor. Thyroid 1997;7:13–19.
100. Wadsworth HL, Chazenbalk GD, Nagayama Y, Russo D, Rapoport B. An insertion in the human thyrotropin receptor critical for high affinity hormone binding. Science 1990;249:1423–1425.
101. Wadsworth HL, Russo D, Nagayama Y, Chazenbalk GD, Rapoport B. Studies on the role of amino acids 38-45 in the expression of a functional thyrotropin receptor. Mol Endocrinol 1992;6:394–398.
102. Kosugi S, Sugawa H, Mori T. Epitope analysis of the thyrotropin receptor, 1997. Mol Cell Endocrinol 1997;128:11–18.
103. Harfst E, Johnstone AP. Characterization of the glutamine synthase amplifiable eukaryotic expression system applied to an integral membrane protein—the human thyrotropin receptor. Anal Biochem 1992;207:80–84.
104. Chazenbalk GD, Jaume JC, McLachlan SM, Rapoport B. Engineering the human thyrotropin receptor ectodomain from a non-secreted form to a secreted, highly immunoreactive glycoprotein that neutralizes autoantibodies in Graves' patients' sera. J Biol Chem 1997;272:18,959–18,965.
105. Huang GC, Collison KS, McGregor AM, Banga JP. Expression of a human thyrotrophin receptor fragment in *Escherichia coli* and its interaction with the hormone and autoantibodies from patients with Graves' disease. J Mol Endocrinol 1992;8:137–144.
106. Seetharamaiah GS, Dallas JS, Patibandla SA, Thotakura NR, Prabhakar BS. Requirement of glycosylation of the human thyrotropin receptor ectodomain for its reactivity with autoantibodies in patients' sera. J Immunol 1997;158:2799–2803.
107. Rapoport B, McLachlan SM, Kakinuma A, Chazenbalk GD. Critical relationship between autoantibody recognition and thyrotropin receptor maturation as reflected in the acquisition of complex carbohydrate. J Clin Endocrinol Metab 1996;81:2525–2533.
108. Morgenthaler NG, Tremble J, Huang G, Scherbaum WA, McGregor AM, Banga, JP. Binding of antithyrotropin receptor autoantibodies in Graves' disease serum to nascent in vitro translated thyrotropin receptor: ability to map epitopes recognised by antibodies. J Clin Endocrinol Metab 1996; 81:700–706.
109. Prentice L, Sanders JF, Perez M, Kato R, Sawicka J, Oda Y, et al. Thyrotropin (TSH) receptor autoantibodies do not appear to bind to the TSH receptor produced in an *in vitro* transcription/translation system. J Clin Endocrinol Metab 1997;82:1288–1292.
110. Dai G, Levy O, Carrasco N. Cloning and characterization of the thyroid iodide transporter. Nature 1996;379:458–460.
111. Smanik PA, Liu Q, Furminger TL, Rhu K, Xing S, Mazzaferri EL, et al. Cloning of the human sodium iodide symporter. Biochem Biophys Res Commun 1996;226:339–345.
112. Morris JC, Bergert ER, Bryant WP. Binding of immunoglobulin G from patients with autoimmune thyroid disease to rat sodium-iodide symporter peptides: evidence for the iodide transporter as an autoantigen. Thyroid 1997;7:527–534.
113. Morris J, Bergert E, Bryant W. Binding of IgG from patients with autoimmune thyroid disease to human sodium-iodine symporter peptides: interspecies variability in the autoimmune response to NIS. Thyroid 1997;7(Suppl 1):234.
114. Endo T, Kogai T, Nakazato M, Saito T, Kaneshige M, Onaya T. Autoantibody against Na$^+$/I$^-$ symporter in the sera of patients with autoimmune thyroid disease. Biochem Biophys Res Commun 1996;224: 92–95.
115. Rees Smith B, Furmaniak J. Editorial: adrenal and gonadal autoimmune diseases. J Clin Endocrinol Metab 1995;80:1502–1505.
116. Betterle C, Greggio NA, Volpato M. Clinical review: autoimmune polyglandular syndrome Type I. J Clin Endocrinol Metab 1998;83:1049–1055.
117. Blizzard RM, Chee D, Davis W. The incidence of parathyroid and other antibodies in the sera of patients with idiopathic hypoparathyroidism. Clin Exp Immunol 1966;1:119–128.
118. Li Y, Song Y-H, Rais N, Connor E, Schatz D, Muir A, et al. Autoantibodies to the extracellular domain of the calcium sensing receptor in patients with acquired hypoparathyroidism. J Clin Invest 1996;97: 910–914.
119. Pearce SHS, Brown EM. Editorial: calcium-sensing receptor mutations: insights into a structurally and functionally novel receptor. J Clin Endocrinol Metab 1996;81:1309–1311.

120. Freichel M, Zinklorenz A, Holloschi A, Hafner M, Flockerzi V, Raue F. Expression of a calcium-sensing receptor in a human medullary thyroid carcinoma cell line and its contribution to calcitonin secretion. Endocrinology 1996;137:3842–3848.
121. Sepe V, Lai M, Shattock M, Foxon R, Collins P, Bottazzo GF. Islet-related autoantigens and the pathogenesis of insulin-dependent diabetes mellitus. In: Leslie RDG, ed. Molecular Pathogenesis of Diabetes Mellitus, vol. 22. Karger, Basel, 1997, pp. 68–89.
122. Bottazzo GF, Florin-Christensen A, Doniach D. Islet cell antibodies in diabetes mellitus with autoimmune polyendocrine deficiency. Lancet 1974;ii:1279–1283.
123. Christie MR. Islet cell autoantigens in type 1 diabetes. Eur J Clin Invest 1996;26:827–838.
124. Mennuni C, Santini C, Lazzaro D, Dotta F, Farilla L, Fierabracci A, et al. Identification of a novel type 1 diabetes-specific epitope by screening phage libraries with sera from pre-diabetic patients. J Mol Biol 1997;268:599–606.
125. Bingley PJ, Bonifacio E, Williams AJK, Genovese S, Bottazzo GF, Gale EAM. Prediction of IDDM in the general population—strategies based on combinations of autoantibody markers. Diabetes 1997;46:1701–1710.
126. Baekkeskov S, Nielsen JH, Marner B, Bilde T, Ludvigsson J, Lernmark A. Autoantibodies in newly diagnosed diabetic children immunoprecipitate human pancreatic islet cell proteins. Nature 1982;298:167–169.
127. Baekkeskov S, Aanstoot H-J, Christgau S, Reetz A, Solimena M, Cascalho M, et al. Identification of the 64K autoantigen in insulin-dependent diabetes as the GABA-synthesizing enzyme glutamic acid decarboxylase. Nature 1990;347:151–156.
128. Ellis TM, Atkinson MA. The clinical significance of an autoimmune response against glutamic acid decarboxylase. Nature Med 1996;2:148–153.
129. Lernmark A. Glutamic acid decarboxylase—gene to antigen to disease. J Int Med 1996;240:259–277.
130. Bu D-F, Erlander MG, Hitz BC, Tillakaratne NJK, Kaufman DL, Wagner-McPherson CB, et al. Two human glutamate decarboxylases, 65-kDa GAD and 67-kDa GAD, are each encoded by a single gene. Proc Natl Acad Sci USA 1992;89:2115–2119.
131. Erlander MG, Tobin AJ. The structural and functional heterogeneity of glutamic acid decarboxylase: a review. Neurochem Res 1991;16:215–226.
132. Namchuk M, Lindsay L, Turck CW, Kanaani J, Baekkeskov S. Phosphorylation of serine residues 3, 6, 10, and 13 distinguishes membrane anchored from soluble glutamic acid decarboxylase 65 and is restricted to glutamic acid decarboxylase 65α. J Biol Chem 1997;272:1548–1557.
133. Rowley MJ, Mackay IR, Chen Q-Y, Knowles WJ, Zimmet PZ. Antibodies to glutamic acid decarboxylase discriminate major types of diabetes mellitus. Diabetes 1992;41:548–551.
134. Ohta M, Obayashi H, Takahashi K, Kitagawa Y, Nakano K, Matsuo S, et al. A simple solid-phase radioimmunoassay for glutamic acid decarboxylase (GAD) antibodies in patients with diabetes mellitus. J Clin Biochem Nutr 1996;20:139–148.
135. Kaufman DL, Erlander MG, Clare-Salzier M, Atkinson MA, Maclaren NK, Tobin AJ. Autoimmunity to two forms of glutamate decarboxylase in insulin-dependent diabetes mellitus. J Clin Invest 1992;89:283–292.
136. Petersen JS, Hejnæs KR, Moody A, Karlsen AE, Marshall MO, Høier-Madsen M, et al. Detection of GAD_{65} antibodies in diabetes and other autoimmune diseases using a simple radioligand assay. Diabetes 1994;43:459–467.
137. Grubin CE, Daniels T, Toivola B, Landin-Olsson M, Hagopian WA, Li L, et al. A novel radioligand binding assay to determine diagnostic accuracy of isoform-specific glutamic acid decarboxylase antibodies in childhood IDDM. Diabetologia 1994;37:344–350.
138. Hagopian WA, Karlsen AE, Gottsätter A, Landin-Olsson M, Grubin CE, Sundkvist G, et al. Quantitative assay using recombinant human islet glutamic acid decarboxylase (GAD65) shows that 64K autoantibody positivity at onset predicts diabetes type. J Clin Invest 1993;91:368–374.
139. Aanstoot H-J, Sigurdsson E, Jaffe M, Shi Y, Christgau S, Grobbee D, et al. Value of antibodies to GAD_{65} combined with islet cell cytoplasmic antibodies for predicting IDDM in a childhood population. Diabetologia 1994;37:917–924.
140. Lühder F, Schlosser M, Mauch L, Haubruck H, Rjasanowski I, Michaelis D, et al. Autoantibodies against GAD_{65} rather than GAD_{67} precede the onset of type 1 diabetes. Autoimmunity 1994;19:71–80.
141. Lühder F, Woltanski K-P, Mauch L, Haubruck H, Kohnert K-D, Rjasanowski I, et al. Detection of autoantibodies to the 65-kD isoform of glutamate decarboxylase by radioimmunoassay. Eur J Endocrinol 1994;130:575–580.

142. Matsuba T, Yano M, Abiru N, Takino H, Akazawa S, Nagataki S, et al. Expression of recombinant human glutamic acid decarboxylase (GAD) in myeloma cells and enzyme-linked immunosorbent assay (ELISA) for autoantibodies to GAD. J Biochem 1997;121:20–24.
143. Powell M, Prentice L, Asawa T, Kato R, Sawicka J, Tanaka H, et al. Glutamic acid decarboxylase autoantibody assay using ^{125}I-labelled recombinant GAD$_{65}$ produced in yeast. Clin Chim Acta 1996; 256:175–188.
144. Ohta M, Obayashi H, Takahashi K, Kitagawa Y, Nakano K, Matsuo S, et al. Radioimmunoprecipitation assay for glutamic acid decarboxylase antibodies evaluated clinically with sera from patients with insulin-dependent diabetes mellitus. Clin Chem 1996;42:1975–1978.
145. Falorni A, Ackefors M, Carlberg C, Daniels T, Persson B, Robertson J, et al. Diagnostic sensitivity of immunodominant epitopes of glutamic acid decarboxylase (GAD65) autoantibodies in childhood IDDM. Diabetologia 1996;39:1091–1098.
146. Richter W, Jury KM, Loeffler D, Manfras BJ, Eiermann TH, Boehm BO. Immunoglobulin variable gene analysis of human autoantibodies reveals antigen-driven immune response to glutamate decarboxylase in type 1 diabetes mellitus. Eur J Immunol 1995;25:1703–1712.
147. Jury KM, Loeffle, D, Eiermann TH, Ziegler B, Richter W. Evidence for somatic mutation and affinity maturation of diabetes associated human autoantibodies to glutamate decarboxylase. J Autoimmunity 1996;9:371–377.
148. Madec A-M, Rousset F, Ho S, Robert F, Thivolet C, Orgiazzi J, et al. Four IgG anti-islet human monoclonal antibodies isolated from a type 1 diabetes patient recognize distinct epitopes of glutamic acid decarboxylase 65 and are somatically mutated. J Immunol 1996;156:3541–3549.
149. Daw K, Ujihara N, Atkinson M, Powers AC. Glutamic acid decarboxylase autoantibodies in stiff-man syndrome and insulin-dependent diabetes mellitus exhibit similarities and differences in epitope recognition. J Immunol 1996;156:818–825.
150. Björk E, Velloso LA, Kämpe O, Karlsson FA. GAD autoantibodies in IDDM, stiff-man syndrome and autoimmune polyendocrine syndrome type I recognize different epitopes. Diabetes 1994;43:161–165.
151. Seissler J, Bieg S, Yassin N, Mauch L, Northemann W, Boehm BO, et al. Association between antibodies to the MR 67,000 isoform of glutamate decarboxylase (GAD) and type 1 (insulin-dependent) diabetes mellitus with coexisting autoimmune polyendocrine syndrome type II. Autoimmunity 1994;19:231–238.
152. Tuomi T, Björses P. Falorni A, Partanen J, Perheentupa J, Lernmark A, et al. Antibodies to glutamic acid decarboxylase and insulin-dependent diabetes in patients with autoimmune polyendocrine syndrome type I. J Clin Endocrinol Metab 1996;81:1488–1494.
153. Maclaren NK, Atkinson MA. Insulin-dependent diabetes mellitus: the hypothesis of molecular mimicry between islet cell antigens and microorganisms. Mol Med Today 1997;February:76–83.
154. Volpé R. The autoimmune endocrinopathies—the complexities continue to ravel. Trends Endocrinol Metab 1997;8:59–63.
155. Bonifacio E, Christie MR. Tyrosine phosphatase-like proteins as autoantigens in insulin-dependent diabetes mellitus: the targets for 37/40k antibodies. Diabetes Nutr Metab 1996;9:183–187.
156. Pietropaolo M, Hutton JC, Eisenbarth GS. Protein tyrosine phosphatase-like proteins: link with IDDM. Diabetes Care 1997;20:208–214.
157. Notkins AL, Lu J, Li Q, VanderVegt FP, Wasserfall C, Maclaren NK, et al. IA-2 and IA-2β are major autoantigens in IDDM and the precursors of the 40 kDa and 37 kDa tryptic fragments. J Autoimmunity 1996;9:677–682.
158. Lan MS, Modi WS, Xie H, Notkins AL. Assignment of the IA-2 gene encoding an autoantigen in IDDM to chromosome 2q35. Diabetologia 1996;39:1001–1003.
159. Notkins AL, Zhang B, Matsumoto Y, Lan MS. Comparison of IA-2 with IA-2b and with six other members of the protein tyrosine phosphatase family: recognition of antigenic determinants by IDDM sera. J Autoimmunity 1997;10:245–250.
160. Hatfield ECI, Hawkes CJ, Payton MA, Christie MR. Cross reactivity between IA-2 and phogrin/IA-2β in binding of autoantibodies in IDDM. Diabetologia 1997;40:1327–1333.
161. Powell M, Chen S, Tanaka H, Masuda M, Beer C, Rees Smith B, et al. Autoantibodies to IA-2 in IDDM —measurements with a new immunoprecipitation assay. J Endocrinol 1997;155(Suppl 2):P27.
162. Palmer JP, Asplin CM, Clemons P, Lyen K, Tatpati O, Raghu PK, et al. Insulin antibodies in insulin-dependent diabetics before insulin treatment. Science 1983;222:1337–1339.
163. Porte D, Halter JB. The endocrine pancreas and diabetes mellitus. In: Williams R, ed. Textbook of Endocrinology. W.B. Saunders, Philadelphia, 1981, pp. 716–843.

164. Bell GI, Swain WF, Pictet R, Cordell B, Goodman HM, Rutter WJ. Nucleotide sequence of a cDNA clone encoding human preproinsulin. Nature 1979;282:525–527.
165. Bell GI, Pictet RL, Rutter WJ, Cordell B, Tischer E, Goodman HM. Sequence of the human insulin gene. Nature 1980;284:26–32.
166. Greenbaum CJ, Palmer JP, Kuglin B, Kolb H, Participating Laboratories. Insulin autoantibodies measured by RIA methodology are more related to IDDM than those measured by ELISA. J Clin Endocrinol Metab 1992;74:1040–1044.
167. Addison T. On the constitutional and local effects of disease of the suprarenal capsules. A collection of the published writings of the late Thomas Addison MD, Physician to Guy's Hospital, London London 1868 New Sydenham Society Reprinted in Medical Classics 1937;2:244–293.
168. Anderson JR, Goudie RB, Gray KG, Timbury GC. Preliminary communication. Autoantibodies in Addison's disease. Lancet June 1957;1:1123–1124.
169. Blizzard RM, Kyle M. Studies of the adrenal antigens and antibodies in Addison's disease. J Clin Invest 1963;42:1653–1660.
170. Betterle C, Pedini B, Presotto F. Serological markers of Addison's disease. In: Bhatt HR, James VHT, Besser GM, Bottazzo GF, Keen H, eds. Advances in Thomas Addison's Diseases. Journal of Endocrinology Ltd, Bristol, 1994, pp. 67–84.
171. Anderson JR, Goudie RB, Gray K, Stuart-Smith DA. Immunological features of idiopathic Addison's disease: antibodies to cells producing steroid hormones. Clin Exp Immunol 1968;3:107–117.
172. Bottazzo GF, Mirakian R, Drexhage HA. Adrenalitis, oophoritis and autoimmune polyglandular disease. In: Rich RR, Fleisher TA, Shearer WT, Schwartz BD, Strober W, ed. Clinical Immunology Principles and Practice. St. Louis, Mosby-Year Book, 1996, pp. 1523–1536.
173. Furmaniak J, Talbot D, Reinwein D, Benker G, Creagh FM, Rees Smith B. Immunoprecipitation of human adrenal microsomal antigen. FEBS 1988;231:25–28.
174. Baumann-Antczak A, Wedlock N, Bednarek J, Kiso Y, Krishnan H, Fowler S, et al. Autoimmune Addison's disease and 21-hydroxylase. Lancet 1992;340:429–430.
175. Winqvist O, Karlsson A, Kämpe O. 21-hydroxylase, a major autoantigen in idiopathic Addison's disease. Lancet 1992;339:1559–1562.
176. Bednarek J, Furmaniak J, Wedlock N, Kiso Y, Baumann-Antczak A, Fowler S, et al. Steroid 21-hydroxylase is a major autoantigen involved in adult onset autoimmune Addison's disease. FEBS 1992;309:51–55.
177. Song Y-H, Connor EL, Muir A, She JX, Zorovich B, Derovanesian D, et al. Autoantibody epitope mapping of the 21-hydroxylase antigen in autoimmune Addison's disease. J Clin Endocrinol Metab 1994;78:1108–1112.
178. Uibo R, Aavik E, Peterson P, Perheentupa J, Aranko S, Pelkonen R, Krohn KJE. Autoantibodies to cytochrome P450 enzymes P450scc, P450c17 and P450c21 in autoimmune polyglandular disease types I and II and in isolated Addison's disease. J Clin Endocrinol Metab 1994;78:323–328.
179. Uibo R, Perheentupa J, Ovod V, Krohn KJE. Characterization of adrenal autoantigens recognized by sera from patients with autoimmune polyglandular syndrome (APS) type I. J Autoimmunity 1994;7:399–411.
180. Miller WL. Clinical review 54. Genetics, diagnosis, and management of 21-hydroxylase deficiency. J Clin Endocrinol Metab 1994;78:241–246.
181. Azziz R, Dewailly D, Owerbach D. Clinical review 56. Nonclassic adrenal hyperplasia: current concepts. J Clin Endocrinol Metab 1994;78:810–815.
182. Wilson RC, Mercado AB, Cheng KC, New MI. Steroid 21-hydroxylase deficiency: genotype may not predict phenotype. J Clin Endocrinol Metab 1995;80:2322–2329.
183. White PC, New MI, Dupont B. Structure of human steroid 21-hydroxylase genes. Proc Natl Acad Sci USA 1986;83:5111–5115.
184. Trowsdale J, Ragoussis J, Campbell RD. Map of the human MHC. Immunology Today 1991;12:443–446.
185. Kominami S, Ochi H, Kobayashi Y, Takemori S. Studies on the steroid hydroxylation system in adrenal cortex microsomes. J Biol Chem 1980;255:3386–3394.
186. Bumpus JA, Dus KM. Bovine adrenocortical microsomal hemeproteins P-450$_{17\alpha}$ and P-450$_{C-21}$. Isolation, partial characterization and comparison to P-450scc. J Biol Chem 1982;257:12,696–12,704.
187. Hsu LC, Hu MC, Cheng HC, Lu JC, Chung B. The N-terminal hydrophobic domain of P450c21 is required for membrane insertion and enzyme stability. J Biol Chem 1993;268:14,682–14,686.
188. Picado-Leonard J, Miller WL. Cloning and sequence of the human gene for P450c17 (steroid 17α-hydroxylase/17,20 lyase): similarity with the gene for P450c21. DNA 1987;6:439–448.

189. Lin D, Zhang L, Chiao E, Miller WL. Modeling and mutagenesis of the active site of human P450c17. Mol Endocrinol 1994;8:392–402.
190. Colls J, Betterle C, Volpato M, Prentice L, Rees Smith B, Furmaniak J. Immunoprecipitation assay for autoantibodies to steroid 21-hydroxylase in autoimmune adrenal disease. Clin Chem 1995;41:375–380.
191. Falorni A, Nikoshkov A, Laureti S, Grenbäck E, Hulting A-L, Casucci G, et al. High diagnostic accuracy for idiopathic Addison's disease with a sensitive radiobinding assay for autoantibodies against recombinant human 21-hydroxylase. J Clin Endocrinol Metab 1995;80:2752–2755.
192. Chen S, Sawicka J, Betterle C, Powell M, Prentice L, Volpato M, et al. Autoantibodies to steroidogenic enzymes in autoimmune polyglandular syndrome, Addison's disease and premature ovarian failure. J Clin Endocrinol Metab 1996;81:1871–1876.
193. Söderbergh A, Winqvist O, Norheim I, Rorsman F, Huseby ES, Dolva O, et al. Adrenal autoantibodies and organ-specific autoimmunity in patients with Addison's disease. Clin Endocrinol 1996;45:453–460.
194. Peterson P, Uibo R, Peränen J, Krohn K. Immunoprecipitation of steroidogenic enzyme autoantigens with autoimmune polyglandular syndrome type I (APS I) sera; further evidence for independent humoral immunity to P450c17 and P450c21. Clin Exp Immunol 1997;107:335–340.
195. Tanaka H, Perez MS, Powell M, Sanders JF, Sawicka J, Chen S, et al. Steroid 21-hydroxylase autoantibodies: measurements with a new immunoprecipitation assay. J Clin Endocrinol Metab 1997;82:1440–1446.
196. Wedlock N, Asawa T, Baumann-Antczak A, Rees Smith B, Furmaniak J. Autoimmune Addison's disease. Analysis of autoantibody binding sites on human steroid 21-hydroxylase. FEBS 1993;332:123–126.
197. Asawa T, Wedlock N, Baumann-Antczak A, Rees Smith B, Furmaniak J. Naturally occurring mutations in human steroid 21-hydroxylase influence adrenal autoantibody binding. J Clin Endocrinol Metab 1994;79:372–376.
198. Nikishkov A, Lajic S, Holst M, Wedell A, Luthman H. Synergistic effect of partially inactivating mutations in steroid 21-hydroxylase deficiency. J Clin Endocrinol Metab 1997;82:194–199.
199. Tanaka H, Asawa T, Powell M, Chen S, Rees Smith B, Furmaniak J. Autoantibody binding to steroid 21-hydroxylase—effect of five mutations. Autoimmunity 1997;26:253–259.
200. Hu MC, Hsu LC, Hsu NC, Chung B. Function and membrane topology of wild-type and mutated cytochrome P450c21. Biochem J 1996;316:325–329.
201. Furmaniak J, Kominami S, Asawa T, Wedlock N, Colls J, Rees Smith B. Autoimmune Addison's disease—evidence for a role of steroid 21-hydroxylase autoantibodies in adrenal insufficiency. J Clin Endocrinol Metab 1994;79:1517–1521.
202. Boscaro M, Betterle C, Volpato M, Fallo F, Furmaniak J, Rees Smith B, et al. Hormonal responses during various phases of autoimmune adrenal failure: no evidence for 21-hydroxylase enzyme activity inhibition *in vivo*. J Clin Endocrinol Metab 1996;81:2801–2804.
203. Volpato M, Prentice L, Chen S, Betterle C, Rees Smith B, Furmaniak J. A study of the epitopes on steroid 21-hydroxylase recognized by autoantibodies in patients with or without Addison's disease. Clin Exp Immunol 1998;111:422–428.
204. Winqvist O, Gustafsson J, Rorsman F, Karlsson FA, Kämpe O. Two different cytochrome P450 enzymes are the adrenal antigens in autoimmune polyendocrine syndrome type I and Addison's disease. J Clin Invest 1993;92:2377–2385.
205. Richter W, Northemann W, Müller M, Böhm O. Mapping of an autoreactive epitope within glutamate decarboxylase using a diabetes-associated human monoclonal autoantibody and an epitope cDNA library. Hybridoma 1996;15:103–108.
206. Betterle C, Volpato M, Rees Smith B, Furmaniak J, Chen S, Zanchetta R, et al. II. Adrenal cortex and steroid 21-hydroxylase autoantibodies in children with organ-specific autoimmune diseases: markers of high progression to clinical Addison's disease. J Clin Endocrinol Metab 1997;82:939–942.
207. Betterle C, Volpato M, Rees Smith B, Furmaniak J, Chen S, Greggio NA, et al. I. Adrenal cortex and steroid 21-hydroxylase autoantibodies in adult patients with organ-specific autoimmune diseases: markers of low progression to clinical Addison's disease. J Clin Endocrinol Metab 1997;82:932–938.
208. Krohn K, Uibo R, Aavik E, Peterson P, Savilahti K.; Identification by molecular cloning of an autoantigen associated with Addison's disease as steroid 17α-hydroxylase. Lancet 1992;339:770–773.
209. Chung B, Picado-Leonard J, Haniu M, Bienkowski M, Hall PF, Shivley JE, et al. Cytochrome P450c17 (steroid 17α-hydroxylase/17,20 lyase): cloning of human adrenal and testis cDNAs indicates the same gene is expressed in both tissues. Proc Natl Acad Sci USA 1987;84:407–411.
210. Peterson P, Krohn KJE. Mapping of B cell epitopes on steroid 17α-hydroxylase, an autoantigen in autoimmune polyglandular syndrome type I. Clin Exp Immunol 1994;98:104–109.

211. Chung B-C, Matteson KJ, Voutilainen R, Mohandas TK, Miller WL. Human cholesterol side-chain cleavage enzyme, P450scc: cDNA cloning, assignment of the gene to chromosome 15, and expression in the placenta. Proc Natl Acad Sci USA 1986;83:8962–8966.
212. Velloso LA, Winqvist O, Gustafsson J, Kämpe O, Karlsson FA. Autoantibodies against a novel 51 kDa islet antigen and glutamate decarboxylase isoforms in autoimmune polyendocrine syndrome type I. Diabetologia 1994;37:61–69.
213. Rorsman F, Husebye ES, Winqvist O, Björk E, Karlsson FA, Kämpe O. Aromatic-L-amino-acid decarboxylase, a pyridoxal phosphate-dependent enzyme, is a β-cell autoantigen. Proc Natl Acad Sci USA 1995;92:8626–8629.
214. Husebye ES, Gebre-Medhin G, Tuomi T, Perheentupa J, Landin-Olsson M, Gustafsson J, et al. Autoantibodies against aromatic L-amino acid decarboxylase in autoimmune polyendocrine syndrome type I. J Clin Endocrinol Metab 1997;82:147–150.
215. Winqvist O, Gebre-Medhin G, Gustafsson J, Martin E, Lundkvist Ö, Karlsson FA, et al. Identification of the main gonadal autoantigens in patients with adrenal insufficiency and associated ovarian failure. J Clin Endocrinol Metab 1995;80:1717–1723.
216. Winqvist O, Söderbergh A, Kämpe O. The autoimmune basis of adrenocortical destruction in Addison's disease. Mol Med Today 1996;July:282–289.
217. Arif S, Vallian S, Farzaneh F, Zanone MM, James SL, Pietropaolo M, et al. Identification of 3β-hydroxysteroid dehydrogenase as a novel target of steroid cell autoantibodies: association of autoantibodies with endocrine autoimmune disease. J Clin Endocrinol Metab 1996;81:4439–4445.
218. Peterson P, Perheentupa J, Krohn KJE. Detection of candidal antigens in autoimmune polyglandular syndrome type I. Clin Diag Lab Immunol 1996;3:290–294.
219. Betterle C, Volpato M, Greggio AN, Presotto F. Type 2 polyglandular autoimmune disease (Schmidt's syndrome). J Pediat Endocrinol Metab 1996;9:113–123.
220. Weetman AP. Editorial review. Autoantigens in Addison's disease and associated syndromes. Clin Exp Immunol 1997;107:227–229.
221. Betterle C, Rossi A, Dalla Pria S, Artifoni A, Pedini B, Gavasso S, et al. Premature ovarian failure: autoimmunity and natural history. Clin Endocrinol 1993;39:35–43.
222. Wheatcroft NJ, Toogood AA, Li TC, Cooke ID, Weetman AP. Detection of antibodies to ovarian antigens in women with premature ovarian failure. Clin Exp Immunol 1994;96:122–128.
223. Wheatcroft N, Weetman A. Is premature ovarian failure an autoimmune disease? Autoimmunity 1997;25:157–165.
224. Anasti JN, Flack MR, Froehlich J, Nelson LM. The use of human recombinant gonadotropin receptors to search for immunoglobulin G-mediated premature ovarian failure. J Clin Endocrinol Metab 1995;80:824–828.
225. Lambert A, Weetman AP, McLoughlin J, Wardle C, Sunderland J, Wheatcroft N, et al. A search for immunoglobulins inhibiting gonadal cell steroidogenesis in premature ovarian failure. Hum Reprod 1996;11:1871–1876.
226. Roitt IM. Essential Immunology, 7th ed. Blackwell Scientific, Oxford, 1991, pp. 305–324.
227. Jacobson DL, Gange SJ, Rose NR, Graham NMH. Short analytical review—epidemiology and estimated population burden of selected autoimmune diseases in the United States. Clin Immunol Immunopathol 1997;84:223–243.

9 The Immunology of Human Autoimmune Thyroid Disease

Robert Volpé, MD, FRCP(C), FACP, FRCP

CONTENTS
>   INTRODUCTION
>   BRIEF OUTLINE OF IMMUNOGENETICS IN AITD
>   POSSIBLE AVENUES FOR PATHOGENESIS OF AITD
>   THE QUESTION OF THE INVOLVEMENT OF THE TARGET CELL,
>   THYROID ANTIGENS, AND MICROORGANISMS
>   IN THE PATHOGENESIS OF AITD
>   T LYMPHOCYTES IN AITD
>   CYTOKINES AND OTHER MOLECULES
>   B LYMPHOCYTES AND THYROID AUTOANTIBODIES IN AITD
>   REMISSIONS OF GD
>   IMMUNOLOGICAL ASPECTS OF THE THERAPY FOR GD
>   NATURAL COURSE OF AUTOIMMUNE THYROIDITIS
>   AND MODIFICATION WITH THERAPY
>   EXTRATHYROIDAL MANIFESTATIONS OF GD
>   REFERENCES

INTRODUCTION

The present chapter is devoted to a discussion of human autoimmune thyroid disease, but will draw on animal (primarily murine) evidence whenever appropriate. Moreover, one preceding chapter (Chapter 4) deals with experimental models, and still another chapter (Chapter 2) discusses immunoregulation in such models. The term autoimmune thyroid disease (or actually diseases) (AITD) includes several conditions with widely disparate clinical and laboratory expression *(1,2)*. However, there is a common thread linking their autoimmune etiology(ies), which unites them all under the above generic term, and this interelationship is reflected by the well-known progression from one disorder to another in some patients *(3)*. Moreover, in addition to those entities that may strictly fall under that heading, there are other thyroid conditions (e.g., subacute thyroiditis, nontoxic nodular goitre, and papillary thyroid carcinoma) that are not primary autoimmune diseases, but nevertheless may manifest (secondary) immunologic disturbances (see Table 1) *(1)*; these will be briefly discussed below.

From: *Contemporary Endocrinology: Autoimmune Endocrinopathies*
Edited by: R. Volpé © Humana Press Inc., Totowa, NJ

Table 1
Classification of Thyroid Diseases with Immunological Aspects[a]

AITDs
Autoimmune hyperthyroidism (GD, Parry's disease, Basedow's disease, Flagiani's disease)
Autoimmune thyroiditis
HT *(Struma lymphomatosa)*
Fibrous variant
Lymphocytic thyroiditis of childhood and adolescence
Postpartum thyroiditis
At least some cases of silent thyroiditis
Atrophic thyroiditis
Asymptomatic or minimal autoimmune thyroiditis
Nonimmune thyroid diseases with secondary immune responses
Subacute De Quervain's thyroiditis
Papillary carcinoma of thyroid
Nodular goiter

[a]Reprinted with permission from ref. *(1)*.

The first AITD, namely Graves' disease (GD) (Parry's disease, Basedow's disease, autoimmune hyperthyroidism) is defined as a form of hyperthyroidism associated with a diffuse hyperplastic goiter, resulting from the stimulation of the thyroid-stimulating hormone (TSH) receptor (TSHR) by a TSHR antibody, now known as thyroid-stimulating antibody (TSAb); associated extrathyroidal manifestations, such as exophthalmos (Graves' ophthalmopathy), are frequently noted, whereas pretibial myxoedema (Graves' dermopathy) and a form of clubbing of the fingers (thyroid acropachy) are uncommon accompaniments *(1)*. (The extrathyroidal manifestations of Graves' disease are discussed in Chapter 10). The second AITD, autoimmune thyroiditis, was initially described by Hashimoto *(4)* in 1912. He reported four women with goiters in whom the thyroid gland appeared to have been transformed into lymphoid tissue, *lymphomatosen veranderung*; the histological examination of the thyroid gland showed atrophy of parenchymal cells, diffuse lymphocytic infiltration, fibrosis, and an increase in oxyphilic (Hurthle) cells. These patients had been euthyroid until thyroidectomy, whereupon hypothyroidism supervened. Many decades later, thyroid autoantibodies were described in patients with this condition *(1)*, ultimately leading to the currently universally accepted view that the disorder is autoimmune in nature. Table 1 lists the variants of autoimmune thyroiditis (in addition to the "classic" Hashimoto's Thyroiditis [HT]). In the "chronic fibrous thyroiditis" variant, fibrosis predominates, and lymphocytic infiltration is less marked. In lymphocytic thyroiditis of childhood and adolescence, Hurthle cells, fibrosis, and germinal centres are less evident than in the adult form, and thyroid antibodies are often absent or present in lower titers. Postpartum thyroiditis is a transient condition occurring after pregnancy; it is frequently associated with a hyperthyroid phase followed by a hypothyroid phase, or a hypothyroid phase occurring *de novo*, and it usually resolves spontaneously, although perhaps incompletely, thereafter. It may however culminate in a chronic form. (*See* Chapter 11.) In silent (painless) thyroiditis (unrelated to pregnancy), as in postpartum thyroiditis, the thyroid gland is infiltrated with lymphocytes, but germinal centres and Hurthle cells are generally absent. This condition runs a course similar to postpartum thyroiditis, usually to recovery, but with frequent recurrences. In "idiopathic myxoedema" or atrophic thyroiditis, the thyroid is atrophied either from total destruction of thyroid parenchyma or from the presence of TSH-blocking antibodies. In minimal or occult thyroiditis, the degree of lymphocytic infiltration is less marked, with either no evidence of clinical thyroid dysfunction or with subclinical (compensated) hypothyroidism. There appear to be subtle genetic and/or pathogenetic differences between these variants; as mentioned above, however, they also share many similarities and thus deserve to be included under the generic term autoimmune thyroiditis *(1)*.

Autoimmune thyroiditis has been diagnosed much more frequently in the past two generations, when compared to earlier years. Dayan *(5)* has recently published a review of the prevalence of autoimmune thyroiditis; among adult women, approx 40% have some lymphocytic infiltration in their thyroid glands, and 10–15% have detectable thyroid autoantibodies. About 5–10% of women have raised TSH values, but obvious clinical hypothyroidism is observed in only 1% *(5)*. The prevalence increases with age, but about 45% of elderly females have some degree of thyroidal lymphocytic infiltration *(6,7)*. The apparent recent increase in prevalence may in part be owing to improved means of recognition and awareness, but may also be a result of an actual increased number of afflicted cases, probably owing to the increased iodine consumption that has characterized the Western world in the past 60 years *(1,2)*. About 1% of the population has or has had GD *(8)*. (Prevalence is dealt with in detail in Chapter 6). Males are much less commonly afflicted. Dayan *(5)* argues cogently that autoimmune thyroiditis is almost as "normal" as osteoporosis in women, and progresses actively at all stages, although at such a slow rate that only those who reach the higher level of the disease pyramid in early adulthood will develop clinical sequelae before the time that they die.

The overlap between GD and autoimmune thyroiditis has long been recognized. Indeed both disorders frequently aggregate in the same family. There are several reports of identical twins in which one has GD and the other has autoimmune thyroiditis. Indeed both conditions can coexist within the same thyroid gland; in such circumstances, the clinical expression will depend on which disease predominates *(1)*. Moreover, one condition can culminate in the other *(1,9–15)*. Nevertheless, GD and Hashimoto's disease cannot be considered merely opposite ends of a spectrum of the same disease, since there are genetic and pathogenetic differences between them, marking them as separate entities *(16)*.

As mentioned above, there are genetic, pathogenetic, serological, and clinical similarities and differences between the entities described above. The disturbance(s) in immunoregulation (*see* Chapters 1 and 2), which leads to AITD, is partly genetic *(16)* and partly environmental in nature *(1,2)*. AITD and those other autoimmune diseases with which AITD may be associated (e.g., insulin-dependent diabetes mellitus, pernicious anemia, vitiligo, myesthenia gravis, Addison's disease, and so forth) tend to aggregate in families, and more than one of these maladies may occur concomitantly within the same patient or her/his family *(1)*. The modes of inheritance do not follow simple genetic rules, and environmental factors, such as stress *(17,18)*, infection, trauma, drugs, smoking *(19)*, irradiation, nutrition (including iodine intake) *(2,20)*, pregnancy, and aging *(21)*, may distort the penetrance and expressivity of these conditions (by acting on the immune system) *(1)*. There is a strong female preponderance in most of these autoimmune diseases, including AITD *(1,2)*, which may partially relate to the influence of one gene on another *(22)*, but the predominant relationship is to hormonal factors *(23–26)*; these are discussed in a separate chapter (Chapter 7). The influence of the major histocompatibility complex (MHC) genes (in humans, termed the human leukocyte antigen [HLA] system) *(27)* and other genes is described in detail in Chapter 3, and will only be briefly discussed here in relation to AITD.

BRIEF OUTLINE OF IMMUNOGENETICS IN AITD

An increased frequency of HLA-DR3 in Caucasian patients with GD and atrophic thyroiditis is a well-known observation, but in goitrous HT, an increased frequency of HLA-DR5 has been reported *(27,28)*. Studies of restriction fragment-length polymorphisms (RFLP) of DR_β, DQ_α, DQ_β, and DP_α and DP_β in GD have shown a significant linkage disequilibrium between DR3 and DX_α, but this was considered representative of a generalized linkage disequilibrium between the two alleles and not specific for GD *(29)*. A study of RFLP among HLA-DR3 positive subjects with GD, disseminated lupus erythematosus, and normal persons showed no significant differences among the various groups *(30)*.

A further significantly increased frequency of HLA-DQA1*0501 has recently been observed among GD patients, even after exclusion of DR3-positive subjects *(31)*. These findings suggest that HLA-DQA1*0501 or a closely related unknown gene confers susceptibility for GD. However, the associations between HLA alleles and GD remain weak, suggesting only a minor role for HLA genes in susceptibility, and this is even more cogent for HT (*see* Chapter 3). First, there appear to be differences between various reports of HLA associations in HT. One such study showed an increased frequency of HLA-DR5, HLA-DR4, HLA-DR4/DR5 heterozygosity, DQw3 (DQw3.1 + 3.2 + 3.3), (DQw3.1), and DQA2 LL in HT as compared to controls *(32)*. Farid el al. *(33)* have shown an increased prevalence of HLA-DRw52 in 80% of patients with HT, as opposed to 54% in the control population. A study in the UK using RFLP and polymerase chain reaction (PCR)-based techniques showed an increased association of HT with HLA-DQB1*0201 (DQw2). It would appear from all of these studies that HLA-encoded genes confer only weak susceptibility to HT. Although it appears evident that genes other than MHC play roles in inducing AITD, studies of T-lymphocyte receptor genes and thyroperoxidase genes, at least, have failed to show such an association *(29,35)*. Specific susceptibility genes for GD have been recently identified on chromosome 14, in the region of 14q24.3-31 *(36)*. The CTLA-4 gene, which is in linkage disequilibrium with the CD28 gene, is associated with both GD and HT *(37,38)*. In Japanese patients additionally, it would appear that the 180-bp allele of the TSH recepror microsatellite is also associated with a susceptibility locus for AITD *(39)*. Tomer et al. *(40)* have recently reviewed this topic. Other candidate genes are discussed in Chapter 3.

It is nevertheless difficult to escape the conclusion that the HLA system (which is essential for antigen processing and presentation) does constitute a factor in the pathogenesis of these disorders. The presentation of antigen by these HLA class I and class II genes is central to the development of these conditions (including the disturbance in target cell function) initiating a complex interplay among the antigen(s) on and from the target cells, the antigen-presenting cells (APCs), the CD4 helper/inducer T lymphocytes, T-effector cells, and CD8 suppressor (regulatory)/cytotoxic T lymphocytes. The production by these then activated T lymphocytes of interferon γ (IFN-γ), as well as certain cytokine patterns (i.e., T_H1 and T_H2 cells), the importance of certain adjunctive molecules (e.g., intercellular adhesion molecules [ICAM] *[41]*, heat-shock proteins [hsp] *[42,43]*, CD40 *[44]*, Ctla4 *[45]*, and so forth, are all important in coordinating the immune response), B lymphocytes, and antibodies. This complex interaction makes it likely that several genetic loci are involved in the development of AITD, each making an indepen-

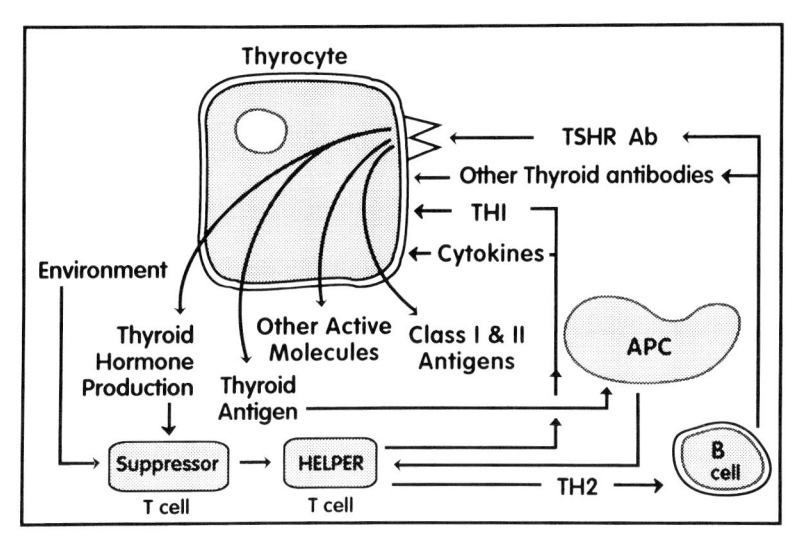

Fig. 1. The pathogenesis of AITD. The author's hypothesis for the pathogenesis of AITD is depicted schematically. The thyrocyte is considered initially normal, but becomes a victim to immunological events. AITD is considered a genetically induced disturbance in specific antigen presentation (by APCs), such that regulatory (suppressor) T lymphocytes are not adequately activated. This genetic abnormality is further amplified by environmental factors (e.g., stress, infection, drugs, smoking, aging) acting on the immune system, which appear necessary to reduce immunoregulation further, in order to worsen the immune dysfunction. There is consequent increased helper T-lymphocyte response, with T_H1 activity causing direct thyrocyte damage (via cytokines), whereas T_H2 activity predisposes to thyroid autoantibody production. Thyrotrophin-receptor antibodies (TSHRAb) include TSAb, which is the proximate cause of GD, and which in turn stimulates the thyrocyte to produce increased amounts of thyroid hormones and thyroid antigens, and also enhances cytokine-induced thyrocyte class I and II antigen expression, and the expression of "other molecules," e.g., ICAM-1, CTLA-4, hsps, prostaglandin E1, and so forth, all of which interact with the immune system.

dent, but interdependent, variable contribution (3). Several candidate genes are being considered for appropriate roles. The production of various elements as mentioned above by the immune system will then provoke the target cell to express molecules of various types, including HLA class I (46,47) and class II antigens (46), ICAM-1, hsp, various cytokines, and autoantigens, which will further modify the immune response (1,2) (see Fig. 1). Hormonal and environmental factors further modify the immune response, as previously mentioned. Although there is a wealth of literature on the immune response, controversy still abounds about the autoimmune process, the role of the target cell and the antigen(s), the importance of antigen presentation (is it abnormal?), and the frequently proposed posssible involvement of microorganisms in these events (48,49).

POSSIBLE AVENUES FOR PATHOGENESIS OF AITD

Theoretical possibilities that would account for the development of organ-specific or antigen-specific autoimmune disease would include

1. An antigenic stimulus (however initiated, including molecular mimicry) precipitating and/or sustaining the disorder—either involving actual infection of the target cells or involving nonthyroidal infections with microorganisms with "superantigens" or with antigens displaying homology(ies) with target cell antigens (48).

2. A precipitating antigenic stimulus, but in a person with an additional underlying immune abnormality.
3. Abnormal antigen-specific induction of subsets of T lymphocytes because of abnormal antigen-presenting gene(s), resulting in an operational disorder within the T lymphocytes (the primary defect would then be in the APCs, e.g., macrophages, dendritic cells) *(50)*; this would relate to abnormalities in HLA-related and other genes (*see* Chapter 3).
4. Mutation of appropriate T or B lymphocytes to form abnormal clone(s) of lymphocyte interactive with a particular target organ—these would be autonomous and not subject to normal immunoregulation.
5. A specific, but partial, inherent defect in immunoregulation, probably owing to reduced specific induction (by specific antigen) of regulatory (suppressor) T lymphocytes resulting from an abnormality of antigen presenting gene(s) in APCs. In the latter hypothesis, favored by the author *(1,51)*, all that would be additionally necessary to precipitate the particular disease would be:
    a. The presence of the antigen without any need for it to be abnormal in quantity or quality.
    b. The availability of the antigen via an APC, e.g., the macrophage and/or dendritic cell.
    c. The appearance and availability of target cell-directed helper T and B lymphocytes with the necessity of a second, costimulatory signal for CD4$^+$ cell activation derived from a set of receptor-ligand interactions *(52)* (in addition to the first signal of MHC class II molecule plus antigenic epitope delivered to the T-cell receptor), and additional perturbations of the immune system from such environmental stresses as have already been mentioned, which would be superimposed, and thus additive, on the partial antigen-specific abnormality.

There is new evidence against the notion that the thyroid cell can directly present its antigens to T lymphocytes via thyrocyte MHC expression (at least at the initiation of the autoimmune process) *(46)*, although this point is controversial, and this will be considered below. Further elaboration of the available evidence follows.

THE QUESTION OF THE INVOLVEMENT OF THE TARGET CELL, THYROID ANTIGENS, AND MICROORGANISMS IN THE PATHOGENESIS OF AITD

Over several years, we have argued (and continue to do so) that there is no significant intrinsic abnormality in the thyrocyte, or in the thyroid autoantigens, which would be a requirement for the initiation of AITD *(51)*. Many other investigators hold differing views. For example, Wilkin *(53,54)* suggests that autoimmunity could be considered a physiological response of a normal immune system to autoantigen released in an inflammatory response to virus infection or another antigen expressed in the target tissue. A viral or microbial antigen with homology to an autoantigen (molecular mimicry) might initiate production of autoantibodies that crossreact with the autoantigen, with a subsequent immune response reacting with the corresponding autologous cell structures. Tomer and Davies *(48)* described several potential avenues whereby infection might induce AITD, but provided no evidence that would make a convincing case for any of them (*see* following sections for further discussion). Despite this lack of evidence, the same group *(55)* proposed that AITD is "probably induced by an external insult, such as an infection, with consequent thyrocyte HLA-DR expression leading to the development of AITD." Wick et al. *(56)* and Rose et al. *(57)* have further shown evidence in the obese strain (OS) chicken that there is a genetic abnormality of the thyroid cell, which, they argue, is a *sine qua non* for the development of AITD, although these investigators recognize the additional requirement of an abnormality of the immune system. The author has argued elsewhere against these proposals regarding thyrocyte or thyroid antigenic abnormalities *(51)*, or a role for microbial initiation (at least as related to human AITD), and will briefly repeat these objections below. Indeed, there is evidence that thyrocyte class I and class II expression, far from participating in the early phases of the pathogenesis (as suggested by Kohn et al. *[58]* and Bottazzo et al. *[59]*), are secondary phenomena resulting in anergy instead, i.e., is protective *(46,60,61)*, at least in the initial phase of the disease. This will be discussed further below.

Possible Involvement of Viruses in the Pathogenesis of AITD

The most obvious example of what appears (almost certainly) to be a viral infection of the thyroid gland is Subacute De Quervain's thyroiditis. The clinical and laboratory features of this entity have been thoroughly described elsewhere *(1,62)*. There are many descriptions of the immunological and serological phenomena that appear during the course of this illness, only to disappear gradually as the inflammatory lesions subside; these include the appearance of thyroid autoantibodies (including TSHR antibodies) and thyrocyte HLA-DR expression in at least a minority of patients *(1,51)*. However, AITD only rarely follows. Thus, two points should be made from these observations. First, the lymphocytes in normal persons have the genes and capacity to produce thyroid autoantibodies, including TSHR antibodies (also including TSAb) in response to the increased release of thyroid antigen from the inflamed and damaged thyroid cells. Second, this excess antigenic release into the immune system will not itself lead to AITD. For that to occur, an abnormality of the immune system is required (and it will be argued later that no abnormality of the target cell or the amount or nature of the autoantigen is then necessary).

Bottazzo et al. *(59)* first reported "aberrant" expression of class II antigen (HLA-DR) on the AITD thyrocyte cell surfaces, which they subsequently proposed *(63)* to be owing to viruses that stimulated intrathyroidal T lymphocytes to produce IFN-γ; this in turn would induce thyrocytes to express HLA-DR, thus be able to present antigen directly, and, hence, induce AITD. (We will argue below that the ability of the thyrocyte to present antigen is very limited, and that there is dissociation between thyrocyte HLA-DR expression, and the ability to induce thyroid autoantibody production.) Indeed transfection of thyroid cells in culture by viral vectors has been reported to induce weak thyrocyte HLA-DR expression, although not at the magnitude observed in AITD *(64,65)*. Moreover, Ciampiolillo et al. *(66)* had demonstrated the presence of HIV *gag* sequences by Southern blot analysis in the thyroid glands of GD, but not normal glands or thyroid neoplasms. Wick et al. *(67,68)* have reported that antibodies against the *gag* 2 protein of the human foamy virus binds to GD thyroids, as well as to retrobulbar fibroblasts from Graves' ophthalmopathy. Lagaye et al. *(69,70)* have reported the presence of HTLV-1 *gag*-related sequences in leukocyte DNA from patients with Graves' disease and insulin-dependent diabetes mellitus (IDDM), and humane spumaretrovirus-related sequences in leukocyte DNA from patients with Graves' disease. Jaspan et al. *(71)* have described the presence of antibodies to a human intracisternal type A retrovirus in over 85% of patients with Graves' disease, and have suggested that a viral particle might be an important, even essential, ingredient in the pathogenesis of this disorder. It has also been suggested that hepatitis C might precipitate AITD *(72)*; a high frequency of thyroid antibodies have been found in patients with that condition *(73)*.

However there is much evidence against the theory that viruses induce AITD. First, BB rats (named from Biobreeding Laboratories) raised in a cesarean-induced germ-free (gnotobiotic) environment still develop insulin-dependent diabetes (and AITD) despite being free of viruses *(74)*. Second, the presence of HIV *gag* sequences in the thyroid glands could not be confirmed by two other groups *(75,76)*. Third, the presence of foamy virus (spumaretrovirus, HSRV) sequences could not be demonstrated in three other centers in GD thyroid tissues or peripheral blood leukocytes in frequencies greater than normal control subjects *(77–80)*. In relation to hepatitis C, Metcalfe et al. *(81)* failed to confirm any association between that condition and AITD. Finally, in relation to the finding of Jaspan et al. *(71)* of antibodies against a human intracisternal type A retrovirus, those authors failed to take into account the possibility that the viral particle might have crossreactivity with a thyrocyte membrane antigen, such as the TSHR, and the antiviral antibodies so reported may actually only reflect the latter. Mowat *(82)* has pointed out that virus infections stimulate IFN-α and β production, whereas IFN-γ can be produced only by mitogenic or antigenic stimulation of primed lymphocytes. Moreover, if AITD thyrocyte HLA-DR expression was a result of virus infection of the thyroid cells, it would not be expected that thyrocyte HLA-DR would quickly disappear from those cells in tissue culture *(83)* or after xenografting of AITD tissue into nude mice *(84,85)*, as indeed it does.

Evidence is now overwhelming that thyrocyte HLA-DR expression is not a primary inductive phenomenon in AITD, but is a secondary process, i.e., secondary to the production of IFN-γ by activated intrathyroidal helper T lymphocytes sensitized to thyroid antigen *(1,2)*. Iwatani et al. *(86)* have shown that the expression of HLA-DR antigen on thyroid cells in culture depends on the presence of not only helper T cells, but also on monocytes. If either of these two types of cells are removed from the preparation, thyrocyte HLA-DR expression is prevented *(86)*. Moreover, there is nothing unique about the response of the AITD thyroid cells to IFN-γ or other cytokines (e.g., tumor necrosis factor α, TNF-α), since normal thyroid tissue responds at least as well as or better than AITD thyroid tissue when treated with these agents, both in terms of HLA-DR expression and ICAM-1 expression *(87,88)*. The expression of these molecules on the thyrocytes depends entirely on the local cytokine environment, which in turn is dependent on the local immunocyte infiltration, and hence is a secondary phenomenon *(1,2)*. The role of thyrocyte HLA-DR expression on thyroid antigen presentation will be discussed below. It might be added that the immune response as observed in papillary carcinoma of the thyroid (partly constitutive) differs markedly from that of AITD *(89)*, and it is possible that similar mechanisms might underlie the immune response in nontoxic nodular goiter.

Involvement of Bacterial Infection in the Pathogenesis of AITD?

As mentioned above, it has been suggested that microorganisms, including those of bacterial origin, may play a role in the induction of AITD *(90,91)*. Although several organisms have been suggested, the greatest focus has been on *Yersinia enterocolitica* (Y.e.) *(90)*. Indeed, evidence of crossreactivity between antigens from these microorganisms and thyroid cell membrane antigens (including TSHR) has been reported *(92,93)*, although two groups (including our own) have recently failed to confirm this *(94,95)*. If there is indeed crossreactivity between bacterial and thyroid antigens (molecular mimicry), this should certainly not automatically lead to the conclusion that such homology plays any role in the induction of AITD; in fact, the evidence suggests otherwise. For example, in a study of patients with active Y.e. infections, there were frequently TSHR antibodies (some with thyroid-stimulating properties), yet there were no examples of thyroid dysfunction *(96)*. Furthermore, although immunization of experimental animals with Y.e. led to the development of TSHR antibodies in the animals, the thyroid histology remained normal *(97)*. Thus, unusual or excessive antigen presentation, even if the antigen has homology with human thyroid antigens, does not appear to be sufficient to induce AITD. The situation seems analogous to that of subacute thyroiditis, where there is a transient, appropriate response (of a normal immune system) to the liberation of antigen, but AITD does not follow *(51)*. Thus, once again, AITD depends upon an abnormal immune system.

Is an Intrinsic Abnormality of the Thyrocyte Necessary to Induce AITD?

Several investigators who have studied the obese strain (OS) chicken model of spontaneous hereditary AITD have stressed the similarities to human AITD *(55,56,98,99)*. However, these workers have found a genetic abnormality of the OS chicken thyroid cell, which, it is claimed, is an important ingredient in the development of AITD in that strain *(55,56)*. This is manifested by thyroid autonomy, an increased thyroidal uptake of iodide, and increased thyrocyte expression of HLA-DR in response to IFN-γ. (Thyroiditis-susceptible rats also show an increased thyrocyte expression of HLA-DR in response to IFN-γ *[100]*). These authors have analogized that these observations ought to be applicable to the human condition.

However, the evidence points in the opposite direction, since no such abnormalities can be demonstrated in humans with AITD. Both in patients in remission after antithyroid drug treatment for GD and in AITD xenografts in nude mice, the thyroid cells can be demonstrated to be functioning normally, under normal physiological control, and with normal suppressibility with exogenous thyroid hormone *(1,78,101)*. Moreover, human AITD thyroid cells in tissue culture *(75)* or in vivo in nude mouse xenografts do not respond in an excessive manner to IFN-γ either alone or in combination with TNF-α, in terms of HLA-DR expression *(87,88)*. One can only conclude that the human AITD thyroid cells are intrinsically normal with no evidence of a genetic thyrocyte abnormality.

Are Thyroid Autoantigens Abnormal?

There is no convincing evidence that there are alterations of the thyroid autoantigens that are of immunological significance *(102,103)*. However it must be mentioned that Cuddihy et al. *(104)* and Bohr et al. *(105)* have reported that there is an increase in the number of mutations at codon 52 in the extracellular domain of the TSHR (which changes threonine to proline) on the thyroid cells in GD, such that about 18% of GD patients manifest this finding. However, about 12% of normal persons show the same alteration, thus marking it as a simple polymorphism of no immunogenic significance, very unlikely to be involved in the etiology of GD. Perhaps the increase in this polymorphism in GD may be owing to prolonged stimulation of the TSHR by TSAb. In any event, Watson et al. *(106)* could not confirm this association.

Recently, an interesting report has appeared describing the induction of Graves'-like disease in mice by immunization with fibroblasts transfected with the human thyrotropin receptor and a class II molecule *(107)*. The authors interpreted the findings to suggest that class II molecules on target cells expressing the TSHR can induce anti-TSHR antibodies capable of stimulating the thyroid. However, whether thyroid cells, rather than fibroblasts, can act as APCs in the presence of class I and II expression is a moot point, as will be discussed below.

AITD appears to be primarily a disorder of immunoregulation, with the organ dysfunction resulting from an antigen-specific attack mounted by inadequately suppressed (and thus activated) lymphocytes directed toward antigen(s) on specific cellular targets, i.e., thyrocytes, with production of various cytokines (e.g., IFN-γ) acting on the target cell at close range *(1)*. Certainly the antigen must be available and presented to the T lymphocytes (*see* next section) for this activation and assault to occur. There is now evidence that TSHR circulates normally in solubilized form *(108–112)*, and thyroperoxidase (TPO) and thyroglobulin (Tg) are equally available to the immune system. As mentioned, although there is no evidence of any significant abnormalities of these antigens that would result in AITD, nevertheless, the epitopes of these antigens that are operative in a given individual appear to vary widely. The presentation of antigen requires expression of class I and class II (HLA-D) antigens on the APCs; these include monocytes, macrophages, and dendritic cells *(2)*. The thyrocytes also express class I and class II antigens; whether this permits the thyroid cell actually to present antigen will be the subject of the following discussion. It is certainly evident that thyrocyte expression of HLA-DR results from cooperation of local APCs, and infiltrating sensitized and activated CD4 T lymphocytes in producing the IFN-γ, which in turn induces class I and II antigen on the thyroid cells *(46,61,86,113)*.

This is a secondary event, occurring after the initiation of the immune assault *(1,2)*. (It had been suggested that the thyroid cell could be damaged by some external stimulus *[48,55]*, e.g., infection, and then express class I and class II antigens as a consequence *[58]*, thus precipitating AITD, but this notion does not withstand close scrutiny *[51]*.) Rather, the evidence is consistent with the idea that the thyroid cell is initially normal, and expresses molecules, such as class I and II, ICAM-1, and hsp as consequences of the immune disturbance *(46,61,112)*. Kawai et al. *(61)* and Yue et al. *(46)* have shown evidence that both class I and class II expression by thyrocytes in AITD results from cytokine stimulation by infiltrating lymphocytes; removal of those lymphocytes results in diminution of the thyrocyte class I and class II expression. Moreover, IFN-γ, which does stimulate thyrocyte class I and II expression, does not significantly increase thyroid autoantibody production. Indeed IFN-γ will even increase thyrocyte class I and II expression in normal thyroid tissue, but no thyroid antibody production results *(46,61)*. Thus, there is complete dissociation between the expression of thyrocyte class I and II vs thyroid autoantibody production, allowing the conclusion that such expression does not contribute to the pathogenesis of AITD. This evidence is thus not consistent with the hypothesis advanced by Kohn's group *(58)*.

As discussed above, the notion that the primary event might be infective is entirely speculative; on the contrary, the author would argue that the thyroid cell is a passive captive to immunological events, and was initially and intrinsically normal *(51)*. As mentioned above, AITD thyroid tissue xenografted into nude mice reverts functionally, immunologically, and histologically to normal as a result of removing the immune environment *(84,85,87,88)*. Evidence will be presented below supporting the postulate that AITD represents a disorder in immunoregulation, resulting from a partial defect in antigen-specific immunosuppression combined with nonspecific environmental factors, which also play on the immune system *(1,51)*. (*See* Fig. l.)

T LYMPHOCYTES IN AITD

Since the early 1970s, it has been clear that T lymphocytes play a central role in the development of GD and autoimmune thyroiditis *(114)*. Ahmann and Burman *(115)* and Bagnasco and Pesce *(15)* have summarized the roles that these cells play in these disorders. Indeed, removal of or inhibiting T lymphocytes from the autoimmune lesion will ameliorate the pathological and serological abnormalities *(116,117)*. Many reports attest to the sensitization of (primarily CD4) AITD T lymphocytes to intact thyroid cells or specific thyroid antigens, such as Tg, TPO, or *(118–123)*. Current studies have focused on determining which epitope(s) of these antigenic molecules is the particular binding and active site(s) for the thyroid-specific T cells as well as, or perhaps differing from, that for the thyroid autoantibodies. The evidence thus far indicates that these epitopes vary from patient to patient *(2,122,123)*, presumably owing to antigenic spreading.

There has also been interest in the possibility that only one, or at most a few T-cell clones may be involved at the outset of AITD, as shown by the restricted usage of T-cell receptor (TCR) V genes by autoreactive T lymphocytes. In this regard, Davies et al. *(124,125)* have reported limited variability of TCR Vα and Vβ genes in hyperthyroid GD intrathyroidal T cells, and similar but less marked results for TCR Vα genes for autoimmune thyroiditis. This finding might be considered surprising given the proclivity of an autoimmune lesion to recruit an expanded population of nonspecific T-lymphocyte clones into the affected tissue over time, coupled with the difficulty in attempting to study AITD within just a few days after onset *(126)*. In this context, McIntosh et al. *(127)* have failed to confirm the findings of Davies et al. *(124,125)*. However, McIntosh et al. *(128)* have shown evidence for restricted accumulation of CD8$^+$ T cells in HT (in the absence of CD4$^+$ T-cell restriction).

Studies of the numbers and function of peripheral blood T cells in AITD have been divided into those relating to CD4 and to CD8 cells, since their functions and responses are quite different, and often contrary *(120)*. In earlier years, CD4$^+$ cells were considered helper/inducer cells, whereas CD8$^+$ cells were considered suppressor/cytotoxic cells. However, the phenotypes do not, after all, relate directly to function. Although therefore under different circumstances the phenotype of suppressor (regulatory) T cells may vary, nevertheless in humans, CD8 cells can be clearly shown to contain suppressor activity *(116)*. Moreover, CD8 + CD11b+ cells have suppressor activity, and a few NK cells, but no cytotoxic activity *(129,130)*. They may therefore be characterized as suppressor (regulatory) T lymphocytes; fortunately, studies of suppressor function and the activation of the latter cells in vitro parallel results using CD8$^+$ cells, and thus, CD8$^+$ cells may be employed in experiments as "suppressor" T cells under appropriate circumstances *(131)*. Studies of "suppressor" T cells have been of two quite different types, namely, those of generalized (nonspecific) suppressor T cells and, conversely, observations of antigen-specific suppressor T-cell function *(1)*.

Although clonal deletion in the thymus of autoreactive T lymphocytes plays an important role in the development of tolerance to self-antigens, many autoreactive T lymphocytes reach the periphery where they remain unresponsive to the self-antigen *(132)*. Both "anergy" and active suppression have been postulated to fulfill this role. Anergic T lymphocytes can certainly be identified in the periphery, but this cannot account for the observation that adoptive transfer of T lymphocytes from mice tolerant to a given antigen reduces the immune response to that same antigen in syngeneic recipients *(133)*. The best explanation for this observation is that T lymphocytes exist that can suppress immune responses.

The previous scepticism regarding the nature or even existence of suppressor (regulatory) T lymphocytes has now been largely laid to rest *(134)*. There is increasing evidence favoring a role for these cells in preventing autoimmune diseases, and for a deficient function of these same cells in causing these disorders, as recently reviewed *(134–137)*. Indeed, there is evidence that in normal animals, T lymphocytes exist, which prevent thyroid autoimmunity *(136,137)*. Although the final molecular pathway for such suppression may be via cytokines (e.g., T_H2 cells) *(138)*, the important point is the cellular source and stimulus of such cytokine production. (T_H2 cells secrete IL-4, IL-5, and IL-10, and thus inhibit autoimmune processes.)

Several reports have described a reduction in the number, activation, and function of nonspecific suppressor T lymphocytes during the hyperthyroid phase of GD, tending to normalize as thyroid function improves *(139–141)*. Thus, in one study, after 1 yr following ^{131}I therapy, suppressor cell numbers had returned to normal, even when TSAb was still strongly positive *(140)*. The values also return to normal with antithyroid drug therapy *(139)*. With some exceptions, results usually are normal in euthyroid autoimmune thyroiditis *(139–141)*. One report also showed a reduction in nonspecific suppressor T cells in toxic nodular goiter (a nonimmune form of hyperthyroidism), but less marked than in GD *(142)*, suggesting that hyperthyroidism has to be severe and perhaps prolonged to have such an effect. Indeed, an inverse correlation has been observed between the number of nonspecific suppressor T cells and the serum triiodothyronine concentrations *(140)*. Thus, the reduction in nonspecific suppressor T lymphocytes does not seem to be a primary or specific event, and appears to be secondary to the hyperthyroidism itself; however, by its additive effect (superimposed on the antigen-specific defect in suppressor T-cell function, specific and fundamental for AITD—*see* next paragraph), it may act to perpetuate and amplify the disease. Moreover, environmental factors, such as stress *(17,18,143–158)*, infection, trauma, drugs *(159,160)*, smoking *(19)*, nutrition *(2)* and aging *(21,161)*, may have similar adverse effects on nonspecific suppressor T-lymphocyte function and, thus, precipitate the disorder by a similar additive effect. There is considerable literature regarding the effect of various physical and emotional stresses on the immune system in general and on GD specifically *(17,18, 143–158,161)*. Many articles attest to an increased frequency of stresses prior to onset of GD *(143–158)*. However, Gray and Hoffenberg *(162)* were unable to document any such increase; this actually should not be surprising, since patients susceptible to GD may not require any unusual additive stress; "ordinary" stresses superimposed on an already abnormal immune system might suffice to disturb immunoregulation.

These effects on nonspecific suppressor T-lymphocyte function must be considered quite separately from results of studies on antigen-specific suppressor T-cell function, although as mentioned, there can be an additive action exerted by these two types of cells. First, the idea that there could be an antigen-specific disturbance in suppressor T lymphocytes seems more rational than that of a generalized abnormality in suppressor T-cell function; the latter would result in multiple clinical disorders of immunoregulation and, thus, would not be in accord with genetic observations in which relatives of the AITD propositi also usually have only AITD, rather than other autoimmune disorders *(16)*. There are now several studies indicating the presence of an organ-specific defect in suppressor T-lymphocyte function in AITD, in which the observations do not relate to the thyroid function of the patient (i.e., whether the patient is hyperthyroid, hypothyroid, or euthyroid) (summarized in *134,135*). More recently, it has been demonstrated that thyroid-specific antigens (Tg and TPO) activate AITD CD8$^+$ (or CD8 + CD11b+ "pure" suppressor) cells significantly less than similar cells from normal donors; the AITD CD8$^+$ (or CD8 + CD11b+) cells also responded less to the thyroid-specific antigens when compared to irrelevant antigens, whereas normal and AITD cells reacted equally to the irrelevant antigens *(131)*. Moreover, TSHR antigen will not activate GD CD8$^+$ T lymphocytes as well as control CD8$^+$ cells (from normal persons, HT, nontoxic goiter, and IDDM *[163]*). Conversely, glutamic acid decarboxylase (GAD-65), the putative autoantigen of the pancreatic islet β cells involved in IDDM, will not activate IDDM CD8$^+$ cells as much as GD or normal CD8$^+$ cells *(163)*. In animal models, there is also increasing evidence for an antigen-specific suppressor T-lymphocyte abnormality in AITD in several studies (summarized in *134,135*). The antigen specific suppressor T-lymphocyte disturbance (which is partial or relative) may well be owing to a defect in specific antigen presentation (presumably because of a disturbance in antigen-presenting gene[s]), resulting in reduced specific suppressor cell activation. Since there is no convincing evidence for any alteration of the antigen(s), AITD appears to be primarily a disorder of immunoregulation, with the organ dysfunction resulting from an antigen-specific attack mounted by inadequately suppressed (and thus activated) T_H1 and T_H2 (*see* next paragraph) lymphocytes directed against their specific antigen(s) on the target cells (Fig. 1). This immune attack additionally depends on many other complex elements, including the environmental factors mentioned earlier, the availability of the antigen(s) via the APCs, the nature of the APCs and antigen processing and presenting genes, the production of various cytokines and their action on the target cells and the immune system, and the role of various immune-reactive molecules produced by the immune and target cells following the initiation of the immune assault. Some of these aspects will be discussed below.

CYTOKINES AND OTHER MOLECULES

It is apparent that the immunological disturbance is based on the presentation of antigen by APCs (e.g., monocytes, macrophages, dendritic cells, and possibly, thyrocytes *[see below]*) and the response of T and B lymphocytes. These cellular interactions depend on a variety of participitating molecules (e.g., CD40 *[44]*, Ctla4 *[45]*) that facilitate the response. In addition, the production of various cytokines by elements of the immune system in a coordinated fashion and at close range to the target cell constitutes essential ingredients in completing the pathophysiological picture. Helper T lymphocytes are divisible into T_H1 and T_H2 subsets depending on their pattern of cytokine production; T_H1 cells release IFN-γ, TNF-α, and interleukin 2 (IL-2), and are inflammatory in effect, whereas T_H2 cells "help" B lymphocytes by primarily producing IL-4, IL-5, and IL-6 *(2)*. Although these cytokines have certain effects on the thyroid cells (*see* next paragraph), they do not seem to have much influence on thyroid function in vitro *(164)*, although they do interfere with TSH stimulation *(165,166)*.

IL-1 is considered to be a costimulatory molecule, is released by APCs after interaction with T lymphocytes, and is necessary for the activation of resting T cells *(132,133)*.

IFN-γ is released by CD4+ cells in response to antigen *(118,119)* (and mitogen) *(86)*, is the major stimulus for thyrocyte HLA-DR and ICAM-1 expression, which thus occurs secondarily result of the initiation of the immune assault *(16,168)* (despite the arguments of some that these are primary pathogenetic events) *(48,53–55,59,63)*. (These molecules disappear from thyrocytes when the immune environment is removed either in tissue culture or in nude mice, and can be restored by addition of appropriate cytokines *[87,88,168]*.) The significance of adhesion molecules in AITD has been extensively discussed by Bagnasco and Pesce *(15)*; readers are referred to that excellent article. It has also been thought that thyrocyte HLA-DR expression resulted in an ability of the thyroid cells to function as APCs and thus express antigen; however, this may not be correct. Earlier contrary evidence may have been the result of the contamination of even a few macrophages in the thyroid cell preparations *(169)*. Indeed, it is possible that thyrocyte HLA-DR expression may exert a protective effect, as we had suggested a few years ago *(170)*, and which has been recently reiterated and amplified by Weetman *(171)*. Tandon et al. *(172)* and Teng et al. *(173)* have shown that thyroid cells do not express B7-1 or B7-2, even after stimulation with IFN-γ and other cytokines. B7-1 and B7-2 are the most well-characterized costimulators, and bind to CD28 or CTLA-4 receptors on the T lymphocytes. Failure to provide this second signal results in T-cell anergy, rather than stimulation *(174)*. Indeed, as mentioned above, our own recent data indicate a dissociation between thyrocyte class I and class II expression vs the production of thyroid antibodies; in particular, an IFN-γ-induced rise in thyrocyte class I and II expression is not accompanied by a significant increase in thyroid autoantibody production *(46,61)*. However, the expression of thyrocyte class II expression may be double-edged under different circumstances; it may prevent the local initiation of an autoimmune process, but if the response is already established by conventional APCs, thyrocyte class II expression might then help to activate the T cells by cooperation with infiltrating professional APCs *(3,15,20,175)*. The effect of TNF-α, a macrophage product, may enhance the action of IFN-γ *(89)*. It is, however, questionable whether any additional antigen-presenting capacity supplied by thyroid cells would have much impact on the evolution of AITD, particularly since the stimulation of T lymphocytes produced by thyroid cells in those experiments in which it has been observed seems to be relatively weak *(3,20)*.

Various other molecules are important in the development of AITD. These include lymphocyte function-associated antigens (LFA-1, LFA-2, LFA-3), which act as accessory molecules increasing the binding of T cells to APCs *(15,176)*. The expression of ICAM-1 by thyroid cells, which does not occur normally, is obvious in AITD, interacting with LFA-1 and, thus, enhancing lymphocyte activation *(15,177–179)*. As mentioned above, the appearance of thyrocyte ICAM-1 in AITD is clearly a secondary event *(168)*. The same comments could be made for thyrocyte hsp-72, which is also expressed in AITD, but not in normal thyroid cells. It likewise disappears in AITD thyroid xenografts in the nude mouse, marking it as a secondary phenomenon. Such expression may have some immunomodulatory effects in increasing binding of immunoglobulin *(180)*. Thyroid cells can produce some other immunologically active molecules as a result of cytokine stimulation or complement attack; these include prostaglandin-E2, IL-6, and IL-8, thus, further increasing thyrocyte-immunocyte "signaling" *(181)*.

At this time, the precise roles and nature of the participation of cytokines are yet to be completely illuminated; although the subject of intense study, much remains to be learned.

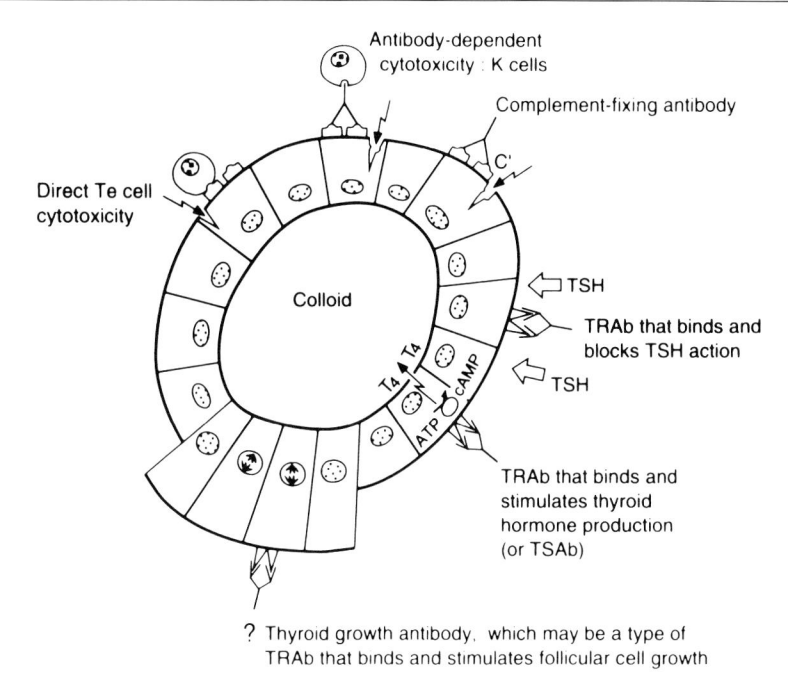

Fig. 2. Composite diagram of a thyroid follicle showing possible immune effector mechanisms in AITD. Cytotoxic mechanisms include direct cytotoxicity by sensitized effector T_H1 (Te) cells, antibody-dependent cytotoxicity by killer (K) cells armed with thyroid autoantibody, and cell lysis by complement-fixing thyroid autoantibody. The various types of TSHR antibodies (TRAb) have different mechanisms of action. One type binds to TSHR and blocks TSH from binding and stimulating the receptor. Another type, TSAb binds to and stimulates the receptor, resulting in excess thyroid hormone production. Thyroid growth-promoting and inhibiting antibodies have been demonstrated by some workers, but are still controversial. Reproduced with permission from ref. *(182a)*.

B LYMPHOCYTES AND THYROID AUTOANTIBODIES IN AITD

Once activated, self-reactive CD4+ helper T lymphocytes can induce autoreactive B lymphocytes to be recruited into the thyroid gland where they interact with target thyroid autoantigen(s), and, as a consequence, produce thyroid autoantibodies. The three most important autoantigens include the TSHR, TPO, and Tg. The nature of the B-lymphocyte responses and the mechanisms involved have been detailed by Weetman *(60)*. Of particular interest, the B lymphocytes recruited into the thyroid are not antigen-specific; their apparent antigen specificity results from delivery of cytokines by antigen-specific T cells interacting with B cells and class II MHC molecules locally at the site of the thyrocytes.

The various antibodies that may be found in AITD and their possible functions are depicted in Fig. 2. TSAb has received the most attention because it acts to stimulate thyroid cells, resulting in hyperthyroidism; it is an antibody directed against epitope(s) on the extracellular domain of the TSHR and is an agonist of TSH; functionally, it stimulates the thyroid cells for several hours compared to the short duration of TSH stimulation *(1)*. The original test for long-acting thyroid stimulator (LATS) was an in vivo guinea pig and later mouse bioassay.

Table 2
Thyroid Stimulating Antibody (TSAb)

Antibody to TSHR that stimulates receptor (and thyrocyte) in a manner indistinguishable from TSH, but with a much longer duration
Positive in approx 95% of patients with GD
Also positive in some cases of silent and subacute thyroiditis, and following acute *Yersiniosis* (crossreactivitity)
Declines in third trimester of pregnancy, and rebounds thereafter
If still high in late pregnancy, may produce fetal and neonatal GD
Rises further after ^{131}I therapy for GD for several months
Usually (not invariably) declines with antithyroid drug (ATD) therapy
If positive after ATD course, relapse of GD almost invariable
Positive test helps to diagnose euthyroid exophthalmos

Of course, it is now obvious that LATS was actually TSAb and is an antibody to the TSHR; in addition, other antibodies to the TSHR have also been described *(1)*. Since some of these antibodies are not stimulatory, the term TSAb should be employed to refer only to those antibodies that stimulate increased cAMP in thyroid cells. The radioligand assay that measures the binding of IgG to the TSHR (by inhibition of the binding of labeled TSH) is generally referred to as thyrotrophin binding inhibitory immunoglobulin, TBII. Although in GD TBII usually does equate to TSAb, some IgGs positive in the TBII will not stimulate thyroid cells, and some even inhibit TSH activity in vitro and in vivo (thyrotrophin stimulation-blocking antibody, TSBAb), thus being capable of causing or contributing to hypothyroidism. This most typically is associated with atrophic hypothyroidism *(1)*. It also has been associated with transient neonatal hypothyroidism owing to passive transfer to the fetus *(1)*.

Using assays measuring the generation of cAMP in human or FRTL-5 thyrocytes, several laboratories have demonstrated TSAb in the sera of about 95% of patients with untreated GD (Table 2). TSAb in pregnant women may rise in the first trimester, but usually declines in the third trimester and may even temporarily disappear; however, if the levels are initially very high, even a considerable drop may leave the TSAb still markedly abnormal throughout pregnancy. In such instances, there is a very real possibility of fetal and neonatal hyperthyroidism, which can be a serious illness. It is a result of placental passive transfer of the antibody, which thus gradually clears over several weeks in the newborn; therefore, treatment is necessary only for this length of time. Following delivery, maternal TSAb might rebound to higher levels again, sometimes leading to postpartum GD. TSAb declines in most patients with long-term antithyroid drug therapy and may become negative; although this, along with regression of the goiter might suggest that the patient is in remission, sometimes the latter is short-lived, and the disease then recurs. However, conversely, it is a virtual certainty that the continued presence of TSAb is associated with a high relapse rate following discontinuance of such medication. TSAb will become further elevated following ^{131}I treatment for several months as a result of radiation-induced release of thyroid antigens, including TSHR, and will then decline *(1)*. TSAb has been reported to appear transiently with liberation of membrane antigens in subacute or silent thyroiditis *(51)*, or owing to molecular mimicry following acute Yersiniosis *(96)*; in the latter patients, however, there was no evidence of thyroid dysfunction (Table 2) *(96)*.

Other thyroid antibodies that are useful clinically include TPO (microsomal) and Tg antibodies of IgG class *(1)*. A high titer of Tg antibody, a noncomplement-fixing antibody, is found in about 55% of patients with HT and 25% of patients with GD. It occurs less often in patients with thyroid carcinoma and other (nonthyroidal) autoimmune disease. TPO antibodies (complement-fixing) are found much more commonly in AITD compared to Tg antibodies, and have a much closer relationship with thyroid dysfunction and abnormal histology. They are detectable in about 95% of patients with HT, 90% of those with "idiopathic myxoedema," and 80% of patients with GD; 72% of patients positive for TPO antibodies manifest some degree of thyroid dysfunction. In terms of case finding and cost reductions, performance of Tg antibodies is hardly necessary; one study has shown that TPO antibody was the only positive test in 64% of all patients with positive tests, whereas Tg antibody was the only positive test in 1% *(182)*. Thus, the widespread practice of performing both tests increases the costs without an offsetting diagnostic gain *(182)*. Even low titers of TPO antibody correlate with thyroidal lymphoid infiltration *(1)*. High titers are highly suggestive of AITD, and very high titers are virtually diagnostic of AITD; conversely, a minority of AITD patients have only low titers or undetectable thyroid autoantibodies. Low titers are also noted in some cases of subacute thyroiditis, nontoxic goiter, and papillary thyroid carcinoma. When TPO antibodies are detected in women before or in early pregnancy, these tend to predict subsequent postpartum thyroiditis; in addition, these antibodies rise higher transiently concomitantly with the functional disturbances that accompany postpartum thyroiditis. Thyroid antibodies in patients with HT with high TSH values will generally fall with thyroxine TSH-suppressive therapy. They will also usually decline in GD patients treated with antithyroid drugs *(1)*. The nature of these thyroid autoantibodies and their interacting antigenic epitopes have been reviewed elsewhere *(60,100,103,183,184)*. Antibodies directed against the thyroid hormones may also be detected in patients with AITD *(1)*, but will not be discussed further in this space. Likewise, natural IgM Tg antibodies, frequently found in healthy persons, will not be further discussed *(60)*.

Antinuclear antibodies and autoantibodies to a few other organ antigens, such as gastric antigens, islet cell antigens, and others, are found more commonly in AITD as compared to the normal population *(1)*. This does not reflect antigenic crossreactivity, but rather may signify the inheritance of more than one disease susceptibility gene situated in close proximity to one another. Antibodies against certain bacteria, such as Y.e. have been reported in AITD. This appears to arise from an artifact of homology between thyroid and bacterial antigens, but does not necessarily imply or signify the presence or relevance of actual bacterial infection *(1,51)*.

REMISSIONS OF GD

More than one type of clinical remission occurs in GD *(1)*. Destruction of sufficient thyroid parenchyma with ^{131}I or thyroidectomy may prevent recurrence. Conversely, spontaneous continuous immunological thyroid destruction owing to concomitant HT may bring about euthyroidism or even hypothyroidism. Hypothyroidism may ensue from a change in the nature of a TSHR antibody from a stimulating to a blocking antibody. In contrast, another important type of remission is one in which all immunological stigmata of the disease disappear, including the goiter, thyroid antibodies, TSAb, and evidence of sensitization of T lymphocytes *(185)*.

This form of remission may occur only in patients with a less severe defect in immunoregulation; in such patients, hyperthyroidism may have been precipitated by some environmental insult adversely influencing the immune system, converting a previously occult specific regulatory T-lymphocyte defect to an overt one. This is then reversible when the environmental disturbance disappears, and the adverse effect on the immune system of hyperthyroidism itself is vitiated by restoration of euthyroidism by appropriate treatment (antithyroid drugs, ^{131}I, or thyroidectomy) *(1)*. Moreover, rest, the passage of time, the recovery from infection, the use of sedation, and other nonspecific measures each will serve to permit the partially disturbed immunoregulatory system to be restored to its previous functional efficiency *(1)*.

Those persons with a presumed severe defect would not be expected to undergo immunological remission, no matter how long their antithyroid drugs were continued. Only those remissions associated with spontaneous or iatrogenic thyroid destruction wouuld occur in this group *(1)*.

IMMUNOLOGICAL ASPECTS OF THE THERAPY FOR GD

Despite greatly improved understanding of the immune basis of GD, there have been few substantive changes in its management over the past generation. However, the selection of patients for specific therapies and the nature of effects of different treatments have benefited from our new knowledge.

First, it had been claimed that the antithyroid drugs are themselves immunosuppressive *(186,187)*. However, it was difficult to reconcile this notion with the fact that many patients continue to display immunological activity throughout the course of therapy, no matter what dosage of antithyroid drug is used, and no matter how well hyperthyroidism is controlled *(188)*. This is not in accord with an expected pharmacological effect of these agents, in which a dose-response should impact on the immune system, but did not: recent studies have failed to show differing effects on a variety of immune parameters from high- vs low-dose antithyroid drug regimens; control of hyperthyroidism was the crucial factor affecting these parameters *(185–191)*. Thus, the normalization of thyroid hormone levels is attended by normalization of the suppressor/helper T-cell ratio *(188–192)*, reduced activation of CD4+ helper T cells *(121)*, normalized solubilized IL-2 *(193)*, solubilized CD8 *(194)*, and soluble ICAM-1 *(195)*. In any event, because of the relatively short duration of action of these agents, it is difficult to comprehend how a long-term remission would persist after cessation of therapy. The action of antithyroid drugs on thyroid cells (not directly on immune cells), normalizing all thyroid functions and restoring euthyroidism, would far better explain remissions; drug effects on thyroid hormone production and other thyroid cellular activities then reduce "thyrocyte immunocyte signalling," restoring the previous (precarious) state of immunoregulation, tending to result in a remission *(196,197)*.

The use of ^{131}I therapy for GD *de novo* also is associated with immunological perturbations, namely, a transient rise in TSAb and other thyroid autoantibodies, followed by an ultimate decline. This is almost certainly owing to the liberation of thyroid antigens from the damaged thyroid parenchyma, stimulating the already disturbed immune system *(1)*. Indeed, this effect may be additive to an already-present intrinsic tendency toward autoimmune destruction, leading to an even higher incidence of hypothyroidism. The factors involved in leading to post-^{131}I hypothyroidism are listed in Table 3.

Table 3
Factors Leading to Hypothyroidism after ^{131}I Treatment for GD

Direct destruction of thyroid cells by radiation damage
Interference of thyrocyte mRNA synthesis; thus cells cannot replicate
Increased liberation of thyroid antigen by ^{131}I-damage to an already abnormal immune system increases immune response and immune damage
Natural propensity for GD to progress to HT

Finally, subtotal thyroidectomy is often associated with a decline in TSAb activity, perhaps because most of the offending thyroid-committed lymphocytes are removed with the gland. Recurrences after surgery would have to be associated with sufficient remaining thyroid parenchyma to be able to respond to TSAb and sufficient remaining thyroid-committed lymphocytes to mount the immune attack *(1)*.

NATURAL COURSE OF AUTOIMMUNE THYROIDITIS AND MODIFICATION WITH THERAPY

The thyroid functional state and serology can vary markedly over time, even with temporary or permanent remissions *(1)*. This is particularly evident in subclinical or minimal autoimmune thyroiditis. Although a full explanation of these variations is as yet forthcoming, it seems obvious that the variations are in the immune system, secondarily affecting thyroid function. These perturbations in immunoregulation likely reflect the "milieu interieure" or immune environment, i.e., influences from the environment on a day-to-day basis. Nevertheless, there is some tendency for autoimmune thyroiditis to go on gradually to more severe destruction, consistent with the known effect of aging on the immune system *(21,127)*. In subclinical hypothyroidism associated with thyroid autoantibodies, about 5%/yr will go on to overt hypothyroidism *(1)*. About 45% of elderly women will have demonstrable autoimmune thyroiditis *(1)*. Males have a much lower incidence.

On this basis, it is relatively easy to comprehend the general outline of the pathogenesis of postpartum thyroiditis. In the latter part of pregnancy, all autoimmune phenomena are inhibited by a number of possible factors, all perhaps tied teleologically to a need not to reject the fetus. Following delivery, there is a reversal of these alterations. This will be dealt with in detail in Chapter 11, and thus will not be further discussed in this section.

Another interesting environmental factor influencing the natural history of autoimmune thyroiditis is that of iodine intake. There is considerable evidence that iodine adversely affects thyroid function and antibodies in those with occult or overt AITD, and can certainly abruptly precipitate hypothyroidism in susceptible persons *(1,2,59)*. This may be brought about by at least two mechanisms, namely, by increasing the immunogenicity of Tg, and by reducing the conversion of iodide to organic iodine. The increased iodide intake over the past generations almost certainly has been a major factor in markedly increasing the prevalence of autoimmune thyroiditis during this era.

Thyroid hormone therapy of course constitutes rational treatment for patients with hypothyroidism *(198)*, and this has an added advantage beyond merely normalizing thyroid function in those whose hypothyroidism is the result of autoimmune thyroiditis. In those patients with elevated TSH levels, such therapy was able to reduce thyroid autoantibody titers, almost certainly owing to a consequent reduction in thyroid antigen presentation via reduced thyrocyte stimulation *(1)*. Since it is known that increased TSH stimulates increased thyrocyte HLA-DR expression and increased thyroid antigenic expression, it may be inferred that reduced TSH induced by thyroxine therapy will do the reverse *(1)*. Theoretically, this effect should also reduce the autoimmune pathological process, although this desirable effect has not actually been documented.

EXTRATHYROIDAL MANIFESTATIONS OF GD

This topic will be covered in Chapter 10.

REFERENCES

1. Volpé R. Autoimmune Diseases of the Endocrine System. CRC, Boca Raton, 1990, pp. 1–364.
2. Weetman AP, McGregor AM. Autoimmune thyroid disease: further developments in our understanding. Endocr Rev 1994;15:788–830.
3. Weetman AP. Recent progress in thyroid autoimmunity. Thyroid Today 1996;19(2):1–9.
4. Hashimoto H. Zur Kenntniss der lymphomatosen Veranderung der Schilddruse (Struma lymphomatosa). Arch Klin Chir 1912;97:219–248.
5. Dayan CM. The natural history of autoimmune thyroiditis: how normal is autoimmunity? Proc Roy Coll Physicians Edinburgh 1996;26:419–433.
6. Okayasu I, Hara Y, Nakamura K, Rose NR. Racial and age-related differences in incidence and severity of focal autoimmune thyroiditis. Am J Clin Pathol 1994;101:698–702.
7. Williams ED, Doniach I. The post-mortem incidence of focal thyroiditis. J Pathol Bacteriol 1962;83:55–264.
8. Tunbridge WMG, Evered DC, Hall R, Appleton D, Brewis M, Clark F, et al. The spectrum of thyroid disease in a community: the Whickham survey. Clin Endocrinol 1977;7:481–493.
9. Dayan CM, Daniels GH. Chronic autoimmune thyroiditis. N Engl J Med 1996;335:99–107.
10. Kurihara H, Sasaki J, Takamatsu M. Twenty cases of Hashimoto disease changing to Graves' disease. In: Nagataki S, Mori T, Torizuka K, eds. 80 Years of Hashimoto Disease. Elsevier Science, Amsterdam, 1993, pp. 249–253.
11. Sugrue D, McEvoy M. Feely J, Drury MI. Hyperthyroidism in the land of Graves': results of treatment by surgery, radio-iodine and carbimazole in 837 cases. Q J Med 1980;49:51–61.
12. Wood LC, Ingbar SH. Hypothyroidism as a late sequel in patients with Graves' disease treated with anti-thyroid agents. J Clin Invest 1979;64:1426–1439.
13. Volpé R. The natural history of autoimmune thyroid disease. Clin Exp Thyroidology 1988;1:31–41.
14. Hedley AJ, Young RE, Jones SJ, Alexander WD, Bewsher PD. Anti-thyroid drugs in the treatment of Graves' disease: longterm followup of 434 patients. Clin Endocrinol (Oxford) 1989;31:209–218.
15. Bagnasco M, Pesce G. Autoimmune thyroid disease: immunological model and clinical problem. Fundam Clin Immunol 1996;4:7–27.
16. Nagataki S, Yamashita S, Tamai H. Immunogenetics of autoimmune endocrine disease. In: Volpé R, ed. Autoimmune Diseases of the Endocrine System. CRC, Boca Raton, 1990, pp. 51–72.
17. Plotnikoff N, Murgo A, Faith R, Wybran J. Stress and immunity. CRC, Boca Raton, 1991, pp. 1–558.
18. Glaser R, Kiecolt-Glaser JK. Handbook of human stress and immunity. Academic, San Diego and London, 1994, pp. 1–414.
19. Holt PG. Immune and inflammatory function in cigarette smokers. Thorax 1987;42:241–249.
20. Weetman AP. Autoimmune thyroiditis: predisposition and pathogenesis. Clin Endocrinol (Oxford) 1992;36:307–323.
21. Hirokawa K. Understanding the mechanism of the age-related decline in immune function. Nutrition Rev 1992;50:361–366.
22. Wachtel SS, Koo GC, Boyce EA. Evolutionary conservation of HY male antigen. Nature 1975;254:270–274.
23. Nelson JL, Steinberg AD. Sex steroids, autoimmunity and autoimmune disease. In: Berczi I, Kovacs K, eds. Hormones and Immunity. MTP, Lancaster, England, 1987, pp. 93–119.
24. Olsen NJ, Watson MB, Henderson GS, Kovacs WJ. Androgen deprivation induces phenotypic and functional changes in the thymus of adult male mice. Endocrinology 1991;129:2471–2476.

25. Viselli SM, Stanziale S, Shults K, Kovacs WJ, Olsen NJ. Castration alters peripheral immune function in normal male mice. Immunology 1995;84:337–342.
26. Olsen NJ, Kovacs WJ. Gonadal steroids and immunity. Endocr Rev 1996;17:369–383.
27. Svejgaard A, Platz P, Ryder LR. HLA and endocrine disease. In: Volpé R, ed. Autoimmunity in Endocrine Disease. Marcel Dekker, New York, 1985, pp. 93–107.
28. Farid NR, Bear JC. The human major histocompatibility complex and endocrine disease. Endocr Rev 1981;2:50–86.
29. Mangklabruks A, Cox N, DeGroot LJ. Genetic factors in autoimmune thyroid disease analyzed by restriction fragment length polymorphisms of candidate genes. J Clin Endocrinol Metab 1991;73: 236–244.
30. Garcia-Ameijeiras A, Gladman DD, Chan JYC, Volpé R. Studies of restriction fragment length polymorphism of DR and DQ genes in HLA-DR3 positive patients with Graves' disease or systemic lupus erythematosus. Clin Invest Med 1993;16:326–332.
31. Yanagawa T, Mangklabruks A, Chang YB, Okamoto Y, Fisfalen ME, Curran PG, et al. Human histocompatibility leukocyte antigen DQA*0501 allele associated with genetic susceptibility to Graves' disease in a Caucasian population. J Clin Endocrinol Metab 1993;76:1569–1574.
32. Badenhoop K, Schwarz G, Walfish PG, Drummond V, Usadel KH, Bottazzo GF. Susceptibility to thyroid autoimmune disease: molecular analysis of HLA-D region genes identifies new markers for goitrous Hashimoto's thyroiditis. J Clin Endocrinol Metab 1990;71:1131–1137.
33. Farid NR, Shi Y, Zou M, Stenzky V, Zhonglin W, Stephens HAF, et al. Immunogenetics of Hashimoto disease: the 11th Histocompatibility Workshop experience. In: Nagataki S, Mori T, Torizuka K eds. Eighty Years of Hashimoto Disease, Excerpta Medica, International Congress Series 1028, Elsevier, Amsterdam, 1993, pp. 31–36.
34. Tandon N, Zhang L, Weetman AP. HLA associations with Hashimoto's thyroiditis. Clin Endocrinol 1991;34:383–386.
35. McLachlan S. Editorial: The genetic basis of autoimmune thyroid disease: time to focus on chromosomal loci other than the major histocompatibility complex (HLA in man). J Clin Endocrinol Metab 1993;77:605A–605C.
36. Tomer Y, Barbesino G, Keddache M, Greenberg DA, Concepcion ES, Davies TF. Mapping of major suscepitbilty loci (GD-1 & GD-2) for Graves' disease to chromosome #14q. J Invest Med 1997;45: 251A (Abstract).
37. Yanagawa T, Hidaka Y, Guimaraes V, Soliman M, DeGroot LJ. CTLA-4 gene polymorphism associated with Graves' disease in a Caucasian population. J Clin Endocrinol Metab 1995;80:41–45.
38. Kotsa K, Watson PF, Weetman AP. A CTLA-4 gene polymorphism is associated with both Graves' disease and autoimmune hypothyroidism. Clin Endocrinol 1997;46:551–554.
39. Sale MM, Akamizu T, Howard TD, Yokota T, Nakao K, Mori T, et al. Association of autoimmune thyroid disease with a microsatellite marker for the thyrotropin receptor gene and CTLA-4 in a Japanese population. Proc Assoc Am Physicians 1997;109:453–461.
40. Tomer Y, Barbesino G, Greenberg D, Davies TF. The immunogenetics of autoimmune diabetes and autoimmune thyroid disease. Trends Endocrinol Metab 1997;8:63–70.
41. Zheng RQH, Abney ER, Grubeck-Loebenstein B, Dayan C, Maini RN, Feldmann M. Expression of intercellular adhesion molecule-l and lymphocyte function-associated antigen-3 on human thyroid epithelial cells in Graves' and Hashimoto's diseases. J. Autoimmunity 1990;3:727–736.
42. Ratanachaiyavong S, Demaine AG, Campbell RD, McGregor AM. Heat shock protein 70 and complement C4 genotypes in patients with hyperthyroid Graves' disease. Clin Exp Immunol 1991;84: 48–52.
43. Trieb K, Sztankay A, Hermann M, Gratzl R, Szabo J, Jindal S, et al. Do heat shock proteins play a role in Graves' disease? Heat shock protein-specific T-cells from Graves' disease thyroids do not recognize thyroid epithelial cells. J Clin Endocrinol Metab 1993;77:528–535.
44. Resetkova E, Kawai K, Enomoto T, Foy TM, Noel RJ, Volpé R. Antibody to gp39, the ligand for CD40, significantly inhibits humoral responses for Graves' thyroid tissues xenografted into severe combined immunodeficient (SCID) mice. Thyroid 1996;6:267–273.
45. Waterhouse P, Penninger JM, Timms E, Wakeham A, Shahinian A, Lee KP, et al. Lymphoproliferative disorders with early lethality in mice deficient in Ctla-4. Science 1995;270:985–988.
46. Yue SJ, Enomoto T, Matsumoto Y, Kawai K, Volpé R. Thyrocyte class I and class II expression are secondary phenomena and do not contribute to the pathogenesis of autoimmune thyroid disease. Thyroid 1998;8:755–763.

47. Saji M, Moriarity J, Ban T, Singer D, Kohn LD. Major histocompatibility complex Class I gene expression in rat thyroid cells is regulated by hormones, methimazole, and iodide as well as interferon. J Clin Endocrinol Metab 1992;75:871–878.
48. Tomer Y, Davies TF. Infection, thyroid disease and autoimmunity. Endocr Rev 1993;14:107–120.
49. Krieg AM, Steinberg AD. Review: retroviruses and autoimmunity. J Autoimmunity 1990;3:137–166.
50. Delemarre FGA, Simons PJ, Drexhage HA. Histomorphological aspects of the development of thyroid autoimmune diseases: consequences for our understanding of endocrine ophthalmopathy. Thyroid 1996;6:369–377.
51. Volpé R. A perspective on human autoimmune thyroid disease: is there an abnormality of the target cell which predisposes to the disorder? Autoimmunity 1992;12:3–9.
52. Geppert TD, Davis LS, Gur H, Wacholt MC, Lipsky PE. Accesory cell signals involved in T-cell activation. Immunol Rev 1990;117:5–66.
53. Wilkin TJ. Receptor autoimmunity in endocrine disorders. N Engl J Med 1990;323:1318–1324.
54. Wilkin TJ. The primary lesion theory of autoimmunity: a speculative hypothesis. Autoimmunity 1990;7:225–235.
55. Martin A, Davies TF. T cells in human autoimmune thyroid disease: emerging data shows the lack of need to invoke suppressor T cell problems. Thyroid 1992;2:247–261.
56. Wick G, Muller PU, Kuhn L, Lefkovits I. Molecular analysis of genetically determined target cell abnormalities in spontaneous autoimmune thyroiditis. Immunobiology 1990;181:414–429.
57. Rose NR, Bacon LD, Sundick RS, Kong YM. The role of genetic factors in autoimmunity. In: Meischer PA, Bolis L, Gorini S, Lambo TA, Nossal GJV, Torrigiani G, eds. The Menarini Series of Immunopathology—First Symposium on Organ-Specific Autoimmunity. Schwabe, Basel, Switzerland, 1978, pp. 225–233.
58. Kohn LD, Giuliani C, Montani V, Napolitano G, Ohmori M, Ohta M, et al. Anti-receptor autoimmunity. In: Rayner D, Champion BR, eds. Thyroid Autoimmunity. RG Landes Co., Austin, TX, 1995, pp. 116–169.
59. Bottazzo GF, Pujol-Borell R, Hanafusa T, Feldmann M. Role of aberrant HLA-DR expression and antigen presentation in induction of endocrine autoimmunity. Lancet 1983;2:1115–1119.
60. Weetman AP. Autoimmune thyroiditis: predisposition and pathogenesis. Clin Endocrinol 1992;36:307–323.
61. Kawai K, Enomoto T, Togun R, Resetkova E, Volpé R. The longterm effect of human interferon alpha and interferon gamma on xenografted human thyroid tissue in severe combined immunodeficient and nude mice. Proc Assoc Am Physicians 1997;109:126–135.
62. Volpé R. Subacute thyroiditis. In: Burrow GN, Oppenheimer J, Volpé R, eds.Thyroid Function and Disease. Saunders, Philadelphia, 1989, pp. 179–190.
63. Bottazzo GF, Mirakian R, De Lazzari F, Mauerhoff T, Todd I, Pujol-Borrel R. Autoimmune endocrine/organ specific disorders: clinical diagnostic relevance and novel approach to pathogenesis. In: Berczi I, Kovacs K, eds. Hormones and Immunity. MTP, Norwell, MA, 1987, pp. 296–311.
64. Gaulton GN, Stein ME, Safko B, Stadecker MJ. Direct induction of Ia antigen on murine thyroid-derived epithelial cells by reovirus. J Immunol 1989;142:3821–3825.
65. Neufeld BS, Platzer M, Davies TF. Reovirus induction of MHC Class II antigen in rat thyroid cells. Endocrinology 1980;124:543–545.
66. Ciampiolillo A, Mirakian R, Schulz T, Vittoria M, Buscema M, Pujol-Borrell R, et al. Retrovirus-like sequences in Graves' disease: implications for human autoimmunity. Lancet 1989;2:1096–1099.
67. Wick GB, Grubeck-Loebenstein B, Trieb K, Kalischnig A, Aguzzi A. Human foamy virus antigens in thyroid tissue of Graves' disease patients. Int. Arch. Allergy Immunol. 1992;99:153–156.
68. Wick GB, Trieb K, Aguzzi A, Recheis H, Anderl H, Grubeck-Loebenstein B. Possible role of human foamy virus in Graves' disease. Intervirology 1993;35:101–112.
69. Lagaye S, Vexiau P, Morozov V, Guenebaut-Claudet V, Tobaly-Tapiero J, Canivet M, et al. Detection of HTLV-1 gag related sequences in leucocyte DNA from patients with polyendocrinopathies (Basedow-Graves' disease and insulin-dependent diabetes). C R Acad Sci 1991;III.312:309–315.
70. Lagaye S, Vexiau P, Morozov V, Guenebaut-Claudet V, Tobaly-Tapiero J, Canivet M, et al. Human spumaretrovirus-related sequences in the DNA of leukocytes from patients with Graves' disease. Proc Natl Acad Sci USA 1992;89:10,070–10,074.
71. Jaspan JB, Sullivan K, Garry RF, Lopez M, Wolfe M, Clejan S, et al. The interaction of a Type A retroviral particle and class II human leukocyte antigen susceptibility genes in the pathogenesis of Graves' disease. J Clin Endocrinol Metab 1996;81:2271–2279.

72. Tran A, Quaranta JF, Beusnel C, Thiers V, De Souza M, Francois E, et al. Hepatitis C virus and Hashimoto's thyroiditis. Eur J Med 1992;1:116–118.
73. Quaranta JF, Tran A, Régnier D, Letestu R, Beusnel C, Fuzibet JG, et al. High prevalence of antibodies to hepatitis C virus (HCV) in patients with antithyroid antibodies. J Hepatol 1993;18:136–138.
74. Rossini AA, Williams RM, Mordes JP, Appel C, Like AA. Spontaneous diabetes in the gnotobiotic BB/W rat. Diabetes 1979;28:1031,1032.
75. Tominaga T, Katamine S, Namba H, Yokoyama N, Nakamura S, Morita S, et al. Lack of evidence of the presence of human immunodeficiency virus type 1-related sequences in patients with Graves' disease. Thyroid 1991;1:307–314.
76. Humphrey M, Baker JR, Carr E, Wartofsky L, Mosca J, Drabick JJ, et al. Absence of retroviral sequences in Graves' disease. Lancet 1991;337:17–18.
77. Yanagawa T, Ito K, Kaplan EL, Ishikawa N, DeGroot LJ. Absence of association between human Spumaretrovirus and Graves' disease. Thyroid 1995;5:379–382.
78. Heneine W, Musey VC, Sinha SD, Landay A, Northrup G, Khabbaz R, et al. Absence of evidence for human Spumaretrovirus sequences in patients with Graves' disease. J Acquir Immun Defic Dis Hum Retrovirol 1995;9:99–100.
79. Newmann-Haefelin D, Fleps U, Renne R, Schweizer M. Foamy viruses. Intervirology 1993;35:196–207.
80. Schweizer M, Turek R, Reinhardt M, Neumann-Haefelin D. Absence of foamy virus DNA in Graves' disease. AIDS Res Hum Retroviruses 1994;10:601–605.
81. Metcalfe RA, Ball G, Kudesia G, Weetman AP. Failure to find an association between hepatitis C virus and thyroid autoimmunity. Thyroid 1997;7:421–424.
82. Mowat WM. Interferon and Class II antigen expression in autoimmunity. Lancet 1986;2:283.
83. Aguayo J, Michaud P, Iitaka M, Row VV, Volpé R. Lack of effect of methimazole on thyrocyte cell surface antigen expression. Autoimmunity 1989;2:133–143.
84. Kasuga Y, Matsubayashi S, Sakatsume Y, Miller N, Jamieson C, Volpé R. Effects of long term, high dosage bovine thyrotropin administration on human thyroid tissues from patients with Graves' disease and normal subjects xenografted into nude mice. Endocr Pathol 1990;1:220–227.
85. Kasuga Y, Matsubayashi S, Sakatsume Y, Akasu F, Jamieson C, Volpé R. The effect of xenotransplantation of human thyroid tissue following radioactive iodine ablation on thyroid function in the nude mouse. Clin Invest Med 1991;14:277–281.
86. Iwatani Y, Gerstein HC, Iitaka M, Row VV, Volpé R. Thyrocyte HLA-DR expression and interferon gamma production in autoimmune thyroid tissue. J Clin Endocrinol Metab 1986;63:695–707.
87. Kasuga Y, Matsubayashi S, Sakatsume Y, Miller N, Jamieson C, Volpé R. Effects of recombinant human interferon gamma on human thyroid tissues from patients with Graves'disease and normal subjects transplanted into nude mice. J Endocrinol Invest 1990;1:220–227.
88. Kasuga Y, Matsubayashi S, Akasu F, Miller N, Jamieson C, Volpé R. Effects on recombinant human interleukin-2 and tumor necrosis factor alpha with or without interferon gamma on human thyroid tissues from Graves' disease and normal subjects xenografted into nude mice. J Clin Endocrinol Metab 1991;97:133–138.
89. Kawai K, Resetkova E, Enomoto T, Fornasier V, Volpé R. Is HLA-DR and ICAM-1 expression constitutive in papillary thyroid cancer?: comparative studies of human thyroid xenografts in SCID and nude mice. J Clin Endocrinol Metab 1998;83:157–164.
90. Wenzel B, Heeseman J, Wenzel KW, Schrieber EC. Antibodies to plasmid-encoated protein of enteropathic Yersinia in patients with autoimmune thyroid disease. Lancet 1988;1:56.
91. Ingbar SH, Weiss M, Cushing GW, Kasper DL. A possible role for bacterial antigen in the pathogenesis of autoimmune thyroid disease. In: Pinchera A, Ingbar SH, McKenzie JM, Fenzi GF, eds. Thyroid Autoimmunity. Plenum, New York, 1987, pp. 35–42.
92. Heyma P, Harrison LC, Robins-Browne R. Thyrotropin binding sites on Yersinia enterocolitica recognized by immunoglobulins from humans with Graves' disease. Clin Exp Immunol 1986;64:249–254.
93. Burman KD, Lukes YG, Gemiski P. Molecular homology between the human TSH receptor and *Yersinia enterocolitica* [Abstract]. Thyroid 1991;(Suppl 1):S–62.
94. Arscott P, Rosen ED, Koenig RJ, Kaplan MM, Ellis T, Thompson N, et al. Immunoreactivity to *Yersinia enterocolitica* antigens in patients with autoimmune thyroid disease. J Clin Endocrinol Metab 1992;75:295–300.
95. Resetkova E, Notenboom R, Arreaza G, Mukuta T, Yoshikawa N, Volpé R. Seroreactivity to bacterial antigens is not a unique phenomenon in patients with autoimmune thyroid disease in Canada. Thyroid 1994;4:269–274.

96. Wolf MW, Misaki T, Bech K, Tvede M, Silra JE, Ingbar SH. Immunoglobulins of patients recovering from *Yersinia enterocolitica* infections exhibit Graves'-like activity in human thyroid membranes. Thyroid 1991;1:315–320.
97. Sakata S, Matsuda M, Komaki T, Kojima N, Yabuuci E, Miura K. Production of anti-TSH receptor antibodies in rats by immunization with *Yersinia enterocolitica*. Abstract 12-18-073, in Proceedings of the 8th International Congress of Endocrinology, Kyoto, July 17–23, 1988.
98. Wick G. The role of the target organ in the development of autoimmune diseases exemplified in the obese strain chicken model for human Hashimoto disease. Exp Clin Endocrinol Diabetes 1996; 104(Suppl 3):1–4.
99. Sundick RS, Bagchi N, Brown TR. The obese strain chicken as a model for human Hashimoto's thyroiditis. Exp Clin Endocrinol Diabetes 1996;104(Suppl 3):4–6.
100. Lahat N, Hirose W, Davies TF. Enhanced induction of thyroid cell MHC Class II antigen expression in rats highly responsive to thyroglobulin. Endocrinology 1989;124:1754–1759.
101. Volpé R, Kasuga Y, Akasu F, Morita T, Resetkova E, Arreaza G. The use of the SCID mouse and nude mouse as models for the study of human autoimmune thyroid disease. Clin Immunol Immunopathol 1993;67:93–99.
102. Dawe K, Hutchings P, Champion B, Cooke A, Roitt IR. Autoantigens in thyroid disease. Springer Semin Immunopathol 1993;14:285–307.
103. Ludgate M, Vassart G. The molecular genetics of three thyroid autoantigens: thyroglobulin, thyroid peroxidase and the thyrotrophin receptor. Autoimmunity 1990;7:201–211.
104. Cuddihy RM, Dutton CM, Bahn RS. A polymorphism in the extracellular domain of the thyrotropin receptor is highly associated with autoimmune thyroid disease in females. Thyroid 1995;5:89–95.
105. Bohr URM, Behr M, Loos U. A heritable point mutation in an extracellular domain on the TSH receptor involved in the interaction with Graves' immunoglobulins. Biochem Biophys Acta 1993;1216: 504–508.
106. Watson PF, French A, Pickerill AP, McIntosh RS, Weetman AP. Lack of association between a polymorphism in the coding region of the thyrotropin receptor and Graves' disease. J Clin Endocrinol Metab 1995;80:1032–1035.
107. Shimojo N, Kohno Y, Yamaguchi KI, Kikuoka SI, Hoshioka A, Niimi H, et al. Induction of Graves'-like disease in mice by immunization with fibroblasts transfected with the thyrotropin receptor and a class II molecule. Proc Natl Acad Sci USA 1996;93:11,074–11,079.
108. Murakami M, Myashita K, Monden T, Yamada M, Iriuchijima T, Mori M. Evidence that a soluble form of TSH receptor is present in the peripheral blood of patients with Graves' disease. In: Nagataki S, Mori T, Torizuka K, eds. Eighty Years of Hashimoto Disease. Excerpta Medica, International Congress Series 1028, Elsevier, Amsterdam, 1993, pp. 683–685.
109. Murikami M, Myashita K, Yamada M, Iriuchijima T, Mori M. Characterization of human thyrotropin receptor peptide-like immunoreactivity in perpheral blood of Graves' disease. Biochem Biophys Res Commun 1992;186:1074–1080.
110. Hunt N, Wiley KP, Northemann W, Leidenberger F. The thyrotropin receptor of Graves' disease exists as a soluble receptor in the thyroid and serum. J Endocrinol Invest 1992;15(Suppl 2):80 (Abstract).
111. Hunt N, Wiley KP. Alternative splicing of the human TSH receptor: a possible role of the soluble TSH receptor in the aetiology of Graves' disease. In: Reinwein D, Weinheimer B, eds. Schilddruse 1993. Therapie der hyperthyreose. Walter de Gruyter, Berlin, 1994, pp. 10–12.
112. Arreaza G, Yoshikawa N, Mukuta T, Resetkova E, Barsouk A, Nishikawa M, et al. Expression of intercellular adhesion molecule-1 (ICAM-1) on human thyroid cells from patients with autoimmune thyroid disease; study of thyroid xenografts in nude and severe combined immunodeficient mice and treatment with FK-506. J Clin Endocrinol Metab 1995;80:3724–3734.
113. Weetman AP, Volkman DJ, Burman KD, Margolick JB, Petrick P, Weintraub BD, et al. The production and characterization of thyroid derived T cell lines in Graves' disease and Hashimoto's thyroiditis. Clin Immunol Immunopath 1986;39:139–150.
114. Volpé R, Edmonds MW, Lamki L, Clarke PV, Row VV. The pathogenesis of Graves' disease: a disorder of delayed hypersensitivity? Mayo Clin Proc 1972;47:824–836.
115. Ahmann A, Burman KD. Role of T lymphocytes in autoimmune thyroid disease. In: Wall JR, ed. Autoimmune thyroid disease. Endocrinol Metab Clin North Am 1987;16:287–326.
116. Yoshikawa N, Arreaza G, Morita T, Mukuta T, Resetkova E, Akasu F, et al. Effect of removing human Graves' thyroid xenografts after eight weeks in nude mice and rexenografting them into SCID mice. J Clin Endocrinol Metab 1994;78:367–374.

117. Yoshikawa N, Arreaza G, Mukuta T, Resetkova E, Miller N, Jamieson C, et al. Effect of FK-506 on xenografted human thyroid tissue in severe combined immunodeficient mice. Clin Endocrinol 1994; 41:31–39.
118. Aguayo J, Sakatsume Y, Jamieson C, Row VV, Volpé R. Nontoxic nodular goiter and papillary thyroid carcinoma are not associated with peripheral blood sensitization to thyroid cells. J Clin Endocrinol Metab 1989;68:145–149.
119. Sakatsume Y, Matsubayashi S, Kasuga Y, Aguayo J, Row VV, Volpé R. Lack of response of peripheral blood mononuclear cells to thyroid microsomal antigen in nontoxic nodular goiters. Regional Immunol 1990;3:42–45.
120. Sakatsume Y, Matsubayashi S, Kasuga Y, Miller N, Jamieson C, Volpé R. CD4 cells from patients with autoimmune thyroid disease secrete interferon gamma after stimulation with thyroid microsomal antigen: CD8 cells suppress this secretion. J Endocrinol Invest 1990;13:717–726.
121. Akasu F, Kasuga Y, Matsubayashi S, Carayon P, Volpé R. Studies of CD4+ helper/inducer T lymphocytes in autoimmune thyroid disease. Thyroid 1991;l:215–227.
122. Tandon N, Freeman M, Weetman AP. T cell responses to synthetic peroxidase peptides in autoimmune thyroid disease. Clin Exp Immunol 1991;86:56–60.
123. Nagayama Y, Rapoport B. Thyroid stimulatory autoantibodies in different patients with autoimmune thyroid disease do not all recognize the same components of the human thyrotrophin receptor: Selective role of receptor amino acids Ser 25-Glu 30. J Clin Endocrinol Metab 1992;75:1425–1430.
124. Davies TF, Martin A, Concepcion ES, Graves P, Cohen L, Ben-Nun A. Evidence of limited variability of antigen receptors on intrathyroidal T cells in autoimmune thyroid disease. N Engl J Med 1991; 325:238–244.
125. Davies TF, Concepcion ES, Ben-Nun A, Graves PN, Tarjan G. T cell receptor V gene use in autoimmune thyroid disease: direct assessment by thyroid aspiration. J Clin Endocrinol Metab 1993;76: 660–666.
126. Navarrete C, Bottazzo GF. In search of TCR restriction in autoreactive T cell in human autoimmunity: why is it so elusive? Clin Exp Immunol 1993;91:189–192.
127. McIntosh RS, Watson PF, Pickerill AP, Davies R, Weetman AP. No restriction of intrathyroidal T cell receptor Valpha families in the thyroid of Graves' disease. Clin Exp Immunol 1993;91:147–152.
128. McIntosh RS, Watson PF, Weetman AP. Analysis of the T cell receptor Valpha repertoire in Hashimoto's thyroiditis: evidence for the restricted accumulation of CD8+ T cells in the absence of CD4+ T cell restriction. J Clin Endocrinol Metab 1997;82:1140–1166.
129. Landay A, Gartland GL, Clement LT. Characterization of a phenotypical subpopulation of Leu-2 cells that suppresses T cell proliferative responses. J Immunol 1983;131:2757–2761.
130. Clement LT, Dagg MK, Landay A. Characterization of human lymphocyte subpopulations: alloreactive cytotoxic T-lymphocyte precursor and effector cells are phenotypically distinct from Leu-2+ suppressor cells. J Clin Immunol 1984;4:395–402.
131. Yoshikawa N, Morita T, Resetkova E, Arreaza G, Carayon P, Volpé R. Reduced activation of suppressor T lymphocytes by specific antigens in autoimmune thyroid disease. J Endocrinol Invest 1993; 15:609–617.
132. Iwatani Y, Amino N, Miyai K. Peripheral self-tolerance and autoimmunity: the protective role of expression of Class II histocompatibility antigens on non-lymphoid cells. Biomed Pharmacother 1989; 43:593–605.
133. Dorf ME, Kuchroo V, Collins M. Suppressor T cells: some answers but more questions. Immunol. Today 1992;13:241–243.
134. Volpé R. Suppressor T lymphocyte dysfunction is important in the pathogenesis of autoimmune thyroid disease. Thyroid 1993;3:345–350.
135. Volpé R. Immunoregulation in autoimmune thyroid disease. Thyroid 1994;4:373–377.
136. Chen X, Shelton J, McCullagh P. Suppression of anti-thyrocyte autoreactivity by the lymphocytes of normal fetal lambs. J Autoimmunity 1995;8:539–559.
137. Chen X, McCullagh P. Expression and regulation of anti-thyroid autoimmunity directed against cultivated rat thyrocytes. J Autoimmunity 1995;8:521–538.
138. Herold KC, Quintans J. Immunological mechanisms causing autoimmune endocrine disease. In: DeGroot LJ, ed. Endocrinology, 3rd ed., vol. 3. WB Saunders, Philadelphia, 1995, pp. 2990–3012.
139. Volpé R, Row VV. Role of antigen specific suppressor T lymphocytes in the pathogenesis of autoimmune thyroid disease. In: Walfish PG, Wall JR, Volpé R, eds. Autoimmunity and the Thyroid. Academic, Orlando, FL, 1984, pp. 79–94.

140. Gerstein HC, Rastogi B, Iwatani Y, Iitaka M, Row VV, Volpé R. The decrease in nonspecific lymphocytes in female hyperthyroid Graves' disease is secondary to the hyperthyroidism. Clin Invest Med 1987;10:337–344.
141. Chan JYC, Walfish PG. Activated (Ia+) T lymphocytes and their subsets in autoimmune thyroid disease: analysis by dual laser flow microfluorocytometry. J Clin Endocrinol Metab 1986;62:403–409.
142. Grubeck-Loebenstein B, Derfler K, Kassal H, Knapp W, Krisch K, Liszka K, et al. Immunological features of nonimmunogenic hyperthyroidism. J Clin Endocrinol Metab 1985;60:150–155.
143. Parry CH. Collections from the Unpublished Medical Writings of the Late Caleb Hillier Parry, vol. 2, Underwood, London, 1825, pp. 111–128.
144. Hennemann G. Historical aspects about the development of our knowledge of morbus Basedow. J Endocrinol Invest 1991;14:617–624.
145. Ferguson-Rayport SM. The relation of emotional factors to the recurrence of Graves' disease. Can MAJ 1956;15:993–998.
146. Gibson JC. Emotions and the thyroid gland: a critical appraisal. J. Psychosomatic Res 1962;6:93–99.
147. Hadden DR, McDevitt DG. Environmental stress and thyrotoxicosis. Lancet 1974;2:577–578.
148. Harris T, Creed F, Brugha TS. Stressful life events and Graves' disease. Br J Psychol 1992;161:535–541.
149. Hobbs JR. Stress and Graves' disease. Lancet 1992;339:427–428.
150. Kung AW. Life events, daily stresses and coping in patients with Graves' disease. Clin Endocrinol 1995;42:303–308.
151. LeClere J, Weryha G. Stress and autoimmune endocrine disease. Horm Res 1989;31:90–93.
152. Morillo E, Gardner LI. Bereavement as an antecedent factor in the thyrotoxicosis of childhood: four case studies with survey of possible metabolic pathways. Psychosomatic Med 1979;41:545–555.
153. Petticrew M. Stress and Graves' disease. Lancet 1992;339:427.
154. Rosch PJ. Stress and Graves' disease. Lancet 1992;339:428.
155. Rosch PJ. Stressful life events and Graves' disease. Lancet 1993;342:566–567.
156. Shlomo YB, Chaturvedi N. Stress and Graves' disease. Lancet 1992;339:427.
157. Sonino N, Girelli ME, Boscaro M, Fallo F, Busnardo B, Fava GA. Life events in the pathogenesis of Graves' disease: a controlled study. Acta Endocrinol (Copenhagen) 1993;128:293–296.
158. Wimsa B, Adami HO, Bergstrom R, Gamstedt A, Dahlberg P, Adamson U, et al. Stressful life events and Graves' disease. Lancet 1991;338:1475–1479.
159. Brown DM, Lowman JT. Thyrotoxicosis occurring in two patients on prolonged high dose6s of steroids. N Engl J Med 1964;270:278–281.
160. McDougall IR, Greig WR, Gray HW, Smith JFB. Thyrotoxicosis developing during cyclophosphamide therapy. Br Med J 1971;4:275–276.
161. Weinberg K, Parkman R. Age, the thymus, T lymphocytes. N Engl J Med 1995;332:182–183.
162. Gray J, Hoffenberg R. Thyrotoxicosis and stress. Q J Med 1985;54:153–160.
163. Mukuta T, Yoshikawa N, Arreaza G, Resetkova E, Leushner J, Song YH, et al. Activation of T cell subsets by synthetic TSH receptor peptides and recombinant glutamate decarboxylase in autoimmune thyroid disease and insulin dependent diabetes mellitus. J Clin Endocrinol Metab 1995;80:1264–1272.
164. McLachlan SM, Taverne J, Atherton MC, Cooke A, Middleton S, Pegg CAS, et al. Cytokines, thyroid autoantibody synthesis and thyroid cell survival in culture. Clin Exp Immunol 1990;79:175–181.
165. Nagayama Y, Izumi M, Ashizawa K, Kiriyama T, Yokoyama N, Morita S, et al. Inhibitory effect of interferon gamma on the response of human thyrocytes to thyrotropin stimulation: relationship between the response to TSH and the expression of DR antigen. J Clin Endocrinol Metab 1987;64:949–953.
166. Kennedy RL, Jones TH. Cytokines in endocrinology: their roles in health and disease. J Endocrinol 1990;129:167–178.
167. Dinarello CA. The biology of interleukin-1. Chem Immunol 1992;9:27–66.
168. Arreaza G, Yoshikawa N, Resetkova E, Mukuta T, Barsuk A, Muellin C, et al. Expression of intercellular adhesion molecule-l on human thyroid cells before and after xenografting in nude and severe combined immunodeficient mice. J Clin Endocrinol Metab 1995;80:3724–3731.
169. Kabel PJ, Voorbij JAM, De Haan M, Van Der Gaag, RD, Drexhage HA. Intrathyroidal dendritic cells. J Clin Endocrinol Metab1988;66:199–207.
170. Iwatani Y, Iitaka M, Row VV, Volpé R. Effect of HLA-DR positive thyrocytes on in vitro thyroid autoantibody production. Clin Invest Med 1988;11:279–285.
171. Weetman AP. Review: Antigen presentation in the pathogenesis of autoimmune endocrine disease. J Autoimmunity 1995;8:305–312.

172. Tandon N, Metcalfe RA, Barnett D, Weetman AP. Expression of the costimulatory molecule B7/BB1 in autoimmune thyroid disease. Q J Med 1994;87:231–236.
173. Teng WP, You X, Shan ZY, Volpé R. Effects of human interferon-alpha on human peripheral blood mononuclear cells and human thyrocytes. Proc 70th Meeting, American Thyoid Assoc. Colorado Springs, Oct 15–19, 1997, Abstract 91. Thyroid 1997;7(Suppl 1):S-46.
174. Janeway CA Jr, Bottomly K. Signals and signs for lymphocyte responses. Cell 1994;76:275–285.
175. Matsuoka N, Eguchi K, Kawakami A, Tsuboi M, Nakamura H, Kimura H, et al. Lack of B7-1/BB1 and B7/B70 expression on thyrocytes of patients with Graves' disease. Delivery of costimulatory signals from bystander professional antigen presenting cells. J Clin Endocrinol Metab 1996;81:4137–4143.
176. Dustin ML, Springer TA. Role of lymphocyte adhesion receptors in transient interactions and cell locomotion. Ann Rev Immunol 1991;9:27–66.
177. Weetman AP, Cohen SB, Makgoba MW, Borysiewicz LK. Expression of an intracellular adhesion molecule, ICAM-l, by human thyroid cells. J Endocrinol 1989;122:185–191.
178. Zheng RQH, Abney ER, Grubeck-Loebenstein B, Dayan C, Maini RN, Feldmann M. Expression of intercellular adhesion molecule-1 and lymphocyte function-associated antigen-3 on human thyroid epithelial cells in Graves' and Hashimoto's diseases. J Autoimmunity 1990;3:727–736.
179. Tandon N, Makgoba MW, Gahmberg CG, Weetman AP. The expression and role in T cell adhesion on LFA-3 and ICAM-2 on human thyroid cells. Clin Immunol Immunopathol 1992;64:30–35.
180. Heufelder AE, Goellner JR, Wenzel BE, Bahn RS. Immunohistochemical detection and localization of a 72-kilodalton heat shock protein in autoimmune thyroid disease. J Clin Endocrinol Metab 1993;77:528–535.
181. Weetman AP. The immunomodulatory effects of antithyroid drugs. Thyroid 1994;4:145–146.
182. Nordyke RA, Gilbert FI, Miyamoto LA, Fleury KA. The superiority of antimicrosomal over antithyroglobulin antibodies for detecting Hashimoto's thyroiditis. Arch Int Med 1993;153:862–865.
182a. Strakosch C, Wenzel B, Volpé R. Immunology of autoimmune thyroid disease. N Engl J Med 1982;307:1499–1507.
183. Chazenbalk GD, Portolano S, Russo D, Hutchison JS, Rapoport B, Mclachlan S. Human organ-specific autoimmune disease. Molecular cloning and expression of an autoantibody gene repertoire for a major autoantigen reveals an antigenic immunodominant region and restricted immunoglobulin gene usage in the target organ. J Clin Invest 1993;92:62–74.
184. Weetman AP. Thyroid peroxidase as an antigen in autoimmune thyroidits. Clin Exp Immunol 1990;80:1–3.
185. How J, Topliss DJ, Strakosch C, Lewis M, Row VV, Volpé R. T lymphocyte sensitization and suppressor T lymphocyte defect in patients long after treatment for Graves' disease. Clin Endocrinol 1983;18:61–72.
186. Weetman AP, McGregor AM, Hall R. Evidence for an effect of antithyroid drugs on the natural history of Graves' disease. Clin Endocrinol 1984;21:163–167.
187. Ratanachaiyawong S, McGregor AM. Immunosuppressive effects of antithyroid drugs. Clin Endocr Metab 1985;14:449–466.
188. Volpé R, Karlsson FA, Jansson R, Dahlberg PA. Thyrostatic drugs act through modulation of thyroid cell activity to induce remissions in Graves' disease. Acta Endocrinol 1987;115(Suppl 218):305–311.
189. Reinwein D, Benker G, Lazarus JH, Alexander WD, the European Multicentre Study Group on Antithyroid Drug treatment. A prospective randomized trial of antithyroid drug dose in Graves' disease therapy. J Clin Endocrinol Metab 1993;76:1516–1521.
190. Escobar-Morreale HF, Serrano-Gotarredona J, Villar LM, Garcia-Robles R, Gonzalez Porque P, et al. Methimazole has no dose-related effect on the serum concentrations of soluble Class I major histocompatibility complex antigens, soluble interleukin-2 receptor, and beta-2 microglobulin in patients with Graves' disease. Thyroid 1996;8:29–36.
191. Paschke R, Vogg M, Kristoferitsch R, Aktuna D, Wawschinek O, Eber O, et al. Methimazole has no dose-related effect on the intensity of the intrathyroidal autoimmune process in relapsing Graves' disease. J Clin Endocrinol Metab 1995;80:2470–2474.
192. Totterman TH, Karlsson FA, Bengtsson M, Mendel-Hartvig I. Induction of circulating activated suppressor-like T cells by methimazole therapy for Graves' disease. N Engl J Med 1987;316:5–22.
193. Koukkou E, Panayiotidis P, Alevizou-Terzaki V, Thalassinos N. High levels of serum soluble interleukin-2 receptors in hyperthyroid patients: correlation with serum thyroid hormones and independence from the etiology of the hyperthyroidism. J Clin Endocrinol Metab 1991;73:771–776.

194. Watanabe M, Amino N, Hochito K, Watanabe K, Kuma K, Iwatani Y. Opposite changes in serum soluble CD8 in patients at the active stages of Graves' and Hashimoto's diseases. Thyroid 1997;7:743–748.
195. Escobar-Morreale HF, Serrano J, Sancho JM, Varela C. Soluble intercellular adhesion molecule-1 and Graves' disease. Thyroid 1997;7:801–803.
196. Volpé R. Immunoregulation in autoimmune thyroid disease. N Engl J Med 1987;316:44–46.
197. Volpé R. Evidence that the immunosuppressive effects of anti-thyroid drugs are mediated through actions on the thyroid cell, modulating thyrocyte-immunocyte signalling: a review. Thyroid 1994;4:217–223.
198. Toft AD. Thyroxine therapy. N Engl J Med 1994;31:174–180.

10 Thyroid-Associated Ophthalmopathy and Dermopathy

Anthony P. Weetman, MD, DSc

CONTENTS

INTRODUCTION
PATHOLOGY
PREDISPOSING FACTORS
IMMUNOLOGICAL FEATURES
THERAPEUTIC ASPECTS
THYROID DERMOPATHY
REFERENCES

INTRODUCTION

Nomenclature and Clinical Signs

Various names have been given to the eye signs associated with autoimmune thyroid disease—Graves' ophthalmopathy, endocrine exophthalmos, ophthalmic Graves' disease, and so on—but the term thyroid-associated ophthalmopathy (TAO) is now generally accepted as the best, providing recognition that the condition is not always associated with Graves' disease. The major clinical signs are shown in Table 1 and Fig. 1. Fortunately TAO does not cause problems of diplopia or loss of visual fields in the majority of patients, but the impact of having bulging eyes and periorbital swelling on the patient's sense of well-being is often underestimated, and even the grittiness and discomfort that are common and among the early features of TAO prove irksome to many patients with Graves' disease.

A number of classification schemes have been proposed, but the older of these failed to take into account clinical activity and did not recognize the different ways TAO may progress. As a result, the various International Thyroid Associations have prepared a statement on the measurements and assessments recommended for the classification of patients with TAO *(1)*. The recommendations include:

1. Measurement of lid fissure.
2. Formal documentation of exposure keratitis.
3. Quantitation of extraocular muscle function.
4. Exophthalmometry or CT/MR-based measurement of proptosis.

From: *Contemporary Endocrinology: Autoimmune Endocrinopathies*
Edited by: R. Volpe © Humana Press Inc., Totowa, NJ

Table 1
Main Clinical Features of TAO[a]

Class	Signs and symptoms	Approximate frequency[b]
0	No physical signs or symptoms	40%
I	Only signs (lid lag, lid retraction), no symptoms	60%
II	Soft tissue involvement (periorbital edema) with symptoms	40%
III	Proptosis (3 mm or more)	20%
IV	Extraocular muscle dysfunction, causing diplopia	10%
V	Corneal involvement (stippling, ulceration, clouding, or necrosis)	<5%
VI	Sight loss (optic neuropathy)	1%

[a] This is the so-called NOSPECS classification system (1), which is a useful mnemonic, but is not optimal for objective assessment.

[b] In patients with Graves' disease; patients with TAO often have multiple signs.

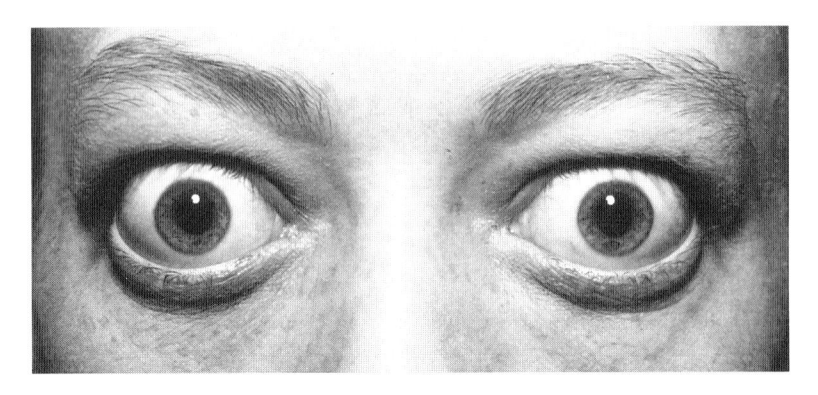

Fig. 1. Typical appearance of moderate TAO, showing lid retraction, proptosis, and periorbital edema.

5. Documentation of visual acuity, visual fields, and color vision.
6. Use of an activity score.
7. Self-assessment by the patient of the status of the eye signs and symptoms.

The value of producing a clinical activity score, derived from such a classification scheme, is underlined by the evident utility of the score in predicting the outcome of immunosuppressive treatment (2). In this survey, disease activity and not duration was the key determinant of outcome.

Relationship to Other Thyroid Disorders

The question of whether TAO is a separate disease from thyroid autoimmune disease, although closely related, has vexed investigators for decades. The presence of TAO in euthyroid individuals is in favor of TAO being a separate entity, but closer analysis of such individuals reveals varying subtle degrees of thyroid involvement. In a detailed review of the literature, comprising 589 euthyroid individuals with TAO, 50% had an abnormal thyroid on examination, 62% failed to suppress radioiodine uptake with T_3, 50% had a blunted thyroid stimulating hormone (TSH) response to thyrotropin releasing hormone (TRH), and 47% had thyroid antibodies. Overall, 89% had at least one thyroid abnormality. It is possible that our present assays are not sensitive enough to pick up low-grade abnormalities in the remaining 11%. Furthermore, TAO may be clinically evident for years before the onset of Graves' disease in some patients, although the two disorders occur within a year of each other in around two-thirds of cases. Therefore, those few TAO patients who are euthyroid and have no evidence of thyroid involvement on detailed testing could later develop thyroid autoimmunity, and only prolonged follow-up studies will determine if this is so.

In a recent survey of 120 North American TAO patients, 90% had Graves' disease, 1% had primary myxedema, 3% Hashimoto's thyroiditis, and 6% were euthyroid at presentation *(3)*. This population-based study reflects well previous estimates of the frequency of thyroid disorders in TAO *(4)*. Symptoms and signs of TAO are clinically apparent in only 50–60% of Graves' disease patients and in far fewer patients with autoimmune hypothyroidism, which has also fueled the debate about the relationship between the orbital and the thyroid diseases. It is clear, however, that more subtle evidence of TAO can be found in 40–80% of Graves' disease patients without clinical features of TAO, using imaging techniques, such as ultrasound or CT and MR scanning, to demonstrate extraocular muscle enlargement *(4,5)*. Together with those who have clinical evidence, this means that TAO is present in at least 90% of patients with Graves' disease, and it is possible that some orbital involvement, insufficient to be detected by current imaging, is present in the remainder. Much less is known about occult TAO in autoimmune hypothyroidism. In conclusion, TAO is so closely linked to thyroid autoimmunity that the orbital autoimmune process is almost certainly part of the same underlying autoimmune response as that in the thyroid (*see also* Chapter 9). The much clearer association with Graves' disease than with autoimmune hypothyroidism indicates that only a subset of that latter patients have this shared autoimmune response, which presumably is the same as that in Graves' disease.

With regard to more general epidemiology, a bimodal peak incidence rate has been found by some *(5)*, but not others *(6)*; peak incidence on average is around 45–50 yr in women and 5 yr later in men. Men are overrepresented in those Graves' disease patients with severe TAO, compared to those without obvious TAO, and patients older than 50–60 are also more likely to have severe disease *(5,6)*. Finally, euthyroid patients have fewer features of TAO than patients with abnormal thyroid function (either hypo- or hyperthyroidism) *(7)*. Different mechanisms may underlie this observation, including an association with immunological activity and the adverse effect of hypothyroidism on glycosaminoglycan production (*see* Cytokines and Fibroblast Responses).

The natural history of the disease is generally for a period of worsening, followed by stabilization after 2–3 yr, but in some patients, severe complications occur many years after the initial onset; vascular factors or fibrosis may produce these changes *(8)*. On the other hand, around 20% of patients have substantial, spontaneous improvement in eye signs 1–2 yr after onset, and a further 40% improve to a lesser degree *(9)*. Such observations clearly affect evaluation of treatment studies that do not include suitable control groups.

PATHOLOGY

Extraocular Muscles

Gross examination of affected orbits, as well as sequential imaging, show that the extraocular muscles are the first and main structures to be affected in TAO *(10,11)*. The muscles are enlarged by a combination of edema, secondary to glycosaminoglycan (GAG) accumulation, lymphocytic infiltration, and fibrosis. All extraocular muscles are

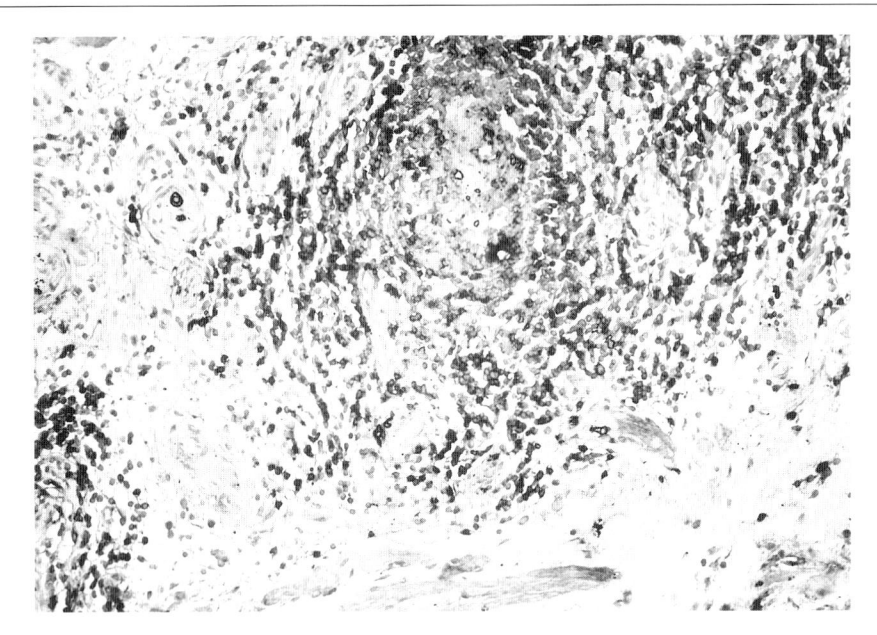

Fig. 2. Section of extraocular muscle from an untreated patient with TAO, stained with an MAb against CD45 R0, showing that the majority of infiltrating lymphocytes are activated/memory T cells. Muscle cells (bottom of picture) are intact, but separated by edema (original magnification ×400).

affected by these changes, but there is often asymmetry, with the medial and inferior recti showing the most pronounced changes. The lymphocytic infiltrate is primarily lymphocytic, with some macrophages and plasma cells, and is both diffuse and focal, particularly around blood vessels where mast cells also occur. The fibroblasts in the interstitium are enlarged and increased in number, and associated with GAG and collagen deposition. The majority component of the GAG accumulation is hyaluronate *(12)*. The resulting muscle swelling is responsible for the clinical features shown in Table 1. In particular, optic neuropathy is caused by compression of the nerve at the apex of the orbit, and those patients with minimal proptosis, but acute muscle enlargement, are still at risk. This is because patients whose orbital anatomy permits a greater degree of proptosis have, to some extent, decompression of the orbital contents.

Later, the lymphocytic infiltrate appears to diminish, although this may be the result of immunomodulatory treatment as well as time. Fibrous bundles compress and atrophy; dense scarring is a feature of burnt-out disease that results in impaired muscle action. Changes within the muscle cells themselves, even by electron microscopy, are not a feature of the early stages of TAO, and any degeneration is believed to be the result of later fibrosis *(10,13)*. Another late and inconsistent feature is fatty infiltration of the muscles.

Immunohistochemical analysis of the lymphocytic infiltrate (Fig. 2) shows that this is predominantly composed of $CD4^+$ and $CD8^+$ T cells, many of which are activated *(13,14)*. The interstitial cells, most likely fibroblasts, express HLA class II and intercellular adhesion molecule-1 (ICAM-1), particularly in the early phase of disease, and the vascular endothelial cells are activated, as shown by expression of E-selectin (ELAM-1) and vascular cell adhesion molecule-1 *(14–16)*. The muscle cells, in contrast, do not express class II or adhesion molecules.

In summary, the extraocular muscles are the key tissues affected by the disease process in TAO, but it is the interstitial fibroblasts, rather than the muscle cells themselves, which are the main cellular targets. The muscles become swollen by a predominantly T-cell lymphocytic infiltrate and edema, secondary to GAG accumulation. Later, fibrosis and fatty infiltration also affect muscle function, but in the early stages of the disease, it is the muscle swelling that produces proptosis, periorbital edema, diplopia, and optic neuropathy.

Other Tissues

The levator palpebrae superioris muscle is affected by a distinct pathological process in TAO, comprising muscle fiber enlargement with minimal evidence of inflammatory changes *(17)*. In common with the extraocular muscles, the fibers are in an edematous matrix; fibrosis and fatty infiltration are less commonly found. It remains unclear how much this hypertrophy of the muscle fibers contributes to the lid lag and retraction of TAO, and how it is caused. However, the description of a unique pathology in the upper eyelid of TAO patients accounts for the increased frequency and severity of these signs in TAO compared to other hyperthyroid states, in which β-adrenergic stimulation of the eyelid is the only cause of lid retraction.

The retrobulbar adipose tissue is often increased in TAO and contributes to proptosis. In some patients, without prominent extraocular muscle involvement, this increase in fat volume has been proposed to result from enlargement of the superior rectus muscle, which reduces venous outflow from the orbit *(18)*. Such venous obstruction may also contribute to the changes seen in more typical patients with generalized extraocular muscle involvement. Even less commonly, patients with apparent TAO have inflammation in the orbital fat in the absence of any muscle enlargement *(19)*, but a detailed analysis of such cases has not been performed.

Intracranial herniation of orbital fat through the superior ophthalmic fissure is an important imaging feature that associates strongly with the presence of optic neuropathy in TAO, especially in the context of apical crowding *(20)*. This emphasizes the importance of the retrobulbar adipose tissue in TAO, and further work is necessary to determine whether changes in this compartment are all secondary to a primary autoimmune response in the extraocular muscles. In support of a related autoimmune process is the description of lymphocytic infiltration in retrobulbar tissues from TAO patients, composed predominantly of $CD4^+$ and $CD8^+$ T cells, in association with expression of HLA-DR and ICAM-1 on adipose cells *(21)*.

Finally, the lacrimal gland may be involved with similar connective tissue changes to those seen in the extraocular muscles *(10)*. There is a variable lymphocytic infiltrate, and fibrosis tends to be mild, so that the glandular structures are rarely affected.

PREDISPOSING FACTORS

Immunogenetics

Many attempts have been made to determine whether Graves' disease patients with TAO differ immunogenetically from those with clinically evident TAO, and some of the conflicting results that have arisen may stem from differences in the criteria used for diagnosing the presence or severity of TAO. Indeed, the basis for such studies can be questioned, since the majority of clinically unaffected Graves' disease patients will have subclinical disease *(5)* and penetrance is incomplete, as shown by the late onset of complications in some patients *(8)*. However, by comparing patients with the most severe TAO (e.g., requiring orbital surgery) with clinically unaffected subjects with Graves' disease, the effect of candidate genes on exacerbating the orbital autoimmune response might be determined.

Initial studies focused on HLA class I and II genes, and a significant increase in HLA-Bw35 was reported in 14 patients with severe TAO responding to corticosteroids when compared to controls, and those with severe disease who did not respond to steroids *(22)*. However, there was only a weak association between Bw35 and severe TAO overall, and this has not been reproduced *(23)*. Others have reported a highly significant association of TAO with HLA-DR3, greater than in Graves' disease without obvious TAO, and a complex effect of HLA-DR7, which appeared to enhance the risk for TAO in HLA-B8-negative Graves' patients and protect against it in the absence of HLA-B8 *(24)*. A subsequent study from the same group failed to find any difference between Graves' patients with and without ophthalmopathy in the frequency of HLA-B8 and DR3 *(25)*, but a negative association was observed with HLA-DR4. However, there were no differences in HLA class I and DR gene frequencies in other surveys, including one using molecular typing methods *(23,26)*. HLA-DPB1*0201 appears to be reduced in Caucasian patients with severe TAO compared to controls and Graves' disease without TAO *(27)*. This has been confirmed in Japanese patients with TAO who were hyperthyroid; HLA-DPw2 was significantly lower than in controls, but patients without clinical TAO did not differ from the control population *(28)*.

Only a limited number of other candidate genes have been proposed for susceptibility to Graves' disease, and there have been no positive associations with TAO. An increase in blood group P in TAO patients *(23)* has not been confirmed *(29)*. The low frequency of TAO in Asian patients with Graves' disease suggests the effect of some genetic susceptibility factor, but this remains to be identified *(30)*.

Nongenetic Factors

There are more men with severe TAO in Graves' disease populations than expected, and this disorder also occurs in older patients *(5,6)*, suggesting the influence of a culmulative environment factor. These epidemiological results seem to be explained by the adverse effects of smoking, first reported in a small series of patients *(31)* and subsequently confirmed by many groups (reviewed in *32*). The relative risk conferred by smoking is around 3. A dose effect is apparent, and the risk is most clearly related to current rather than lifetime tobacco consumption *(33)*. Smoking has no race-specific effect and remains associated with TAO in Asians with a low prevalence of TAO *(30)*. The possible reasons for this association are discussed below. No other environmental factors have been shown to influence the initiation of TAO. As in so many aspects of TAO, the absence of an animal model has slowed progress, preventing a detailed exploration of the influence of candidate environmental factors on the orbital autoimmune process.

IMMUNOLOGICAL FEATURES

The most widely accepted hypothesis to explain the clinical and pathological features of TAO is that autoreactive lymphocytes in the extraocular muscles are stimulated by an autoantigen that is the same as or is crossreactive with an autoantigen in the thyroid *(34,35)*.

This leads to fibroblast stimulation, most likely cytokine-mediated, and hence, GAG and collagen production. The key questions are the nature of the autoantigen and the mechanism by which fibroblast stimulation occurs. Linked to these issues is controversy over the role of autoantibodies in the pathogenesis of TAO, and this will be considered first.

Autoantibodies

CONVENTIONAL THYROID AUTOANTIBODIES

A number of studies have examined the levels of thyroid autoantibodies in patients with TAO to determine whether patients with Graves' disease and severe TAO can be distinguished serologically from those without clinical evidence of TAO, and to identify or exclude potential crossreactive autoantigens. This second aim has the drawback that the absence of particular autoantibodies does not preclude a reaction against the target autoantigen at the T-cell level; in addition, localized production of autoantibodies in the orbit could have pathological effects without being detectable in serum.

In agreement with older studies reviewed elsewhere *(4)*, a detailed evaluation of 63 patients with severe TAO found that 88% had TSH receptor (TSHR) antibodies, 60% had thyroid peroxidase (TPO) antibodies, and 25% had thyroglobulin (Tg) antibodies *(36)*. These frequencies did not differ significantly from Graves' disease patients without TAO, but in the Tg antibody-positive subgroup of TAO patients, the antibody response was shifted to the IgG_4 subclass (suggesting a more chronic response), and the levels of TSHR antibody were higher. The basis for such a subdivision of TAO patients is unclear, since Tg antibody-positive TAO patients do not appear clinically distinct.

The low frequency of Tg antibodies in TAO patients suggests, but does not prove that autoreactivity against this autoantigen is unlikely to be important in initiating TAO. Early studies, particularly those generating Tg monoclonal antibodies (MAb), which crossreacted with eye muscle membranes *(37,38)*, indicated that Tg may be important because of crossreactivity with a similar or identical orbital autoantigen. The description of homology between acetylcholinesterase (AChE) and Tg, and a shared epitope identified by screening a thyroid cDNA library, makes AChE a candidate orbital antigen *(39)*. However, there is no clear relationship between AChE and Tg antibodies, and the presence of AChE antibodies is not restricted to patients with TAO *(40,41)*. This does not exclude crossreactivity between the two antigens at the T-cell level as a pathogenic mechanism in TAO, but transfer of AChE antibodies to rats produces an autoimmune preganglionic sympathectomy *(42)*. Therefore, it is likely that either cell-mediated or humoral autoimmunity would induce an autonomic neuropathy rather than extraocular muscle pathology in humans.

As discussed below (The TSHR as an Autoantigen in TAO), considerable interest has been aroused in the TSHR as a critical crossreactive antigen *(43)* and studies that have examined TSHR antibodies in TAO have an important bearing on this suggestion. Using the assay for TSHR binding inhibitory immunoglobulins (TBII), no association was found between antibody levels and the severity or duration of TAO, nor with response to immunotherapy *(44)*. This has been confirmed recently *(45,46)*, but when TSHR-stimulating antibodies (TSAb) were measured, there was a correlation between the presence of eye disease and its activity (estimated by MR imaging), and the level of TSAb *(45)*. Furthermore, all five patients with TAO and hypothyroidism in one study had both TBII and TSAb, indicating some relationship between TSHR antibodies and TAO *(47)*.

More euthyroid and hypothyroid patients are clearly needed to be certain of these results, and the lack of correlation between TBII levels and TAO means that any association is likely to be with reactivity against unique TSHR epitopes only recognized by TSAb. At present, the best conclusion seems to be that TSHR reactivity is a very frequent finding in TAO patients, but present data using modern assays are inadequate to assess whether it is universal.

Eye Muscle Autoantibodies

There have been many attempts to identify specific eye muscle antibodies in TAO patients, particularly using the ELISA and immunoblot techniques *(48–58)*. The lack of agreement between these studies, which are summarized in Table 2, is in part owing to differences in the substrate used (human or porcine extraocular muscle or orbital connective tissue), methodology, and the level of binding designated as positive. The ELISA suffers from the heterogeneity of proteins contained in any muscle extract and detects antibodies of low affinity whose pathological relevance is uncertain. Immunoblotting utilizes gel fractionation to overcome the first of these drawbacks, but suffers from the problems arising with denaturation of proteins, making it appropriate only for antibodies that do not depend on recognition of conformational determinants. In addition, immunoblotting is relatively insensitive, and the presence or absence of bands depends on the time of exposure, for radiolabeled or chemiluminescent methods, or incubation in substrate, for enzyme-based methods.

Although eye muscle antibodies reacting in the ELISA methods were initially believed to be site-specific *(48)*, subsequent studies showed that there was crossreactivity with skeletal muscle, thyroid and liver *(49–51,53)*. Detailed analysis by radioimmunoassay (RIA) revealed that this was, in part, owing to antibodies in TAO sera against myosin, actin, and acetylcholine receptor *(59)*. Although in several studies the frequency of eye muscle antibodies was higher in Graves' disease patients with TAO, compared to those without TAO, the frequency of antibodies in TAO has never approached 100%, and in some series, there has been little difference between these patient groups and controls (Table 2). As well as reflecting an orbital autoimmune process, patients with TAO may have a more intense intrathyroidal autoimmune response, and the ELISA results could reflect a nonspecific set of autoantibodies or the production of antibodies secondary to extraocular muscle injury.

Although immunoblotting has failed to reveal specific autoantibodies in several studies *(50,51,53,58)*, Wall and colleagues have consistently detected antibodies against a 64-kDa protein in up to 75% of patients with active TAO, as well as less frequent antibodies against 55-kDa and 95-kDa proteins *(52,55)*. The frequency of 64-kDa antibodies in controls is disputed, with a low frequency in the latter studies, but a higher frequency (although lower titer) in others *(54)*, suggesting that these are natural autoantibodies. The identification of a 64-kDa protein, called 1D, by screening an eye muscle cDNA library with sera from patients with autoimmune thyroid disease suggested a candidate autoantigen *(60)*. Despite initial evidence that antibodies against this protein are associated with TAO, being found in 71% of patients with recent-onset disease, antibodies were also found in 24% of controls and 1D was unable to absorb out 64-kDa reactivity in immunoblots *(61)*. Others have found the highest frequency of 1D antibodies in Hashimoto's thyroiditis and a widespread tissue distribution of this autoantigen, making it unlikely to have any major role in TAO *(62)*.

Table 2
Summary of Results Using ELISA and Immunoblotting to Detect Eye Muscle Autoantibodies[a]

Study	Antigen and source	ELISA	Immunoblot	Comment
Atkinson et al. (48)	Porcine EM	+	ND	Ab in 64% TAO+ and 5% GD TAO−
Kadlubowski et al. (49)	Porcine EM	ND[b]	ND	Ab in 25% GD sera, independent of TAO
Ahmann et al. (50)	Porcine EM	+	+	Ab in 42% TAO+ and 23% GD TAO−; multiple antigens by immunoblot
Schifferdecker et al. (51)	Human EM	+	+	Ab in 10% TAO+ and 14% GD TAO−; no disease-specific antigens by immunoblot
Salvi et al. (52)	Human EM	ND	+	64-kDa protein recognized by 55% TAO+ sera and not by controls; reactivity also against 50, 58, and 85-kDa proteins
Weightman and Kendall-Taylor (53)	Porcine EM	ND	+	Multiple antigens; 64-kDa reactivity in controls
Kendler et al. (54)	Human EM	ND	+	64-kDa reactivity in 30–38% of sera, including controls
Salvi et al. (55)	Porcine EM	ND	+	64-kDa reactivity in active TAO; 55- and 95-kDa reactivity in many of these patients
Chang et al. (56)	Porcine EM	ND	+	55-kDa reactivity in 47% of GD sera with CT evidence of TAO and in 11% of controls; 64-kDa reactivity in TAO and controls
Hiromatsu et al. (57)	Rat EM	ND	+	64-kDa reactivity in 71% of TAO sera and 35% of Hashimoto's sera
Tandon et al. (58)	Porcine and Human EM	+	+	No differences between TAO and controls for IgG antibodies

[a] Ab = antibodies; EM = eye muscle; ND = not done; GD = Graves' disease.
[b] Based on radioimmunoassay.

Further evidence for involvement of a 64-kDa autoantigen has come from purification by solubilization of porcine eye muscle membranes and isoelectric focusing under nondenaturing conditions. Using this material in immunoblots, reactive antibodies were found in 64% of patients with TAO, 38% with Graves' disease, but clinically absent in TAO, 11% with Hashimoto's thyroiditis, and 13% of healthy controls *(63)*. Many of the positive sera also reacted in an assay of antibody-dependent cell-mediated cytotoxicity (ADCC) using human eye muscle cells, but there was no significant correlation between the two tests, suggesting the existence of two separate antibody–antigen systems. Further analysis has shown the absence of this solubilized 64-kDa protein in skeletal muscle, and such site specificity, linked with expression in thyroid tissue *(52)*, makes the antigen of particular significance to the understanding of TAO *(64)*. It is still unclear why so many other groups have been unable to detect a high frequency of 64-kDa antibodies in TAO (Table 2), and it is only with the cloning of this protein that these discrepancies will be resolved and the role of the 64-kDa protein in TAO will be clarified.

Fibroblast Antibodies

If fibroblasts are the main target cell in the autoimmune process causing TAO, it makes sense to look for antibodies to fibroblasts; by culturing such cells, a relatively homogeneous population can be used in assays, thereby overcoming the problems associated with crude extraocular muscle antigen preparations. Of course, the presence of such antibodies does not necessarily imply that these have a pathogenic role, but would support the involvement of fibroblasts in the autoimmune response and shed light on the nature of the putative thyroid crossreactive antigen.

In the first such study, fibroblasts derived from retrobulbar connective tissue and from skin were used to perform immunoblots, and antibodies against a 23-kDa protein were found in 56% of Graves' disease sera, irrespective of TAO, and were also present in 15% of normal controls *(65)*. Using whole fibroblasts coated to ELISA plates, no TAO-specific IgG binding could be detected, but by immunoblotting, fibroblast proteins of 80 and 92-kDa were recognized by significantly more TAO patients than controls *(58)*. No 23-kDa binding was found. In addition, IgA class antibodies binding to whole fibroblasts in ELISA were present in more TAO sera than controls and these were particularly obvious in patients with TAO and dermopathy (*see* Thyroid Dermopathy *below*), reacting with both dermal and orbital fibroblasts *(66)*. By immunoblotting, these IgA antibodies recognized a 54-kDa protein in dermal fibroblasts and a 66-kDa protein in retrobulbar fibroblasts. The antigens appeared to be crossreactive, and also were crossreactive with proteins derived from thyroid. This involvement of IgA rather than IgG class antibodies has previously been observed in an ELISA based on eye muscle cytosol extract as substrate *(67)*, but it is unclear if it was a fibroblast-derived protein in the substrate, which gave these results. Others have found no increased binding of IgG to porcine or human retrobulbar fibroblasts by ELISA *(68)*.

In summary, fibroblast antibodies have been detected by various assays at increased frequency in TAO sera, yet also occur in some control sera. IgA class fibroblast antibodies seem to be the most specific, but the retrobulbar fibroblasts are not antigenically unique, sharing expression of autoantigens with dermal fibroblasts.

Other Antibodies

Several other techniques have been employed to detect eye muscle-specific antibodies in TAO. Antibodies capable of mediating ADCC have already been mentioned *(63)* and contrast with the failure of these antibodies to fix complement *(69)*. Although this was suggested to be because of IgG$_3$ subclass predominance, antibodies binding to eye muscle membranes in ELISA are mainly IgG$_1$ and IgG$_2$, with little IgG$_3$ *(58)*. Patients with Hodgkin's disease treated with mantle irradiation are at risk of developing Graves' disease, and eye muscle ADCC has been reported in such patients, although in the absence of TAO and other thyroid or 64-kDa eye muscle antibodies *(70)*. Although it is tempting to speculate that such ADCC may signal an early autoimmune response triggered by thyroid damage, it could equally suggest lack of disease specificity with this assay.

Two novel autoantibodies have been described by Kendall-Taylor and colleagues. The first set, termed eye muscle-stimulating antibodies, was detected by the ability of IgGs prepared from TAO sera to stimulate proliferation of porcine extraocular myoblasts *(71)*. There was a significant correlation between these antibodies and those binding to extraocular muscle membranes in an ELISA, but not with conventional thyroid antibodies, nor with clinical severity of TAO. It is difficult to envisage how such antibodies would operate in pathogenesis since the extraocular muscles are not hyperplastic, but a role is possible in the hypertrophy of the levator palpebrae muscle (although there is no firm evidence for or against hyperplasia in this site). The second set of antibodies inhibited binding of insulin-like growth factor 1 (IGF-1) to orbital fibroblasts, and IgGs with this activity were found in 52% of Graves' sera, when compared to controls *(72)*. The majority of strongly positive sera were from patients with TAO, but unfortunately, no information was provided about the correlation between these antibodies and those stimulating myoblast proliferation. Given the wide distribution of IGF-1 and its receptor, a discreet effect on orbital tissue in TAO is hard to imagine for IGF-1 receptor antibodies.

A more radical approach to studying eye muscle antibodies is to produce immunoglobulin heavy- and light- chain libraries from the orbital tissues of TAO patients, on the grounds that B cells infiltrating these sites will be enriched for autoantibody-producing cells. Such libraries could then be used to construct phage display systems that would allow screening of candidate autoantigens. Despite evidence for restricted variable gene usage (for IgG heavy and κ light chains), compatible with clonal B-cell expansion in the orbital tissue *(73)*, this technique has not been pursued. The fact that IgA heavy chains can also be amplified from TAO orbital tissue at least supports the involvement of this class of antibodies in TAO *(74)*.

T-Cell-Mediated Immune Responses

A major problem bedeviling research on TAO, in the absence of an animal model, is the difficulty of accessing the orbital tissues. Even when possible, biopsy is usually late in the disease process and after administration of immunomodultory treatment. As a consequence, the peripheral blood is often used as a source of T cells for study of cell-mediated responses, but this compartment may only reflect poorly (if at all) what is happening in the orbit. The difficulties are further compounded by the concurrent thyroid autoimmunity, and nonspecific changes in the blood may reflect either or both responses.

CIRCULATING T CELLS

The simplest, but least informative analysis is of circulating T-cell phenotypes. A reduced proportion of CD8$^+$ T cells is frequent in Graves' disease, whereas euthyroid patients with severe TAO had elevated circulating CD8$^+$ numbers, which returned to normal after successful treatment with corticosteroids *(75)*. CD4$^+$ T-cell numbers were normal in this study, although a subsequent re-examination and review of subset distribution in euthyroid TAO found a significant increase in CD4+ T cells, and no significant changes in CD8+ T cells *(76)*. The change in CD4+ cells correlated with the severity of TAO. The phenotypes of infiltrating T cells in the orbit is discussed in the Extraocular Muscles section.

Circulating NK cell activity is suppressed in euthyroid patients with TAO, yet normal in Graves' disease without clinical TAO, and this defect seemed to be owing to impaired release of a soluble factor *(77)*. It is difficult to see how this defect fits with what is known about the disease pathogenesis. More clearly defined soluble markers of cell-mediated immunity have also been studied in the sera of TAO patients. In euthyroid TAO patients, soluble ICAM-1, interleukin-2 (IL-2) receptor, and IL-1 receptor antagonist (RA) are all elevated in a proportion of patients and decline with successful treatment *(78–80)*. Notably, patients who smoked had lower levels of IL-1 RA and a worse therapeutic outcome than nonsmokers, suggesting that the adverse effects of smoking could be mediated through suppression of this important regulatory molecule.

T-Cell Functional Studies

Early studies are reviewed in detail elsewhere *(81)*. Only weak circulating T-cell proliferative responses occur in response to human or porcine eye muscle membranes in TAO; the most consistent results appeared after CD8+ T-cell depletion in response to proteins of 25–50 kDa *(82)*. In this study, 1D-reactive T cells were not found in TAO patients. In a complicated series of experiments, circulating T cells from TAO patients were stimulated by autologous fibroblasts, but the numbers were too small for statistical analysis *(83)*. A more comprehensive study, involving orbital T cells expanded in vitro, has also shown that fibroblasts can stimulate autologous T cells in TAO, in this case CD8+ T-cell lines *(84)*. Of great interest is the fact that only one of the four lines studied was cytotoxic, but all released interferon γ (IFN-γ), IL-4, and IL-10. This is compatible with the model of pathogenesis based on cytokine-mediated fibroblast proliferation. Although the necessary period of culture may have altered the T cells' behavior and, therefore, the results cannot be generalized, this approach opens up the possibility of identifying a fibroblast autoantigen critical to TAO.

In some contrast to these results, expansion of TAO retrobulbar T cells, under different culture condition, led to a predominance of cytotoxic T cells in T-cell lines, with more CD8+ cells than in peripheral blood-derived lines *(85)*. These cytotoxic T cells had a T_H1-like cytokine profile, secreting IL-2, IFN-γ, and tumor necrosis factor (TNF), and the results were similar to those obtained with intrathyroidal T cells in Hashimoto's thyroiditis. However, the absence of any antigen specificity data restricts the importance of these observations, since cytotoxicity was evaluated by killing of a mastocytoma cell line and thus is NK-cell-like; the pathogenic relevance of this in vivo is unknown.

Two other recent studies have studied cultured orbital T cells, and in both, the T-cell lines were predominantly CD4+ *(86,87)*. One set of T cells responded to proteins of 6–10 kDa derived from autologous adipose tissue and connective tissue, and similar proteins were present in thyroid, suggesting a shared autoantigen *(85)*. In the other study, responses to extracts of extraocular muscle and thyroid were observed with two T-cell lines, both of which also responded to TSHR, implicating this as an autoantigen *(87)*.

Another new approach has been to analyze T-cell receptor (TCR) variable (V) region gene usage by the infiltrating T cells, utilizing the techniques of reverse transcriptase-polymerase chain reaction (RT-PCR). Demonstration of restricted heterogeneity of V gene usage suggests clonal expansion, most likely of specific autoreactive T cells. Two studies from the same group have found restricted Vα and Vβ gene usage in extraocular muscle and orbital connective tissue derived from patients with acute, severe TAO *(88,89)*. Greater diversity of Vβ usage and loss of Vα restriction was found in samples from patients with more chronic disease *(88)*. Moreover, similar TCR restriction was present in thyroid, retrobulbar tissues, and pretibial skin in two patients with Graves' disease, TAO, and dermopathy, suggesting sharing of T cells at these sites *(89)*. Reproduction of these results is awaited, particularly since quantitative results are very difficult to achieve with this method, and the perforce limited muscle sample size available from patients with acute TAO may not reflect the entire orbital process. Nonetheless, these results, and the others detailed in this section, indicate the power of modern techniques to begin analysis of the retrobulbar immune response, and are compatible with a major role for T cells, possibly stimulated by fibroblast autoantigens, which remain to be characterized. The consequences of these are discussed in the next section.

Cytokines and Fibroblast Responses

In the absence of muscle cell destruction, and given the primary role for GAG accumulation in pathogenesis *(12)*, current research is focused on the interaction between extraocular muscle fibroblasts and the inflammatory infiltrate. The pattern of cytokine production is complex, and divergent results are probably explicable through differences in disease stage and tissues sampled. Immunoreactivity for IL-1α, TNF-α, and IFN-γ was found in five of six samples from TAO retrobulbar connective and fatty tissue, all of which had a mononuclear infiltrate, although the fibroblasts themselves were shown to be producing IL-1 *(90)*. The more sensitive RT-PCR technique has allowed small biopsies to be tested, and IL-2, IL-4, IL-5, and IL-10 could all be amplified from a single extraocular muscle specimen, whereas IL-2, IL-4, and IL-10 were found in some, but not all connective tissue specimens, and IFN-γ could not be detected *(91)*.

A more extensive study of 12 eye muscle specimens taken from 5 patients with chronic TAO demonstrated IL-1α, IL-2, and IL-10 in 25%, IL-4, IL-8, and TNF-α in 67%, and IL-6 and IL-15 in 42 and 33%, respectively *(87)*. IL-1β, IL-12, IL-13, and IFN-γ were not detected but T cells derived by culture from extraocular muscles produced IFN-γ, as well as IL-4 and IL-10 in vitro. The demonstration of cytokine mRNA and protein in retrobulbar tissue in TAO, even in chronic disease, often previously treated with steroids, has led to further work examining how such cytokines could affect fibroblast function.

IL-1, transforming growth factor (TGF)-β, TNF-α, and IFN-γ all stimulate GAG synthesis, predominantly hyaluronate, by fibroblasts *(92–94)*, and differences in responses between retrobulbar and dermal fibroblasts suggest that the apparent site specificity of the autoimmune process in TAO could be owing to qualitative differences in the behavior of orbital fibroblasts (Table 3). Hypoxia also enhances basal and cytokine-stimulated GAG synthesis by fibroblasts, which could explain the adverse effects of smoking *(94)* in addition to the previously mentioned effects on IL-1RA synthesis *(80)*; indeed it is possible these two activities are related. Other factors may also be involved in fibroblast activation, including IGF-1 *(95)* and prostaglandin E_2 *(96)*, but these have been less well characterized. Particular attention has focused on thyroid hormones, since of course hypothyroidism is associated with generalized myxedema and GAG accumulation *(12)*.

Table 3
Characteristics of Retrobulbar and Dermal Fibroblasts[a]

Characteristic	Fibroblast course Retrobulbar	Dermal	References
GAG synthesis induced by			
IFN-γ	+	0	93,94
IL-1	++	+	94
GAG synthesis inhibited by			
T_3	+	++	97
Dexamethasone	+	++	97
DNA synthesis induced by			
IL-1	–	+	94
TNF	0	+	94
PGE_2-induced morphologic and impedance change	+[b]	NT	96
Monosialoganglioside content	+	++	98
HLA-DR expression induced by IFN-γ	+[b]	+[c]	99
hsp expression	+[b]	+[c]	99

[a]NT = not tested; – = inhibition; 0 = no effect; + = stimulation; ++ = strong stimulation.
[b]Response enhanced in TAO, but not normal retrobulbar fibroblasts.
[c]Response enhanced in dermopathy, but not normal dermal fibroblasts.

T3 undoubtedly inhibits GAG production by fibroblasts, and therefore there are strong theoretical grounds for avoiding hypothyroidism in patients with TAO. Retrobulbar fibroblasts appear to be less susceptible to T3-mediated effects than those from other sites, but unfortunately, the same applies to the suppression of GAG synthesis by glucocorticoids (97), which may explain in part the failure of steroid treatment in some patients.

A variety of other properties have been described in retrobulbar fibroblasts that are qualitatively or quantitatively unique (Table 3). Of these, increased expression of HLA-DR in response to IFN-γ, and basal and induced expression of heat-shock protein (hsp)-70, are different in fibroblasts derived from patients with TAO when compared to normals (99,100). The reason for this change in behavior with disease, which persists through several passages in culture, is unknown. As described above (Pathology), fibroblasts express HLA-DR in TAO and also express hsp-70 (101); only a single report has identified DR and hsp expression in the muscle cells themselves in TAO (102), and the reasons for this difference is unknown, although disease duration may be one factor. The expression of hsp by fibroblasts clearly implies that they are under stress, and is presumably the result of exposure to cytokines, reactive oxygen metabolites, and other phlogistic molecules. It is also possible that HLA-DR expression by fibroblasts allows antigen presentation to T cells, which could exacerbate the autoimmune process, although in the absence of evidence of costimulatory molecule expression, this is probably not sufficient to initiate autoimmunity.

Another mechanism whereby fibroblasts may interact with the immune system is suggested by observations on the rheumatoid synovium, which demonstrate that fibroblasts actively inhibit T-cell apoptosis, via an integrin interaction and also possibly by production of hyaluronate (103). Such inhibition, occurring in the orbital tissues, could contribute to the lymphocyte infiltration seen in untreated disease, rather than this simply being the result of recruitment via migration through activated endothelial cells (104). A summary of the probable pathogenic mechanisms in TAO is shown in Fig. 3.

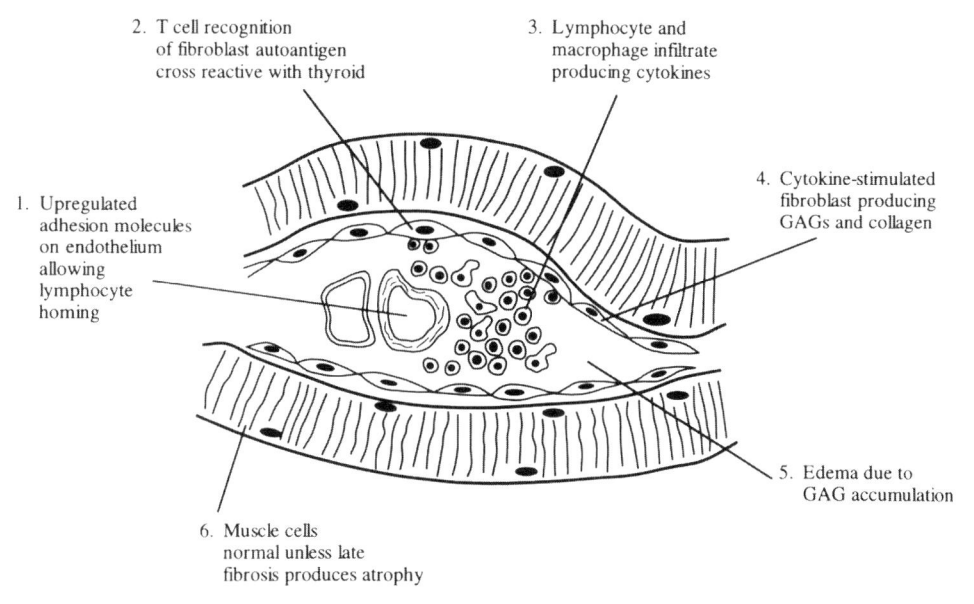

Fig. 3. Probable mechanisms in the pathogenesis of TAO.

The TSHR as an Autoantigen in TAO

The main unsolved problem in TAO is the identity of the autoantigen, presumed to be crossreactive with thyroid, which causes TAO. Much of the work on extraocular muscle and other autoantibodies described in Autoantibodies has been directed at determining what the antigen might be, and it is apparent that there are several potential, but poorly characterized candidates whose cloning will allow a proper assessment of any role they may have. Of the well-characterized candidates, the TSHR has emerged as the strongest contender and is worth further consideration.

Analysis of TSHR autoantibodies in TAO patients (Conventional Thyroid Autoantibodies) provides inconclusive support for involvement, particularly since the autoimmune response in TAO seems likely to depend on T-cell rather than B-cell responses. Despite initial reports that TSHR antibodies in TAO patients' sera can stimulate fibroblasts *(105)*, these results have not been reproduced, and neither TSH nor TSHR antibodies can stimulate GAG synthesis by fibroblasts in vitro *(106–108)*. Thus, any involvement of the TSHR in TAO seems unlikely to be antibody-mediated, but the presence of the receptor in the orbit might allow TSHR-specific T cells, activated in the thyroid, to mount an autoimmune response. It is difficult to accommodate the failure of the thyroid to accumulate GAG and become edematous in such a scenario, since the crossreactive T cells are presumably present in the thyroid, but site-specific differences in fibroblast behavior (Table 3) could account for this.

Despite such problems, many groups have searched for TSHR in orbital tissues using RT-PCR, and the results remain confusing, particularly because different conditions and primers have been used for PCR *(108,109)* and variable or unspecified fat contamination of specimens has occurred: adipose cells are known to contain TSHR *(110,111)*. Detailed reviews of these experiments have appeared *(43,109)*, and therefore, only a brief summary of the key studies is given here. Mixed retrobulbar tissue was first shown to express full-length TSHR mRNA transcripts by RT-PCR, but fibroblasts and extraocular muscle

Table 4
Summary of Main Aspects of Management of TAO

Mild disease
  Reassurance and advice (stop smoking; eye protection; sleeping with head elevated)
  Artificial tears and simple eye ointment
  Diuretics
Severe disease
  Corticosteroids (oral or iv)
  Radiotherapy (usually 10 fractionated doses of 2 gy)
  Other immunosuppressive agents (azathioprine, cyclosporine A)
  Intravenous immunoglobulin (IVIG)
  Octreotide
  Plasma exchange
  Orbital decompression
Stable or burnt-out disease
  Correction of diplopia with prisms
  Rehabilitative surgery for diplopia and cosmetically disabling signs; generally needed after decompression

samples were negative *(112)*. Subsequently, part or all of the extracellular domain mRNA has been found in retrobulbar fibroblasts *(113,114)*, whereas others have found only a 1.3-kb variant TSHR transcript in extraocular muscles and one of three retrobulbar fibroblast cell lines *(108)*. More recently, full-length and variant TSHR was detected in extraocular muscle, but not skeletal muscle *(115)*, and a relationship between the quantity of TSHR expression in orbital fat tissue and the severity of TAO was reported *(116)*. Orbital fibroblasts were also positive for TSHR mRNA in this latter report, but it is noteworthy that Northern blot analysis of TSHR mRNA was negative. This raises serious questions about the physiological or immunological relevance of mRNA detectable only by RT-PCR, generally after a considerable number (30–35) of amplification cycles, and suggests that some of the signals could be owing to illegitimate transcription. This is supported by the amplification of Tg, TPO, and even CD25 mRNA from fibroblasts under similar conditions *(117)*.

The demonstration of TSHR protein in the orbit would clearly answer these uncertainties. Murine monoclonal or porcine and rabbit polyclonal antibodies against TSHR peptides have been used to show immunohistochemical staining for TSHR in cultured human retrobulbar fibroblasts, immunoblots of fibroblast proteins, and in situ fibroblasts in orbital tissue sections *(118–120)*. Others, however, have failed to demonstrate TSHR by immunohistochemistry in orbital tissue in TAO, using MAbs against different TSHR peptides *(116)*. More conclusive results will come from the use of human or murine MAbs recognizing conformational epitopes on the TSHR. At present, the TSHR is a clear, but controversial candidate autoantigen in TAO with too many discrepancies in the results to date to be confident that the holy grail of TAO research has been found.

THERAPEUTIC ASPECTS

Many patients require only reassurance and nonspecific treatments to ease their eye symptoms, and when disease is stable, surgery can be used to correct diplopia and restore a more normal appearance (Table 4). These aspects of TAO management are considered in detail elsewhere *(4)*, and this section will focus, although briefly, on two areas of particular immunological interest, namely the effect of treatment for coincident hyperthyroidism on TAO and the responses to immunotherapeutic agents.

Effect of Thyroid Treatment

Many attempts have been made to examine the effect of antithyroid drugs, thyroidectomy and radioiodine on progression of TAO (reviewed in *4*), but these have generally suffered from being retrospective and poorly controlled. Since periods of stabilization and spontaneous remission are unpredictable, the need for appropriate controls is obvious. Fresh interest in this area was aroused by the hypothesis of a crossreactive thyroid/orbital antigen, which when released after destructive thyroid treatment, could trigger or exacerbate TAO, and an assessment of the impact of radioiodine was made *(121)*. In patients with TAO receiving radioiodine, 56% had mild to moderate worsening of periorbital swelling and extraocular muscle function, whereas there was no deterioration in a similar group that also received prophylactic treatment with steroids. In the absence of a control group, untreated with radioiodine, the results of this trial clearly show that steroids are beneficial in TAO, but cannot be taken as proof that radioiodine worsens TAO. A randomized allocation of Graves' patients to the three main treatment modalities showed that 10% of patients receiving medical treatment and 16% having subtotal thyroidectomy experienced the development or worsening of TAO, compared to 33% of those treated with radioiodine *(122)*. Despite randomization, however, there were more smokers in the radioiodine group, and these patients also became hypothyroid more frequently. These factors may have influenced outcome more than the radioiodine itself. Adding antithyroid drugs has no effect on any worsening of TAO after radioiodine *(123)*, but again this study failed to provide a suitable control group from which to judge whether worsening was induced rather than spontaneous. Some have even argued from personal experience that use of radioiodine to ablate the thyroid may be beneficial, and this whole area has been debated extensively *(124)*. At present, the safest conclusion is that TAO may worsen after radioiodine, but only modestly, and then not in the majority. Prophylactic steroids prevent any deterioration, however caused *(121)*, and should be considered in patients with severe TAO, but close follow-up is also acceptable until further data are available.

The idea of thyroid ablation is attractive if the thyroid is an important source of autoantigen or autoreactive T cells *(124)*, and total thyroidectomy has therefore been considered as definitive treatment for Graves' disease patients with TAO, despite the risks of this treatment. The best data to support this concept are retrospective, and do not come from a randomized trial *(125)*. Further work is needed in this area before recommending total thyroidectomy for TAO patients.

Immunomodulatory Treatment

Most patients with Graves' disease and clinical evidence of TAO require no disease-modifying treatment, although this is probably suboptimal and is based more on the blunt therapeutic instruments at our disposal rather than nihilism. If we could predict those patients who will develop congestive TAO, early intervention would seem worthwhile intuitively, and if safe, effective immunomodulatory treatment were available, we would use this earlier and in less severe cases of TAO. Certainly, the development of cytokine antagonists holds out future therapeutic promise *(126)*, and in the distance, autoantigen-based tolerance induction regimens offer the prospect of preventing as well as treating TAO. (*See* Chapter 17.)

However, returning to our current armamentarium, there seems to be a consensus, at least in Europe, that acute, congestive TAO warrants treatments with corticosteroids or radiotherapy, but worsening to optic neuropathy demands more intensive treatment with steroids plus other immunosuppressives or surgical decompression *(127)*. Practice varies from country to country, however, and there are few data to base clear recommendations on. A double-blind, randomized trial of oral prednisone compared to orbital radiotherapy in patients with moderately severe TAO showed equal efficacy, with around half of the patients having a successful outcome; fewer side effects were produced by radiotherapy *(128)*. Open studies of iv methyl prednisolone have shown some benefit, but retrobulbar steroid injection is no more effective than oral prednisone *(129)*. Whatever the steroid regimen, around 20% of patients benefit from surgery after steroid treatment *(129,130)*, emphasizing the need for better treatments. Radiotherapy seems preferable to corticosteroids, at least for some patients *(124,128)*, but is too slow to be useful in optic neuropathy, has limited utility in treating diplopia *(131)*, and the risk of subsequent tumor induction remains uncertain *(132,133)*. There is also controversy over the risks of radiotherapy in diabetic patients with TAO *(127)*. Presumably, at least part of the beneficial effect of radiotherapy is its lympholytic action, which will reduce cytokine production and other orbital autoimmune responses.

The place of other immunomodulatory agents is less clear. Azathioprine is frequently used for its steroid-sparing effect, but offers little benefit used alone *(129)*. Cyclosporine A is effective, in combination with prednisone, in TAO patients who fail to respond to prednisone alone *(134)*. No long-term studies have been performed on the outcome and complications after this. Intravenous immunoglobulin (IVIG) is as effective, but no better than corticosteroids, and although side-effects are lower with IVIG, again no long-term studies are available to prove the safety and prolonged efficacy of this treatment *(135,136)*. The expense of IVIG precludes wider use. Although the benefits of IVIG might seem to support a role for humoral autoimmunity in TAO pathogenesis, such infusions contain a number of soluble immunomodulatory molecules, such as CD4 and CD8, which could readily explain these benefits in a cell-mediated model of pathogenesis.

The long-acting somatostatin analog octreotide is as effective as corticosteroid in reducing symptoms and soft tissue swelling in TAO *(137)*, and scintigraphy using ^{111}In-octreotide predicts those who will benefit from this treatment *(138)*. Presumably the beneficial effects relate to the proposed involvement of IGF-1 in pathogenesis *(95)*. IGF-1 stimulates GAG production by fibroblasts in vitro, compatible with this hypothesis *(139)*, although the proportional contribution IGF-1 makes to fibroblast activation (in comparison to cytokines) is unknown. However, steroids are better than octreotide in reducing extraocular muscle swelling *(137)*, and this, combined with the expense and side effects, makes octreotide of uncertain value in TAO. An open, pilot study of pentoxyifylline reported benefit in 8 of 10 patients, associated with improvement in a number of immunological parameters *(140)*, but confirmation in a randomized study is needed. It has previously been shown that this drug inhibits fibroblast proliferation and GAG production *(141)*, and the development of treatments directed against the fibroblast is a novel addition to existing therapy.

THYROID DERMOPATHY

Although commonly called pretibial myxedema, the term thyroid dermopathy is preferable, since many other anatomical sites can be affected, particularly areas of skin

Chapter 10 / Ophthalmopathy and Dermopathy 263

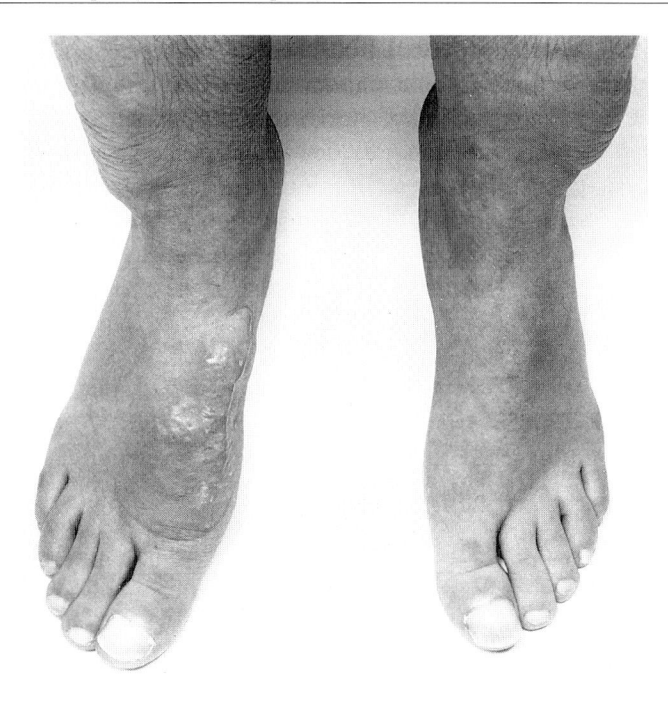

Fig. 4. Typical appearance of pretibial thyroid dermopathy. The patient also has dermopathy over the right foot and acropachy, especially of the big toes.

exposed to trauma *(12)*. Involved skin is indurated and discolored, typically presenting as symmetrical plaques, but sometimes in nodules, and a generalized form resembling elephantasis also occurs (Fig. 4). Almost all patients with thyroid dermopathy have Graves' disease and clinically obvious TAO, but skin involvement is only found in 1% of all Graves' patients *(142)*. A smaller proportion still have thyroid acropachy (nail clubbing), and since such patients generally have dermopathy *(12)*, there seems to be a hierarchy of extrathyroidal complications of Graves' disease from TAO, through dermopathy, to acropachy, with increasing intensity of the underlying pathogenetic process. There has also been a suggestion that clinically obvious dermopathy may be the tip of an iceberg of more generalized and frequent skin involvement in Graves' disease, based on the finding of excess GAGs in biopsies of clinically uninvolved forearm skin *(143)*, but these findings have not been reproduced *(144)* and may have been due to hypothyroidism rather than distinct dermopathy.

The consistent features of thyroid dermopathy are separation of collagen bundles due to GAG deposition in the reticular dermis, a zone of relatively normal collagen in the superficial papillary dermis, and defects in the elastic fibers *(145,146)*. Other conditions, especially stasis dermatitis, mimic dermopathy clinically and can share some of these histological features *(145)*. Although not prominent, lymphocytic infiltration is a feature of dermopathy, and restriction of TCR Vα and Vβ gene usage has been reported in specimens taken from active lesions, suggesting local T-cell clonal expansion *(147)*. Fibroblasts in involved skin express HLA-DR and heat shock proteins *(100,144)*. These features are very similar to the pathological features of TAO and indicate a common etiology, particularly since TCR V gene usage in the orbit and skin is identical in individual patients *(89)*. Although some IgGs from dermopathy patients have been reported to stimulate GAG production by dermal fibroblasts in vitro *(148)*, this has not been the experience of others *(106,107)*. In the experiments showing a stimulating effect *(148)*, IgG was prepared by the relatively crude method of ammonium sulfate precipitation and DEAE-Sephacel chromatography, and the results are therefore most likely explicable by contamination with growth factors, such as IGF-1. Moreover, there was no correlation between fibroblast and thyroid-stimulating activities, so that this stimulation was not mediated via the TSHR.

The simplest explanation for thyroid dermopathy is that it is an extreme form of fibroblast activation occurring via the same T-cell-mediated mechanisms as TAO. The localization to particular areas of skin may relate to trauma and hypoxia, enhancing fibroblast activation *(12,94)*, whereas the differences in behavior between orbital and dermal fibroblasts (Table 3) ensure that only a minority of Graves' patients have a sufficiently strong autoimmune response to produce dermal fibroblast activation. Genetic differences have also been proposed to explain susceptibility to dermopathy, particularly in the distribution of a codon 52 TSHR polymorphism *(149)*, but this has not been confirmed *(150)*. As for TAO, the TSHR is a candidate autoantigen, and receptor mRNA has been detected by RT-PCR in pretibial fibroblasts from patients with dermopathy *(151,152)*. In all 11 patients in which the full-length TSHR was amplified, the sequence did not confirm the proposed codon 52 susceptibility polymorphism *(152)*.

Treatment is often unnecessary, and surgical excision is contraindicated. Corticosteroids, under occlusive dressings, may lead to resolution, but skin atrophy and systemic absorption are problems. Octreotide has been of some benefit in open trials, but in contrast to TAO, ^{111}In-octreotide scintigraphy has no predictive value *(153,154)*.

REFERENCES

1. Wartofsky L. (on behalf of various Thyroid Associations). Classification of eye changes of Graves' disease. Thyroid 1992;2:235–236.
2. Mourits MPh, Prummel MF, Wiersinga WM, Koorneef L. Clinical activity score as a guide in the management of patients with Graves' ophthalmopathy. Clin Endocrinol 1997;47:9-14.
3. Bartley GB. The epidemiological characteristics and clinical course of ophthalmopathy associated with autoimmune thyroid disease in Olmsted County, Minnesota. Trans Am Ophthalmol Soc 1994; 42:477–588.
4. Burch HB, Wartofsky L. Graves' ophthalmopathy: current concepts regarding pathogenesis and management. Endocr Rev 1993;14:747–793.
5. Villadolid MC, Yokoyama N, Izumi M, Nishikawa T, Kimura H, Ashizawa K, et al. Untreated Graves' disease patients without clinical ophthalmopathy demonstrate a high frequency of extraocular muscle (EOM) enlargement by magnetic resonance. J Clin Endocrinol Metab 1995;80:2830–2833.
6. Perros P, Crombie AL, Matthews JNS, Kendall-Taylor P. Age and gender influence the severity of thyroid-associated ophthalmopathy: a study of 101 patients attending a combined thyroid-eye clinic. Clin Endocrinol 1993;38:367–372.
7. Prummel MF, Wiersinga WM, Mourits MPh, Koorneef L, Gerghout A, van der Gaag R. Effect of abnormal thyroid function on the severity of Graves' ophthalmopathy. Arch Intern Med 1990;150: 1098–1101.
8. Chou P-I, Feldon SE. Late onset dysthyroid optic neuropathy. Thyroid 1994;4:213–216.
9. Perros P, Crombie AL, Kendall-Taylor P. Natural history of thyroid associated ophthalmopathy. Clin Endocrinol 1995;42:45–50.
10. Campbell RJ. Immunology of Graves' ophthalmopathy: retrobulbar histology and histochemistry. Acta Endocrinol 1989;121(Suppl 2):9–16.
11. Trokel SL, Jakobiec FA. Correlation of CT scanning and pathological features of ophthalmic Graves' disease. Ophthalmologica 1981;88:553–564.
12. Smith TJ, Bahn RS, Gorman CA. Connective tissue, glycosaminoglycans, and diseases of the thyroid. Endocr Rev 1989;10:366–391.

13. Tallstedt L, Norberg R. Immunohistochemical staining of normal and Graves' extraocular muscle. Invest Ophthalmol Vis Sci 1988;29:175–184.
14. Weetman AP, Cohen S, Gatter KC, Fells P, Shine B. Immunohistochemical analysis of the retrobulbar tissues in Graves' ophthalmopathy. Clin Exp Immunol 1989;75:222–227.
15. Heufelder AE, Bahn RS. Elevated expression in situ of selectin and immunoglobulin superfamily type adhesion molecules in retroocular connective tissues from patients with Graves' ophthalmopathy. Clin Exp Immunol 1993;91:381–389.
16. Pappa A, Calder V, Fells P, Lightman S. Adhesion molecule expression in vivo on extraocular muscles (EOM) in thyroid-associated ophthalmopathy (TAO). Clin Exp Immunol 1997;108:309–313.
17. Small RG. Enlargement of levator palpebrae superioris muscle fibers in Graves' ophthalmopathy. Ophthalmology 1989;96:424–430.
18. Hudson HL, Levin L, Feldon SE. Graves' exophthalmos unrelated to extraocular muscle enlargement. Ophthalmology 1991;98:1495–1499.
19. Hesse RJ. Graves' exophthalmos without muscle involvement. Ophthalmology 1992;99:645 (letter).
20. Birchall D, Goodall KL, Noble JL, Jackson A. Graves' ophthalmopathy: intracranial fat prolapse on CT images as an indicator of optic nerve compression. Radiology 1996;200:123–127.
21. Kahaly G, Hansen C, Felke B, Dienes HP. Immunohistochemical staining of retrobulbar adipose tissue in Graves' ophthalmopathy. Clin Immunol Immunopathol 1994;73:53–62.
22. Sergott RC, Felberg NT, Savino PJ, Blizzard JJ, Schatz NJ, Sanford CA. Association of HLA antigen BW35 with severe Graves' ophthalmopathy. Invest Ophthalmol Vis Sci 1983;24:124–127.
23. Kendall-Taylor P, Stephenson A, Stratton A, Papiha SS, Perros P, Roberts DF. Differentiation of autoimmune ophthalmopathy from Graves' hyperthyroidism by analysis of genetic markers. Clin Endocrinol 1988;28:601–610.
24. Frecker M, Stenszky V, Balazs C, Kozma L, Kraszits E, Farid NR. Genetic factors in Graves' ophthalmopathy. Clin Endocrinol 1986;25:479–485.
25. Frecker M, Mercer G, Skanes VM, Farid NR. Major histocompatibility complex (MHC) factors predisposing to and protecting against Graves' eye disease. Autoimmunity 1988;1:307–315.
26. Weetman AP, So AK, Warner CA, Foroni L, Fells P, Shine B. Immunogenetics of Graves' ophthalmopathy. Clin Endocrinol 1988;28:619–628.
27. Weetman AP, Zhang L, Webb S, Shine B. Analysis of HLA-DQB and HLA-DPB alleles in Graves' disease by oligonucleotide probing of enzymatically amplified DNA. Clin Endocrinol 1990;33:65–71.
28. Inoue D, Sato K, Enomoto T, Sugawa H, Maeda M, Inoko H, et al. Correlation of HLA types and clinical findings in Japanese patients with hyperthyroid Graves' disease: evidence indicating the existence of four subpopulations. Clin Endocrinol 1992;36:75–82.
29. Weetman AP, Poole J. Failure to find an association of blood group P_1 with thyroid-associated ophthalmopathy. Clin Endocrinol 1992;37:423–425.
30. Tellez M, Cooper J, Edmonds C. Graves' ophthalmopathy in relation to cigarette smoking and ethnic origin. Clin Endocrinol 1992;36:291–294.
31. Hagg E, Asplund K. Is endocrine ophthalmopathy related to smoking? Br Med J 1987;295:634–365.
32. Bartalena L, Bogazzi F, Tanda ML, Manetti L, Dell'Unto E, Martino E. Cigarette smoking and the thyroid. Eur J Endocrinol 1995;133:507–512.
33. Pfeilschifter J, Ziegler R. Smoking and endocrine ophthalmopathy: impact of smoking severity and current vs lifetime cigarette consumption. Clin Endocrinol 1996;45:477–481.
34. Weetman AP. Thyroid-associated eye disease: pathophysiology. Lancet 1991;358:25–28.
35. Bahn RS, Heufelder AE. Pathogenesis of Graves' ophthalmopathy. N Engl J Med 1993;329:1468–1475.
36. McLachlan SM, Bahn RS, Rapoport B. Endocrine ophthalmopathy: a re-evaluation of the association with thyroid autoantibodies. Autoimmunity 1992;14:143–148.
37. Kuroki T, Ruf J, Whelan L, Miller A, Wall JR. Antithyroglobulin monoclonal and autoantibodies cross-react with an orbital connective tissue membrane antigen: a possible mechanism for the association of ophthalmopathy with autoimmune thyroid disorders. Clin Exp Immunol 1985;62:361–370.
38. Tao T-W, Cheng P-J, Pham H, Leu S-L, Kriss JS. Monoclonal antithyroglobulin antibodies derived from immunizations of mice with human eye muscle and thyroid membranes. J Clin Endocrinol Metab 1986;63:577–582.
39. Ludgate M, Dong Q, Dreyfus PA, Taylor P, Vassart G, Soreq H. Definition, at the molecular level, of a thyroglobulin-acetylcholinesterase shared epitope: study of its pathophysiological significance in patients with Graves' disease. Autoimmunity 1989;3:167–176.
40. Weetman AP, Tse CK, Randall WR, Tsim KWK, Barnard EA. Acetylcholinesterase antibodies and thyroid autoimmunity. Clin Exp Immunol 1988;71:96–99.

41. Mappouras DG, Philippou G, Haralambous S, Tzartos SJ, Balafas A, Souvatzoglou A, et al. Antibodies to acetylcholinesterase cross-reacting with thyroglobulin in myasthenia gravis and Graves' disease. Clin Exp Immunol 1995;100:336–343.
42. Brimijoin S, Lennon VA. Autoimmune preganglionic sympathectomy induced by acetylcholinesterase antibodies. Proc Natl Acad Sci USA 1990;87:9630–9634.
43. Heufelder AE. Involvement of orbital fibroblast and TSH receptor in the pathogenesis of Graves' ophthalmopathy. Thyroid 1995;5:331–340.
44. Wall JR, Strakosch CR, Fang SL, Ingbar SH, Braverman LE. Thyroid binding antibodies and other immunological abnormalities in patients with Graves' ophthalmopathy: effect of treatment with cyclophosphamide. Clin Endocrinol 1979;10:78–91.
45. Nishikawa M, Yoshimura M, Toyoda N, Masaki H, Yonemoto T, Gondou A, et al. Correlation of orbital muscle changes evaluated by magnetic resonance imaging and thyroid-stimulating antibody in patients with Graves' ophthalmopathy. Acta Endocrinol 1993;129:213–219.
46. Shokeir MO, Pudek MR, Katz S, Rootman J, Kendler DL. The relationship of thyrotropin receptor antibody levels to the severity of thyroid orbitopathy. Clin Biochem 1996;29:187–189.
47. Kasagi K, Hidaka A, Nakamura H, Takeuchi R, Misaki T, Iida Y, et al. Thyrotropin receptor antibodies in hypothyroid Graves' disease. J Clin Endocrinol Metab 1993;76:504–508.
48. Atkinson S, Holcombe M, Kendall-Taylor P. Ophthalmopathic immunoglobulin in patients with Graves' ophthalmopathy. Lancet 1984;ii:374–376.
49. Kadluboswki M, Irvine WJ, Rowland AC. The lack of specificity of ophthalmic immunoglobulins in Graves' disease. J Clin Endocrinol Metab 1986;63:990–995.
50. Ahmann A, Baker JR, Weetman AP, Wartofsky L, Nutman TB, Burman KD. Antibodies to porcine eye muscle in patients with Graves' ophthalmopathy; identification of serum immunoglobulins directed against unique determinants by immunoblotting and enzyme-linked immunosorbent assay. J Clin Endocrinol Metab 1987;64:454–460.
51. Schifferdecker E, Ketzler-Sasse U, Boehm BO, Ronsheimer HB, Scherbaum WA, Schoffling K. Re-evaluation of eye muscle autoantibody determination in Graves' ophthalmopathy: failure to detect a specific antigen by use of enzyme-linked immunosorbent assay, indirect immunofluorescence, and immunoblotting techniques. Acta Endocrinol 1989;121:643–650.
52. Salvi M, Hiromatsu Y, Bernard N, How J, Wall JR. Human orbital tissue and thyroid membrane express a 64kDa protein which is recognised by autoantibodies in serum of patients with thyroid-associated ophthalmopathy. FEBS Lett 1988;232:135–139.
53. Weightman D, Kendall-Taylor P. Cross-reaction of eye muscle antibodies with thyroid tissue in thyroid-associated ophthalmopathy. J Endocrinol 1989;122:201–206.
54. Kendler DL, Huber GK, Rootman J, Davies TF. A 64kDa membrane antigen is a recurrent epitope for natural autoantibodies in patients with Graves' thyroid and ophthalmic diseases. Clin Endocrinol 1991;35:539–547.
55. Salvi M, Bernard N, Miller A, Zhang Z, Gardini E, Wall JR. Presence of antibodies reactive with a 64kDa eye muscle membrane antigen in thyroid-associated ophthalmopathy. Thyroid 1991;1:207–213.
56. Chang TC, Chang TJ, Huang YS, Huang KM, Su RJ, Kao SCS. Identification of autoantigen recognized by autoimmune ophthalmopathy sera with immunoblotting correlated with orbital computed tomography. Clin Immunol Immunopathol 1992;65:161–166.
57. Hiromatsu Y, Sato M, Tanaka K, Shoji S, Nonaka K, Chinami M, et al. Significance of anti-eye muscle antibody in patients with thyroid-associated ophthalmopathy by quantitative Western blot. Autoimmunity 1992;14:9–16.
58. Tandon N, Yan SL, Arnold K, Metcalfe RA, Weetman AP. Immunoglobulin class and subclass distribution of eye muscle and fibroblast antibodies in patients with thyroid-associated ophthalmopathy. Clin Endocrinol 1994;40:629–639.
59. Kadlubowski M, Irvine WJ, Rowland AC. Anti-muscle antibodies in Graves' ophthalmopathy. J Clin Lab Immunol 1987;24:105–111.
60. Dong Q, Ludgate M, Vassart G. Cloning and sequencing of a novel 64kDa antoantigen recognized by patients with autoimmune thyroid disease. J Clin Endocrinol Metab 1991;72:1375–1381.
61. Bernard NF, Nygen TN, Tyutunikov A, Stolarski C, Scalise D, Genovese C, et al. Antibodies against $_1$D, a recombinant 64kDa membrane protein, are associated with ophthalmopathy in patients with thyroid autoimmunity. Clin Immunol Immunopathol 1994;70:225–233.
62. Ross PV, Koenig RJ, Arscott P, Ludgate M, Waier M, Nelson CC, et al. Tissue specificity and serologic reactivity of an autoantigen associated with autoimmune thyroid disease. J Clin Endocrinol Metab 1993;77:433–438.

63. Barsouk A, Wengrowicz S, Scalise D, Stolarski C, Nebes V, Sato M. et al. New assays for the measurement of serum antibodies reactive with eye muscle membrane antigens confirm their significance in thyroid-associated ophthalmopathy. Thyroid 1995;5:195–200.
64. Wall JR, Hayes M, Scalise D, Stolarski C, Nebes V, Kiljanski J, et al. Native gel electrophoresis and isoelectric focusing of a 64-kilodalton eye muscle protein shows that it is an important target for serum autoantibodies in patients with thyroid-associated ophthalmopathy and not expressed in other skeletal muscle. J Clin Endocrinol Metab 1995;80:1226–1232.
65. Bahn RS, Gorman CA, Johnson CM, Smith TJ. Presence of antibodies in the sera of patients with Graves' disease recognizing a 23 kilodalton fibroblast protein. J Clin Endocrinol Metab 1989;69:622–628.
66. Arnold K, Metcalfe RA, Weetman AP. Immunoglobulin A class fibroblast antibodies in patients with Graves' disease and pretibial myxedema. J Clin Endocrinol Metab 1995;80:3430–3437.
67. Molnár I, Balázs CS. Comparative study on IgG and IgA antibodies against human thyroid and eye-muscle antigens in Graves' ophthalmopathy. Acta Med Hungarica 1991;48:13–21.
68. Stover C, Otto E, Beyer J, Kahaly G. Humoral immunity and retrobulbar fibroblasts in endocrine ophthalmopathy. Acta Endocrinol 1992;126:394–398.
69. Dillon J, Zhang Z-Q, Hiromatsu N, Bernard M, Salvi M, Wall JR. Failure to detect complement-mediated antibody-dependent cytotoxicity against human orbital tissue cells in the serum of patients with thyroid-associated ophthalmopathy. Autoimmunity 1989;5:125–132.
70. Ringel MD, Taylor T, Barsouk A, Wall JR, Freter CE, Howard RS, et al. Hodgkin's disease treated with neck radiation is associated with increased antibody-dependent cellular cytotoxicity against human extraocular muscle cells. Thyroid 1997;7:425–432.
71. Perros P, Kendall-Taylor P. Biological activity of autoantibodies from patients with thyroid-associated ophthalmopathy: in vitro effects of porcine extraocular myoblasts. Q J Med 1992;305:691–706.
72. Weightman DR, Perros P, Sherif IH, Kendall-Taylor P. Autoantibodies to IGF-1 binding sites in thyroid associated ophthalmopathy. Autoimmunity 1993;16:251–257.
73. Jaume JC, Portolano S, Prummel MF, McLachlan SM, Rapoport B. Molecular cloning and characterization of genes for antibodies generated by orbital tissue-infiltrating B-cells in Graves' ophthalmopathy. J Clin Endocrinol Metab 1994;78:348–352.
74. McLachlan SM, Prummel MF, Jaume JC, Rapoport B. Immunoglobulin A in Graves' orbital tissue: Deoxyribonucleic acid amplification by polymerase chain reaction. J Endocrinol Invest 1994;17: 247–252.
75. Felberg NT, Sergott RC, Savino PJ, Blizzard JJ, Schatz NJ, Amsel J. Lymphocyte subpopulations in Graves' ophthalmopathy. Arch Ophthalmol 1985;103:656–659.
76. Tyutyunikov A, Raikow RB, Kennerdell JS, Kazim M, Dalbow MH, Scalise D. Re-examination of peripheral blood T cell subsets in dysthyroid orbitopathy. Invest Ophthalmol Vis Sci 1992;33: 2299–2303.
77. Pedersen BK, Perrild H, Feldt-Rasmussen U, Christensen T, Klarlund K, Hansen JM. Suppressed natural killer cell activity in patients with euthyroid Graves' ophthalmopathy. Autoimmunity 1989;2: 291–298.
78. Prummel MF, Wiersinga WM, van der Gaag R, Mourits MP, Koornneef L. Soluble IL-2 receptor levels in patients with Graves' ophthalmopathy. Clin Exp Immunol 1992;88:405–409.
79. Heufelder AE, Bahn RS. Soluble intercellular adhesion molecule-1 (sICAM-1) in sera of patients with Graves' ophthalmopathy and thyroid diseases. Clin Exp Immunol 1993;92:296–302.
80. Hofbauer LC, Mühlberg T, König A, Heufelder G, Schworm H-D, Heufelder AE. Soluble interleukin-1 receptor antagonist serum levels in smokers and non-smokers with Graves' ophthalmopathy undergoing orbital radiotherapy. J Clin Endocrinol Metab 1997;82:2244–2247.
81. Weetman AP. The role of T lymphocytes in thyroid-associated ophthalmopathy. Autoimmunity 1992; 13:69–73.
82. Arnold K, Tandon N, McIntosh RS, Elisei R, Ludgate M, Weetman AP. T cell responses to orbital antigens in thyroid-associated ophthalmopathy. Clin Exp Immunol 1994;96:329–334.
83. Stover C, Otto E, Beyer J, Kahaly G. Cellular immunity and retrobulbar fibroblasts in Graves' ophthalmopathy. Thyroid 1994;4:161–165.
84. Grubeck-Loebenstein B, Trieb K, Sztankay A, Holter W, Anderl H, Wick G. Retrobulbar T cells from patients with Graves' ophthalmopathy are CD8[+] and specifically recognize autologous fibroblasts. J Clin Invest 1994;93:2738–2743.
85. De Carli M, D'Elios MM, Mariotti S, Marcocci C, Pinchera A, Ricci M, et al. Cytolytic T cells with Th1-like cytokine profile predominate in retroorbital lymphocytic infiltrates of Graves' ophthalmopathy. J Clin Endocrinol Metab 1993;77:1120–1124.

86. Otto EA, Ochs K, Hansen C, Wall JR, Kahaly GJ. Orbital tissue-derived T lymphocytes from patients with Graves' ophthalmopathy recognize autologous orbital antigens. J Clin Endocrinol Metab 1996; 81:3045–3050.
87. Pappa A, Calder V, Ajjan R, Fells P, Ludgate M, Weetman AP, Lightman S. Analysis of extraocular muscle-infiltrating T cells in thyroid-associated ophthalmopathy (TAO). Clin Exp Immunol 1997; 109:362–369.
88. Heufelder AE, Herterich S, Ernst G, Bahn RS, Scriba PC. Analysis of retroorbital T cell antigen receptor variable region gene usage in patients with Graves' ophthalmopathy. Eur J Endocrinol 1995;132:266–277.
89. Heufelder AE, Wenzel BE, Scriba PC. Antigen receptor variable region repertoires expressed by T cells infiltrating thyroid, retroorbital and pretibial tissue in Graves' disease. J Clin Endocrinol Metab 81:1996;3733–3739.
90. Heufelder AE, Bahn RS. Detection and localization of cytokine immunoreactivity in retro-ocular connective tissue in Graves' ophthalmopathy. Eur J Clin Invest 1993;23:10–17.
91. McLachlan SM, Prummel MF, Rapoport B. Cell-mediated or humoral immunity in Graves' ophthalmopathy? Profiles of T-cell cytokines amplified by polymerase chain reaction from orbital tissue. J Clin Endocrinol Metab 1994;78:1070–1074.
92. Korducki JM, Loftus SJ, Bahn RS. Stimulation of glycosaminoglycan production in cultured human retroocular fibroblasts. Invest Ophthalmol Vis Sci 1992;33:2037–2042.
93. Smith TJ, Bahn RS, Gorman CA, Cheavens M. Stimulation of glycosaminoglycan accumulation by interferon gamma in cultured human retroocular fibroblasts. J Clin Endocrinol Metab 1991;72:1169–1171.
94. Metcalfe RA, Weetman AP. Stimulation of extraocular muscle fibroblasts by cytokines and hypoxia: possible role in thyroid-associated ophthalmopathy. Clin Endocrinol 1994;40:67–72.
95. Hansson HA, Petruson B, Skottner A. Somatomedin C in pathogenesis of malignant exophthalmos of endocrine origin. Lancet 1986;I:218–219.
96. Smith TJ, Wang H-S, Hogg MG, Henrikson RC, Keese CR, Giaever I. Prostaglandin E_2 elicits a morphological change in cultured orbital fibroblasts from patients with Graves' ophthalmopathy. Proc Natl Acad Sci USA 1994;91:5094–5098.
97. Smith TJ, Bahn RS, Gorman CA. Hormonal regulations of hyaluronate synthesis in cultured human fibroblasts: Evidence for differences between retroocular and dermal fibroblasts. J Clin Endocrinol Metab 1989;69:1019–1023.
98. Berenson CS, Smith TJ. Human orbital fibroblasts in culture express ganglioside profiles distinct from those in dermal fibroblasts. J Clin Endocrinol Metab 1995;80:2668–2674.
99. Heufelder AE, Wenzel BE, Gorman CA, Bahn RS. Detection, cellular localization, and modulation of heat shock proteins in cultured fibroblasts from patients with extrathyroidal manifestations of Graves' disease. J Clin Endocrinol Metab 1991;73:739–745.
100. Heufelder AE, Smith TJ, Gorman CA, Bahn RS. Increased induction of HLA-DR by interferon-γ in cultured fibroblasts derived from patients with Graves' ophthalmopathy and pretibial dermopathy. J Clin Endocrinol Metab 1991;73:307–313.
101. Tanaka K, Hiromatsu Y, Sato M, Inoue Y, Nonaka K. Localization of heat shock protein in orbital tissue from patients with Graves' ophthalmopathy using in situ hybridization. Life Sci 1993;54:355–359.
102. Hiromatsu Y, Tanaka K, Ishisaka N, Kamachi J, Kuroki T, Hoshino T, et al. Human histocompatibility leukocyte antigen-DR and heat shock protein-70 expression in eye muscle tissue in thyroid-associated ophthalmopathy. J Clin Endocrinol Metab 1995;80:685–691.
103. Salmon M, Scheel-Toellner D, Hulssoon AP, Pilling D, Shamsadeen N, Hyde H, et al. Inhibition of T cell apoptosis in the rheumatoid synovium. J Clin Invest 1997;99:439–446.
104. Heufelder AE, Scriba PC. Characterization of adhesion receptors on cultured microvascular endothelial cells derived from the retroorbital connective tissue of patients with Graves' ophthalmopathy. Eur J Endocrinol 1996;134:51–60.
105. Rotella CM, Zonefrati R, Toccafondi R, Valente WA, Kohn LD. Ability of monoclonal antibodies to the thyrotropin receptor to increase collagen synthesis in human fibroblasts: an assay which appears to measure exophthalmogenic immunoglobulins in Graves' sera. J Clin Endocrinol Metab 1986;62:357–367.
106. Tao T-W, Leu S-L, Kriss JP. Biological activity of autoantibodies associated with Graves' dermopathy. J Clin Endocrinol Metab 1989;69:90–99.
107. Metcalfe RA, Davies R, Weetman AP. Analysis of fibroblast-stimulating activity in IgG from patients with Graves' dermopathy. Thyroid 1993;3:207–212.

108. Paschke R, Metcalfe A, Alcalde L, Vassart G, Weetman AP, Ludgate M. Presence of nonfunctional thyrotropin receptor variant transcripts in retroocular and other tissues. J Clin Endocrinol Metab 1994; 79:1234–1238.
109. Paschke R, Vassart G, Ludgate M. Current evidence for and against the TSH receptor being the common antigen in Graves' disease and thyroid associated ophthalmopathy. Clin Endocrinol 1995; 42:565–569.
110. Endo T, Ohta K, Haraguchi K, Onaya T. Cloning and functional expression of a thyrotropin receptor cDNA from rat fat cells. J Biol Chem 1995;270:10,833–10,837.
111. Crisp MS, Lane C, Halliwell M, Wynford-Thomas D, Ludgate M. Thyrotropin receptor transcripts in human adipose tissue. J Clin Endocrinol Metab 1997;82:2003–2005.
112. Feliciello A, Porcellini A, Ciullo I, Bonavolontà G, Avvedimento EV, Fenzi G. Expression of thyrotropin-receptor mRNA in healthy and Graves' disease retro-orbital tissue. Lancet 1993;342:337–338.
113. Heufelder AE, Dutton CM, Sarkar G, Donovan KA, Bahn RS. Detection of TSH receptor RNA in cultured fibroblasts from patients with Graves' ophthalmopathy and pretibial dermopathy. Thyroid 1993;3:297–300.
114. Mengistu M, Lukes YG, Nagy EV, Burch HB, Carr FE, Lahiri S, et al. TSH receptor gene expression in retro-ocular fibroblasts. J Endocrinol Invest 1994;17:437–441.
115. Major BJ, Cures A, Frauman AG. The full length and splice variant thyrotropin receptor is expressed exclusively in skeletal muscle of extraocular origin: a link to the pathogenesis of Graves' ophthalmopathy. Biochem Biophys Res Commun 1997;230:493–496.
116. Hiromatsu Y, Sato M, Inoue Y, Koga M, Miyake I, Kameo J, et al. Localization and clinical significance of thyrotropin receptor mRNA expression in orbital fat and eye muscle tissues from patients with thyroid-associated ophthalmopathy. Thyroid 1996;6:553–562.
117. Aust G, Ludgate M, Weetman AP, Scherbaum WA, Paschke R. Illegitimate transcription of thyroid autoantigens. 10th International Congress. Endocrinology, San Francisco, USA 1996 (Abstract P3-989).
118. Burch HB, Sellitti D, Barnes SG, Nagy EV, Bahn RS, Burman KD. Thyrotropin receptor antisera for the detection of immunoreactive protein species in retroocular fibroblasts obtained from patients with Graves' ophthalmopathy. J Clin Endocrinol Metab 1994;78:1384–1391.
119. Spitzweg C, Joba W, Hunt N, Heufelder AE. Analysis of human thyrotropin receptor gene expression and immunoreactivity in human orbital tissue. Eur J Endocrinol 1997;136:599–607.
120. Stadlmayr W, Spitzweb C, Bichlmair A-M, Heufelder AE. TSH receptor transcripts and TSH receptor-like immunoreactivity in orbital and pretibial fibroblasts of patients with Graves' ophthalmopathy and pretibial myxedema. Thyroid 1997;7:3–12.
121. Bartalena L, Marcocci C, Bogazzi F, Panicucci M, Lepri A, Pinchera A. Use of corticosteroids to prevent progression of Graves' ophthalmopathy after radioiodine therapy for hyperthyroidism. N Engl J Med 1989;321:1349–1352.
122. Tallstedt L, Lundell G, Tørring O, Wallin G, Ljunggren J-G, Blomgren H, et al. Occurrence of ophthalmopathy after treatment for Graves' hyperthyroidism. N Engl J Med 1992;326:1733–1738.
123. Kung AWC, Cheng A. The incidence of ophthalmopathy after radioiodine therapy for Graves' disease: prognostic factors and the role of methimazole. J Clin Endocrinol Metab 1994;79:542–546.
124. DeGroot LJ, Gorman CA, Pinchera A, Bartalena L, Marocci C, Wiersinga WM, et al. Radiation and Graves' ophthalmopathy. J Clin Endocrinol Metab 1995;80:339–349.
125. Winsa B, Rastad J, Åkerström G, Johansson H, Westermark K, Karlsson FA. Retrospective evaluation of subtotal and total thyroidectomy in Graves' disease with and without endocrine ophthalmopathy. Eur J Endocrinol 1995;132:406–412.
126. Tan GH, Dutton CM, Bahn RS. Interleukin-1 (IL-1) receptor antagonist and soluble IL-1 receptor inhibit IL-1 induced glycosaminoglycan production in cultured human orbital fibroblasts from patients with Graves' ophthalmopathy. J Clin Endocrinol Metab 1996;81:449–452.
127. Weetman AP, Wiersinga W. Current management of thyroid-associated ophthalmopathy in Europe. Results of an international survey. Clin Endocrinol 1998;49:21–28.
128. Prummel MF, Mourits MPh, Blank L, Berghout A, Koornneef L, Wiersinga WM. Randomised double-blind trial of prednisone versus radiotherapy in Graves' ophthalmopathy. Lancet 1993;342:949–954.
129. Wiersinga WM. Immunosuppressive treatment of Graves' ophthalmopathy. Thyroid 1992;2:229–233.
130. Bartley GB, Fatourechi V, Kadrmas EF, Jacobsen SJ, Ilstrup DM, Garrity JA, et al. The treatment of Graves' ophthalmopathy in an incidence cohort. Am J Ophthalmol 1996;121:200–206.
131. Wilson WB, Prochoda M. Radiotherapy for thyroid orbitopathy. Effects on extraocular muscle balance. Arch Ophthalmol 1995;113:1420–1425.

132. Snijders-Keilholz A, De Keizer RJW, Goslings BM, Van Dam EWCM, Jansen JThM, Broerse JJ. Probable risk of tumour induction after retro-orbital irradiation for Graves' ophthalmopathy. Radiother Oncol 1996;38:69–71.
133. Blank LECM, Barendsen GW, Prummel MF, Stalpers L, Wiersinga W, Koornneef L. Probable risk of tumor induction after retro-orbital irradiation for Graves' ophthalmopathy. Radiother Oncol 1996; 40:187–189.
134. Prummel MF, Mourits MPh, Berghout A, Krenning EP, van der Gaag R, Koornneef L, et al. Prednisone and cyclosporine in the treatment of severe Graves' ophthalmopathy. N Engl J Med 1989;321:1353–1359.
135. Kahaly G, Pitz S, Müller-Forell W, Hommel G. Randomized trial of intravenous immunoglobulins versus prednisolone in Graves' ophthalmopathy. Clin Exp Immunol 1996;106:197–202.
136. Baschieri L, Antonelli A, Nardi S, Alberti B, Lepri A, Canapicchi R, et al. Intravenous immunoglobulin versus corticosteroid in treatment of Graves' ophthalmopathy. Thyroid 1997;7:579–585.
137. Kung AWC, Michon J, Tai KS, Chan FL. The effect of somatostatin versus corticosteroid in the treatment of Graves' ophthalmopathy. Thyroid 1996;6:381–384.
138. Krassas GE, Dumas A, Pontikides N, Kaltsas Th. Somatostatin receptor scintigraphy and octreotide treatment in paitents with thyroid eye disease. Clin Endocrinol 1995;42:571–580.
139. Imai Y, Odajima R, Inoue Y, Shishiba Y. Effect of growth factors on hyaluronan and proteoglycan synthesis by retroocular tissue fibroblasts of Graves' ophthalmopathy in culture. Acta Endocrinol 1992;126:541–552.
140. Balazs Cs., Kiss E, Vamos A, Molnar I, Farid NR. Beneficial effect of pentoxifylline on thyroid associated ophthalmopathy (TAO): a pilot study. J Clin Endocrinol Metab 1997;82:1999–2002.
141. Chang C-C, Chang T-C, Kao SCS, Kuo Y-F, Chien L-F. Pentoxifylline inhibits the proliferation and glycosaminoglycan synthesis of cultured fibroblasts derived from patients with Graves' ophthalmopathy and pretibial myxoedema. Acta Endocrinol 1993;129:322–327.
142. Fatourechi V, Pajouhi M, Fransway AF. Dermopathy of Graves' disease (pretibial myxedema). Review of 150 cases. Medicine 1994;73:1–7.
143. Wortsman J, Dietrich J, Traycoff RB, Stone S. Pretibial myxedema in thyroid disease. Arch Dermatol 1981;117:635–638.
144. Peacey SP, Flemming L, Messenger A, Weetman AP. Is Graves' dermopathy a generalized disorder? Thyroid 1996;6:1–4.
145. Somiach SC, Helm TN, Lawlor KB, Bergfeld WF, Bass J. Pretibial mucin. Histologic patterns and clinical correlation. Arch Dermatol 1993;129:1152–1155.
146. Matsuoka LY, Wortsman J, Uitto J, Hashimoto K, Kupehella CE, Eng AM, et al. Altered skin elastic fibers in hypothyroid myxedema and pretibial myxedema. Arch Intern Med 1985;145:117–121.
147. Heufelder AE, Bahn RS, Scriba PC. Analysis of T cell antigen receptor variable region gene usage in patients with thyroid-related pretibial dermopathy. J Invest Dermatol 1995;105:372–378.
148. Shishiba Y, Imai Y, Odajima R, Ozawa Y, Shimizu T. Immunoglobulin G of patients with circumscribed pretibial myxedema of Graves' disease stimulates proteoglycan synthesis in human skin fibroblasts in culture. Acta Endocrinol 1992;127:44–51.
149. Bahn RS, Dutton CM, Heufelder AE, Sarkar G. A genomic point mutation in the extracellular domain of the thyrotropin receptor in patients with Graves' ophthalmopathy. J Clin Endocrinol Metab 1994; 78:256–260.
150. Watson PF, French A, Pickerill AP, McIntosh RS, Weetman AP. Lack of association between a polymorphism in the coding region of the thyrotropin receptor gene and Graves' disease. J Clin Endocrinol Metab 1995;80:1032–1035.
151. Chang T-C, Wu S-L, Hsiao Y-L, Kuo S-T, Chien L-F, Kuo Y-F, et al. TSH and TSH receptor antibody-binding sites in fibroblasts of pretibial myxedema are related to the extracellular domain of entire TSH receptor. Clin Immunol Immunopathol 1994;71:113–120.
152. Wu S-L, Chang T-C, Chang T-J, Kuo Y-F, Hsiao Y-L, Chang C-C. Cloning and sequencing of complete thyrotropin receptor transcripts in pretibial fibroblast culture cells. J Endocrinol Invest 1996; 19:365–370.
153. Chang T-C, Kao SCS, Huang KM. Octreotide and Graves' ophthalmopathy and pretibial myxoedema. Br Med J 1992;304:158.
154. Kuyvenhoven JPh, van der Pijl JW, Goslings BM, Wiersinga WM. Graves' dermopathy: does octreotide scintigraphy predict the response to octreotide treatment? Thyroid 1996;6:385–389.

11 Postpartum Autoimmune Endocrine Syndromes

Nobuyuki Amino, MD, *Hisato Tada,* MD, *and Yoh Hidaka,* MD

CONTENTS

INTRODUCTION
THYROID FUNCTION DURING PREGNANCY
AUTOIMMUNE THYROID DISEASE AND PREGNANCY
POSTPARTUM AUTOIMMUNE THYROID DYSFUNCTION
POSTPARTUM AUTOIMMUNE DISEASES
NEONATAL THYROID DISEASE OWING TO ANTIBODY TRANSFER
REFERENCES

INTRODUCTION

Spontaneous fluctuation of endocrine function is frequently observed during the course of autoimmune endocrine diseases. However, little is known concerning the exact aggravating factors. Recently, it has been found that disease is aggravated after pregnancy *(1)* and after attack of allergic rhinitis *(2)*, a typical type I allergy, in autoimmune thyroid diseases. Pregnancy has been described as a successful allograft of foreign tissue, and physiological immunological changes *(3)* influence remarkably the disease course. Many autoimmune diseases occur more commonly in women, often during the childbearing age, and thus, it is very important to elucidate the mechanisms of postpartum onset or aggravation of autoimmune endocrine diseases.

This chapter deals with recent progress in the study of the effects of pregnancy on autoimmune thyroid diseases and describes the various types of postpartum thyroid dysfunction, which are called "postpartum autoimmune endocrine syndromes" *(4)*.

THYROID FUNCTION DURING PREGNANCY

Thyroid function, which is regulated through the hypothalamus–pituitary–thyroid axis, is disturbed by placental hormones during pregnancy (Fig. 1) *(5)*.

Human chorionic gonadotropin (hCG) is composed of an α-subunit that is common in pituitary glycopeptide hormones (thyroid-stimulating hormone [TSH], luteinizing hormone [LH], and follicle-stimulating hormone [FSH]) and a β-subunit that has 46%

From: *Contemporary Endocrinology: Autoimmune Endocrinopathies*
Edited by: R. Volpe © Humana Press Inc., Totowa, NJ

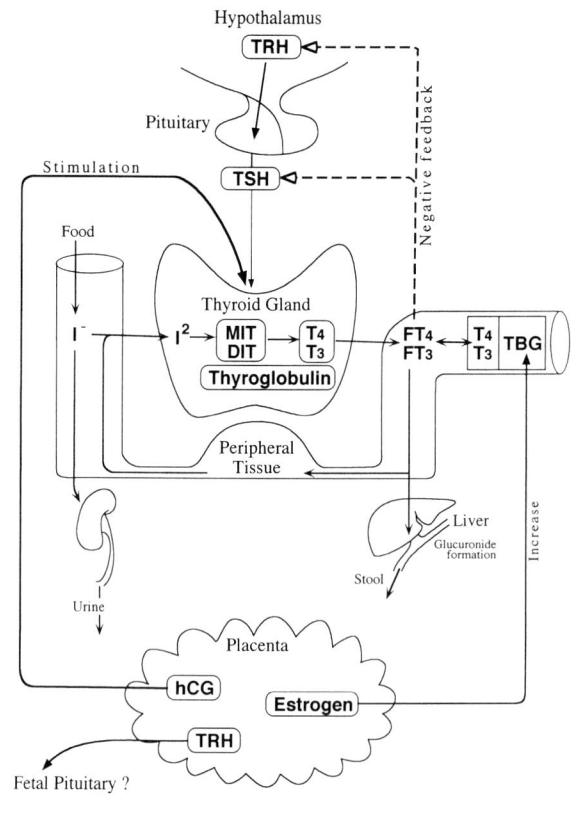

Fig. 1. Regulation of thyroid function during pregnancy. Direct stimulation of the TSH receptor by hCG-induced transient increase of thyroid hormones in early pregnancy. The pituitary–thyroid feedback regulation is kept normal during pregnancy (therefore, TSH may be suppressed in early pregnancy).

homology to TSH in the first 114 amino acid residues (TSH lacks the rest of the 31 amino acids in hCG-β). The similarity of the molecules leads to a weak crossreaction, i.e., hCG can bind to TSH receptor and stimulate thyroid cells *(6–11)*. Thyroid-stimulating activity (TSA) found during early pregnancy was neutralized by treatment with anti-hCG antibody *(12,13)*. Although there is a controversy regarding to whether hCG modifies thyroid function in normal pregnancy *(14,15)*, some researchers consider hCG to be a thyroid-regulatory factor, which may override the hypothalamus–pituitary–thyroid axis in early pregnancy *(13,16)*. Thyroid function is slightly enhanced at 8–12 gestational weeks, when hCG concentrations are highest (Fig. 2). It is estimated that hCG can induce slight enhancement of thyroid function in early pregnancy if hCG is $1/10^4$ as potent as human TSH *(17)*. In particular cases, transient thyrotoxicosis with severe emesis (referred to as "hyperemesis gravidarum") may be observed *(18)*, although this association was not always found *(19)*. Serum TSA in those patients was much higher than that in normal pregnant women, and again it was neutralized by treatment with anti-hCG antibody *(20)* (there is a report in which anti-hCG failed to neutralize TSA *[21]*). The relationship of hCG to hyperemesis is still unknown. However, the severity of vomiting weakly correlated to thyroid function, TSA, and hCG concentration *(18,22)*. Supposing a pathogenic role of hCG, we have proposed a new clinical entity, "gestational thyrotoxicosis" *(20)*, which is induced by asialo-hCG *(23)*.

Chapter 11 / Postpartum Syndromes

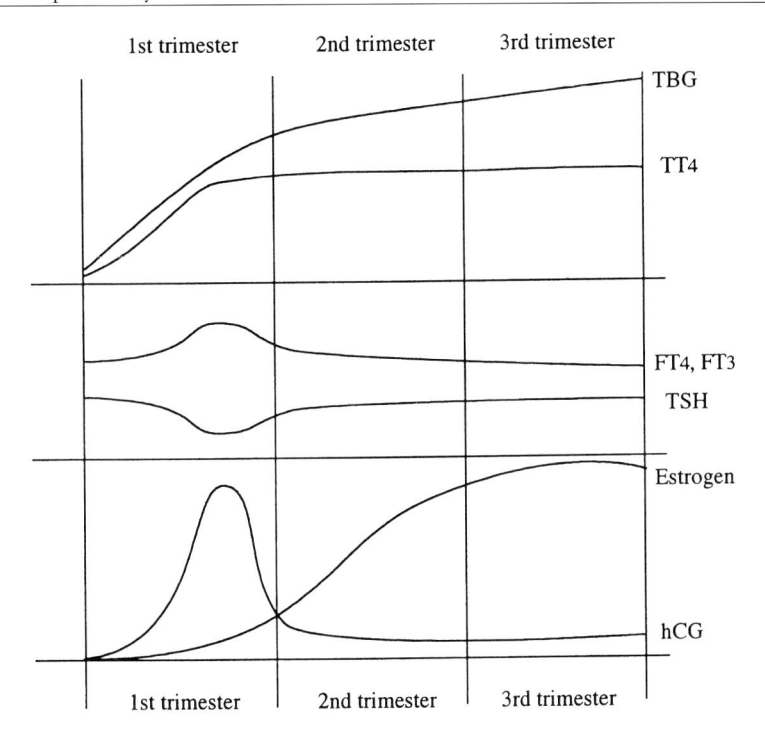

Fig. 2. Changes of serum FT_4, FT_3, TSH, and thyroxine binding globulin (TBG) during pregnancy.

As a consequence of the increase in thyroxine binding globulin (TBG), serum total thyroid hormone levels (TT_4 and TT_3) gradually increase in the first trimester and keep a plateau during the pregnancy. Free T_4 (FT_4), free T_3 (FT_3), and TSH are regulated to keep within normal ranges by the hypothalamus–pituitary–thyroid axis at least after the second trimester (Fig. 2). However, the measurements of FT_4 and FT_3 during pregnancy are sometimes problematic. In many early assay kits, measured values of FT_4 and FT_3 have been reported to decrease gradually in the 2nd–3rd pregnancy *(24)*. This may indicate real hypothyroidism owing to relative iodine deficiency), but is chiefly because those assays were influenced by serum albumin concentration *(25,26)*. The recent assay kits (such as Amerlex-MAB) that are designed to minimize these influences give results as shown in Fig. 2.

Another factor disturbing thyroid function is iodine deficiency. Maternal hypothyroxinemia owing to endemic iodine deficiency *(27)* is suspected to be responsible for impaired fetal psychoneurological development *(28,29)*. Even in the geographic areas where iodine intake is marginal or only mildly deficient, such as in European countries, mothers can become relatively iodine-deficient, since renal iodine clearance increases as gestation proceeds. Mild maternal hypothyroxinemia *(30,31)*, and more frequently, an increase in thyroid volume and serum thyroglobulin, are found in these areas *(32,33)*. In patients with thyroid nodules, an increase in the number and volume of the nodules may be observed *(34)*. An increase in thyroid volume and serum thyroglobulin may also be seen in neonates *(35)*, and iodine supplementation can reduce them both in mother and neonates *(32,33,35)*. However, it is undecided whether iodine supplementation in these areas should be recommended during pregnancy to prevent the risk of maternal and fetal hypothyroidism. In Japan, where iodine intake is rather high, no case of hypothyroxinemia owing to iodine deficiency has been reported.

AUTOIMMUNE THYROID DISEASE AND PREGNANCY

Hyperthyroidism and Pregnancy

Maternal hyperthyroidism is complicated in 0.2% of pregnancies *(36)*. The most common cause of hyperthyroidism during pregnancy is Graves' disease. Others include gestational thyrotoxicosis, often associated with hyperemesis gravidarum *(23)*, toxic nodular goiter, and gestational trophoblastic disease. A clinical or symptomatic diagnosis during gestation may present difficulties, because normal pregnancy may mimic some of the symptoms and signs of thyrotoxicosis, such as heat intolerance, tachycardia, and warm, moist skin. The diagnosis of hyperthyroidism is confirmed by an elevation in FT_4 and/or FT_3 and a suppressed serum TSH. The anti-TSH receptor antibody can be detected in most patients with Graves' disease.

Proper management of Graves' thyrotoxicosis is essential for the prevention of serious maternal, fetal, and neonatal complications. There is a higher incidence of congenital malformations in infants from untreated hyperthyroid mothers with Graves' disease *(37)*. An increase in neonatal mortality, low-birthweight infants, and premature labor are also seen *(38)*. In a report from 1929 before antithyroid therapy became available, total fetal loss rate in hyperthyroid mothers was as high as 48% *(39)*. The risk of thyroid storm may be increased in poorly controlled thyrotoxicosis at the time of labor and delivery. The treatment of choice for thyrotoxicosis in pregnancy is antithyroid drugs. The mothers rendered euthyroid with antithyroid drugs had as low a rate of fetal anomalies as normal mothers *(37)*. Antithyroid drugs cross the placenta and are excreted in breast milk. Propylthiouracil crosses the placenta only about one-fourth as much as methimazole, and is excreted into milk only one-tenth as much, because propylthiouracil is heavily protein-bound *(40)*. Therefore, propylthiouracil is preferred over methimazole for use in pregnancy and lactation. The dosage of the antithyroid drug that maintains maternal FT_4 levels in a mildly thyrotoxic range is appropriate for maintaining the euthyroid status in the fetus *(41)*. Subtotal thyroidectomy is the alternative definitive therapy for Graves' disease in pregnancy. Radioactive iodine is contraindicated during pregnancy, because the fetal thyroid starts to concentrate radioiodine at 12 wk. Cold iodine administration is effective and safe for pregnant women with mild hyperthyroidism, especially in the later stages of pregnancy *(42)*. The use of β-blockers for brief periods for the treatment of hypermetabolic symptoms is not contraindicated in pregnancy.

Graves' disease is aggravated in early pregnancy, ameliorates in the latter half of pregnancy, but often relapses postpartum (Fig. 3) *(43)*. hCG plays a crucial role in the aggravation of Graves' thyrotoxicosis in early pregnancy (Fig. 4) *(44)*. The reason for the postpartum flare-up is presumed to be the result of a rebound in immune surveillance following pregnancy *(45)*. After parturition, patients with Graves' disease do not always show a relapse of Graves' thyrotoxicosis, but destructive thyrotoxicosis may occur as in patients with Hashimoto's thyroiditis. It is important to predict the relapse of Graves' thyrotoxicosis, because treatment is necessary. Most patients with a high FT_4 index in early pregnancy show a recurrence of Graves' thyrotoxicosis after delivery *(45)*.

Hypothyroidism and Pregnancy

Hashimoto's (chronic) thyroiditis is the most common cause of hypothyroidism in women of childbearing age *(46)*. In some women, primary atrophic hypothyroidism is the cause of hypothyroidism. Overt hypothyroidism can cause anovulation and amenor-

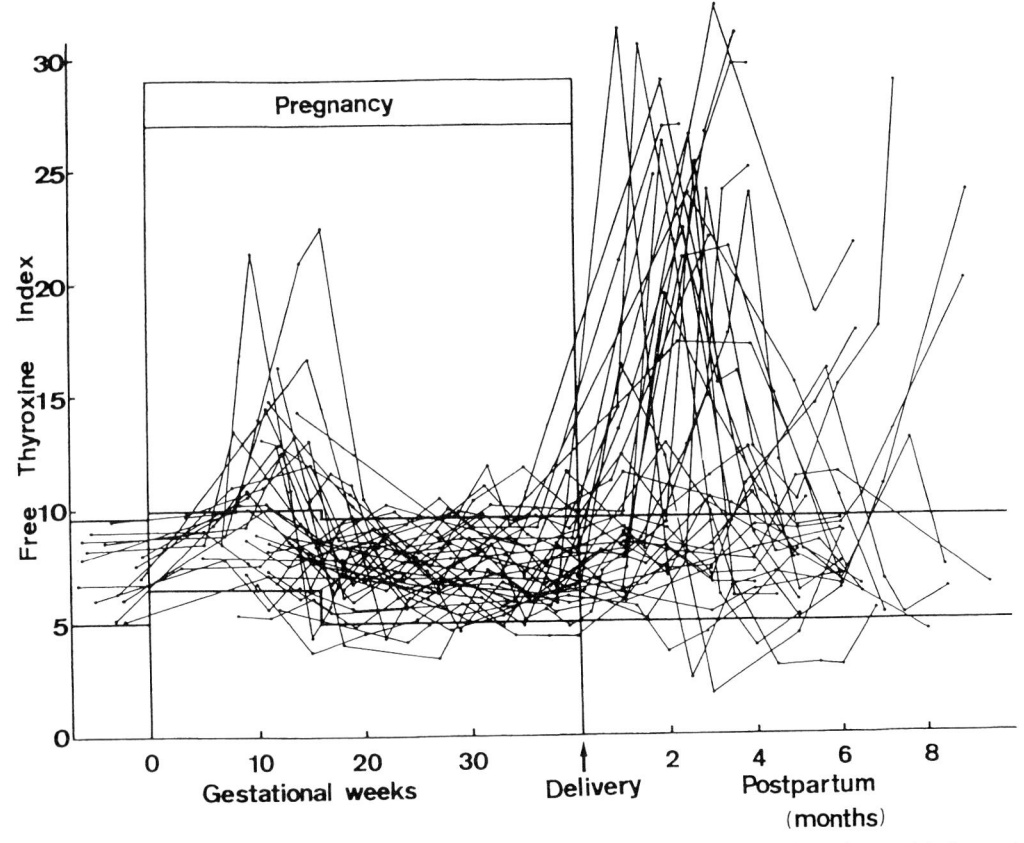

Fig. 3. Spontaneous changes in the serum FT$_4$ index during and after pregnancy in patients with Graves' disease in remission or near remission. Horizontal lines indicate the normal limit of the FT$_4$ index.

rhea, sometimes accompanied by hyperprolactinemia resulting from a feedback increase of TRH. Even latent hypothyroidism, i.e., with slight elevation of TSH and normal serum thyroid hormones, may impair fertility owing to an ovulatory or luteal dysfunction *(47)*. Infertility in hypothyroidism is restored by T$_4$-replacement therapy. An incidence of gestational hypertension and low birthweight is increased in women with hypothyroidism *(48)*.

A latent hypothyroid patient in early pregnancy may not require therapy, since thyroid function would be normalized in late pregnancy. For the patients who are treated with T$_4$-replacement therapy, the replacement should be continued. The dose in the replacement should be determined to keep a normal TSH level. A slight increase in the T$_4$ dose may be necessary in the hypothyroid patients after total thyroidectomy or with atrophic thyroiditis. This is probably because thyroid tissue no longer responds to hCG stimulation and is unable to produce more thyroxine, which is necessary to fill up TBG increased during pregnancy. Reduced peripheral conversion from T$_4$ to T$_3$ during pregnancy may also be of concern *(49–51)*.

Similar to Graves' disease, Hashimoto's thyroiditis spontaneously ameliorates during late pregnancy and is aggravated after delivery. In late pregnancy, TSH becomes significantly lower, and goiter size is reduced compared with those in non- or early pregnancy. Antimicrosomal antibody titers and the count of lymphocytes also show similar serial changes (Fig. 5) *(4)*. After delivery, exacerbation appears in the form of destructive thyrotoxicosis, transient thyrotoxicosis, transient hypothyroidism, or persistent hypothyroidism.

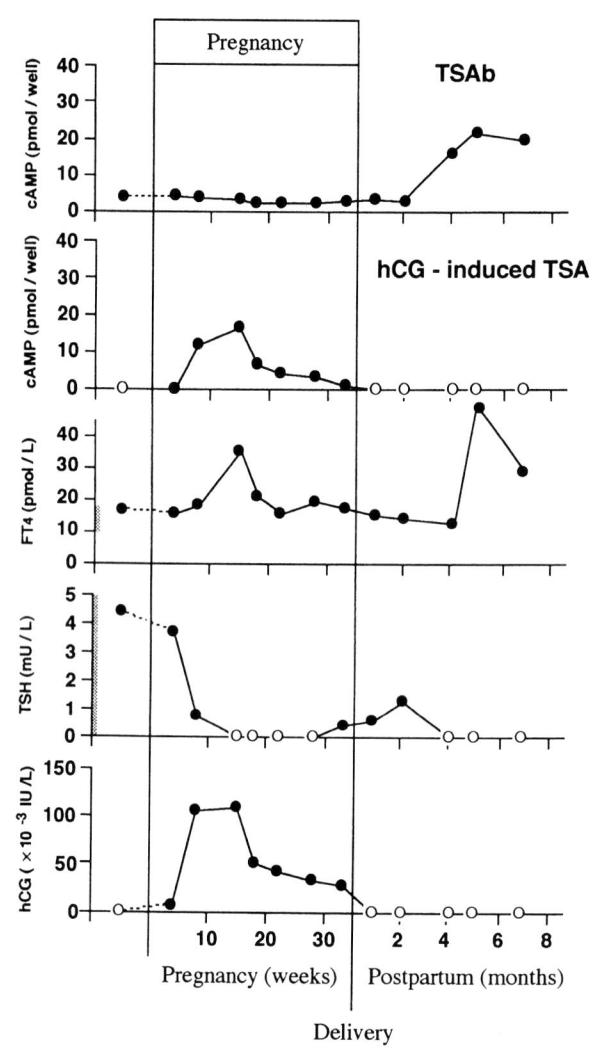

Fig. 4. Serial changes in the serum thyroid-stimulating activities (TSA) owing to TSAb and hCG, FT$_4$, TSH, and hCG in a patient with Graves' disease. Aggravation in early pregnancy was associated with hCG-induced TSA increase, but TSAb showed little change. ○: under the detectable limit.

POSTPARTUM AUTOIMMUNE THYROID DYSFUNCTION

Definition and Classification

In addition to Graves' disease and Hashimoto's disease, which are exacerbated or newly found after parturition, many kinds of thyroid dysfunctions are observed during the postpartum period. Most patients with postpartum thyroid dysfunctions show the positive antithyroid microsomal antibody beforehand. Therefore, we can consider that they had "subclinical autoimmune thyroiditis," which was exacerbated after delivery by the enhancement of immune activities. Thus, postpartum autoimmune thyroid syndrome is defined as any kind of thyroid dysfunction, including Graves' disease and Hashimoto's thyroiditis, newly occurring during the postpartum period from individuals who had experienced no previous thyroid dysfunction *(1)*.

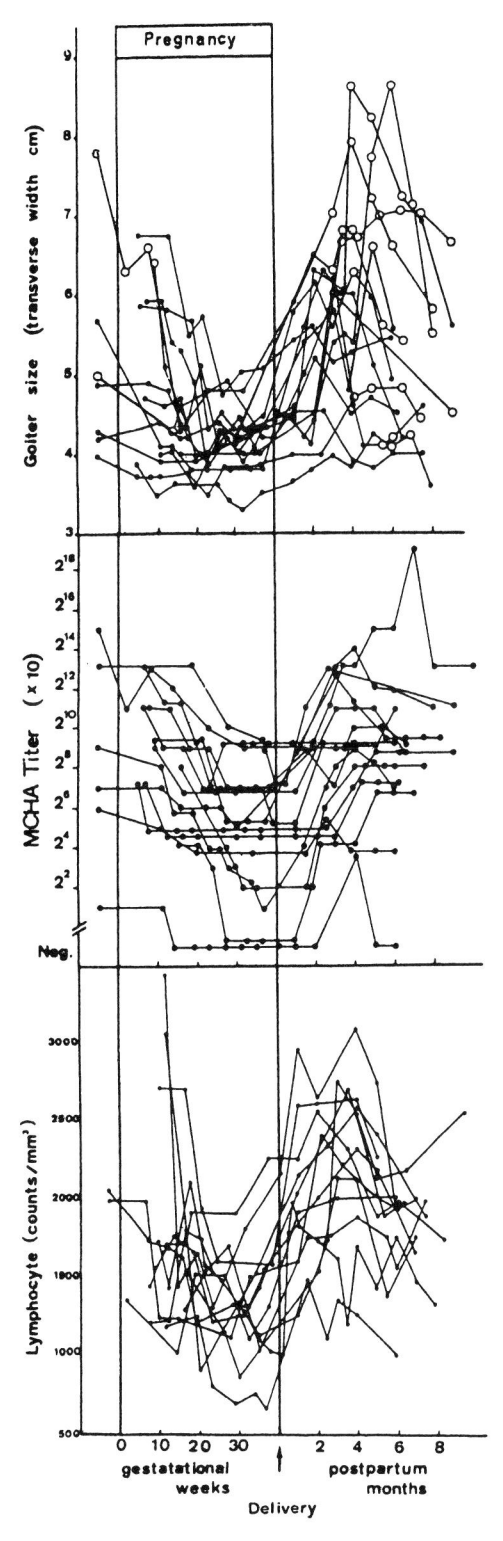

Fig. 5. Serial changes in goiter size, titers of antithyroid microsomal antibody, and the counts of peripheral lymphocytes during pregnancy and postpartum period in patients with Hashimoto's thyroiditis. Open circles denote that TSH was >10mU/L at the time of measurement. MCHA: microsomal hemagglutination antibody.

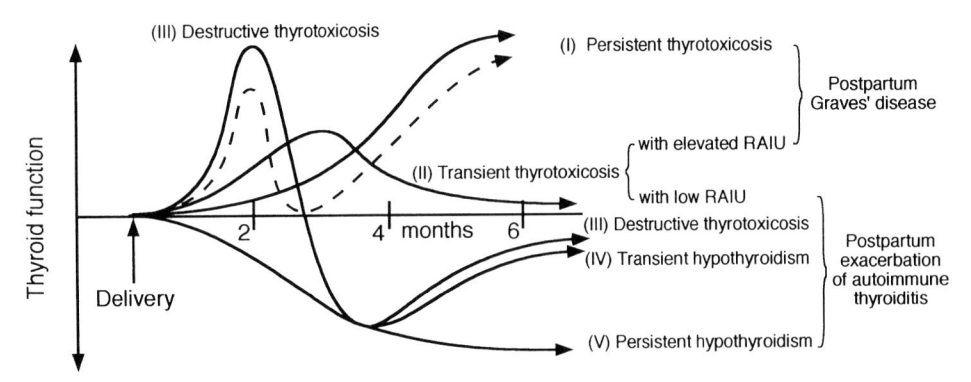

Fig. 6. Various types of postpartum thyroid dysfunction.

Postpartum thyroid dysfunctions were classified by their clinical features—hyperthyroid and/or hypothyroid, and transient or persistent—into five groups, as follows (summarized in Fig. 6).

1. Persistent thyrotoxicosis.
2. Transient thyrotoxicosis.
3. Destructive thyrotoxicosis followed by transient hypothyroidism.
4. Transient hypothyroidism.
5. Persistent hypothyroidism.

Persistent thyrotoxicosis (group I) and a part of transient thyrotoxicosis (group 2) revealed a high radioactive iodine uptake (RAIU), and therefore, they are considered to be Graves' disease. In transient thyrotoxicosis with a high RAIU, the overproduction of thyroid hormones ceases spontaneously within a year. Thyrotoxicosis in postpartum Graves' disease usually occurs at 4–6 mo postpartum.

Most postpartum thyroid dysfunctions occur owing to an exacerbation of autoimmune thyroiditis. They often manifest themselves as transient thyrotoxicosis (destructive thyrotoxicosis). In many cases, destructive thyrotoxicosis develops at 1–3 mo postpartum. Depending on the extent of the destruction, transient hypothyroidism may follow (group 3) or not (group 2, with a low RAIU). Occasionally, Graves' disease occurs closely following, or concomitantly with destructive thyrotoxicosis (dotted line in Fig. 6) *(52)*. When cellular damage occurs slowly, hypothyroidism alone, rather than destructive thyrotoxicosis, may be observed after delivery. In many cases, it is transient (group 4). However, it may last persistently in a few cases (group 5).

Prevalence

The prevalence of postpartum thyroid dysfunctions in the general population is about 5% (1.1–16.7%; Table 1), i.e., one in 20 pregnant women *(1,53–64)*. Thyroid dysfunctions are transient in most cases. However, we should pay more attention to them, since thyroid dysfunction during the postpartum period may negatively affect the quality of life of the mother who must be exhausted taking care of her baby. The prevalence of postpartum Graves' disease (both persistent and transient) is estimated at 11% of those with postpartum thyroid dysfunction and 0.5% of the general population *(65)*. In these types of postpartum thyroiditis, immune status seems quite similar to that in Hashimoto's thyroiditis. Destructive transient thyrotoxicosis (group 2, with a low RAIU + group 3) is the most common form of postpartum thyroid dysfunction, accounting for 50–60% of

Table 1
Prevalence of Postpartaum Thyroid Dysfunction

Year	Author	Country	Prevalence, %
1982	Amino	Japan	5.5
1982	Turney[a]	US	9.0
1984	Jansson	Sweden	6.5
1985	Walfish	Canada	7.1
1986	Freeman	US	1.9
1987	Nikolai	US	6.7
1987	Lervang	Denmark	3.9
1988	Fung	UK	16.7
1990	Rasmussen	Denmark	3.3
1990	Rajatanavin	Thailand	1.1
1991	Roti	Italy	4.8
1991	Löbig	Germany	2.0
1992	Walfish	Canada	6.0
1992	Stagnaro-Green	US	8.8
1992	Kannan[b]	India	7.0
1996	Pizarro[b]	Spain	9.3
1997	Yim[c]	Korea	8.0

[a]Report at American Endocrine Society.
[b]Report at International Congress of Endocrinology.
[c]Report at the Asia-Oceania Thyroid Association Congress.

all postpartum thyroid dysfunction. The rest shows only the hypothyroid phase. However, persistent hyothyroidism is very rare (<0.1%).

Iodine deficiency is not likely to affect the prevalence of postpartum thyroid dysfunction *(66)*, although it may aggravate it *(67)*, and relative iodine deficiency may be prolonged after parturition in breast-feeding mothers, disturbing thyroid status *(68)*.

Diagnosis and Management

Diagnosis of postpartum thyroid dysfunction is rather simple when the patient shows thyroid dysfunction during the postpartum period and positive antithyroid autoantibodies *(69)*. Thyroid dysfunction is most often subclinical, wherein no more than observation is necessary. Clinically, differential diagnosis for overt thyrotoxicosis between Graves' thyrotoxicosis and destructive thyrotoxicosis is essential, although it can usually be ascertained from the time of onset (destructive thyrotoxicosis usually occurs at 1–3 mo after parturition, whereas Graves' disease occurs at 3–6 mo after parturition). The measurement of radioactive iodine uptake is definitive, but might not be preferred for breast-feeding mothers. The serum total T_3/total T_4 ratio (<20 ng/µg) is helpful for the diagnosis of destructive thyrotoxicosis *(70)*. Serial changes of serum thyroglobulin (Tg) concentration may also be helpful, since it increases before the onset of destructive thyrotoxicosis. However, because of the interference by antithyroglobulin antibodies with the conventional measurement system, a new sensitive multisite immunoradiometric Tg assay should be employed for this purpose *(71)*. Markers useful for the differential diagnosis are summarized in Table 2. Even if the diagnosis is once established, patients should be followed up for a year, since Graves' disease may develop following destructive thyrotoxicosis. In the treatment of postpartum Graves' disease, an antithyroid drug may be a good choice for the first-line therapy *(72)*, because:

Table 2
Differential Diagnosis Between Graves' Disease and Postpartum Destructive Thyrotoxicosis

	Graves' disease	Destructive thyrotoxicosis
Onset	3–6 mo postpartum	1–3 mo postpartum
Radioactive iodine uptake	High	Low
Anti-TSH receptor antibody	Positive	Negative in most cases
Eye signs	Yes	No
Total T_3/total T_4 ratio (ng/µg)	>20 in 80% of cases	<20
Serial changes in serum thyroglobulin[a]	<150% increase from a month before the onset	>150% increase from a month befor the onset

[a]Thyroglobulin should be measured with a method not influenced by antithyroglobulin autoantibody (TgAb).

1. Postpartum Graves' hyperthyroidism is often transient.
2. Even in persistent Graves' disease, the patients who were diagnosed early after onset can have their disease easily controlled with an antithyroid drug (65).
3. Mothers may not want to interrupt breast-feeding during radioiodine therapy.

A typical course of postpartum Graves' disease is shown in Fig. 7. The patient became thyrotoxic at 3 mo after delivery. Thyroid-stimulating antibody (TSAb) was continuously positive from early pregnancy and elevated after delivery. On the other hand, thyroid binding inhibitory immunoglobulin (TBII) turned positive only after the onset of thyrotoxicosis. The antithyroid therapy had promptly led to remission (not shown in figure). Radioactive iodine therapy would not be too late to begin a year after the hyperthyroidism appeared persistent and was not controlled with antithyroid drugs.

Hypothyroidism is usually transient, so no therapy is necessary for most cases. Hypothyroidism tends to be transient when the patient is young, and when her goiter enlarges and serum Tg elevates in response to the increase in TSH. For severe hypothyroid symptoms, thyroid hormone replacement is recommended. Usual L-thyroxine (L-T_4) therapy with a gradual reduction in dose may work well, but a recovery of the patient's thyroid function may not be seen explicitly. Alternatively, with triiodothyronine (T_3) therapy, by the time of recovery of thyroid function, the elevation of serum T_4 concentration clearly indicates recovery. In the areas where iodine intake is marginal or mildly deficient, iodine supplementation should be considered for mothers who are breast-feeding and have been hypothyroid during pregnancy (30).

Long-Term Prognosis

In postpartum Graves' hyperthyroidism, there has been little study on long-term prognosis, although we expect better prognosis than "ordinary" Graves' disease because of early diagnosis just after the onset.

In destructive thyrotoxicosis and/or hypothyroidism owing to exacerbation of autoimmune thyroiditis, thyroid dysfunction is transient, and most patients recover to euthyroid spontaneously. Hypothyroidism rarely continues persistently. High titers of antithyroglobulin antibody is a risk factor in persistent hypothyroidism. In the Japanese, hypothyroidism in patients with HLA-DRw9 and/or B51 genotype are likely to be persistent (73). Even though once recovered from hypothyroidism, abnormality in ultrasonography and/or

Chapter 11 / Postpartum Syndromes

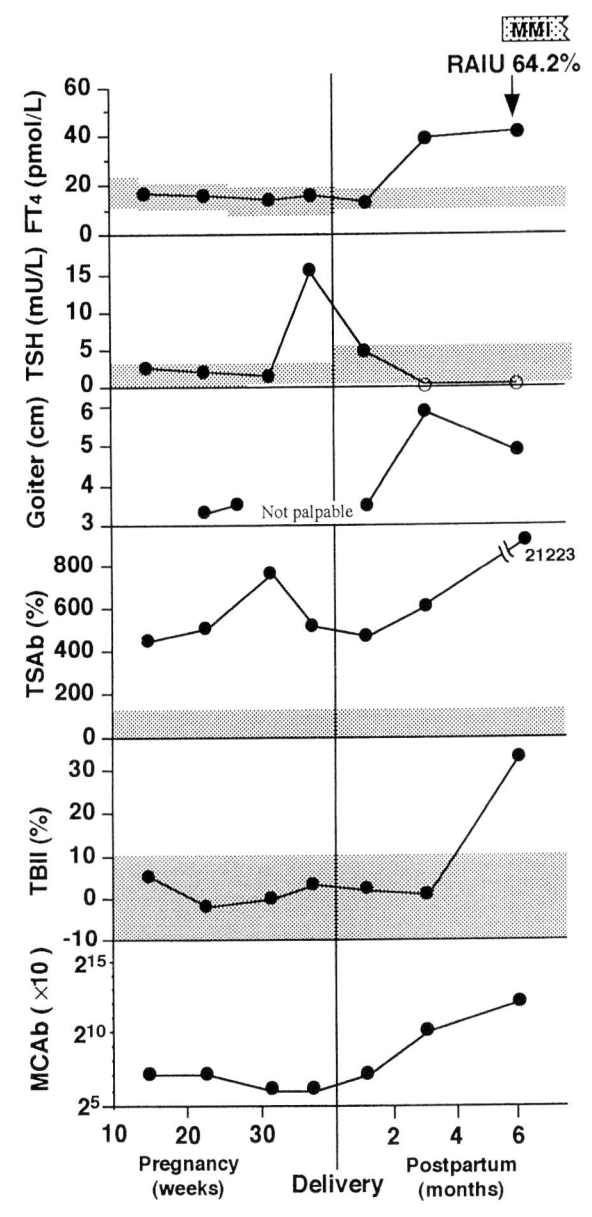

Fig. 7. A case of persistent postpartum Graves' thyrotoxicosis who had positive TSAb in her early pregnancy.

iodide perchlorate discharge tests may long persist *(74,75)*, which may reflect background autoimmune thyroiditis. The later development (after 5 yr or more) of permanent hypothyroidism is found in 1/4 of the patients with postpartum thyroiditis in long-term observation *(76)*. Therefore, they should be followed up at appropriate intervals (every 1–2 yr). High antimicrosomal antibody titre and severity of hypothyroid phase of postpartum thyroiditis were risk factors for later development of permanent hypothyroidism, but there was no association to HLA haplotype or a family history of thyroid disease *(76)*.

Table 3
Postpartum Development of Thyroid Dysfunction
in Patients with Subclinical Autoimmune Thyroiditis

Postpartum thyroid function	Case no.	%	
Normal (euthyroid)	27	38.0	
Dysfunction	44	62.0	
Persistent Graves' thyrotoxicosis	2	2.8	} 7.0
Transient Graves' thyrotoxicosis	3	4.2	
Destructive thyrotoxicosis followed by transient hypothyroidism	23	32.4	} 55.0
Transient thyrotoxicosis alone	7	9.9	
Transient hypothyroidism alone	9	12.7	
Total	71	100	

Prediction of Postpartum Thyroiditis

As mentioned above, postpartum autoimmune thyroid syndrome is briefly characterized as a syndrome of postpartum exacerbation of subclinical autoimmune thyroid disease. Therefore, some immunological abnormalities are observed before the onset of thyroid dysfunction (and therefore, before and during pregnancy). Among these, the measurement of antithyroid microsomal antibody (MCAb) is the most useful marker for the prediction of the occurrence of postpartum thyroid dysfunction. When MCAb is positive, there is always lymphocytic infiltration into the thyroid, and therefore there is "subclinical autoimmune thyroiditis" *(77)*, which may be exacerbated after delivery. Sixty to 70% of women with positive MCAb in early pregnancy develop postpartum thyroid dysfunction *(1)*. Also, the prevalence of the types of thyroid dysfunction developed amoung MCAb-positive pregnant subjects in a prospective study is shown in Table 3. The prevalence of postpartum thyroid dysfunction in the MCAb-negative subjects in early pregnancy is estimated at 1/100 of that in MCAb-positive subjects (Fig. 8), since MCAb is positive in most patients (90%) with autoimmune thyroiditis *(70)*. Other reports say MCAb-positive subjects had 20–23-times relative risk for developing postpartum thyroid dysfunction *(78,79)*. Especially, mothers with high MCAb titer (>5000–10000×) always develop postpartum thyroid dysfunction. Although the measurement of MCAb with semiquantitative particle agglutination tests (MCPA) is simple and cheap, the significance of the screening for postpartum autoimmune thyroid syndrome remains unsettled, probably depending on each country's national health system *(80)*. It may be recommended for all the early pregnant women in Japan, although only for the patients with insulin-dependent diabetes mellitus (IDDM) in some countries. Antithyroid peroxidase antibody (TPOAb) is no better than MCPA for predicting postpartum thyroid dysfunction *(81)*. The initial thyroid volume or changes in volume are not useful indicators of the development of postpartum thyroid dysfunction *(61)*.

Prediction of Postpartum Graves' Disease

Among the groups of postpartum thyroid dysfunction, the onset of Graves' disease is of most interest in clinical practice. Early diagnosis and therapy just at the onset of the disease can lead to early remission *(65)*. As mentioned above, 11.4% of postpartum thyroid dysfunctions (that represents 0.54% of the general population) is Graves' disease.

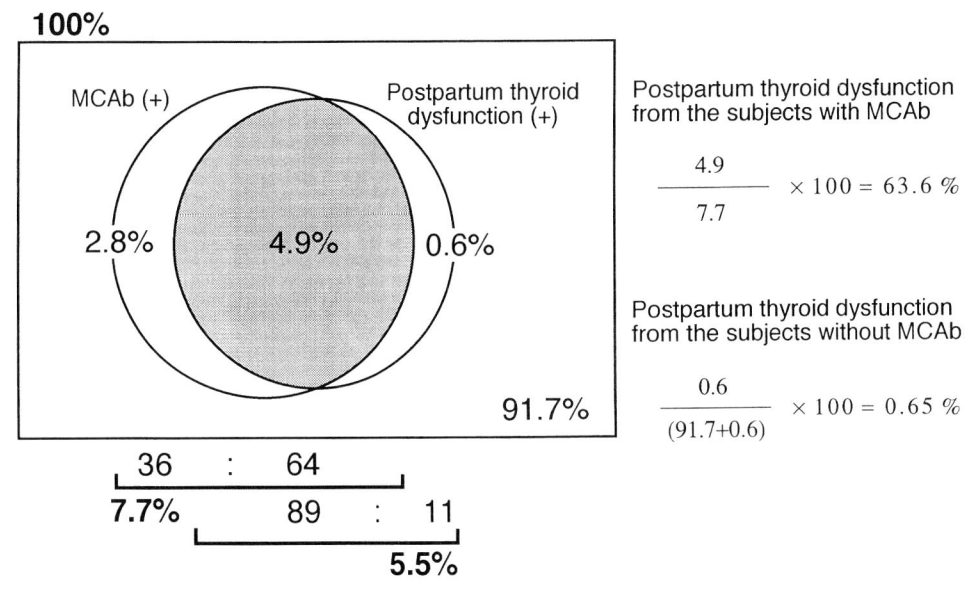

Fig. 8. The prevalence of antithyroid microsomal antibody and the occurence of postpartum thyroid dysfunction among pregnant women in the general population.

Conversely, 40% of Graves' patients 20–39 yr old, who have had one or more deliveries, developed their disease during the postpartum period *(82)*. We can take the stimulating type of the anti-TSH receptor antibody (thyroid-stimulating antibody; TSAb) as a marker for postpartum development of Graves' disease, since TSAb is positive before the onset of Graves' disease *(83)* when measured with a sensitive bioassay *(84)*. Our prospective study *(65)* revealed that the pregnant women with positive TSAb in early pregnancy had an obviously high risk of developing postpartum Graves' disease. Seventy-one pregnant women with positive MCAb in early pregnancy were prospectively observed from early pregnancy to the postpartum period. Among them, seven showed positive TSAb, five (70%) of whom developed postpartum Graves' disease. Thyrotoxicosis in three of those five was transient and spontaneously improved within a year. Graves' disease did not occur in the TSAb-negative subjects (Fig. 9).

Immune Rebound Mechanism

The immune rebound hypothesis explains the enhancement of immune activities after parturition as the rebound from the suppressed immune state. During pregnancy, maternal immune activities are suppressed in order not to reject the baby. Sudden release from the immune suppression at the moment of delivery intensifies immune activities above the normal level, just as the sudden cessation of immunosuppresive drugs gives rise to the exacerbation of autoimmune diseases *(4)*. The serial changes of MCAb titers in pregnant women with Hashimoto's disease (Fig. 5) support this idea. The immune rebound seems to be rather a general phenomenon observed in the postpartum period, since serum levels of immunogloblins *(85)* and counts of lymphocytes and natural killer/killer (NK/K) cell activity *(86)* decrease in late pregnancy, and increase after delivery even in normal pregnant women. Since immunological situations after abortion are similar to those during the postpartum period, postabortional thyroid dysfunction may occur in some cases *(87,88)*.

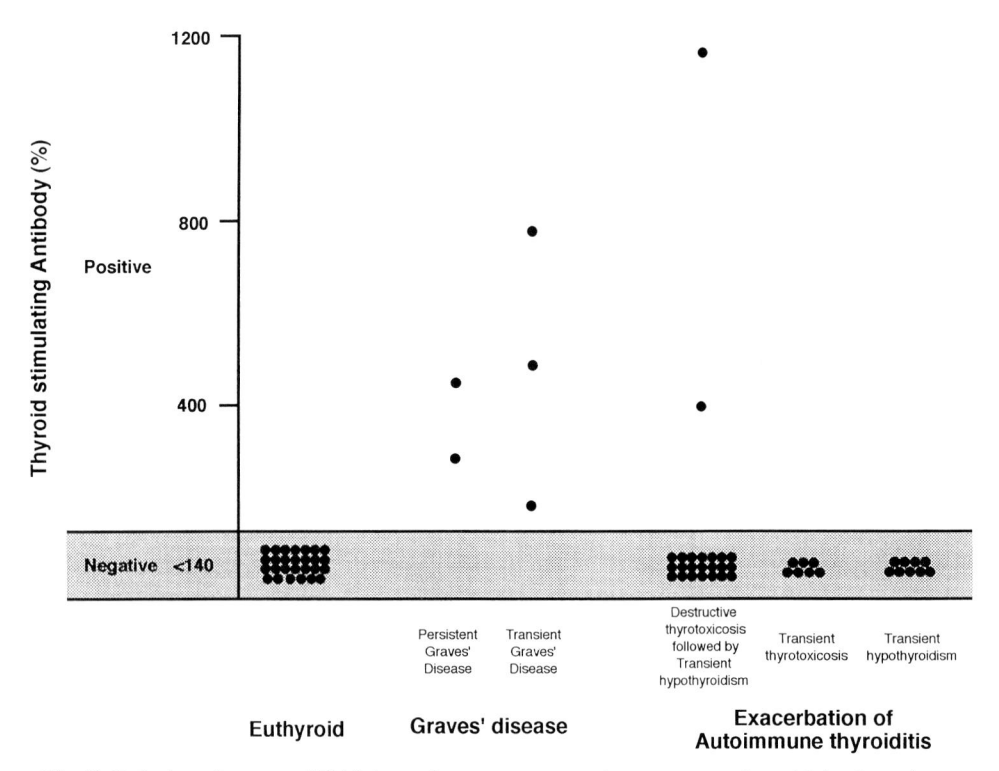

Fig. 9. Relations between TSAb in early pregnancy and postpartum thyroid dysfunctions.

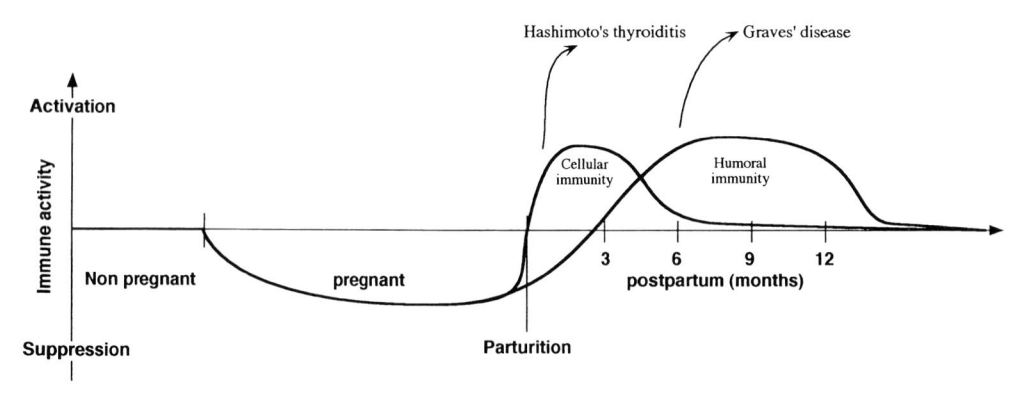

Fig. 10. Immune-rebound hypothesis of postpartum autoimmuine thyroid diseases.

The postpartum rebound of immune activities consists of two phases (Fig. 10). Cytotoxic T (Tc) cells and NK cells increase from 1 to 4 months postpartum (Fig. 11) *(3)*. The enhancement of cellular immunity may exacerbate tissue injury in Hashimoto's thyroiditis. In contrast, CD5+ cells, which produce autoantibodies, increase from 7–10 mo postpartum (Fig. 11) *(3)*. The enhancement of humoral immunity may cause postpartum Graves' disease, which is caused by anti-TSH receptor autoantibodies. Indeed, Hashimoto's thyroiditis is frequently aggravated from 1–3 mo postpartum, and Graves' disease frequently develops or relapses from 3–6 mo postpartum (Fig. 10).

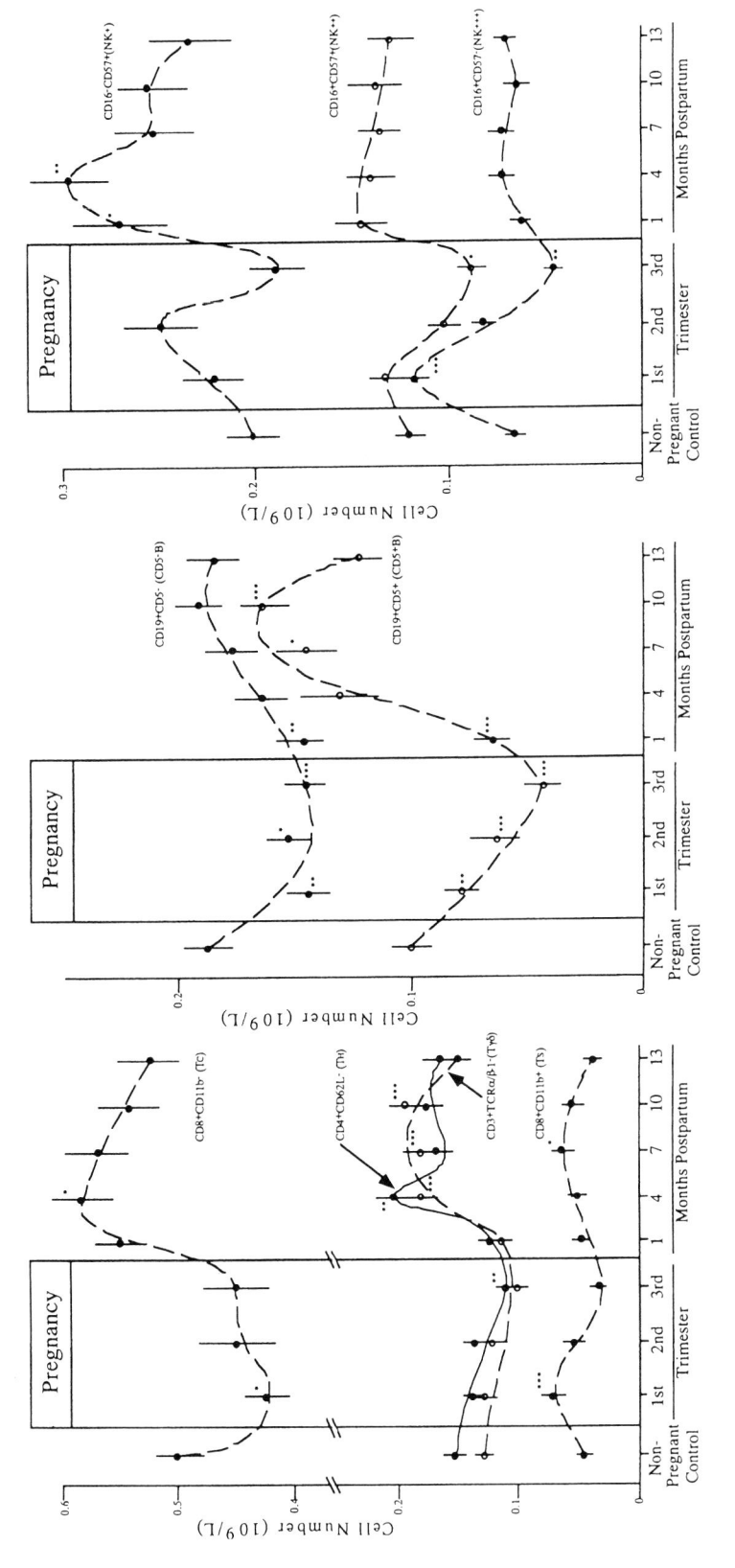

Fig 11. Changes in absolute numbers of peripheral TCRαβ-negative T (Tγδ) cells, helper T (T_H) cells, suppressor T (Ts) cells, cytotoxic T (Tc) cells, CD5⁻ B cells, CD5⁺ B cells, and NK cell subsets during and after pregnancy. *: $P < 0.05$, **: $P < 0.001$, ***: $P < 0.001$ (compared with non-pregnant control).

POSTPARTUM AUTOIMMUNE DISEASES

Postpartum aggravation or onset of autoimmune thyroid diseases through the immune-rebound mechanism is frequently observed as described above. It is well known that autoimmune diseases are often found in women of childbearing age. However, little attention has been paid to the relationship between pregnancy and the onset of autoimmune disease, except autoimmune thyroid disease. It is easy to assume that autoimmune diseases can develop after delivery in many organs.

Lymphocytic autoimmune hypophysitis is a rare disease, but interestingly 30% of the disease developed during the postpartum period in female patients *(89)*. The pituitary may also be the subject of autoimmune damage during the postpartum period. It has long been documented that rheumatoid arthritis is ameliorated during pregnancy and aggravated after delivery *(90)*. The onset of rheumatoid arthritis seems to be suppressed during pregnancy, but conversely, it is increased after delivery, especially the first 3 mo postpartum *(91)*. Postpartum onset of rheumatoid arthritis was found in 0.08% of women in the general population and could be partially predicted by measuring rheumatoid factors in early pregnancy *(92)*. Other diseases are also reported to develop after delivery possibly through the immune-rebound mechanism: postpartum renal failure *(93)* or post-delivery hemolytic-uremic syndrome *(94)*, postpartum idiopathic polymyositis *(95)*, postpartum syndrome with antiphospholipid antibodies *(96)*, postpartum autoimmune myocarditis *(97)*, and others. Puerperal diseases should be carefully examined in relation to autoimmune abnormalities in the affected organs.

NEONATAL THYROID DISEASE OWING TO ANTIBODY TRANSFER

Since maternal IgGs can easily go through placenta and into the baby, the anti-TSH receptor antibody can affect fetal and/or neonatal thyroid function. Thyrotoxicosis may occur only in the fetus if the maternal thyroid has been ablated (as in an operative or radioiodine therapy for Graves' disease), but high levels of anti-TSH receptor antibody persist. High levels of maternal anti-TSH receptor antibody and fetal tachycardia with a heart rate above 160 beats/min suggest fetal hyperthyroidism. In such cases, an antithyroid drug directed toward the fetus should be considered. Neonatal thyroid dysfunction may also be observed in babies whose mothers had considerably high activities of the anti-TSH receptor antibody, referred to as neonatal Graves' disease. Although there is another entity of neonatal hyperthyroidism, i.e., congenital hyperthyroidism owing to activating point mutation in the TSH receptor gene *(98)*, it is very rare, and differential diagnosis might not be difficult.

The pathogenesis of neonatal Graves' diseases is fully "humoral," i.e., passively transferred IgG is responsible for thyroid dysfunction. The anti-TSH receptor antibody, once transferred into the baby, stimulates the baby's thyroid and causes neonatal Graves' disease. The half-lifetime of the anti-TSH receptor antibody in the neonatal circulation is estimated as 13 ± 2.6 d. Therefore, thyroid dysfunction is essentially self-limiting, and it ceases spontaneously after 1–3 mo. Although neonatal Graves' disease is self-limiting, overt hyperthyroidism in the neonate can cause serious heart failure, and result in neonatal death so easily that it should be diagnosed and treated as soon as possible. In a baby from a mother receiving an antithyroid drug that also passes through the placenta, thyrotoxic symptoms may slowly appear on 4–10 d after birth *(99)*. The risk of neonatal Graves' disease can be found beforehand from the mother's high activity of the anti-TSH

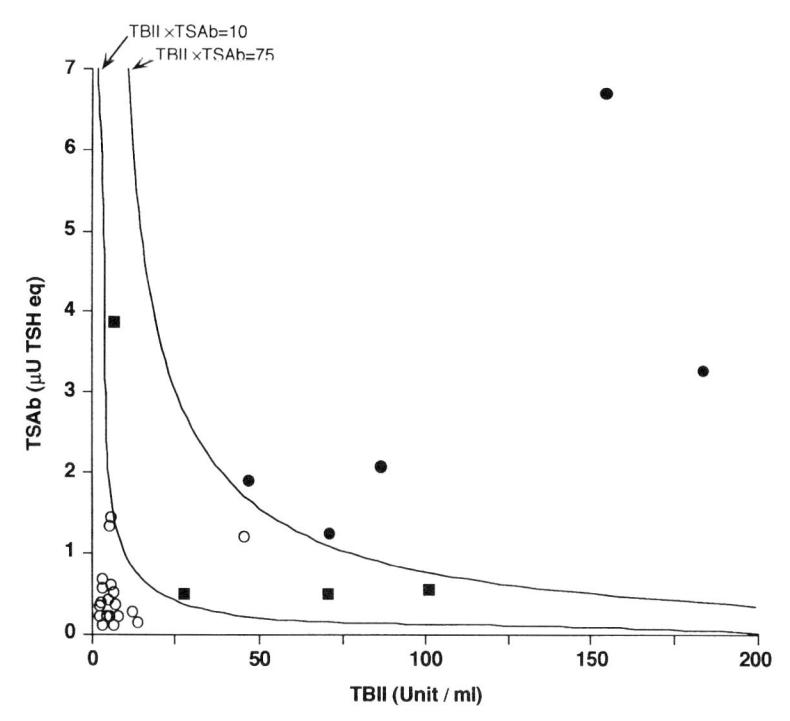

Fig. 12. Prediction of neonatal thyrotoxicosis with the product of TBII and TSAb (BS index). ○: euthyroid; ■: chemical thyrotoxicosis; ●: overt thyrotoxicosis.

receptor antibody in late pregnancy. For the evaluation of risk, the binding-stimulation index (B-S index) was proposed as the numerical product of TBII and TSAb activity *(99)*.

$$\text{B-S index} = \text{TBII (U/mL)} \times \text{TSAb (bTSH μUEq)} \quad (1)$$

Figure 12 shows that thyrotoxicosis in neonates occurred from the area of B-S index >75. Since the actual cutoff value of the index depends on the system of units employed, autoantibody activities are recommended to be expressed in a standardized manner *(100)*, or a cutoff value should be defined in each laboratory according to the method of measurement.

The transfer of the blocking type anti-TSH receptor antibody (thyroid stimulation blocking antibody [TSBAb]) may cause neonatal transient hypothyroidism. Neonatal transient hypothyroidism occurs only in babies whose mothers had extremely high TSBAb activity and had atrophic hypothyroidism *(101)*. It does not occur in babies from mothers with goiterous Hashimoto's disease.

REFERENCES

1. Amino N, Mori H, Iwatani Y, et al. High prevalence of transient postpartum thyrotoxicosis and hypothyroidism. N Engl J Med 1982;306:849–852.
2. Hidaka Y, Amino N, Iwatani Y, Itoh E, Matsunaga M, Tamaki H. Recurrence of thyrotoxicosis after attack of allergic rhinitis in patients with Graves' disease. J Clin Endocrinol Metab 1993;77:1667–1670.
3. Watanabe M, Iwatani Y, Kaneda T, et al. Changes in T, B, and NK lymphocyte subsets during and after normal pregnancy. Am J Reprod Immunol 1997;37:368–377.
4. Amino N, Miyai K. Postpartum autoimmune endocrine syndromes. In: Davies T, eds. Autoimmune Endocrine Disease. John Wiley, New York, 1983, pp. 247–272.

5. Amino N, Tada H, Hidaka Y. Autoimmune thyroid disease and pregnancy. J Endocrinol Invest 1996; 19:59–70.
6. Amir SM, Sullivan RC, Ingbar SH. In vivo responses to crude and purified hCG in human thyroid membranes. J Clin Endocrinol Metab 1980;51:51–98.
7. Azukizawa M, Kurtzman G, Pekary A, Hershman J. Comparison of the binding characteristics of bovine thyrotropin and human chorionic gonadotropin to thyroid plasma membranes. Endocrinology 1977;101:1880–1889.
8. Hoermann R, Broecker M, Grossmann M, Mann K, Derwahl M. Interaction of human chorionic gonadotropin (hCG) and asialo-hCG with recombinant human thyrotropin receptor. J Clin Endocrinol Metab 1994;78:933–938.
9. Kraiem Z, Sadeh O, Blithe DL, Nisula BC. Human chorionic gonadotropin stimulates thyroid hormone secretion, iodide uptake, organification, and adenosine 3',5'-monophosphate formation in cultured human thyrocytes. J Clin Endocrinol Metab 1994;79:595–999.
10. Tomer Y, Huber GK, Davies TF. Human chorionic gonadotropin (hCG) interacts directly with recombinant human TSH receptors. J Clin Endocrinol Metab 1992;74:1477–1479.
11. Yoshimura M, Hershman JM, Pang XP, Berg L, Pekary AE. Activation of the thyrotropin (TSH) receptor by human chorionic gonadotropin and luteinizing hormone in Chinese hamster ovary cells expressing functional human TSH receptors. J Clin Endocrinol Metab 1993;77:1009–1013.
12. Yoshikawa N, Nishikawa M, Horimoto M, et al. Thyroid-stimulating activity in sera of normal pregnant woman. J Clin Endocrinol Metab 1989;69:891–895.
13. Kimura M, Amino N, Tamaki H, Mitsuda N, Miyai K, Tanizawa O. Physiologic thyroid activation in normal early pregnancy is induced by circulating hCG. Obstet Gynecol 1990;75:775–778.
14. Kennedy RL, Darne J, Cohn M, et al. Human chorionic gonadotropin (hCG) may not be responsible for thyroid-stimulating activity (TSA) in normal pregnancy serum. J Clin Endocrinol Metab 1992;72: 258–263.
15. Yoshimura M, Nishikawa M, Yoshikawa N, et al. Mechanism of thyroid stimulation by human chorionic gonadotropin in sera of normal pregnant women. Acta Endocrinol (Copenh) 1991;124:173–178.
16. Ballabio M, Poshychinda M, Ekins RP. Pregnancy-induced changes in thyroid function: role of human chorionic gonadotropin as putative regulator of maternal thyroid. J Clin Endocrinol Metab 1991;73: 824–831.
17. Hershman JM. Role of human chorionic gonadotropin as a thyroid stimulator. J Clin Endocrinol Metab 1991;74:258–259.
18. Goodwin TM, Montoro M, Mestman JH, Pekary AE, Hershman JM. The role of chorionic gonadotropin in transient hyperthyroidism of hyperemesis gravidarum. J Clin Endocrinol Metab 1992;75: 1333–1337.
19. Wilson R, McKillop JH, MacLean M, et al. Thyroid function tests are rarely abnormal in patients with severe hyperemesis gravidarum. Clin Endocrinol (Oxford) 1992;37:331–334.
20. Kimura M, Amino N, Tamaki H, et al. Gestational thyrotoxicosis and hyperemesis gravidarum: possible role of hCG with higher stimulating activity. Clin Endocrinol (Oxford) 1993;38:345–350.
21. Kennedy RL, Darne J, Davies R, Price A. Thyrotoxicosis and hyperemesis gravidarum associated with a serum activity which stimulates human thyroid cells in vitro. Clin Endocrinol (Oxford) 1992;36: 83–89.
22. Mori M, Amino N, Tamaki H, Miyai K, Tanizawa O. Morning sickness and thyroid function in normal pregnancy. Obstet Gynecol 1988;72:355–359.
23. Tsuruta E, Tada H, Tamaki H, et al. Pathogenic role of asialo-hCG in gestational thyrotoxicosis. J Clin Endocrinol Metab 1995;80:350–355.
24. Nissim M, Giorda G, Ballabio M, et al. Maternal thyroid function in early and late pregnancy. Horm Res 1991;36:196–202.
25. Amino N, Nishi K, Nakatani K, et al. Effect of albumin concentration on the assay of serum free thyroxine by equilibrium radioimmunoassay with labeled thyroxine analog (Amerlex Free T_4). Clin Chem 1983;29:321–325.
26. Deam D, Goodwin M, Ratnaike S. Comparison of four methods for free thyroxin. Clin Chem 1991; 37:569–72.
27. Vermiglio F, Lo PV, Scaffidi AG, et al. Maternal hypothyroxinaemia during the first half of gestation in an iodine deficient area with endemic cretinism and related disorders. Clin Endocrinol (Oxford) 1995;42:409–415.

28. Porterfield SP, Hendrich CE. The role of thyroid hormones in prenatal and neonatal neurological development—current perspectives. Endocr Rev 1993;14:94–106.
29. Delange F. The disorders induced by iodine deficiency. Thyroid 1994;4:107–128.
30. Glinoer D, Nayer P, Bourdoux P, et al. Regulation of maternal thyroid during pregnancy. J Clin Endocrinol Metab 1990;71:276–287.
31. Glinoer D, Delange F, Laboureur I, et al. Maternal and neonatal thyroid function at birth in an area of marginally low iodine intake. J Clin Endocrinol Metab 1992;75:800–805.
32. Pedersen KM, Laurberg P, Iversen E, et al. Amelioration of some pregnancy-associated variations in thyroid function by iodine supplementation. J Clin Endocrinol Metab 1993;77:1078–1083.
33. Romano R, Jannini EA, Pepe M, et al. The effects of iodoprophylaxis on thyroid size during pregnancy. Am J Obstet Gynecol 1991;164:482–485.
34. Glinoer D, Soto MF, Bourdoux P, et al. Pregnancy in patients with mild thyroid abnormalities: maternal and neonatal repercussions. J Clin Endocrinol Metab 1991;73:421–427.
35. Glinoer D, De NP, Delange F, et al. A randomized trial for the treatment of mild iodine deficiency during pregnancy: maternal and neonatal effects. J Clin Endocrinol Metab 1995;80:258–269.
36. Burrow GN. The management of thyrotoxicosis in pregnancy. N Engl J Med 1985;313:562–565.
37. Momotani N, Ito K, Hamada N, Ban Y, Nishikawa Y, Mimura T. Maternal hyperthyroidism and congenital malformations in the offspring. Clin Endocrinol 1984;20:695–700.
38. Davis LE, Lucas MJ, Hankins GD, Roark ML, Cunningham FG. Thyrotoxicosis complicating pregnancy. Am J Obstet Gynecol 1989;160:63–70.
39. Gardner-Hill H. Pregnancy complicating simple goitre and Graves' disease. Lancet 1929;1:120–124.
40. Cooper DS. Antithyroid drugs. N Engl J Med 1984;311:1353–1362.
41. Momotani N, Noh J, Oyanaga H, Ishikawa N, Ito K. Antithyroid drug therapy for Graves' disease during pregnancy. N Engl J Med 1986;315:24–28.
42. Momotani N, Hisaoka T, Noh J, Ishikawa N, Ito K. Effects of iodine on thyroid status of fetus versus mother in treatment of Graves' disease complicated by pregnancy. J Clin Endocrinol Metab 1992;75: 738–744.
43. Amino N, Tanizawa O, Mori H, et al. Aggravation of thyrotoxicosis in early pregnancy and after delivery in Graves' disease. J Clin Endocrinol Metab 1982;55:108–112.
44. Tamaki H, Itoh E, Kaneda T, et al. Crucial role of serum human chorionic gonadotropin for the aggravation of thyrotoxicosis in early pregancy in Graves' disease. Thyroid 1993;3:189–193.
45. Amino N, Iwatani Y, Tamaki H. Postpartum autoimmune thyroid syndromes. In: Walfish PG, Wall JR, Volpé R, eds. Autoimmunity and the Thyroid. Academic, Orlando, 1985, pp. 289–314.
46. Amino N, Tada H. Autoimmne thyroid disease/thyroiditis. In: DeGroot LJ, eds. Endocrinology, 3rd ed. W.B. Saunders, Philadelphia, 1995, pp. 726–741.
47. Bohnet HG, Fiedler K, Leidenberger FA. Subclinical hypothyroidism and infertility. Lancet 1981;2: 1278.
48. Leung AS, Millar LK, Koonings PP, Montoro M, Mestman JH. Perinatal outcome in hypothyroid pregnancies. Obstet Gynecol 1993;81:349.
49. Tamaki H, Amino N, Takeoka K, Mitsuda N, Miyai K, Tanizawa O. Thyroxine requirement during pregnancy for replacement therapy of hypothyroidism. Obstet Gynecol 1990;76:230–233.
50. Mandel SJ, Larsen PR, Seely EW, Brent GA. Increased need for thyroxine during pregnancy in women with primary hypothyroidism. N Engl J Med 1990;323:91–96.
51. McDougall IR, Maclin N. Hypothyroid women need more thyroxine when pregnant. J Fam Pract 1995; 41:238–240.
52. Momotani N, Noh J, Ishikawa N, Ito K. Relationship between silent thyroiditis and recurrent Graves' disease in the postpartum period. J Clin Endocrinol Metab 1994;79:285–289.
53. Jansson R, Bernander S, Karlsson A, Zelvin K, Nilsson G. Autoimmune thyroid dysfunction in the postpartum period. J Clin Endocrinol Metab 1984;58:681–687.
54. Walfish P, Chan J. Postpartum hyperthyroidism. Clin Endocrinol Metab 1985;14:417–47.
55. Walfish P, Meyerson J, Provias J, Vargas M, Papsis F. Prevalence and characteristics of post-partum thyroid dysfunction: results of a survey from Toronto, Canada. J Endocrinol Invest 1992;15:265–272.
56. Freeman R, Rosen H, Thysen B. Incidence of thyroid dysfunction in an unselected postpartum population. Arch Intern Med 1986;146:1361–1364.
57. Nikolai TF, Turney SL, Roberts RC. Postpartum lymphocytic thyroiditis. Prevalence, clinical course, and long-term follow-up. Arch Intern Med 1987;147:221–224.

58. Lervang HH, Pryds O, Ostergaard KH. Thyroid dysfunction after delivery: incidence and clinical course. Acta Med Scand 1987;222:369–374.
59. Löbig H, Bohn W, Mau J, Schats H. Prevalence of postpartum thyroiditis in two iodine-deficient regions of Germany. In: Scherbaum W, Bogner U, Weinheimer B, Bottazzo G, eds. Autoimmune Thyroiditis. Springer-Verlag, Berlin, 1991, pp. 185–193.
60. Fung HY, Kologlu M, Collison K, et al. Postpartum thyroid dysfunction in Mid Glamorgan. Br Med J 1988;296:241–244.
61. Rasmussen N, Hornnes P, Hoiter-Madsen M, Feldt-Rasmussen U, Hegedus L. Thyroid size and function in healthy pregnant women with thyroid autoantibodies. Acta Endocrinol (Copenh) 1990;123:395–401.
62. Rajatanavin R, Chailurkit LO, Tirarungsikul K, Chalayondeja W, Jittivanich U, Puapradit W. Postpartum thyroid dysfunction in Bangkok: a geographical variation in the prevalence. Acta Endocrinol (Copenh) 1990;122:283–287.
63. Roti E, Bianconi L, Gardini E, et al. Postpartum thyroid dysfunction in an Italian population residing in an area of mild iodine deficiency. J Endocrinol Invest 1991;14:669–674.
64. Stagnaro-Green A, Roman S, Cobin R, el-Harazy H, Wallenstein S, Davies T. A prospective study of lymphocyte-initiated immunosuppression in normal pregnancy: evidence of a T-cell etiology for postpartum thyroid dysfunction. J Clin Endocrinol Metab 1992;74:645–653.
65. Hidaka Y, Tamaki H, Iwatani Y, Tada H, Mitsuda N, Amino N. Prediction of postpartum onset of Graves' thyrotoxicosis by measurement of thyroid stimulating antibody in early pregnancy. Clin Endocrinol (Oxford) 1994;41:15–20.
66. Othman S, Phillips DI, Lazarus JH, Parkes AB, Richards C, Hall R. Iodine metabolism in postpartum thyroiditis. Thyroid 1992;2:107–111.
67. Kampe O, Jansson R, Karlsson FA. Effects of L-thyroxine and iodide on the development of autoimmune postpartum thyroiditis. J Clin Endocrinol Metab 1990;70:1014–1018.
68. Glinoer D, Lemone M, Bourdoux P, et al. Partial reversibility during late postpartum of thyroid abnormalities associated with pregnancy. J Clin Endocrinol Metab 1992;74:453–457.
69. Amino N, Tada H, Hidaka Y. The spectrum of postpartum thyroid dysfunction: diagnosis, management, and long-term prognosis. Endocr Pract 1996;2:406–410.
70. Amino N, Yabu Y, Miyai K, et al. Defferentiation of thyrotoxicosis induced by thyroid destruction from Graves' disease. Lancet 1978;2:344–346.
71. Hidaka Y, Nishi I, Tamaki H, et al. Differentiation of the postpartum thyrotoxicosis by serum thyroglobulin; Usefulness of the new multi-site immunoradiometric assay. Thyroid 1994;4:275–278.
72. Amino N, Tada H. Postpartum thyroid disease. In: Bardin CW, ed. Current Therapy in Endoctinology and Metabolism, 6th ed. Mosby-Year Book, Philadelphia, 1997, pp. 327–330.
73. Tachi J, Amino N, Tamaki H, Aozasa M, Iwatani Y, Miyai K. Long term follow-up and HLA association in patients with postpartum hypothyroidism. J Clin Endocrinol Metab 1988;66:480–484.
74. Adams H, Jones MC, Othman S, et al. The sonographic appearances in postpartum thyroiditis. Clin Radiol 1992;45:311–315.
75. Creagh FM, Parkes AB, Lee A, et al. The iodide perchlorate discharge test in women with previous post-partum thyroiditis: relationship to sonographic appearance and thyroid function. Clin Endocrinol (Oxford) 1994;40:765–768.
76. Othman S, Phillips DI, Parkes AB, et al. A long-term follow-up of postpartum thyroiditis. Clin Endocrinol (Oxford) 1990;32:559–564.
77. Yoshida H, Amino N, Yagawa K, et al. Association of serum antithyroid antibodies with lymphocytic infiltration of the thyroid gland: studies of seventy autopsied cases. J Clin Endocrinol Metab 1978;46:859–862.
78. Solomon BL, Fein HG, Smallridge RC. Usefulness of antimicrosomal antibody titers in the diagnosis and treatment of postpartum thyroiditis. J Fam Pract 1993;36:177–182.
79. Pop VJ, de Rooy H, Vader HL, D. H, M. S, Komproe IH. Microsomal antibodies during gestation in relation to postpartum thyroid dysfunction and depression. Acta Endocrinol (Copenh) 1993;129:26–30.
80. Hayslip CC, Fein HG, O'Donnell VM, Friedman DS, Klein TA, Smallridge RC. The value of serum antimicrosomal antibody testing in screening for symptomatic postpartum thyroid dysfunction. Am J Obstet Gynecol 1988;159:203–209.
81. Feldt RU, Hoier MM, Rasmussen NG, Hegedus L, Hornnes P. Anti-thyroid peroxidase antibodies during pregnancy and postpartum. Relation to postpartum thyroiditis. Autoimmunity 1990;6:211–214.

82. Tada H, Hidaka Y, Itoh E, et al. Prevalence of postpartum onset of disease within patients with Graves' disease of child-bearing age. Endocr J 1994;41:325–327.
83. Kasagi K, Hatabu H, Tokuda Y, Iida Y, Endo K, Konishi J. Studies on thyrotrophin receptor antibodies in patients with euthyroid Graves' disease. Clin Endocrinol (Oxford) 1988;29:357–366.
84. Tamaki H, Amino N, Aozasa M, Mori M, Tanazawa O, Miyai K. Serial changes in thyroid-stimulating antibody and thyrotropin binding inhibitor immunoglobulin at the time of postpartum occurrence of thyrotoxicosis in Graves' disease. J Clin Endocrinol Metab 1987;65:324–330.
85. Amino N, Tanizawa O, Miyai K, et al. Changes of serum immunoglobulins IgG, IgA, IgM and IgE during pregnancy. Obstet Gynecol 1978;52:415–420.
86. Hidaka Y, Amino N, Iwatani Y, et al. Increase in peripheral netural killer cell activity in patients with autoimmune thyroid disease. Autoimmunity 1992;11:239–246.
87. Amino N, Miyai K, Kuro R, et al. Transient postpartum hypothyroidism: Fourteen cases with autoimmune thyroiditis. Ann Intern Med 1977;87:155–159.
88. Stagnaro-Green A. Post-miscarriage thyroid dysfunction. Obstet Gynecol 1992;80:490–492.
89. Hashimoto K, Takao T, Makino S. Lymphocytic adenohypophysitis and lymphocytic infundibulo-neurohypophysitis. Endocr J 1997;44:1–10.
90. Nelson JL, Østensen M. Pregnancy and rheumatoid arthritis. Rheum Dis Clin North Am 1997;23:195–212.
91. Silman AJ, Kay A, Mitchell H, Brennan P. Timing of pregnancy to the onset of rheumatoid arthritis. Arthritis Rheum 1992;35:152–155.
92. Iijima T, Tada H, Hidaka Y, et al. Prediction of postpartum onset of rheumatoid arthritis. Ann Rhem Dis 1998;57:460–468.
93. Robson JS, Martin AM, Ruckley VA, Macdonald MK. Irreversible post-partum renal failure; A new syndrome. Q J Med 1968;37:423–435.
94. Bohle A. Post-delivery hemolytic-uremic syndrome. Contr Nephrol 1981;25:157–158.
95. Steiner I, Heller LA, Abramsky O, Raz E. Postpartum idiopathic polymiositis. Lancet 1992;339:256.
96. Kochenour NK, Branch DW, Rote NS, Scott JR. A new postpartum syndrome associated with antiphospholipid antibodies. Obstet Gynecol 1986;69:460–468.
97. Yagoro A, Tada H, Hidaka Y, et al. Postpartum onset of acute heart failure possibly due to poatpartum autoimmne myocarditis: a report of three cases. J Intern Med (in press).
98. Kopp P, van SJ, Parma J, et al. Congenital hyperthyroidism caused by a mutation in the thyrotropin-receptor gene. N Engl J Med 1995;332:150–154.
99. Tamaki H, Amino N, Aozasa M, et al. Universal predictive criteria for neonatal overt thyrotoxicosis requiring treatment. Am J Perinatol 1988;5:152–158.
100. Tamaki H, Amino N, Watanabe Y, et al. Radioreceptor assay of anti-TSH receptor antibody activity: Comparison of assays using unextracted serum and immunoglobulin fractions, and standardization of expression of activities. J Clin Lab Immunol 1986;20:1–6.
101. Tamaki H, Amino N, Aozasa M, et al. Effective method for prediction of transient hypothyroidism in neonates born to mothers with chronic thyroiditis. Am J Perinatol 1989;6:296–303.

12 Etiology and Pathogenesis of Human Insulin-Dependent Diabetes Mellitus

Jean-François Bach, MD, DSc

CONTENTS

    INTRODUCTION: LESSONS FROM ANIMAL MODELS
    GENETICS OF HUMAN IDDM
    THE ROLE OF ENVIRONMENTAL FACTORS
    FEATURES OF THE β-CELL-SPECIFIC AUTOIMMUNE RESPONSE
    IMMUNOREGULATION
    CONCLUSIONS
    REFERENCES

INTRODUCTION: LESSONS FROM ANIMAL MODELS

The autoimmune origin of human insulin-dependent diabetes mellitus (IDDM) was suspected in the early 1970s when it was discovered by Bottazzo et al. *(1)* that a majority of IDDM patients harbored islet cell-specific autoantibodies (ICA) at the onset of the disease. We shall see that such autoimmune origin is now firmly established, even if other nonimmunologic factors are also implicated in disease etiology and pathogenesis. Before reviewing the evidence supporting this view, we shall summarize the lessons derived from the study of IDDM animal models, the BioBreeding (BB) rat and especially the nonobese diabetic (NOD) mouse. These studies have brought invaluable information on the mechanisms of the disease, and still represent the major approach for understanding etiology and pathogenesis, as well as for generating new therapeutic strategies.

Autoimmune Origin of IDDM in the NOD Mouse and the BB Rat

THE CENTRAL ROLE OF T CELLS

Compelling evidence demonstrates that IDDM is a T-cell-mediated disease in the NOD mouse and the BB rat. (*See also* Chapter 5.) The disease is associated with an early infiltration of the islets by mononuclear cells, including a majority of T cells (insulitis). T-cell-directed specific immunointervention, notably using anti-T cell monoclonal antibodies (MAbs) (CD3, TCR), totally prevents the onset of the disease and induces a quasi-immediate correction of hyperglycemia when applied in the first days following onset of

From: *Contemporary Endocrinology: Autoimmune Endocrinopathies*
Edited by: R. Volpe © Humana Press Inc., Totowa, NJ

diabetes *(2)*. The disease can be transferred to immunoincompetent syngeneic recipients (scid, irradiated NOD) by infusion of purified T cells or T-cell clones derived from overtly diabetic mice *(3–6)*. C57BL/6 mice, which are not autoimmunity-prone, rapidly develop IDDM when they express a TCR transgene derived from a diabetogenic T-cell clone (inasmuch as they concomitantly express the H-2^{NOD} introduced by repeated backcrossing) *(7,7a)*. The autoreactive specificity of the diabetogenic T cells has been determined for a number of (but not all) diabetogenic T-cell clones.

The role of autoantibodies (that are not found in large amounts in NOD mice and BB rats at variance with human IDDM) appears to be marginal, as suggested by the capacity of the diabetogenic T cells to transfer diabetes in NOD mice rendered agammaglobulinemic by perinatal anti-μ MAb treatment *(8)*. The recent (controversial) observations that B-cell-less NOD mice are protected from diabetes *(9–11)* is more likely explained by the intervention of B cells at the initiation of the autoimmune process (at the level of autoimmunity presentation). This point is, however, complicated by another report indicating that other B cell deficient NOD mice do develop insulitis and diabetes *(12)*.

TARGET AUTOANTIGENS

The pathogenic autoimmune response is driven by β-cell autoantigens. This is suggested by the tight control of the disease predisposition (H-2 molecules present antigenic peptides to T cells). It is also suggested by the restriction of T-cell receptor usage by insulin-reactive T-cell clones, an indication of clonal expansion *(13)*. It has been directly proven by the demonstration that selective β-cell destruction by alloxan induces the exhaustion of diabetogenic T cells (evaluated in a transfer model) *(14)*.

Uncertainty remains though on the nature of the autoantigens that stimulate the pathogenic T cells. Several candidate antigens have been identified on the basis of their capacity to stimulate T-cell proliferation, including insulin, glutamic acid decarboxylase (GAD), heat-shock protein 60 (hsp60), and p69 *(15)*. Much difficulty is met in trying to incriminate one of these antigens as the primary autoantigen. None of these antigens is able to elicit diabetes in nonautoimmune strains. Some insulin-reactive T-cell clones have been shown to transfer diabetes *(16)*, but none of the GAD-reactive T-cell clones has up to now been reported to present such activity *(17)*. Conversely, several of them are able to prevent diabetes onset when injected in NOD mice at an early age in conditions of tolerance induction *(18–22)*. We shall see below that this surprising observation is probably explained by a phenomenon of bystander suppression. It could well be, in fact, that there is not a single triggering (and target) IDDM autoantigen and that several autoantigens can concomitantly or sequentially (but without definite chronology) induce a diabetogenic T-cell response.

EFFECTOR MECHANISMS

The rapid correction mentioned above of hyperglycemia observed after a short-term treatment with a monoclonal anti-T-cell antibody *(2,23)* indicates that the lesion at the origin of β-cell dysfunction is not immediately irreversible. This view is corroborated by the observation that islets collected in recently diagnosed diabetic NOD mice recover most of their capacity to produce insulin when cultured in vitro in the absence of aggressive immune effectors *(24)*. The mechanisms of such T-cell-mediated inflammation are not known, but they probably involve the action of various cytokines.

At a later stage, β cells are finally destroyed. Here again, the underlying mechanisms are elusive. It appears that both CD4 and CD8 T cells can mediate this destruction, since both CD4 *(5)* and CD8 *(25)* T-cell clones can induce full-blown diabetes, but probably both T-cell subsets are required in the spontaneous disease as indicated by transfer experiments *(3,4)*. The role of CD8 cytotoxic T lymphocytes is suggested by several in vitro studies demonstrating the cytotoxic activity against B cells of polyclonal or monoclonal NOD T cells *(25–27)*, as well as by transfer experiments using cytotoxic T-cell clones. It is further suggested by the low incidence of diabetes in perforin-deficient mice *(28)*. A role for cytokine produced by CD4 T cells is also probably important.

In many of these mechanisms, the action of free radicals and NO has been suggested to intervene at a late stage.

Mechanisms of the Rupture of Tolerance to β-Cell Autoantigens

β-cell-specific T cells can be demonstrated at an early age in NOD mice (3–5 wk) as illustrated by the lymphocyte proliferation induced by islet cell extracts or biochemically defined antigens, notably GAD *(18,19)*. It is only 2–3 mo later, however, that diabetogenic T cells appear (in transfer experiments) and overt diabetes emerges. The absence of progression to destructive insulitis during this phase is supported by the absence of disease acceleration provided by partial pancreatectomy performed at a young age *(29)*. Compelling evidence indicates that this clinically silent prediabetic stage is under the control of CD4 regulatory T cells. Diabetes transfer is only obtained in syngeneic prediabetic mice if this host is immunoincompetent (neonate *[3]*, NOD-scid *[6]*, irradiated adult thymectomized *[4]*, or CD4 cell depleted *[30]*). Diabetes onset is accelerated by thymectomy performed at 3 wk of age *(31)* or by cylophosphamide treatment *(32)*. Finally, diabetes can be prevented by infusion of CD4 T cells *(33)* or CD4 T-cell clones *(34)* derived from prediabetic donors.

The mechanisms of this active tolerance and of its cessation in the weeks preceding diabetes onset are not clear. One may assume that regulatory cytokines play an important role as suggested by diabetes prevention or even regression afforded by IL-4 therapy (systemic administration *[35]*, transgenic mice *[36,37]*, gene therapy [Yamamoto et al., in preparation]), but limited evidence has been brought so far directly showing the responsibility of this or other cytokines. *In situ* intraislet detection of IL-4 or other TH2 cytokines has proven to be disappointing with the exception of an isolated report *(38)*, and no evidence of disease acceleration after gene deletion or antibody-mediated neutralization of IL-4 or IL-10 has been reported. Transforming growth factor β (TGF-β) perhaps plays a major role as suggested by its production by a suppressor clone *(34)*. It also remains to be understood why this putative cytokine-mediated regulation declines at 3–4 mo of age. The possible role of an early natural killer (NK) T-cell deficiency in NOD mice could provide a possible explanation *(39,40)*, but the NK T cells would not be in this hypothesis the regulatory cells themselves, since one can physically separate NK T cells, which are CD62L$^-$ and the regulatory T cells that are CD62L$^+$ *(40a)*.

Other mechanisms could be involved in the rupture of self-tolerance to β-cell autoantigens.

1. A β-cell abnormality (intrinsic or extrinsic) that enhances the immunogenicity of one or several of its molecular constituents. Viral-induced inflammation could be involved, but has never been clearly demonstrated.
2. Stimulation by a microbe whose constituents crossreact with some β-cell antigen(s) (mimicry).
3. Nonspecific triggering of TH1 cells as afforded by mechanisms leading to interleukin 12 (IL-12) production (IL-12 treatment accelerates disease onset in NOD mice) *(41)*.

Conversely the genetically programmed rupture of tolerance to β-cell autoantigen(s) can be slowed down or even prevented in a number of ways, including various bacterial or viral infections (pathogen-free NOD mice [our unpublished observations], and BB rats *[42]* show exacerbated disease incidence and severity), β-cell autoantigen administration *(18–22)*, complete Freund's adjuvant *(43,44)*, or anti-CD3 antibody treatment *(2)*, all procedures that probably act through cytokine production.

Etiology

The etiology of diabetes in NOD mice or BB rats is not known. As just mentioned, environmental factors probably play an important role (either positive or negative), but no particular etiologic agent has been clearly identified.

In any case, the genetic predisposition to the disease is clearly established. The major histocompatibility complex (MHC) and, more particularly, class II genes play the central role, but many other genes are also important. More than 15 of these diabetes predispositions genes have been unraveled *(45)*. Very few of these genes have been identified, and much remains to be known concerning their functions and their interactions. Incidentally, the NOD mouse does not harbor the best possible set of predisposing genes, since it also possesses some protector genes, such as the Fcγ receptor III gene *(46)* and since the expression of a diabetogenic T-cell receptor transgene on the C57BL/6 background provides a more rapid emergence of the disease than in the NOD background *(7a)*.

GENETICS OF HUMAN IDDM

Heredity

Human IDDM is a hereditary disease, as illustrated by the disease concordance rate in siblings (7%) and parent–child combinations (5%) *(15)*. The concordance rate in monozygotic twins is more difficult to evaluate with precision, since its evaluation is based on smaller samples that are severely biased (concordant twin pairs show up more easily than discordant ones). One may assume, however, that this concordance rate is approx 35–55% *(47)*, which indicates a penetrance of this order, even if by definition twin pairs who possess all predisposing genes, but are concordant for disease protection are not recognized.

An interesting, but still unexplained case has been made for a higher transmission of disease predisposition by diabetic fathers than diabetic mothers *(48)*.

One may also mention that the disease incidence considerably varies all around of the world, a phenomenon that is partly, but probably not exclusively explained by environmental factors *(see below)*. Thus, the Japanese show a very low disease incidence, whereas the Scandinavian show a very high one.

HLA Genes

IDDM association with human leukocyte antigen (HLA) genes has been known for a very long time *(49)*. It was rapidly observed that the disease is associated with HLA DR3 and DR4 and that, conversely, disease incidence is significantly lower in HLA DR2 subjects. The emergence of genotyping after polymerase chain reaction (PCR) amplification has provided more precise analysis of this association *(50,51)*.

As far as the DR4 haplotype is concerned, the main predisposing allele could in fact be DQB1*0302, which is in tight linkage disequilibrium with DR4. Interestingly, the various DR4 subtypes modulate DQB1*0302 predisposing effect: some of them reinforce it (i.e., DRB1*0401, DRB1*0402, DRB1*0405), whereas others lead to a dominant protection (DRB1*0403, DRB1*0404) *(52)*. Surprisingly, anti-GAD antibodies are rather associated with the usually protective DRB1*0403 and DRB1*0404 alleles *(53)*.

As far as DR3 is concerned, one has to distinguish the direct association of DR3 (or DQB1*0201, which is closely linked to it) and genes present in the ancestral A1B8DR3 haplotype, which could intervene independently of DR3. Evidence in this direction has been collected by Dawkins' group *(54)*, pointing to a predisposing gene located between HLA B and tumor necrosis factor (TNF) present in the ancestral haplotype, but involved in the disease predisposition independently of DR3 (as illustrated by patients showing only part of the ancestral haplotype). Studies are in progress to characterize this new locus.

Much interest had been raised by the observations that diabetic patients rarely show an aspartic acid residue on position 57 of their DQβ chain *(55)*. This is interesting, because this position is central for peptide binding by the DQβ molecule. However, this non-Asp genotype does not provide higher relative risk than DR3 and DR4.

One should also note that at variance with the postulated codominance of the IDDM predisposing HLA genes, homozygosity, for either DR3 or DR4 can be associated with an increased relative risk, in some populations *(53)*. It is not clear if DR3/4 heterozygosity, which is associated with the highest risk, implicates cumulative or synergistic effect of the two genes and if transcomplementation, which does occur in some subjects, is an important factor.

One should finally mention the recent renewed interest in HLA class I genes. HLA A24 appears to be associated with early onset of the disease *(56)* and rapid loss of remaining endogenous insulin production after diabetes onset *(57)*. Its frequency is increased in diabetic subjects independently of a linkage disequilibrium with DR3 or DR4, but not in ICA+ relatives of diabetics. These data suggest that whereas DR3 and DR4 genes (which are associated with ICA positivity) are already used in the first stage of the disease (insulitis and ICA positivity), HLA A24 is used at the time of disease progression toward diabetes *(58)*, posing the question of the involvement of class I-restricted CD8 T cells in the β-cell lesion.

Taken together with data obtained in animal models, these observations indicate that both MHC class I and class II antigen molecules are required for β-cell autoantigen peptide presentation to T cells. An important point will be to determine which β-cell-specific peptides are bound by the various HLA molecules mentioned above. Two important approaches have been undertaken to answer this question: (1) the study of the fine specificity and restriction of β-cell antigen-specific T-cell clones *(59–61)* and (2) HLA-peptide binding studies either in vitro *(62)* or in vivo using transgenic mice expressing DR4 *(63)* or other HLA class II human HLA genes.

A last important issue is that of HLA-associated protection. The protection afforded by DR2 or better DQB1*0602 is a very strong one (quasi-absolute, even in the presence of DR3 or DR4) *(64)*. It is reminiscent of diabetes protection observed in transgenic NOD mice expressing non-NOD MHC class II genes *(65,66)*. It will be important to determine these mechanisms of negative association. One would like to know if it involves the same kind of active protection as demonstrated in the transgenic mice just mentioned (the protection can be abrogated by cyclophosphamide therapy and is transferable by T cells). If it were the case, one could envision the possibility that regulatory T cells (TH2 or others) recognize different β-cell peptides in the context of different MHC molecules.

Alternatively, as initially suggested by Nepom and Erlich *(67)*, protective molecules could capture the diabetogenic peptides and withdraw them from predisposing HLA molecules. Other mechanisms could also be involved, such as variable level of expression of HLA molecules depending on HLA alleles or a role for nonconventional class I or class II molecules, notably those coded by alleles present on the ancestral haplotype.

Non-HLA Genes

This decade has been associated with rapidly increasing knowledge concerning non-MHC genes. Their involvement was apparent when considering the difference in disease concordance rate between monozygotic twins (35%) and HLA identical siblings (15%) *(15)*. The emergence of new technologies enabling the rapid screening of the genome raised immense hopes. Essentially using the microsatellite approach, Todd and Wicker followed by several laboratories described a number of disease-predisposing genes that were localized on the mouse and human genomes for the NOD mouse *(45)* and human IDDM *(68)*, respectively. The genes in question remain still unidentified at the present time, except the insulin *(69,70)* and perhaps CTLA4 *(71,72)* genes in humans and the IL-2 gene in the mouse. The precise mapping and final identification of these genes will prove difficult, since these genes probably do not show mutations that would have allowed their rapid positioning. Their contribution to disease predisposition could mostly rely on the fortuitous combination of their polymorphisms: each polymorphism is common in the general population and devoid of any direct deleterious effect when present alone in the absence of the other predisposing gene polymorphisms. The case of CTLA4 is a good illustration of this complexity. As just mentioned, the CTLA4 gene polymorphism is associated with IDDM *(71,72)*, but one cannot exclude that the predisposing gene is close to CTLA4, but distinct from it. NOD mouse genetic segregation data also show that the CTLA4 area is associated with disease predisposition. We have shown that the CTLA4 gene shows an abnormally low expression in the NOD mouse (Garchon et al., in preparation), which would fit with possible loss of regulatory function of this gene in IDDM. However, study of several recombinant strains has indicated that the CTLA4 locus could be separated from the disease-predisposing chromosome area (Garchon et al., in preparation). However, one can exclude the CTLA4 gene as the disease-predisposing gene; it is still possible that the incriminated gene regulates CTLA4 expression (regulatory gene?).

The problem is complicated by the existence of protective genes mentioned above recently shown to exist in the NOD mouse itself, namely the Fcγlll receptor gene *(46)* and gene(s) present in NOD mice, but absent in C57BL/6 mice, which explain the higher incidence and more rapid occurrence of diabetes in transgenic mice expressing a diabetogenic T-cell receptor (TCR) on the C57BL/6, rather than on the NOD background *(7a)*. The best approach, as used by Wicker, probably consists of generating congenic mice lacking a restricted critical chromosomal area recognized to be predisposing to the disease. One may also hope that the study of diabetes genetics will be simplified by the usage of transgenic mice expressing one of the disease effectors, such as a TCR, from diabetogenic clones as mentioned above.

One might have expected from the high disease concordance rate in siblings from diabetic patients (7%) that only few non-MHC genes are involved in disease predisposition. It was a great surprise to realize that at least 15 genes are involved in the predisposition to IDDM. Such a multiplicity of predisposition genes may be explained in several ways:

1. Only a few of the identified genes play a significant role (major genes) contrasting with the trivial role of minor genes.
2. Some genes play a major role, but their frequency in the general population is very high, hence their absence of discriminating effect.
3. Different genes are used by different patients, which is a less likely hypothesis since the identification of the predisposing genes is based on the combination of data derived from multiple families.

In any case, this diversity of predisposition genes will complicate the understanding of their role in disease pathogenesis and will render their use in disease prediction somewhat difficult.

THE ROLE OF ENVIRONMENTAL FACTORS

Epidemiology

Two important facts emerge from the study of IDDM epidemiology: (1) There has been a clear increase in disease incidence over the last 25 yr *(73)*, particularly in highly developed countries. Such increase parallels a similar augmentation noted for other immunologically mediated diseases, such as multiple sclerosis or asthma. (2) The disease prevalence varies from country to country in a considerable manner. These variations are organized in the Northern hemisphere along a North–South gradient with a much higher disease prevalence in northern countries in both America and Europe *(74)* (with the interesting exception of less-well-developed eastern countries). This gradient is also seen for multiple sclerosis and Crohn's disease. Sardinia is an intriguing exception to this gradient for both IDDM and multiple sclerosis *(75)*. Additionally, in a given country, there appears to be a tendency for lower disease incidence in subjects leaving in areas with highest population density *(76)*. No definitive explanation has been provided for this very striking distribution. The role of genetic factors cannot be excluded. It is however difficult to consider them as playing an exclusive role in view of the wide range of disease incidence observed over such a large area. The role of environmental factors is more plausible. The strict negative correlation noted between the pathogen weight and the disease incidence in NOD mice (our unpublished results) and BB rats *(42)* (only specific pathogen free NOD mice show a disease incidence > 80%, whereas a number of bacterial or viral infections nonspecifically protect from the disease) suggests that infections may protect through a mechanism of antigenic competition *(77)*. The mirror image of the European distribution of antihepatitis A virus antibody carriers (taken as a marker of a contamination by a common water-borne virus) is also suggestive of this hypothesis *(77)*, as well as the negative correlation noted between IDDM incidence and frequency of childhood infections *(78)*. One may assume that the better hygiene and the lower average temperature in Northern countries explain the lower rate of infectious contaminations.

Epidemiologic studies have revealed other interesting, but unconfirmed trends: lower incidence of IDDM in breast-fed children (an observation fitting with the increased incidence of diabetes in diabetes-prone animals fed with cow's milk, in BB rats *[79]*, but not in the NOD mouse *[80]*), and the seasonal increase of IDDM incidence with a particular role for Coxsackie virus infections *(81,82)*.

This latter argument had received less consideration in the last few years when it was realized that the β-cell specific autoimmune response begins many years before diabetes onset, making less important the role of acute infections preceding by a few weeks of the disease onset. This idea should be revisited with the notion that a trigger mechanism (e.g., infectious disease) could induce the progression from insulitis to clinically overt diabetes.

Models for the Triggering Role of Viruses

Independently of these potential nonspecific protective role, viruses could play a central positive role in the disease pathogenesis according to at leat four mechanisms.

1. A virus could induce nonspecific inflammation of β cells (through the production of various cytokines). This inflammation could enhance the immunogenicity of β-cell constituents. An increase in the intra-islet cytokines and of β-cell expression MHC class I and class II molecules has indeed been reported in recently diagnosed diabetics *(83,84)*. It remains to be demonstrated that these changes precede the autoimmune β-cell attack and are not secondary to the T-cell-mediated β-cell targeted response.
2. A virus could induce the expression of neoantigens (that are encoded by the virus genome) according to the model of hepatitis B. The RIP SV40 transgenic mice expressing the SV40 T antigen in β cells illustrates this model *(85)*.
3. Viral proteins (or antiviral antibodies) can share sequences with β-cell autoantigens. This has been observed for Coxsackie B virus and glutamic acid decarboxylase (GAD) *(86–88)*. This crossreactive (mimicry) epitope could bypass T-cell tolerance to β-cell autoantigens and give rise to a β-cell-specific bona fide autoimmune response.
4. Finally, viruses, notably retroviruses, could also act as superantigens. This mechanism has been recently documented for a retrovirus isolated from a series of diabetic patients *(89)*. This virus known to be a superantigen for Vβ7+ T cells could explain the TCR Vβ7 gene-restricted usage by CD4 T cells observed in CD4 cells eluted from the pancreas of recently diagnosed diabetic patients *(90)*. It is conceivable that stimulation of such T cells triggers the β-cell-specific autoimmune response.

FEATURES OF THE β-CELL-SPECIFIC AUTOIMMUNE RESPONSE

Autoantibodies

The first description of islet-specific autoantibodies was performed by Bottazzo et al. *(1)* using indirect immunofluorescence (islet cell antibodies [ICAs]). ICAs appear several years before diabetes onset, and their presence in relatives to diabetic patients is highly predictive of the risk of developing the disease, particularly when high titers are present (>1/40) *(91)*. However, even when using the most sensitive techniques, 10–20% of patients remain ICA-negative.

A major effort has been devoted over the last 10 yr to dissect the antibody specificities that contribute to ICA positivity and more generally that are associated with IDDM (even in ICA-negative cases).

Antibodies to GAD that are also found in the Stiffman syndrome (at even higher titers than in IDDM) *(92)* represent a significant fraction of these antibodies *(93,94)*. They do not seem, however, to be as tighly associated with ICAs or to IDDM onset in recently diagnosed diabetic patients.

Antibodies to insulin *(95)* or to IA-2 *(96–100)*, a tyrosine phosphatase, are more consistently associated with the disease progression, but they are less commonly observed. It is the combination of the presence of several of these antibodies that provides the best disease prediction *(101,102)*. The presence of the three antibodies *(103)* to chemically defined antigens is associated with a risk >90% of IDDM development within 5 yr of follow-up, but many patients reach the diabetic stage without showing the three antibodies. For the present time, it is still difficult to say whether one can definitively substitute the three chemically defined antibodies to ICAs, although this has been suggested by several groups on a firm basis.

Other autoantibody specificities include gangliosides (antiganglioside antibodies appear to be a very significant constituent of ICAs) *(104)*, carboxypeptidase H *(105)*, and p69 *(106,107)*, a protein crossreactive with cow albumin *(108)*.

There are still few data on the isotype of these various antibodies. Some studies have been performed to elucidate the fine epitope specificies that they recognize, but knowledge of these B epitopes is probably not as essential as that of the T epitope (to be discussed below), since autoantibodies are not thought to play a central role in disease pathogenesis.

β-Cell-Specific T Cells

The islets of recently diagnosed diabetics are infiltrated by mononuclear cells *(109)* that comprise both cells of the macrophage/monocyte lineage and lymphoid cells of B and T origin. Among T cells, the prevalence of CD4 and CD8 T cells has been the subject of controversial reports *(83,90)* probably explained by the small number of specimens studied.

Circulating T cells react to β-cell antigens (porcine fetal islet cells, islet cell extracts, insulin, or GAD) *(110 113)*, but the proliferative response is usually not intense and not clearly different from that observed with normal lymphocytes *(114)*.

A few positive reports have, however, been published using fetal islets *(110)* and GAD *(111–113)*. In the latter case, a negative correlation was observed between the GAD-specific T-cell response and the titer of anti-GAD antibodies *(115,116)*, but this observation was not corroborated by another study *(117)*.

Interesting data have been obtained on the study of GAD-specific T-cell lines (and T-cell clones) *(59–61)*. Dominant epitopes could be made evident with usually the recognition of a single (dominant) epitope for T-cell lines derived from each individual patient. It remains, however, that different epitopes were identified in different patients even when they shared HLA alleles. It is interesting to note that one of the most commonly involved epitope corresponds to the "mimicry" epitope shared with the Coxsackie B virus sequence *(88)*. Concerning insulin reactivity, it has proven difficult to bring direct evidence for increased T-cell proliferation in response to insulin or its peptides independently of insulin treatment. It is interesting, however, that when newly diagnosed diabetics are treated with insulin, insulin-reactive cells show a more restricted range of specificities to insulin epitopes *(116)*.

hsp60 also induces proliferation of peripheral blood lymphocytes *(118)* from diabetic patients. The selective response of hsp-specific T-cell lines to defined peptides (including p277) was observed.

IMMUNOREGULATION

Some evidence has been reported suggesting the existence of an imbalance of T-cell subsets in recently diagnosed patients or in prediabetic subjects (identified by the presence of anti-β-cell autoantibodies).

Thus, an increase in CD4/CD8 T-cell ratio has been reported *(119)* as well as a decrease in IL-4 production by double-negative CD4⁻CD8⁻ Vα24+ T cells, the human counterpart of murine NK T cells mentioned above *(120,121)*.

Indirect evidence for the existence of an immune dysregulation in diabetes is provided by the abnormally common observation of extrapancreatic autoantibodies or autoimmune disease other than IDDM observed in both NOD mice *(122)* and up to 10% of type I human diabetics. The presence of these autoantibodies (or diseases, notably thyroid diseases) defines the type 1b subset, which is more frequently found in females after the age of 25. Efforts made to delineate selective genetic markers (HLA, CTLA4) for type 1b diabetes have not been fully successful, even if some trends could be noted.

CONCLUSIONS

The autoimmune origin of human IDDM is now established on a firm basis that does not anymore only rely on the similarity with animal models. The genetic and environmental factors predisposing to the disease are progressively unraveled. All this rapidly progressing knowledge opens considerable perspectives for the immunotherapy and even better immunoprevention (*see* Chapter 17). Genetic and immunologic markers allow a fairly precise identification of patients at risk of IDDM, and several therapies can be thought of, including autoantigen or anti-T-cell antibody-induced tolerance. It will also be important to delineate further the scope of the disease: a significant fraction (10%) of noninsulin-dependent diabetes mellitus cases appears to be related to a slow autoimmune attack (as supported by the presence of anti-islet antibodies and frequent progression to insulin dependency) *(123–126)*, posing the question of a new classification of clinical diabetes (autoimmune vs nonautoimmune diabetes).

REFERENCES

1. Bottazzo GF, Florin-Christensen A, Doniach D. Islet-cell antibodies in diabetes mellitus with autoimmune polyendocrine deficiencies. Lancet 1974;2:1279–1283.
2. Chatenoud L, Thervet E, Primo J, Bach JF. Anti-CD3 antibody induces long-term remission of overt autoimmunity in nonobese diabetic mice. Proc Natl Acad Sci USA 1994;91:123–127.
3. Bendelac A., Carnaud C, Boitard C, Bach JF. Syngeneic transfer of autoimmune diabetes from diabetic NOD mice to healthy neonates. Requirement for both L3T4+ and Lyt-2+ T cells. J Exp Med 1987;166: 823–832.
4. Miller BJ, Appel MC, O'Neil JJ, Wicker LS. Both the Lyt-2+ and L3T4+ T cell subsets are required for the transfer of diabetes in nonobese diabetic mice. J Immunol 1988;140:52–58.
5. Haskins K, McDuffie M. Acceleration of diabetes in young NOD mice with a CD4+ islet-specific T cell clone. Science 1990;249:1433–1436.
6. Christianson SW, Shultz, LD, Leiter EH. Adoptive transfer of diabetes into immunodeficient NOD-scid/scid mice. Relative contributions of CD4+ and CD8+ T-cells from diabetic versus prediabetic NOD.NON-Thy-1a donors. Diabetes 1993;42:44–55.
7. Katz JD, Wang B, Haskins K, Benoist C, Mathis D. Following a diabetogenic T cell from genesis through pathogenesis. Cell 1993;74:1089–1100.
7a. Gonzalez A, Katz JD, Mattei MG, Kikutani H, Benoist C, Mathis D. Genetic control of diabetes progression. Immunity 1997;7:873–883.
8. Bendelac A, Boitard C, Bedossa P, Bazin H, Bach JF, Carnaud C. Adoptive T cell transfer of autoimmune nonobese diabetic mouse diabetes does not require recruitment of host B lymphocytes. J Immunol 1988;141:2625–2628.
9. Noorchashm H, Noorchashm N, Kern J, Rostami SY, Barker CF, Naji A. B-cells are required for the initiation of insulitis and sialitis in nonobese diabetic mice. Diabetes 1997;46:941–946.

10. Serreze DV, Chapman HD, Varnum DS, Hanson MS, Reifsnyder PC, Richard SD, et al. B lymphocytes are essential for the initiation of T cell-mediated autoimmune diabetes: analysis of a new "speed congenic" stock of NOD.Ig mu(null) mice. J Exp Med 1996;184:2049–2053.
11. Akashi T, Nagafuchi S, Anzai K, Kondo S, Kitamura D, Wakana S, et al. Direct evidence for the contribution of B cells to the progression of insulitis and the development of diabetes in non-obese diabetic mice. Int Immunol 1997;9:1159–1164.
12. Yang M, Charlton B, Gautam AM. Development of insulitis and diabetes in B cell-deficient NOD mice. J Autoimmunity 1997;10:257–260.
13. Simone E, Daniel D, Schloot N, Gottlieb P, Babu S, Kawasaki E, et al. T cell receptor restriction of diabetogenic autoimmune NOD T cells. Proc Natl Acad Sci USA 1997;94:2518–2521.
14. Larger E, Becourt C, Bach JF, Boitard C. Pancreatic islet beta cells drive T cell-immune responses in the nonobese diabetic mouse model. J Exp Med 1995;181:1635–1642.
15. Bach JF. Insulin-dependent diabetes mellitus as an autoimmune disease. Endocr Rev 1994;15:516–542.
16. Daniel D, Gill RG, Schloot N, Wegmann D. Epitope specificity, cytokine production profile and diabetogenic activity of insulin-specific T cell clones isolated from NOD mice. Eur J Immunol 1995;25:1056–1062.
17. Schloot NC, Daniel D, Norbury-Glaser M, Wegmann DR. Peripheral T cell clones from NOD mice specific for GAD65 peptides: lack of islet responsiveness or diabetogenicity. J Autoimmunity 1996;9:357–363.
18. Kaufman DL, Clare-Salzler M, Tian J, Forsthuber T, Ting GSP, Robinson P, et al. Spontaneous loss of T-cell tolerance to glutamic acid decarboxylase in murine insulin-dependent diabetes. Nature 1993;366:69–72.
19. Tisch R, Yang XD, Singer SM, Liblau RS, Fugger L, McDevitt HO. Immune response to glutamic acid decarboxylase correlates with insulitis in non-obese diabetic mice. Nature 1993;366:72–75.
20. Elias D, Cohen IR. Peptide therapy for diabetes in NOD mice. Lancet 1994;343:704–706.
21. Muir A, Peck A, Clare-Salzler M, Song YH, Cornelius J, Luchetta R, et al. Insulin immunization of nonobese diabetic mice induces a protective insulitis characterized by diminished intraislet interferon-gamma transcription. J Clin Invest 1995;95:628–634.
22. Zhang ZJ, Davidson L, Eisenbarth G, Weiner HL. Suppression of diabetes in nonobese diabetic mice by oral administration of porcine insulin. Proc Natl Acad Sci USA 1991;88:10,252–10,256.
23. Sempe P, Bedossa P, Richard MF, Villa MC, Bach JF, Boitard C. Anti-alpha/beta T cell receptor monoclonal antibody provides an efficient therapy for autoimmune diabetes in nonobese diabetic (NOD) mice. Eur J Immunol 1991;21:1163–1169.
24. Strandell E, Eizirik DL, Sandler S. Reversal of beta-cell suppression in vitro in pancreatic islets isolated from nonobese diabetic mice during the phase preceding insulin-dependent diabetes mellitus. J Clin Invest 1990;85:1944–1950.
25. Wong FS, Visintin I, Wen L, Flavell RA, Janeway CA. CD8 T cell clones from young nonobese diabetic (NOD) islets can transfer rapid onset of diabetes in NOD mice in the absence of CD4 cells. J Exp Med 1996;183:67–76.
26. Hayakawa M, Yokono K, Nagata M, Hatamori N, Ogawa W, Miki A, et al. Morphological analysis of selective destruction of pancreatic beta-cells by cytotoxic T lymphocytes in NOD mice. Diabetes 1991;40:1210–1217.
27. Nagata M, Santamaria P, Kawamura T, Utsugi T, Yoon JW. Evidence for the role of CD8+ cytotoxic T cells in the destruction of pancreatic beta-cells in nonobese diabetic mice. J Immunol 1994;152:2042–2050.
28. Kagi D, Odermatt B, Seiler P, Zinkernagel RM, Mak TW, Hengartner H. Reduced incidence and delayed onset of diabetes in perforin-deficient nonobese diabetic mice. J Exp Med 1997;186:989–997.
29. Itoh A, Maki T. Protection of nonobese diabetic mice from autoimmune diabetes by reduction of islet mass before insulitis. Proc Natl Acad Sci USA 1996;93:11053–11056.
30. Sempe P, Richard MF, Bach JF, Boitard C. Evidence of CD4+ regulatory T cells in the non-obese diabetic male mouse. Diabetologia 1994;37:337–343.
31. Dardenne M, Lepault F, Bendelac A, Bach JF. Acceleration of the onset of diabetes in NOD mice by thymectomy at weaning. Eur J Immunol 1989;19:889–895.
32. Yasunami R, Bach JF. Anti-suppressor effect of cyclophosphamide on the development of spontaneous diabetes in NOD mice. Eur J Immunol 1988;18:481–484.
33. Boitard C, Yasunami R, Dardenne M, Bach JF. T cell-mediated inhibition of the transfer of auto-immune diabetes in NOD mice. J Exp Med 1989;169:1669–1680.

34. Han HS, Jun HS, Utsugi T, Yoon JW. Molecular role of TGF-beta, secreted from a new type of CD4+ suppressor T cell, NY4.2, in the prevention of autoimmune IDDM in NOD mice. J Autoimmunity 1997;10:299–307.
35. Rapoport MJ, Jaramillo A, Zipris D, Lazarus AH, Serreze DV, Leiter EH, et al. Interleukin 4 reverses T cell proliferative unresponsiveness and prevents the onset of diabetes in nonobese diabetic mice. J Exp Med 1993;178:87–99.
36. Mueller R, Krahl T, Sarvetnick N. Pancreatic expression of interleukin-4 abrogates insulitis and autoimmune diabetes in nonobese diabetic (NOD) mice. J Exp Med 1996;184:1093–1099.
37. Mueller R, Bradley LM, Krahl T, Sarvetnick N. Mechanism underlying counterregulation of autoimmune diabetes by IL-4. Immunity 1997;7:411–418.
38. Fox CJ, Danska JS. IL-4 expression at the onset of islet inflammation predicts nondestructive insulitis in nonobese diabetic mice. J Immunol 1997;158:2414–2424.
39. Gombert JM, Herbelin A, Tancrede-Bohin E, Dy M, Carnaud C, Bach JF. Early quantitative and functional deficiency of NK1(+)- like thymocytes in the NOD mouse. Eur J Immunol 1996;26:2989–2998.
40. Gombert JM, Tancrede-Bohin E, Hameg A, Leite-de-Moraes MC., Vicari A, Bach JF, et al. IL-7 reverses NK1+ T cell-defective IL-4 production in the non-obese diabetic mouse. Int Immunol 1996;8:1751–1758.
40a. Herbelin A, Gombert JM, Lepault F, Bach JF, Chatenoud L. Mature mainstream TCR alpha beta(+)CD4(+) thymocytes expressing L-selectin mediate "activate tolerance" in the nonobese diabetic mouse. J Immunol 1998;161:2620–2628.
41. Trembleau S, Penna G, Bosi E, Mortara A, Gately MK, Adorini L. Interleukin 12 administration induces T helper type 1 cells and accelerates autoimmune diabetes in NOD mice. J Exp Med 1995;181:817–821.
42. Like AA, Guberski DL, Butler L. Influence of environmental viral agents on frequency and tempo of diabetes mellitus in BB/Wor rats. Diabetes 1991;40:259–262.
43. Sadelain MW, Qin HY, Lauzon J, Singh B. Prevention of type I diabetes in NOD mice by adjuvant immunotherapy. Diabetes 1990;39:583–589.
44. Calcinaro F, Gambelunghe G, Lafferty KJ. Protection from autoimmune diabetes by adjuvant therapy in the non-obese diabetic mouse: The role of interleukin-4 and interleukin-10. Immun Cell Biol 1997;75:467–471.
45. Wicker LS, Todd JA, Peterson LB. Genetic control of autoimmune diabetes in the NOD mouse. Annu Rev Immunol 1995;13:179–200.
46. Luan JJ, Monteiro RC, Sautes C, Fluteau G, Eloy L, Fridman WH, et al. Defective Fc gamma RII gene expression in macrophages of NOD mice—genetic linkage with up-regulation of IgG1 and IgG2b in serum. J Immunol 1996;157:4707–4716.
47. Lo SS, Tun RY, Hawa M, Leslie RD. Studies of diabetic twins. Diabetes Metab Rev 1991;7:223–238.
48. Warram JH, Krolewski AS, Gottlieb MS, Kahn CR. Differences in risk of insulin-dependent diabetes in offspring of diabetic mothers and diabetic fathers. N Engl J Med 1984;311:149–152.
49. Nerup J, Platz P, Andersen OO, Christy M, Lyngsoe J, Poulsen JE, et al. HL-A antigens and diabetes mellitus. Lancet 1974;2:864–866.
50. Caillat-Zucman S, Garchon HJ, Timsit J, Assan R, Boitard C, Djilali-Saiah I, et al. Age-dependent HLA genetic heterogeneity of type 1 insulin-dependent diabetes mellitus. J Clin Invest 1992;90:2242–2250.
51. Baisch JM, Weeks T, Giles R, Hoover M, Stastny P, Capra JD. Analysis of HLA-DQ genotypes and susceptibility in insulin-dependent diabetes mellitus. N Engl J Med 1990;322:1836–1841.
52. Harfouch-Hammoud E, Timsit J, Boitard C, Bach JF, Caillat-Zucman S. Contribution of DRB1*04 variants to predisposition to or protection from insulin dependent diabetes mellitus is independent of DQ. J Autoimmunity 1996;9:411–414.
53. Caillat-Zucman S, Djilali-Saiah I, Timsit J, Bonifacio E, Sepe V, Collins P, et al. Insulin dependent diabetes mellitus (IDDM): 12th International Histocompatibility Workshop study. In: Charron D, ed. Genetic Diversity of HLA. Functional and Medical Implication. EDK, Sevres, 1997, pp. 389–398.
54. Degli-Esposti MA, Abraham LJ, McCann V, Spies T, Christiansen FT, Dawkins RL. Ancestral haplotypes reveal the role of the central MHC in the immunogenetics of IDDM. Immunogenetics 1992;36:345–356.
55. Todd JA, Bell JI, McDevitt HO. HLA-DQ beta gene contributes to susceptibility and resistance to insulin-dependent diabetes mellitus. Nature 1987;329:599–604.
56. Mizota M, Uchigata Y, Moriyama S, Tokunaga K, Matsuura N, Miura J, et al. Age-dependent association of HLA-A24 in japanese IDDM patients. Diabetologia 1996;39:371–373.

57. Nakanishi K, Kobayashi T, Murase T, Nakatsuji T, Inoko H, Tsuji K, et al. Association of HLA-A24 with complete beta-cell destruction in IDDM. Diabetes 1993;42:1086–1093.
58. Honeyman MC, Harrison LC, Drummond B, Colman PG, Tait BD. Analysis of families at risk for insulin-dependent diabetes mellitus reveals that HLA antigens influence progression to clinical disease. Mol Med 1995;1:576–582.
59. Bach JM, Otto H, Nepom GT, Jung G, Cohen H, Timsit J, et al. High affinity presentation of an autoantigenic peptide in type I diabetes by an HLA class II protein encoded in a haplotype protecting from disease. J Autoimmunity 1997;10:375–386.
60. Lohmann T, Leslie RDG, Londei M. T cell clones to epitopes of glutamic acid decarboxylase 65 raised from normal subjects and patients with insulin-dependent diabetes. J Autoimmunity 1996;9:385–389.
61. Endl J, Otto H, Jung G, Dreisbusch B, Donie F, Stahl P, et al. Identification of naturally processed T cell epitopes from glutamic acid decarboxylase presented in the context of HLA-DR alleles by T lymphocytes of recent onset IDDM patients. J Clin Invest 1997;99:2405–2415.
62. Godkin A, Friede T, Davenport M, Stevanovic S, Willis A, Jewell D, et al. Use of eluted peptide sequence data to identify the binding characteristics of peptides to the insulin-dependent diabetes susceptibility allele HLA-DQ8 (DQ 3.2). Int Immunol 1997;9:905–911.
63. Patel SD, Cope AP, Congia M, Chen TT, Kim E, Fugger L, et al. Identification of immunodominant T cell epitopes of human glutamic acid decarboxylase 65 by using HLA-DR(alpha1*0101,beta1*0401) transgenic mice. Proc Natl Acad Sci USA 1997;94:8082–8087.
64. Pugliese A, Gianani R, Moromisato R, Awdeh ZL, Alper CA, Erlich HA et al. HLA-DQB1*0602 is associated with dominant protection from diabetes even among islet cell antibody-positive first-degree relatives of patients with IDDM. Diabetes 1995;44:608–613.
65. Slattery RM, Miller JF, Heath WR, Charlton B. Failure of a protective major histocompatibility complex class II molecule to delete autoreactive T cells in autoimmune diabetes. Proc Natl Acad Sci USA 1993;90:10,808–10,810.
66. Singer SM, Tisch R, Yang XD, McDevitt HO. An Abd transgene prevents diabetes in nonobese diabetic mice by inducing regulatory T cells. Proc Natl Acad Sci USA 1993;90:9566–9570.
67. Nepom GT, Erlich H. MHC class-II molecules and autoimmunity. Annu Rev Immunol 1991;9:493–525.
68. Merriman TR, Todd JA. Genetics of insulin-dependent diabetes; Non-major histocompatibility genes. Horm Metab Res 1996;28:289–293.
69. Bell GI, Horita S, Karam JH. A polymorphic locus near the human insulin gene is associated with insulin-dependent diabetes mellitus. Diabetes 1984;33:176–183.
70. Bennett ST, Wilson AJ, Cucca F, Nerup J, Pociot F, McKinney PA, et al. IDDM2-VNTR-encoded susceptibility to type 1 diabetes: dominant protection and parental transmission of alleles of the insulin gene-linked minisatellite locus. J Autoimmunity 1996;9:415–421.
71. Nistico L, Buzzetti R, Pritchard LE, Van Der Auwera B, Giovannini C, Bosi E, et al. The CTLA-4 gene region of chromosome 2q33 is linked to, and associated with, type 1 diabetes. Hum Mol Genet 1996;5:1075–1080.
72. Marron MP, Raffel LJ, Garchon HJ, Jacob CO, Serrano-Rios M, Larrad MTM, et al. Insulin-dependent diabetes mellitus (IDDM) is associated with CTLA4 polymorphisms in multiple ethnic groups. Hum Mol Genet 1997;6:1275–1282.
73. Schoenle EJ, Molinari L, Bagot M, Semadeni S, Wiesendanger M. Epidemiology of IDDM in Switzerland. Increasing incidence rate and rural-urban differences in Swiss men born 1948–1972. Diabetes Care 1994;17:955–960.
74. Green A, Gale EAM, Patterson CC. Incidence of childhood-onset insulin-dependent diabetes mellitus: the EURODIAB ACE study. Lancet 1992;339:905–909.
75. Bottazzo GF, Cossu E, Cirillo R, Loviselli A, Velluzzi F, Mariotti S, et al. Sardinia: a battlefield approach to type I diabetes epidemiology. Horm Res 1997;48:64–66.
76. Patterson CC, Carson DJ, Hadden DR. Epidemiology of childhood IDDM in Northern Ireland 1989–1994: low incidence in areas with highest population density and most household crowding. Diabetologia 1996;39:1063–1069.
77. Bach JF. Predictive medicine in autoimmune diseases: from the identification of genetic predisposition and environmental influence to precocious immunotherapy. Clin Immunol Immunopathol 1994;72:156–161.
78. Gibbon C, Smith T, Egger P, Betts P, Phillips D. Early infection and subsequent insulin dependent diabetes. Arch Dis Child 1997;77:384–385.
79. Elliott RB, Martin JM. Dietary protein: a trigger of insulin-dependent diabetes in the BB rat? Diabetologia 1984;26:297–299.

80. Paxson JA, Weber JG, Kulczycki A. Cow's milk-free diet does not prevent diabetes in NOD mice. Diabetes 1997;46:1711–1717.
81. Yoon JW. Role of viruses in the pathogenesis of IDDM. Ann Med 1991;23:437–445.
82. Frisk G, Diderholm H. Antibody responses to different strains of coxsackie B4 virus in patients with newly diagnosed type I diabetes mellitus or aseptic meningitis. J Infect 1997;34:205–210.
83. Bottazzo GF, Dean BM, McNally JM, MacKay EH, Swift PG, Gamble DR. In situ characterization of autoimmune phenomena and expression of HLA molecules in the pancreas in diabetic insulitis. N Engl J Med 1985;313:353–360.
84. Foulis AK, Farquharson MA, Meager A. Immunoreactive alpha-interferon in insulin-secreting beta cells in type 1 diabetes mellitus. Lancet 1987;2:1423–1427.
85. Adams TE, Alpert S, Hanahan D. Non-tolerance and autoantibodies to a transgenic self antigen expressed in pancreatic beta cells. Nature 1987;325:223–228.
86. Atkinson MA, Bowman MA, Campbell L, Darrow BL, Kaufman DL, MacLaren NK. Cellular immunity to a determinant common to glutamate decarboxylase and coxsackie virus in insulin-dependent diabetes. J Clin Invest 1994;94:2125–2129.
87. Lonnrot M, Hyoty H, Knip M, Roivainen M, Kulmala P, Leinikki P, et al. Antibody cross-reactivity induced by the homologous regions in glutamic acid decarboxylase (GAD(65)) and 2C protein of coxsackievirus B4. Clin Exp Immunol 1996;104:398–405.
88. Bach JM, Otto H, Jung G, Cohen H, Boitard C, Bach JF, et al. Identification of mimicry peptides based on structural motifs of epitopes derived from 65-kDa glutamic acid decarboxylase. Eur J Immunol 1998;28:1902–1910.
89. Conrad B, Weissmahr RN, Boni J, Arcari R, Schupbach J, Mach B. A human endogenous retroviral superantigen as candidate autoimmune gene in type I diabetes. Cell 1997;90:303–313.
90. Conrad B, Weidmann E, Trucco G, Rudert WA, Behboo R, Ricordi C, et al. Evidence for superantigen involvement in insulin-dependent diabetes mellitus aetiology. Nature 1994;371:351–355.
91. Bingley PJ, Bonifacio E, Williams AJK, Genovese S, Bottazzo GF, Gale EAM. Prediction of IDDM in the general population: Strategies based on combinations of autoantibody markers. Diabetes 1997;46:1701–1710.
92. Solimena M, Folli F, Aparisi R, Pozza G, de Camilli P. Autoantibodies to GABA-ergic neurons and pancreatic beta cells in stiff-man syndrome. N Engl J Med 1990;322:1555–1560.
93. Hagopian WA, Karlsen AE, Gottsater A, Landin-Olsson M, Grubin CE, Sundkvist G, et al. Quantitative assay using recombinant human islet glutamic acid decarboxylase (GAD65) shows that 64K autoantibody positivity at onset predicts diabetes type. J Clin Invest 1993;91:368–374.
94. Atkinson MA, Kaufman DL, Newman D, Tobin AJ, MacLaren NK. Islet cell cytoplasmic autoantibody reactivity to glutamate decarboxylase in insulin-dependent diabetes. J Clin Invest 1993;91:350–356.
95. Palmer JP, Asplin CM, Clemons P, Lyen K, Tatpati O, Raghu PK, et al. Insulin antibodies in insulin-dependent diabetics before insulin treatment. Science 1983;222:1337–1339.
96. Wiest-Ladenburger U, Hartmann R, Hartmann U, Berling K, Bohm BO, Richter W. Combined analysis and single-step detection of GAD65 and IA2 autoantibodies in IDDM can replace the histochemical islet cell antibody test. Diabetes 1997;46:565–571.
97. Roll U, Ziegler AG. Combined antibody screening for improved prediction of IDDM—modern strategies. Exp Clin Endocrinol Diabetes 1997;105:1–14.
98. Christie MR, Roll U, Payton MA, Hatfield ECI, Ziegler AG. Validity of screening for individuals at risk for type I diabetes by combined analysis of antibodies to recombinant proteins. Diabetes Care 1997;20:965–970.
99. Lu J, Li Q, Xie H, Chen ZJ, Borovitskaya AE, MacLaren NK, et al. Identification of a second transmembrane protein tyrosine phosphatase, ia-2 beta, as an autoantigen in insulin-dependent diabetes mellitus: precursor of the 37-kda tryptic fragment. Proc Natl Acad Sci USA 1996;93:2307–2311.
100. Bonifacio E, Lampasona V, Genovese S, Ferrari M, Bosi E. Identification of protein tyrosine phosphatase-like IA2 (islet cell antigen 512) as the insulin-dependent diabetes-related 37/40K autoantigen and a target of islet-cell antibodies. J Immunol 1995;155:5419–5426.
101. Verge CF, Gianani R, Kawasaki E, Yu LP, Pietropaolo F, Chase HP, et al. Number of autoantibodies (against insulin, GAD or ICA512/IA2) rather than particular autoantibody specificities determines risk of type I diabetes. J Autoimmunity 1996;9:379–383.
102. Verge CF, Gianani R, Kawasaki E, Yu L, Pietropaolo M, Jackson RA, et al. Prediction of type I diabetes in first-degree relatives using a combination of insulin, GAD, and ICA512bdc/IA-2 autoantibodies. Diabetes 1996;45:926–933.

103. Gorus FK, Goubert P, Semakula C, Vandewalle CL, de Schepper J, Scheen A, et al. IA-2-autoantibodies complement GAD(65)-autoantibodies in new-onset IDDM patients and help predict impending diabetes in their siblings. Diabetologia 1997;40:95–99.
104. Dotta F, Falorni A, Tiberti C, Dionisi S, Anastasi E, Torresi P, et al. Autoantibodies to the GM2-1 islet ganglioside and to GAD-65 at type 1 diabetes onset. J Autoimmunity 1997;10:585–588.
105. Castano L, Russo E, Zhou L, Lipes MA, Eisenbarth GS. Identification and cloning of a granule autoantigen (carboxypeptidase-H) associated with type I diabetes. J Clin Endocrinol Metab 1991;73:1197–1201.
106. Pietropaolo M, Castano L, Babu S, Buelow R, Kuo YL, Martin S, et al. Islet cell autoantigen 69 kD (ICA69). Molecular cloning and characterization of a novel diabetes-associated autoantigen. J Clin Invest 1993;92:359–371.
107. Miyazaki I, Gaedigk R, Hui MF, Cheung RK, Morkowski J, Rajotte RV, et al. Cloning of human and rat p69 cDNA, a candidate autoimmune target in type 1 diabetes. Biochim Biophys Acta 1994;1227:101–104.
108. Karjalainen J, Martin JM, Knip M, Ilonen J, Robinson BH, Savilahti E, et al. A bovine albumin peptide as a possible trigger of insulin-dependent diabetes mellitus. N Engl J Med 1992;327:302–307.
109. Gepts W, Lecompte PM. The pancreatic islets in diabetes. Am J Med 1981;70:105–115.
110. Honeyman MC, Cram DS, Harrison LC. Glutamic acid decarboxylase 67-reactive T cells: a marker of insulin-dependent diabetes. J Exp Med 1993;177:535–540.
111. Harrison LC, Chu SX, de Aizpurua HJ, Graham M, Honeyman MC, et al. Islet-reactive T cells are a marker of preclinical insulin-dependent diabetes. J Clin Invest 1992;89:1161–1165.
112. Atkinson MA, Kaufman DL, Campbell L, Gibbs KA, Shah SC, Bu DF, et al. Response of peripheral-blood mononuclear cells to glutamate decarboxylase in insulin-dependent diabetes. Lancet 1992;339:458–459.
113. Durinovic-Bello I, Hummel M, Ziegler AG. Cellular immune response to diverse islet cell antigens in IDDM. Diabetes 1996;45:795–800.
114. Roep BO. T-cell responses to autoantigens in IDDM—The search for the holy grail. Diabetes 1996;45:1147–1156.
115. Harrison LC, Honeyman MC, de Aizpurua HJ, Schmidli RS, Colman PG, Tait BD, et al. Inverse relation between humoral and cellular immunity to glutamic acid decarboxylase in subjects at risk of insulin-dependent diabetes. Lancet 1993;341:1365–1369.
116. Schloot NC, Roep BO, Wegmann D, Yu L, Chase HP, Wang T, et al. Altered immune response to insulin in newly diagnosed compared to insulin-treated diabetic patients and healthy control subjects. Diabetologia 1997;40:564–572.
117. Hummel M, Durinovic-Bello I, Ziegler AG. Relation between cellular and humoral immunity to islet cell antigens in type 1 diabetes. J Autoimmunity 1996;9:427–430.
118. Abulafia-Lapid R, Elias D, Raz I, Keren-Zur Y, Atlan H, Cohen IR. T cell responses of IDDM patients and healthy individuals to human hsp60 and its peptides. 1998 (Abstract).
119. Chatenoud L, Volpini W, Timsit J, Boitard C, Bach JF. Aberrant distribution of CD4 and CD8 lymphocyte subsets in recent-onset IDDM patients. Effect of cyclosporin. Diabetes 1993;42:869–875.
120. Berman MA, Sandborg CI, Wang ZS, Imfeld KL, Zaldivar F, Dadufalza V, et al. Decreased IL-4 production in new onset type I insulin- dependent diabetes mellitus. J Immunol 1996;157:4690–4696.
121. Wilson SB, Kent SC, Patton KT, Orban T, Jackson RA, Exley M, et al. Extreme Th1 bias of invariant V-alpha-24J-alpha-Q T cells in type 1 diabetes. Nature 1998;391:177–186.
122. Damotte D, Colomb E, Cailleau C, Brousse N, Charreire J, Carnaud, C. Analysis of susceptibility of NOD mice to spontaneous and experimentally induced thyroiditis. Eur J Immunol 1997;27:2854–2862.
123. Zavala AV, Fabiano de Bruno LE, Cardoso AI, Mota AH, Capucchio M, Poskus E, et al. Cellular and humoural autoimmunity markers in type 2 (non-insulin-dependent) diabetic patients with secondary drug failure. Diabetologia 1992;35:1159–1164.
124. Tuomi T, Groop LC, Zimmet PZ, Rowley MJ, Knowles W, MacKay IR. Antibodies to glutamic acid decarboxylase reveal latent autoimmune diabetes mellitus in adults with a non-insulin-dependent onset of disease. Diabetes 1993;42:359–362.
125. Groop L, Groop PH, Koskimies S. Relationship between B-cell function and HLA antigens in patients with type 2 (non-insulin-dependent) diabetes. Diabetologia 1986;29:757–760.
126. Irvine WJ, Sawers JS, Feek CM, Prescott RJ, Duncan LJ. The value of islet cell antibody in predicting secondary failure of oral hypoglycaemic agent therapy in diabetes mellitus. J Clin Lab Immunol 1979;2:23–26.

13   Autoimmune Adrenocortical Failure

Hemmo A. Drexhage, MD, PhD

CONTENTS

    INTRODUCTION
    EPIDEMIOLOGY
    MACROSCOPIC PATHOLOGY AND HISTOPATHOLOGY
        OF AUTOIMMUNE ADDISON'S DISEASE
    HUMORAL AUTOIMMUNE RESPONSE AND ANTIGENS
    CELL-MEDIATED AUTOIMMUNE RESPONSES AND ANTIGENS
    IMMUNOGENETIC ASPECTS
    ANIMAL MODELS OF AUTOIMMUNE ADDISON'S DISEASE
    THE ETIOLOGY AND PATHOGENESIS OF ADDISON'S DISEASE
    CONCLUSIONS
    ACKNOWLEDGMENTS
    REFERENCES

INTRODUCTION

In 1849, Thomas Addison described a group of patients who died with severe anemia *(1)*. At autopsy, in three of these patients, the adrenals were diseased. This observation provided the first evidence of a clinical picture resulting from a dysfunction of the adrenal glands. He reported the full classical description of clinical adrenocortical failure in 1855 in his monograph "On the constitutional and local effects of disease of the suprarenal capsules" *(2)*.

Addison's disease is a chronic disorder of the adrenal cortex, characterized by deficient production of adrenocortical hormones together with increased secretion of anterior pituitary adrenocorticotrophic hormone (ACTH).

Clinically, adrenocortical insufficiency induces a variety of signs and symptoms that include muscle weakness, fatigue, weight loss, gastrointestinal complaints (nausea, vomiting, diarrhea), hypotension, electrolyte disturbances (hyponatremia and hyperkalemia), and often skin hyperpigmentation (ACTH effect) or hypopigmentation (the disease is occasionally accompanied by vitiligo *[3,4]*).

In the past (the times of Thomas Addison), tuberculous involvement of the adrenals was the more common cause of chronic acquired adrenoprivic hypocorticalism, but the overall decrease in the prevalence of tuberculosis in the Western countries has resulted

From: *Contemporary Endocrinology: Autoimmune Endocrinopathies*
Edited by: R. Volpe © Humana Press Inc., Totowa, NJ

in a relative increase in the "idiopathic" form of atrophy of the adrenals. Idiopathic Addison's disease is a rare disorder that can be treated quite adequately by replacement therapy with glucocorticoids and mineralocorticoids. However, an adrenal crisis can occur, either spontaneously or precipitated by stress, in any subject whose cortisol output is too low for the demand *(5,6)*. An Addisonian crisis is potentially fatal, and stress factors precipitating disease include e.g., infection, trauma, surgery, and general anesthesia. Even a seemingly simple viral cold can trigger an Addisonian crisis, which can lead to death within 1 or 2 d. Therefore, it is important to understand the etiology and pathogenesis of Addison's disease, investigate animal models of this condition, and identify useful disease markers that can help in recognizing individuals at risk.

EPIDEMIOLOGY

Worldwide, tuberculosis still accounts for the highest number of cases of adrenal insufficiency in the world, with a prevalence of approx 100/million. However in "developed" countries, idiopathic atrophy has increased to over 75% of the cases, tuberculosis still being the second most frequent cause responsible for up to sometimes 15–20% of cases *(7,8)*. In a recent series in the Netherlands, the cause of Addison's disease in 91 collected cases was idiopathic in 83 (91.2%) and tuberculosis in 6 (6.6%) *(9)*. Other known, but rare causes of adrenal insufficiency *(5)* include malignant destruction, lymphomatous infiltration, amyloidosis, sarcoidosis, hemachromatosis, hemorrhage owing to trauma, or toxemia of pregnancy, and adrenal infections, such as candidiasis, histoplasmosis, coccidioidomycosis, and cytomegalovirus, these infections now mostly known as superinfections caused by HIV infection.

The prevalence of the idiopathic form of Addison's disease has been estimated at 30–60/million in European and North American populations, and its prevalence is highest in the fourth decade of life; there is also a marked female preponderance *(10)*.

Considerable evidence suggests that idiopathic adrenal atrophy is an autoimmune disease. The histopathology of the affected adrenals resembles that of other organs that are proven targets of autoimmune disease (thyroiditis, insulitis). Autoimmune responses to adrenocortical antigens have now been detected in patients with idiopathic Addison's disease, various adrenal antigens have been characterized on the molecular level, and animal models have been experimentally obtained. However, a transfer of clinical disease by antibodies and/or T cells (a prerequisite for the proof of the autoimmune genesis of a clinical disease *(11)* has not been performed successfully. Collectively, the evidence, even though not completely satisfactory, clearly points to an autoimmune nature of idiopathic Addison's disease. For this reason, the term "autoimmune" will mostly be used in this chapter.

MACROSCOPIC PATHOLOGY AND HISTOPATHOLOGY OF AUTOIMMUNE ADDISON'S DISEASE

Macroscopy

In autoimmune Addison's disease, the adrenal glands are reduced in weight to in general 1.2–2.5 g each (normal range, 4–5 g each), both cortices being narrowed and largely replaced by fibrous tissue *(12)*. The macroscopic appearance closely resembles the original description of the adrenal glands in one of Addison's own patients: "The two supra-renal capsules appeared exceedingly small and atrophied; the right one was natural firm; the left deformed by contraction; each adherent to surrounding parts by dense areolar tissue; the section gave a pale and homogeneous aspect; it presented a fibrous tissue, fat and cells about the size of white blood corpuscles" *(2)*. Indeed the adrenal glands are often very difficult to recognize or may be missing altogether, being substituted by adipose and fibrotic tissue. In such cases, remnants may be found by dissection of the adrenal veins, following these vessels to their entrance into the remains of the gland. However, in spite of these precautions, it has also been reported that adrenal tissue could not be found anymore *(13)*, though classically it is assumed that the medulla is spared by the destructive process that apparently attacks predominantly the cortex in the autoimmune form of Addison's disease. This in contrast to tuberculous adrenalitis, where the entire gland is affected.

Microscopy

The microscopic histopathological examination of postmortem adrenal specimens provides strong evidence that autoimmunity plays a pivotal role in idiopathic Addison's disease, i.e., the presence of a diffuse and focal infiltration of the cortex by lymphoid cells. The normal architecture of the zonae glomerulosa, fasciculata, and reticularis is completely distorted and almost all cells have disappeared. The remaining cortical cells are dispersed in a scarce and delicate fibrous tissue, as single cells or in small clusters *(12)*.

A finding that was reported quite early, but perhaps has not been given adequate attention, is the presence of small "regeneration" nodules, especially near the capsule. Kiefer *(14)* was the first to describe one such case with numerous nodules. Saphir and Binswanger *(15)* were second to observe the presence of such nodules in one patient, who had no clinical symptoms up to a few days before death, that occurred suddenly after appendectomy. Various other authors have since then reported nodule formation in Addison's disease *(16–18)*, and both hyperplasia and hypertrophy can be observed in adrenals from patients with idiopathic Addison's disease. Scattered islands of cells may be seen in the cortex as well as large, well-circumscribed adenoma-like nodules, without typical zonal division of the parenchyma. At times, the hyperplastic nodules are seen to extend far into the periglandular fat. Their cells resemble those of the zona fasciculata, less often those of the zona glomerulosa. The nodules may have a bizarre appearance and sometimes are huge, with deeply pigmented cytoplasm and large hyperchromatic nuclei. Inflammatory infiltrates may be present within the nodules or at their periphery.

What is the cause of these nodules? The hypertrophy of the cells has been attributed to the effects of raised plasma ACTH levels *(19)*. However, the consequences of increased ACTH stimulation should be diffuse, as observed after administration of high amounts of ACTH or in bilateral adrenocortical hyperplasia. Are immune cells causing the nodular adrenocortical hyperplasia and hypertrophy as well as atrophic changes? The nodules are somewhat similar to those described in familial micronodular Cushing's syndrome *(20, 21)*. Foci of lymphocytes are observed in the vicinity of these nodules *(20,22)*. Antibodies stimulating adrenocortical cells have been detected in the circulation of patients with micronodular Cushing's syndrome *(20,21)*, and it has been suggested that hyperplasia and hypertrophy of adrenocortical cells might reflect a local activity of infiltrated immune cells and their products (cytokines and antibodies; *see* also *below*). Such local activity of immune cells might also occur in autoimmune Addison's disease, where the histopathology (atrophy alone or in combination with hyperplasia and hypertrophy) could depend on the balance of local inhibition vs local stimulation by the components of the immune system (cells and/or their products) accumulated in the adrenal cortex.

Indeed a cortical inflammatory infiltrate is present in idiopathic Addison's disease, with a high prevalence of small lymphocytes. Plasma cells and macrophages are also present, but in fewer numbers. The adrenal medulla is usually intact or infiltrated by some lymphoid cells. The chronic cortical infiltrate is mostly diffuse, but in some areas, lymphocytes may form aggregates (foci) of various dimensions. Germinal centers are seldom present. Although such diffuse infiltrate is thus highly suggestive for an autoimmune character of the disease, it is not conclusive proof of autoimmune Addison's disease. Similar, but mainly focally arranged infiltrates can also be observed at postmortem examination in non-Addisonian cases. The initial extensive study of Petri and Nerup *(23)* confirmed the presence of a diffuse lymphocytic inflammation with disappearance of the epithelial cells of the adrenal cortex in idiopathic Addison's disease. However, the authors also observed small clusters of lymphocytes in 15 and 19% of their controls, i.e., adrenal glands from two autopsy series of 413 and 161 individuals, respectively, without previously reported signs or symptoms of Addison's disease. Hayashi et al. *(24)* also studied the histological appearance of the adrenal cortex in a series of autopsies of individuals who died without Addison's disease. The series, in this case, was analyzed separately in young and old individuals. In 110 (63%) of 174 autopsy specimens of those who died at the "old" age of over 60 yr, the authors found a mainly focally arranged mononuclear cell infiltration of varying degrees within the adrenal cortex, whereas such focal infiltration was observed less frequently in young cases, that is, in only 4 (7%) of 54 autopsy specimens of persons aged <49 yr. In addition, the severity of the infiltration was graded, and 13 out of 14 adrenals examined and scored as having diffuse and severely infiltrating lesions were found in autopsies of the elderly subjects all aged over 70 yr. Wulffraat *(25)* did similar findings in a series of 60 consecutive autopsies of individuals who died without clinically overt adrenal disease. He found focal mononuclear cell infiltration in the adrenal cortex in 22 cases (35%) where the mean age of the group identified with these infiltrations was 72 yr. In the subjects without adrenal infiltrations, the mean age was younger (62 yr). Is it possible that older individuals start to develop a mild form of autoimmune cortical adrenalitis, without (sub)clinical signs of adrenal failure and without (detectable) autoantibody production, and are these focal infiltrates instrumental in the nodule development often seen in the aged adrenal cortices?

Using immunohistochemical techniques, Hayashi et al. *(24)* found that in their non-Addisonian autopsy cases, 80% of the mononuclear cells present in the adrenal focal infiltrates were CD3-positive T lymphocytes. Of these T lymphocytes, 70% were CD4, and 12.5% were CD8 T cells. Twenty-four percent of the CD4-positive cells were activated T lymphocytes, as judged by positive staining for the expression of interleukin-2 (IL-2) receptors. CD22-positive cells (pan-B cells) comprised only 5% of the infiltrated cells. These B lymphocytes, however, were found dispersed throughout the adrenal cortex. The authors did indeed regard the presence of the focal T-lymphoid cell infiltrates in elderly persons as a possible presign of adrenal autoimmunity. Also in Wulffraat's *(25)* autopsy series, lymphoid cell infiltrations were mainly foci of CD4-positive T cells and lymphoid follicle-like B cell structures were absent. Single CD8-positive cells were scattered throughout the cortex. Almost 50% of the infiltrated lymphoid cells were human leucocyte antigen (HLA) class II-positive.

It is regrettable that reports on immunohistochemical studies, aimed at the fine characterization of the severe diffuse and large focal mononuclear infiltrates in the adrenal cortex from patients with active autoimmune Addison's disease, are still lacking. The spontaneously occurring cases of Addison's disease in dogs and cats *(see below)* may be helpful to obtain such detailed immunohistochemical studies *(26)*. A further immunohistological indication for an autoimmune process most likely underlying the pathogenesis of idiopathic Addison's disease has come from another postmortem study, in which a detailed analysis of infiltrated cells was not performed, but in which it was reported that almost all the cortical cells spared by the destructive process were HLA class II positive (8 of 14 cases examined) *(27)*. The phenomenon of "inappropriate" expression of HLA molecules by autoimmune target cells (which normally do not express these products) was first shown for thyrocytes of patients with autoimmune thyroid disease, and it is now a recognized histopathologic feature of tissues affected by autoimmunity *(28)*. Such inappropriate expression of HLA molecules by endocrine cells is the consequence of the in vivo production of cytokines (e.g., interferon-gamma [IFN-γ], tumor necrosis factor [TNF]) by infiltrated immune cells *(29)*. However, in the case of the adrenal gland, the zona reticularis contains cells that do under normal conditions express HLA class II products *(30)*. The question for the adrenal thus remains "What induces such HLA class II expression?" Are again the small foci of infiltrated immune cells relevant in this respect?

HUMORAL AUTOIMMUNE RESPONSE AND ANTIGENS

Addison's Disease in Isolation and as Part of Polyglandular Autoimmune Syndromes

Autoimmune Addison's disease seldom develops in isolation. In about 50% of cases, the disease manifests itself clinically as a single disease, but in the other half of patients several glands and organs are affected *(31)*. In 1926, Schmidt reported the presence of a simultaneous lymphocytic infiltration of the thyroid gland and the adrenal cortex in two patients with Addison's disease *(32)*. This description was the first of what is now called an "autoimmune polyglandular syndrome" (APGS). In 1964, Carpenter et al. *(33)* pointed out that insulin-dependent diabetes mellitus (IDDM) was also frequently present in patients with "Schmidt syndrome." In 1981, a systematic classification of APGS was proposed, with a subdivision into two distinct types of APGS, type I and type II APGS *(34; see* Chapter 15).

In general, type I APGS is relatively rare, but it occurs more frequently in northern European countries *(35)*, which interestingly also have the highest prevalence of other autoimmune diseases, most notably of IDDM *(36)*. The syndrome mainly affects children and has a slight male preponderance. The major criterion for the disease is the associated presence of mucocutaneous candidiasis, hypoparathyroidism, and ectodermal dystrophy. Addison's disease, other autoimmune endocrinopathies, including in particular gonadal failure (clinically often detected at puberty), pernicious anemia, active chronic hepatitis, alopecia, and vitiligo, are also often present. Type I APGS has also been termed autoimmune polyendocrinopathy, candidiasis, ectodermal dystrophy (APECED) *(35; see* Chapter 15).

Type II APGS ("Schmidt syndrome") is more common, with an estimated prevalence of 14–20/million *(37)*. It occurs mainly in the fourth decade of life and has a marked

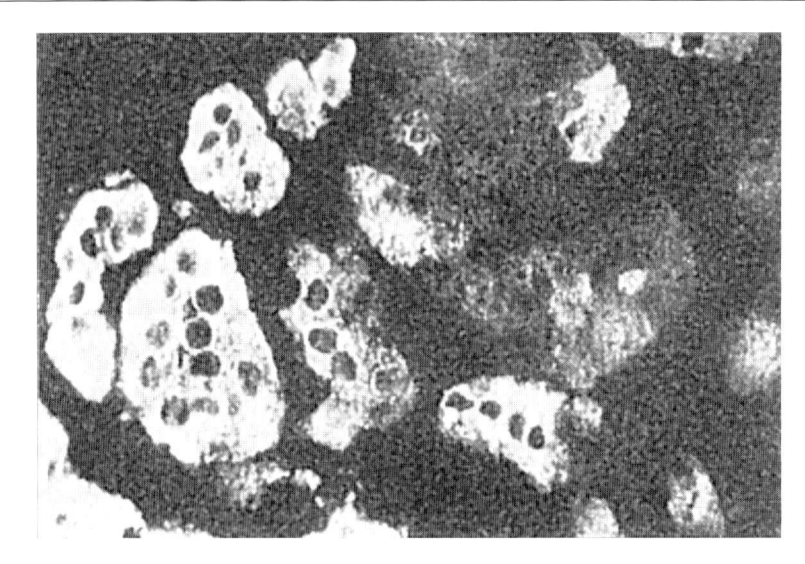

Fig. 1. ACA detected by indirect immunofluorescence on a cryostat section of human adrenal (×900). Note the staining of the cells of the zone glomerulosa, which is predominantly in picture.

female preponderance. It is classically characterized by adrenal failure in association with hypothyroidism although IDDM, Graves' disease, and pernicious anemia are not uniformly excluded. Even when these latter diseases are not clinically manifest, the corresponding organ-specific autoantibodies are nonetheless often present in the patients already affected by Addison's disease, a situation referred to as "positive autoimmune polyendocrine serology" *(38)*.

Antibodies Reacting with Adrenal Cortex Antibodies (ACA) Only and Antibodies Reacting with Cells Producing Steroids in General (Steroid Cell Antibody [St-C-Ab])

The autoantibodies characteristic of autoimmune Addison's disease—be it in isolation or in combination with other endocrine failures—are the ACA or cytoplasmic adrenal antibodies. The discovery of these adrenal autoantibodies in the late 1950s pointed at that time—together with the histopathology of the lesion—to the autoimmune character of idiopathic Addison's disease. The first report described the presence of antibodies to a saline extract of the human adrenal gland by complement fixation in 2 of 10 patients with Addison's disease *(39)*. Subsequently, these findings were confirmed *(40)*, and it soon became apparent that the presence of adrenal antibodies was a good diagnostic tool to differentiate autoimmune Addison's disease from tuberculous adrenal insufficiency (though it has also been reported that around 5% of tuberculous adrenalitis patients are positive for adrenal autoantibodies *[41]*).

Presently, the indirect immunofluorescence (IIF) technique is routinely used. In the technique, cryostat sections of human or monkey adrenal glands are reacted with sera of patients with autoimmune Addison's disease, and ACA are demonstrated by a general reactivity with all three layers of the adrenal cortex (Fig. 1). Sera do not stain the medullary portion of the gland. Interestingly, antibodies that do react with the medullary portion of the adrenals have been described in non-Addisonian patients with IDDM and pre-IDDM *(42)*, with IDDM associated with autoimmune neuropathy *(43)*, and/or with

Table 1
Prevalence of ACA and St-C-Abs as Measured
by Indirect Immunofluorescence in Addisonian and Non-Addisonian Patients

	ACA, %	St-C-Ab, %
Addison's disease		
Isolated cases		
Recent-onset	70–80	10–20
Long-standing	20–30	1–5
With ovarian failure	90-100	80–90
In the context of APGS type I	90-100	60–80
In the context of APGS type II	70–80	30–40
Autoimmune endocrine disease, but no Addison's disease		
APGS type I	20–30	10–20
Thyroiditis and/or IDDM	1–2	<1
Healthy individuals		
Normal population	0.2–0.8	<0.2
First-degree relatives of Addisonian patients	1–3	n.d.
Unselected infertility/amenorrhea	<1	<1

possible abnormalities of the glucose contraregulatory hormone pathway (44). ACA as detected in the IIF are mainly IgG and fix complement when present in a high titer. They are detected in up to 80% of all patients with idiopathic Addison's disease at diagnosis (Table 1), whether the adrenal insufficiency is in the isolated form or in association with other endocrine diseases (45). However, with time, the prevalence of these antibodies falls to about 30% in isolated adrenal insufficiency, but tends to be unchanged for several years in the serum of patients with adrenal insufficiency associated with the autoimmune polyglandular syndromes, especially when the disease develops in young children in the context of type I APGS (45). In adults with type II APGS, these antibodies are detected more frequently among females than among males.

ACA have also been found to occur in 0.2–0.8% of normal healthy control individuals without overt or subclinical (i.e., "positive autoimmune polyendocrine serology") related endocrine- or organ-specific autoimmune manifestations. Although there is a trend for the presence of these antibodies to increase with age (as do the focal lymphocytic cortical adrenal infiltrates—see before), the rarity of these antibodies in healthy individuals reinforces the high specificity of these antibodies for the presence of present or future autoimmune Addison's disease. As is the case for islet reactive antibodies in prediabetics and for thyroperoxidase (TPO) antibodies in prethyroiditis patients, ACA in non-Addisonian patients are risk factors for a later development of clinically overt Addison's disease. The predictive value of ACA in non-Addisonian patients varies, and depends on age and other concomitant disease. Non-Addisonian children who already suffer from type I APGS and are positive for ACA (reported prevalences are 40–50% of type 1 APGS cases) almost invariably progress to Addison's disease in a period of approx 10 yr time (45). Adults without APGS type 1, but ACA-positive have a cumulative risk for Addison's disease of around 30% in 10 yr time (45). Especially high titres and antibodies fixing the complement components C5-C9 represent an additional risk (46).

The natural history of Addison's disease progresses through four different stages of adrenal cortex hypofunction (47); in stage 1, an increase in plasma renin activity is associated with a normal or low-serum aldosterone level, which suggests that initially the zona glomerulosa is affected. After several months or years, a dysfunction of the zona fasciculata becomes evident, which is manifested at first by a decrease in the plasma cortisol response to ACTH (stage 2), followed by an increased plasma ACTH level (stage 3) and finally by a decreased plasma cortisol level and overt clinical symptoms (stage 4). In general, more than 50% of apparently healthy individuals with ACA have some biochemical evidence of cortico-adrenal impairment. Nevertheless, it has also been reported that ACA in some patients without a clinical Addison's disease can disappear spontaneously or after corticosteroid therapy with restoration of the previous impaired adrenal function *(48)*.

A proportion of ACA crossreacts in IIF assays with cytoplasmic antigens of other steroid-producing cells, such as those present in the testis, the ovary, and the placenta *(49)*. Except for patients who have suffered from spermatic cord torsion, there is invariably an association between the presence of such St-C-Ab and that of ACA. In other words, St-C-Abs can only be detected in IIF in the presence of ACA. St-C-Abs can be distinguished from ACA by preabsorption tests with homogenates of any of the steroid-producing target organs, whereas ACA recognize exclusively the adrenal gland.

Originally, St-C-Ab were found in two males affected by Addison's disease, but without clinically overt hypogonadism *(49)*. Subsequently, these antibodies were detected in almost all female Addisonian patients with primary amenorrhea and in around 60% of those with secondary amenorrhea *(50)*. Patients with primary or secondary amenorrhea who are positive for St-C-Ab almost never revert to fertility. However, in one case, this reversion has exceptionally occurred, and the patient, after a prolonged period of amenorrhea, conceived and delivered a healthy baby *(51)*.

In the absence of overt hypogonadism, St-C-Ab have been described in about 15–25% of patients with clinical or latent Addison's disease *(52)*. St-C-Ab are seen most frequently in those patients who also have one or more additional endocrine diseases. However, heterogeneity does exist between type I and type II APGS in relation to the production of St-C-Ab. More than 60% of patients with type I APGS and Addison's disease have St-C-Ab. This high prevalence of St-C-Ab explains the common association with gonadal failure seen in this group, especially in females. Pediatricians should seek St-C-Ab in prepubertal ACA-positive patients in order to avoid misdiagnoses of autoimmune oöphoritis at the time of puberty, especially if the patient presents with unexplained gonadal dysfunction. In contrast, St-C-Abs are only present in about 30% of patients with type II APGS *(52)*.

The Autoantigens Recognized by ACA and St-C-Abs

Considerable progress has been made with regard to the identification of the target antigens of the cytoplasmic ACA and St-C-Abs *(53)*. The adrenal cytochrome p450 enzyme 21 hydroxylase (21-OH, which converts 17-α-progesterone and progesterone into 11-deoxycortisol and deoxycorticosterone) is the major autoantigen recognized by autoantibodies present in patients with Addison's disease *(54,55)*, either in the form of isolated adrenal failure, type II APGS, or in ACA-positive individuals without overt Addison's disease (*see* Chapter 8).

In type I APGS, autoantibodies could be detected, which were directed to two other members of the cytochrome p450 enzyme family, namely, to the p450 side-chain cleavage enzyme (p450 scc) and to 17-α-hydroxylase *(56–58)* (17-α-OH). In addition, antibodies were found to a 51-kDa islet protein *(59)*. After some controversies and following comparison with St-C-Ab, it is now clear that 17-α-OH and p450 scc are the major components of St-C-Abs measured by IIF *(60)*. Indeed of the steroidogenic p450 enzymes, 21-OH is adrenal-specific, 17-α-OH is expressed in both adrenal and gonadal tissues, whereas p450 scc is present in adrenal, gonads, and placenta. Autoantibody reactivity against other steroidogenic enzymes has been studied, but none of the sera of Addisonian patients was found to react with 11 β hydroxylase, 3β-hydroxysteroid dehydrogenase, aromatase, or adrenodoxin *(61–63)*. The earlier-mentioned 51-kDa autoantigen in type 1 APGS has turned out to be the enzyme aromatic *l*-amino decarboxylase (AADC) *(64)*. This enzyme has a wide tissue distribution, and is particularly present in islets, liver, granulosa cells, and placenta. Autoantibodies to AADC are associated with the chronic active autoimmune hepatitis and vitiligo of type I APGS *(64)*.

Two different immunoprecipitation assays (IPA) for the detection of autoantibodies to 21-OH (21-OH-Abs) have presently been developed, one based on ^{35}S-labeled 21-OH produced in an in vitro transcription-translation system *(65,66)*, and the other based on ^{125}I-labelled recombinant 21-OH produced in yeast *(67)*. These tests are highly sensitive and specific, and a good agreement was found between 21-OH Abs measured by these two assays and ACA by IIF *(60,61,65,67,68)*. The assays based on 21-OH labeled with ^{125}I have in comparison to the ^{35}S-labeled 21-OH as advantage that they will be more convenient and easy to use in routine clinical laboratories. It must be noted also that some investigators *(69)* have found some discrepancies between the presence of 21-OH Abs and ACA. To avoid further discrepancies on adrenal autoantibody measurements, an international standardization should be performed *(47)*.

Pathogenic Role of p450 Enzyme Autoantibodies

Evidence for a direct pathogenic role of the antibodies directed to the p450 enzymes in ovarian and adrenal failure is weak. Antibody preparations from Addisonian patients can inhibit in vitro the activity of 21-OH in the conversion of progesterone to deoxyprogesterone *(70)*, and likewise, antibodies to 17-α-OH and p450scc *(57)* can inhibit enzyme activity in gonadal cells. However, it remains difficult to envisage how the autoantibodies gain access to the intracytoplasmic enzymes in the in vivo situation. It is also of note that sera of patients with APGS type I and Addison's disease, positive for ACA and St-C-Abs in high titer, are cytotoxic for cultured granulosa cells in the presence of complement *(71)*. Such complement-dependent antibody cytotoxicity could be one of the immune mechanisms leading to autoimmune adrenal and ovarian failure. The antibodies may, however, also be the consequence of primarily macrophage-mediated, T-cell-mediated, or other forms of endocrine cellular destruction. The latter is, for instance, seen with as yet ill-defined ovarian antibodies detectable in ELISA after iatrogenically induced premature ovarian failure *(72)*.

Antibodies Blocking Adrenal Function and Growth

Some autoantibodies have the ability to bind to cell membrane receptors. These "receptor antibodies" are able to mimic the action of stimulating hormones if they have an affinity similar to the hormone itself for the specific binding site. This mechanism underlies the hyperthyroidism and goiter formation in patients with Graves' disease, where thyroid-stimulating immunoglobulins bind specifically to the thyroid-stimulating hormone (TSH) receptor (TSHR) on thyrocytes and stimulate thyroid cells by inducing the same effects as pituitary TSH, although escaping the physiologically negative feedback mechanism with the pituitary gland *(73)*. On the other hand, autoantibodies, which similarly interact with hormonal or other ligand receptors, but block the action of the corresponding stimulating hormones, have also been described. Such blocking receptor antibodies include antibodies to the acetylcholine receptor *(74)*, the TSHR *(75,76)*, and the insulin receptor *(77)*.

Bigazzi was the first to speculate that blocking antibodies may also play a role in the pathogenesis of idiopathic Addison's disease *(13)*. One such patient, who was found to have ACTH-blocking antibodies, was described by Kendall-Taylor et al. *(78)*. We extended these findings by searching for the presence of similar adrenal-blocking antibodies in a series of 25 patients with idiopathic Addison's disease *(79)*. Guinea pig adrenal segments were cultured, as described by Chayen et al. *(80)*, in the presence of ACTH in combination with various concentrations of patients' IgG added to the culture system. Subsequently, the cortisol level present in the culture medium was assayed by radioimmunoassay (RIA) and the activity and DNA synthesis of the adrenal cells were measured using cytochemical bioassays and Feulgen densitometry on frozen sections of the same cultured adrenal segments. The results clearly demonstrated that many of these sera had IgGs that were able to block both the growth-stimulating and hormone production effects of ACTH. Specifically, IgGs blocking the growth action of ACTH were found in 80% of patients, whereas IgGs blocking the steroidogenic effects of ACTH were detected in 74% of the cases tested. Only two sera had neither growth- nor steroidogenesis-blocking IgG (one was positive for ACA and one was negative). Twenty of the 25 patients tested had ACA, but of the 5 negative for ACA, 4 had blocking antibodies. The implication is that in these latter patients, the adrenal-blocking IgGs were the only serological evidence of the autoimmune nature of the disease.

With regard to the above-described organ culture and cytochemical techniques to detect the growth-blocking and function-blocking antibodies (i.e., the use of guinea pig organ cultures and cytochemical bioassays) it has become clear that particular care must be given to the used detection systems *(81)*. Because the cytochemical bioassays are extremely sensitive, they might also detect effects of impurifications of the used IgG preparations *(81)*. It has also been questioned whether the Feulgen densitometry really measures DNA synthesis *(81)*. Using another assay system employing cultured guinea pig adrenal cells, it was recently reported that at best only 8% of Addisonian patients had blocking IgG, with only minor functional effects *(82)*. Interestingly, with only partially purified IgGs (diethylaminoethyl [DEAE] purification), blocking of cortisol production was found in 41% of Addisonian patients *(82)*. The discrepancies between our earlier *(79)* and this latter set of experiments *(82)* could thus be explained by the difference in experimental conditions, the purity of the used IgG preparations, and by the levels of sensitivity of the two distinct culture assay systems. Therefore, the presence of adrenal blocking antibodies in Addisonian patients is not clear and still questionable, and needs further investigations with renewed approaches.

CELL-MEDIATED AUTOIMMUNE RESPONSES AND ANTIGENS

Cell-mediated immune reactions to adrenal antigens were first described by Nerup and Bendixen in 1969 *(83)*, and since then, several studies have confirmed and extended their initial results *(84)*. Leukocytes obtained from patients with idiopathic Addison's disease have a decreased migration capacity in the presence of adrenal antigens when compared to leukocytes from healthy individuals and patients with tuberculous adrenalitis. Around 50% of patients with idiopathic Addison's disease showed positive results in this test, but the same authors could not observe T-cell proliferation in the blastogenesis assay using their adrenal mitochondrial antigen preparation *(85)*. Later experiments, however, also using T cell blastogenesis as end-point measurement, but triggering the T cells with other adrenal cell fractions, in particular with a fraction of mol wt 18–24 kDa, did show a response in 6/10 Addisonian patients *(86)*. The most recent preliminary experiments on T-cell blastogenesis using the purified antoantigens 21-OH and 17-α-OH coupled to matrices show that none of the T-cell preparations of 16 Addisonian patients reacted with 17-α-OH, but 7/16 did react with 21-OH. Interestingly, the specific T cells recognizing the 21-OH in this latter assay did produce in 1/7 cases tested IFN-γ, but none gave interleukin-4 (IL-4) production (Weetman, personal communication).

Over the past 5–10 yr, it has become clear that the population of CD4+ T cells can functionally be divided into two subsets based on their profile of cytokine production *(87–89)*. One subset predominantly produces IFN-γ, but also IL-2; this is the so-called Th1 subset. The other subset, Th2, produces predominantly IL-4 and IL-5. The functional significance of these different cytokine production profiles is that they represent different T-cell-regulatory actions. Th1 cells and their cytokine products stimulate the cytotoxic action of macrophages and, hence, cell-mediated immunity. Th2 cells and their cytokine products stimulate B cells and, hence, lead to humoral immune responses. It must be noted, however, that the Th1 and Th2 subtypes represent extremes. There are many CD4+ T-cells clones with a cytokine production profile intermediate between Th1 and Th2 cells. The driving of naive CD4+ T cells (Th0 cells) into either the direction of Th1 or Th2 is guided in a complicated network by cytokines, such as IL-1, IL-12, IL-10, IFN-γ, IL-4, and products of the arachidonic acid metabolism *(90–94)*.

A recently developed theory approaches the problem of the control of self-reactivity from the angle of a balance between Th1 and Th2 pathways: endocrine autoimmune diseases characterized by an ultimate failure of the target gland, such as Addison's disease, must according to this theory be viewed as being caused by predominantly Th1-mediated pathways in which the endocrine cells are destroyed by IFN-γ-activated scavenger macrophages. The "Th1-Th2 balance" theory emphasizes the reciprocal relation between the Th1 and Th2 pathways *(88,95)*, and suggests that if the Th1 pathway is diverted into the Th2 pathway, the Th1-mediated autoimmune reactivity is dampened. In essence, tolerance to self is not restored, but the harmful immune reaction to self is diverted to a less harmful one. There are indeed reports on cytokine treatments that are able to induce such a switch from Th1 to Th2 pathways *(96–98)*, resulting in an amelioration of e.g., IDDM in animal models. Circulating antibodies, whose production is switched on by the stimulation of the Th2 cells, apparently contribute little to the damage of such target cells. The question is whether such is also the case in Addison's disease.

Despite its attractivity, the hypothesis that protection from endocrine autoimmune destruction can be achieved by a Th1 to Th2 switch is probably too simplistic. Although earlier data are compelling for a role of Th2 cells in the control of organ-specific autoimmunity, other recent findings (reviewed in *99*) require revision of this model, and suggest that regulatory T-cell populations exist somehow associated with, but distinct from Th2 cells. IL-10-inducible regulatory CD4+ T cells (Tr1 cells) have been described that suppress the proliferation of naive T cells via IL-10 and transforming growth factor-β (TGF-β) production *(100)*. Similar suppressive T cells (Th3 cells) have been obtained from orally tolerized mice and clones of these cells produced TGF-β, but little IL-4 and IL-10 *(101)*. Apart from these two examples of distinct regulatory T cells, examples of yet other regulatory T cells do also exist *(99)*. Although these regulatory CD4+ T cells all have distinct cytokine profiles, they share TGF-β production. This cytokine thus seems to become an important other "suppressive" cytokine apart from IL-4 and IL-10. It must be borne in mind, however, that these "suppressive" cytokines may also have an opposing stimulating effect on immune responses depending on the phase or the milieu of the immune reaction. This notion leaves us again with a complex picture of flexible networks of regulatory T cells governing the immune response via not yet fully understood rules and regulations. Despite these difficulties in pinpointing specific T-suppressor populations, several studies have suggested that patients with Addison's disease in combination with other autoimmune endocrine disorders may have specific defects in their T-cell-mediated suppressive capability *(102,103)*. Similar failures of suppression have also been described in patients with autoimmune thyroid disease and other related conditions *(104,105)*.

In the past Nerup et al. *(85)*—apart from testing patients' leukocytes in migration inhibition assays—also performed intracutaneous delayed-type hypersensitivity (dth) skin tests in Addisonian patients. The dth skin test is the in vivo test for an antigen-specific Th1 reaction. A positive dth response to adrenal antigens that correlated well to the leukocyte migration test was observed *(85)*. Positive results in the latter test were seen more frequently in male patients, but there was no correlation with the presence of ACA, the patient's age, or the duration of the disease. Using peripheral blood mononuclear cells from patients with idiopathic Addison's disease, Ludwig and Schernthaner *(106)* also noted a positive migration inhibition when these cells were incubated not only with crude adrenal extracts, but also with adrenal microsomes. Unexpectedly, however, they also confirmed a reactivity with adrenal mitochondria, a classic nonorgan-specific autoantigen.

In a further support of the concept that T cells are involved in the pathogenesis of Addison's disease, the percentage of circulating "activated" T cells, i.e., T cells expressing HLA class II molecules, was quantified in patients with idiopathic Addison's disease and in controls *(107)*. All control individuals, including one patient with recent-onset adrenal hemorrhage and nine patients with long-standing adrenal insufficiency (five with idiopathic Addison's disease and four studied after bilateral adrenalectomy for Cushing's disease), had normal percentages of activated T cells (up to 3%). In contrast, in five patients with recent-onset Addison's disease, these activated T cells were elevated (7–29%), similar to the rises reported in recent-onset autoimmune thyroid disease *(108)* and IDDM *(109)*.

The Th1 concept of autoimmune endocrine destruction implies that macrophages are also important in the cell-mediated immune destructive reaction toward adrenal cells, if not the only cell killing or silencing the adrenal cell. It has indeed been found that supernatants from lipopolysaccharide-stimulated peritoneal macrophages of C3Heb/Fej mice inhibit ACTH-induced steroidogenesis of rabbit adrenocortical cells in suspension *(110)*. It is likely that the macrophages exert such functions by virtue of their cytokine production. Macrophage-derived and other cytokines (IL-1, IL-6, IFN-γ, TNF) exert several positive and negative actions on the function and growth of various endocrine cells, both in vitro and in vivo *(111)*. Little is known, however, of the effects of cytokines on the adrenal gland and on cortical adrenal cells in particular. In the few studies that have addressed this question, there was no agreement on whether IL-1 has an effect on the function of adrenal cells either in vivo or in in vitro *(112,113)*.

Collectively, there is thus ample evidence to implicate the cell-mediated immune system in the autoreactivity toward adrenal cells in idiopathic Addison's disease, not least because of the diffuse mononuclear cell infiltration present in the diseased glands. Moreover, in an experimental allergic animal model of Addison's disease *(see below)*, transfer of spleen cells from mice immunized with adrenal extracts led both to the development of cortical adrenalitis and to adrenal autoantibodies in the recipients *(114)*. A word of caution is, however, necessary because the T-cell transfers only led to these adrenal microscopic and serologic abnormalities, and not to any development of adrenal failure. Therefore, the ultimate proof of Addison's disease being a T-cell-mediated autoimmune disease has not been given.

IMMUNOGENETIC ASPECTS

Endocrine autoimmune diseases are of multifactorial origin, with various genetic and environmental factors contributing to their development. Of the genes involved the major histocompatability complex (MHC)-linked genes are considered to be the most important ones followed by various other genes coding for other molecules involved in immune regulation (such as e.g., the CTLA-4 gene) and by genes likely involved in the regulation of the metabolism of the target tissue or of antigen expression (such as e.g., the insulin gene in IDDM).

With regard to the MHC-linked genes, there is a general consensus for Addison's disease that the major association is with HLA-B8 *(115)* and DR3 *(116,117)*, even when Addisonian patients are analyzed separately from those who have other autoimmune disorders *(118)*. The relative risk calculated in genetic terms, however, varies in the different studies with the two European reports indicating a relative risk for HLA-DR3 of approx 3.5 *(116,118)* and the one from the US of 6 *(117)*. In addition, the latter study indicated an association of Addison's disease with HLA-DR4, but this could not be confirmed in the European patients. A recent Italian study indicates an increased prevalence of both HLA-DR3 and HLA-DR5 in Addison patients, HLA-DR3 being predominantly prevalent in APGS type II patients with IDDM, with HLA-DR5 being predominantly prevalent in APGS type II with thyroid autoimmunity *(119)*. Since the association in IDDM is particularly with the HLA-DR3/4-associated HLA-DQB chains that have a nonaspartic amino acid residue at position 57, such latter presence may be a molecular marker of future diabetes development in patients with ACA. On the other hand, the presence of DR-5 may be a risk factor for a future or present complication with thyroiditis.

There is also consensus that there is no HLA-DR3 association in type I APGS *(120)*, despite the strong association with Addison's disease and other classic endocrine autoimmune disorders. The main association in this syndrome has been found with the HLA-A locus, that is, HLA-A28 *(121)*. Recent studies in Finland and Japan have allowed the location of the gene responsible for the condition to chromosome 21, and the investigators have extended their studies by showing that the gene involved is a novel gene, autoimmune regulator (AIRE), encoding a protein containing motifs suggestive of a transcription factor including two zinc-finger (PHD-finger) motifs *(122,123)*. It must also be noted that a recent investigation unexpectedly reported a higher frequency of HLA-DR5 in APGS type I (RR 2.85) *(124)*.

With regard to the CTLA-4 gene (i.e., IDDM12), associations have in particular been reported with IDDM, Graves' disease, and Hashimoto's thyroiditis *(125)*. A special CTLA-4 polymorphism at codon 17 was found with higher frequency in these diseases *(125)*. With regard to Addisonian patients, a higher frequency of this CTLA-4 polymorphism has been reported in a subgroup of patients who are DQα1*0501-positive *(126)*. A preliminary study by Weetman et al. (personal communication) finds frequencies of this polymorphism in around 25–30% of Addison patients. A problem with these findings is, however, the difference of disease-related frequencies with those in various healthy control populations: the background presence of the indicated CTLA-4 polymorphism in the healthy population differs from population to population ranging from 14 (England) to 20 (Norway) percent.

ANIMAL MODELS OF AUTOIMMUNE ADDISON'S DISEASE

Spontaneous Animal Models of Addison's Disease

Until today there has been no description of inbred animal models that spontaneously develop autoimmune adrenal insufficiency. This is in contrast with, for example, IDDM and autoimmune thyroiditis, where animals with such characteristics do exist (e.g., nonobese diabetic [NOD] mice and BioBreeding [BB] rats). Forms of idiopathic Addison's disease do, however, spontaneously develop in dogs and more rarely in cats.

A series of nine cases of adrenal insufficiency in dogs was published in 1966 by Freudiger *(127)*, who calculated that he had observed one case of Addison's disease/ 5000 dogs, a morbidity similar to that reported for hospitalized human patients. Another series of 37 cases of canine Addison's disease has also been published *(128)*, indicating once more that autoimmunity of the adrenals may naturally occur in dogs. In the few cases that have undergone autopsy, atrophy, regeneration of adrenocortical cells, and chronic inflammation of the adrenal cortex have been observed. The origin of adrenal insufficiency in dogs also seems to be of idiopathic, possibly autoimmune origin.

As for other endocrinopathies, little is known about Addison's disease in cats *(129)*. One case of primary adrenal insufficiency was described *(129)* with massive calcifications of both adrenal glands. Peterson et al. *(130)* have diagnosed naturally occurring primary hypoadrenocorticism in 10 cats in a span of 7 yr. Autopsy of four animals has shown complete destruction of both adrenal cortices, with replacement by fibrous connective tissue and/or diffuse infiltration with lymphocytes and a few macrophages.

In conclusion, dogs and cats are capable of spontaneously developing primary hypoadrenocorticism, with a clinical and histopathological picture similar to the one of human idiopathic Addison's disease. It is unfortunate that none of the affected animals has been investigated from an immunological point of view (detailed immunohistology of the lesions, circulating adrenal autoantibodies, delayed-type hypersensitivity reactions, and so forth).

Experimental Allergic Adrenalitis Models

Experimental allergic (autoimmune) adrenalitis has been produced in monkeys, rabbits, guinea pigs, rats, and mice by means of immunization with homogenates of the gland and adjuvants *(131,132)*. Although the microscopic features of lymphocytic infiltration were similar in diseased humans and animals, and although ACA were produced in these animals, the clinical picture of adrenal insufficiency in the animals is benign compared to the more severe symptoms present in humans. In spite of the presence of a chronic inflammatory process, diffuse atrophy of the adrenal cortex combined with regeneration nodules has not been reported in any of these models. Second, there are only two reports suggesting an adrenocortical insufficiency in animals with experimental adrenalitis. Andrada et al. *(133)* detected a decrease in the blood pressure of Lewis rats that had been immunized with rat adrenal extract in complete Freund's adjuvant. Irino and Grollman *(134)* reported failure to gain weight, hypoglycemia during fasting, increased rate of water and salt excretion when placed on a salt-free diet, and a reduced corticosterone content of the blood plasma in adrenal extract-immunized rats. In later studies, there have been no confirmatory tests of primary adrenocortical failure, based on ACTH stimulation, metyrapone test, and RIA of cortisol. Thus, one is left with the suspicion that experimentally induced adrenalitis may have only reproduced some aspects of the human disease, i.e., a secondary autoimmune response to some cytoplasmic (enzymatic?) antigens of adrenocortical cells. The induction of the primary lesions of idiopathic Addison's disease leading to hypocorticism is still a challenge.

Oöphoritis/Adrenalitis Models in Athymic Mice

Neonatal thymectomy in Balb/c and A/J mice at day 3 after birth results in oöphoritis, among other organ-specific autoimmune manifestations, such as thyroiditis, gastritis, and parotitis *(135–137)*. The inflammations are characterized by the presence of T-cell infiltrates in the affected organs and the development of organ-specific antibodies in the serum. There is a strict temporal relationship between the development of the autoimmune syndrome and the day of thymectomy, which has to occur between the 2nd and the 5th d after birth *(138,139)*. An explanation for the phenomenon has been proposed and is based on the premise that self-reactive CD4$^+$ T cells are generated in the thymus throughout life and exported to the periphery. In euthymic animals, autoimmune disease is not observed because these autoreactive CD4$^+$ T cells are controlled by CD4$^+$ T cells with regulatory or suppressor activity. These cells are also generated in the thymus, but only after the first week of life. Therefore, thymectomy at day 3, restricting the T cell repertoire to only effector autoimmune CD4$^+$ T cells, explains the spontaneously occurring autoimmune diseases, because the balance between self-reactive T cells and regulatory T cells tips over to the former.

That animal oöphoritis is directly the result of autoimmune T cells is shown by transfer experiments of CD4$^+$ T cells of thymectomized donors to young recipients, which causes an oöphoritis in these recipients *(139,140)*. This transfer of oöphoritis could be prevented by infusion of CD4$^+$ CD5$^+$ T cells from normal adult mice in an early stage after the transfer of the CD4$^+$ cells of the thymectomized donors.

The histopathological events of the oöphoritis in the thymectomized mice occur in an orderly manner. The oöphoritis is most severe between 4 and 14 wk after thymectomy. This is accompanied by loss of ova and collapse of ovarian follicles. Autoantibodies are detected in the circulation by week 4, with a peak between weeks 7 and 9. Autoantibodies are directed toward oocytes, and in lower titers also to steroid-producing cells (the classical St-C-Abs?), such as to the granulosa cells, the theca cells, and the luteal cells. The inflammation subsides after 14 wk, and the ovary becomes atrophic *(135,137)*. IgG-producing plasma cells are found, but not frequently. The overall picture of the oöphoritis in mice is one of a cell-mediated autoimmune reaction.

Yet another mechanism for the induction of an autoimmune oöphoritis is the transfer of T cells to athymic nude mice. The nude mouse model is characterized by a deficient T-cell function, because the most important function of the thymus, education of T cells to recognize self and nonself properly, cannot take place. When CD4$^+$ CD8$^-$ thymocytes from normal neonatal or adult Balb/c mice are transferred to athymic mice, approx 50–75% of the recipients develop an autoimmune oöphoritis and/or gastritis *(141)*. Neonatal CD4$^+$ splenocytes are also able to transfer the autoimmune diseases, whereas T cells from adult spleen do not *(142)*. However, a fraction of adult spleen CD4$^+$ with a low expression of CD5$^+$ can induce oöphoritis in athymic recipients. The disease-generating CD4$^+$ T cells are of Th1 type. Regulatory T cells that downregulate self-reactive T cells in this animal model are also present, as studied by the combined infusion of neonatal spleen cells that enhance autoimmune oöphoritis and adult spleen cells that inhibit this process *(141)*. The exact nature of these regulatory cells in this animal model is not yet elucidated; however, it is hypothesized that these belong to the Th2 subset of the CD4$^+$ T cells.

The ovarian histopathologies of day 3 thymectomized animals and nude mice that develop an oöphoritis after an adoptive transfer experiment are indistinguishable from each other and compatible with the histological picture of Addison-related oöphoritis; therefore, both might be good models for human oöphoritis in the presence of adrenal autoimmunity/Addison's disease. It is remarkable, however, that the adrenal glands are unaffected in the neonatally thymectomized mice as well as in the T-cell-transferred nude mice, even in the presence of the mouse St-C-Abs. However, modifications of the model, viz immunomodulations using Cyclosprin A after birth, do affect the adrenals *(143)*. Unfortunately, this latter model has hardly been studied in detail yet, though such a model might give important clues to elucidate the mechanisms of the pathogenesis of autoimmune Addison's disease.

THE ETIOLOGY AND PATHOGENESIS OF ADDISON'S DISEASE

The lack of spontaneous animal models of Addison's disease has severely hampered studies on the pathogenesis of the disease. Patients are not numerous and affected tissues difficult to obtain. Patient lymphoid cells and patient sera can only be obtained in the later stages of the disease, and hardly in the subclinical prodromal stages.

In contrast, the pathogenesis of autoimmune thyroiditis and autoimmune insulitis (IDDM) has been studied in detail in the animal models of the spontaneous forms of these autoimmune endocrinopathies, and a synopsis of the outcomes of these studies is given here, assuming that similar etiologic and pathogenetic mechanisms apply for autoimmune adrenal cortical failure. The animal models referred to are the obsese strain of chicken (OS chicken) *(144)*, the BB rat *(145)*, and certain strains of the NOD mouse *(146)*. A word of caution is necessary when trying to extrapolate data obtained in the animal models to the human situation: the animal models clearly show exaggerated and extreme forms of thyroiditis and insulitis, which already differ between the models themselves (let alone from patients), indicating a heterogeneity of the disease process. Therefore, general conclusions drawn on the basis of studies in one animal model should always be verified in other animal models and certainly in human patients.

The animal models of insulitis and thyroiditis indicate that the pathogenesis of the autoimmune failure of an endocrine gland is a multistep process, requiring several genetic and environmental abnormalities to come together before full-blown autoimmune thyroiditis and/or insulitis develops. Therefore, endocrine autoimmune diseases are the outcome of an unfortunate combination of various genetic traits and environmental circumstances that *per se* do not have to be harmful, but can even be advantageous. The following phases in the disease process can be discerned (Fig. 2):

1. An initial phase of an early accumulation of antigen-presenting cells (APC) and accessory cells, particularly of dendritic cells (DCs) and subclasses of macrophages in the endocrine tissue.
2. A later phase of an apparently uncontrolled production of autoreactive $CD4^+$ and $CD8^+$ T cells and of autoantibodies of the IgG class, initially in the draining lymph nodes, but later also in the diseased gland itself.
3. A last phase where the target endocrine tissue becomes susceptible for the autoimmune influence of the generated and locally produced autoreactive T cells and autoantibodies; this may finally result in the destruction of the glandular tissue or its functional and trophic blockade.

The Abnormalities Characteristic of the Afferent Arm of the Autoimmune Response, i.e., Those Related to the Enhanced Early Accumulation of Dendritic Cells and Macrophages in Endocrine Tissue

Blood monocytes are able to mature into various subsets of macrophages as well as into various subsets of DCs *(147)*. DCs are the APC par excellence and the only cells capable of stimulating naive T cells to expand clonally. Macrophages have various functions, ranging from the phagocytosis and degradation of unwanted material, via the regulation of immune responses to factor production for wound healing and remodeling of bone *(148)*. In the thyroids of patients with Graves' disease or Hashimoto's goiter, and in the thyroids and islets of the above-described animal models, increased numbers of MHC class II-positive DCs and specific subsets of macrophages have been described *(146, 149–152)*. In the animal models, an increase in the number of these cells in the future target glands and a local clustering of these cells with T cells are the first signs of a developing autoimmune reaction *(146,153)*. The APC accumulated in the glandular tissues subsequently enter the lymphatics and transport local self-antigens to the draining lymph nodes *(154)*. Indeed the enhanced accumulation of APC in the preautoimmune target glands precedes the clonal expansion of T cells and B cells in the draining lymph nodes *(146,155)*, the production of autoantibodies by these lymph nodes *(146)*, and further signs and symptoms of the later autoimmune disease.

What attracts these DCs and macrophages to the endocrine tissues? Necrosis of thyrocytes owing to viral or bacterial infection *(156,157)* with the concomitant release of self-antigens, or an enhanced release of self-antigens owing to necrosis by toxins and drugs *(146,158,159)* has been described, and such cellular decay causes an attraction of APC to the endocrine tissue. This already indicates the heterogeneity in causal factors at the level of the induction of an endocrine autoimmune disease.

It is also relevant to note that DC and macrophages are normally present in endocrine tissues *(160)* and capable of regulating the growth and function (both in a positive and negative way) of neighboring endocrine cells *(160)*. DCs are normally present in the anterior pituitary and are part of a subgroup of nonendocrine pituitary cells earlier described as "folliculo-stellate cells" *(161)*. It is known that these folliculo-stellate cells regulate the LH release from gonadotrophs and the prolactin release from lactotrophs by virtue of their cytokine production, their production of other signaling molecules (S100,

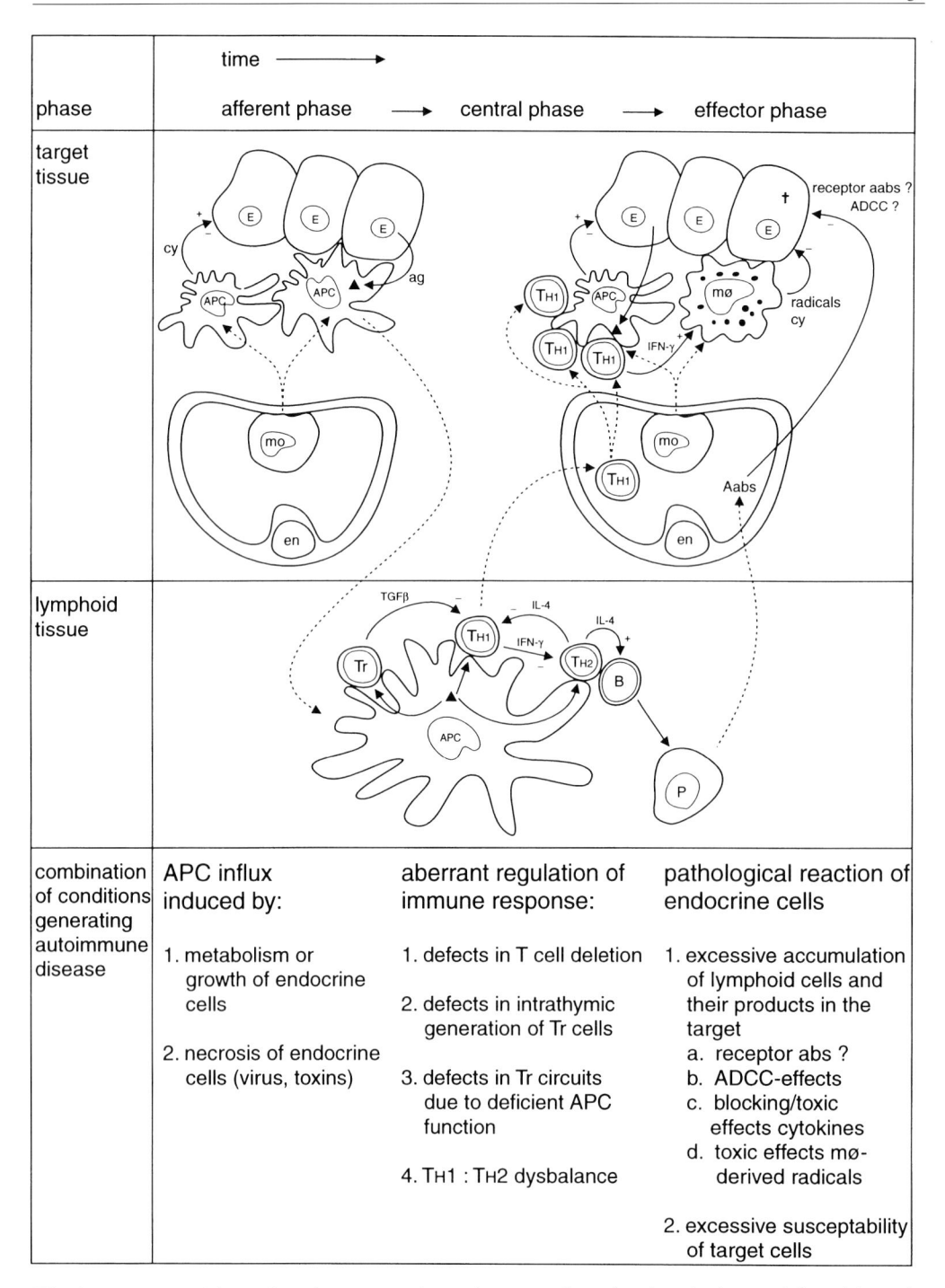

Fig. 2. A cartoon of the various immunopathogenic events that take place in time and that ultimately lead to the glandular failure. *See text* for further explanations. mo, monocyte; en, endothelial cell; APC, antigen-presenting cell; ag, ▲, autoantigen; cy, cytokines; E, endocrine cell; mφ, macrophage; ADCC, antibody-dependent cell-mediated cytotoxicity; P, plasma cell; Th1, T helper 1 cell; Th2, T helper 2 cell; Tr, T-regulator cell; B, B cell; aabs, autoantibodies. +, stimulation; –, suppression; ...., traffic.

platelet-derived growth factor [PDGF], etc.), and by direct cell-to-cell interactions *(161,162)*. Also in the thyroid, DCs and macrophages are normally present in low numbers, and DCs isolated from the spleens of rats are capable of downregulating in vitro the DNA synthesis and thyroxine production from rat thyroid follicles kept in suspension culture *(163)*.

The recognition of a "floating endocrine-regulatory force" of monocyte-derived cells that both play a role in homeostatic processes in normal endocrine glands, but that is also active in the initiation and regulation of immune responses, has implications for the understanding of the induction phase of the endocrine autoimmune reaction: it opens the idea that alterations in the growth and function of an endocrine tissue may necessitate the influx of DCs and macrophages, or in other words, endocrine abnormalities may precede the very early phases of the endocrine autoimmune reaction. Indeed very early abnormalities in the proliferative capability and hormone production of thyrocytes and islet cells have been described in the OS chicken (even in the fetal phase) *(164)*, BB rat *(165)*, and NOD *(166)* mouse. These preautoimmune target cell abnormalities were correctable by a very early prophylactic isohormonal treatment, e.g., an insulin treatment in the case of NOD mouse insulitis *(166)*. It has also become clear that such early corrections of preautoimmune target cell abnormalities lead to a lower influx and activity of DCs and macrophages in the preautoimmune endocrine tissues followed by an attenuation or even blockade of the following autoimmune reaction *(166)*.

Abnormalities Characteristic of the Central Arm of the Autoimmune Response, i.e., the Abnormal Immunoregulation

The initial phase of the glandular accumulation of DCs and accessory types of macrophages is followed by a phase of an apparently uncontrolled clonal expansion of autoreactive effector T and B cells in the draining lymph nodes *(146,155)*. In both the BB rat and the NOD mouse, there are strong indications for various genetically determined immunodysregulations, which lead to an intolerance to self-antigens when they are presented in the lymph node by the incoming APC. These immunodysregulations are partly associated with the presence of particular MHC class I and class II haplotypes, but other genes are also involved (*see* Immunogenetic Aspects). The exact mechanisms for the failure of maintaining tolerance are far from clear. Apparently the genetic makeup characteristic of autoimmune-prone individuals leads to various abnormalities in the function of immune cells involved in tolerance induction and the induction of immunity, such as the DCs, the macrophages, and/or the T cells. Indeed, APC of NOD mice *(167)* and BB rats *(168)* have defects in their capability to stimulate T cells, and in particular T-regulator cells. With regard to such abnormal maturation of immunoregulatory T cells, the BB rat is special in that it lacks a particular regulator population of T cells, the so-called RT6+ cells *(169)*. It is particularly this population that can hardly be stimulated by the DCs of the BB rat *(168)*. The OS strain of chickens also has inborn defects in its T-regulatory cell system *(144)*, as has the neonatally thymectomized BALB/c mouse (*see* Oöphoritis/Adrenalitis Models in Athymic Mice). Whether there are similar (inborn) defects in immunoregulatory cells in the human that lead to an endocrine autoimmune disease needs to be established. There are, however, numerous reports on both numerical and functional deficits in T cells with a suppressive function (*see* above). Also, DC and macrophage defects have been described in patients with autoimmune thyroid disease *(170)* and IDDM *(171)*.

Deficits in immunoregulatory cells do not only exist on an inheritable, genetic basis. They can also be acquired by viral infection. When encephalomyocarditis (EMC) or Kilham rat virus (KRV) viruses infect mice (DBA-2 or SJL mice) or rats (diabetic resistant BB rats), macrophages are affected, leading in the latter model to diabetes *(172)*. Whether similar viruses or retroviruses with an affinity for immune cells are operative in human endocrine autoimmune diseases has been speculated on, but has not yet been proven *(173–178)*.

Abnormalities Characteristic of the Efferent Arm of the Autoimmune Response, i.e., an Enhanced Susceptibility of the Endocrine Cells for the Generated Autoimmune Attack

After the stage of the excessive generation of autoreactive T cells and IgG autoantibodies, yet another factor or factors, at least in the OS chicken, determine whether or not a full-blown autoimmune disease will develop *(144)*. A prerequisite for clinical thyroid failure in this bird is a susceptibility of the target, the thyrocyte, for an autoimmune attack by the generated autoreactive T cells and IgG autoantibodies. Experiments have shown that this susceptibility factor is genetically determined, and it has been speculated that this factor might be an abnormal susceptibility of the thyrocytes for the cytokines produced by the autoreactive immune cells after infiltration. Whether such susceptibility factors are also important in the other animal models and in human disease needs further investigation.

CONCLUSIONS

Considerable progress has been made in the understanding of the pathogenesis of endocrine autoimmune diseases, including Addison's disease. Although the Th1-mediated destruction concept is very fashionable at present, it is likely—taking into account also literature from the 1970s and 1980s—that both humoral and cellular autoimmune mechanisms are involved at the effector level. ACA are found in the majority of idiopathic Addison's cases, and they are good markers of ongoing or imminent Addison's disease. Antibodies to the enzyme 21-OH have appeared to be the major component of ACA, whereas 17-α-OH and p450scc are the major antigens for St-C-Abs that are found in a subgroup of Addisonian patients with an additional risk for autoimmune gonadal dysfunction. The identification of these enzymes as autoantigens now allows the introduction of clinically applicable detection assays for ACA and St-C-Abs. Adrenal antigen-specific T cells do also exist in Addisonian patients, and together with macrophages, they are able to influence adrenal cell growth and function, up to even a destruction of the adrenal cells. Whether "receptor antibodies" contribute to the adrenal failure of Addison's disease still needs to be established.

At the afferent level (induction of the autoimmune reaction) and at the level of the actual immunodysregulations leading to the excessive production of autoantibodies and effector T cells, many questions still remain. A few years ago, there existed mostly a "monistic" approach to these problems, i.e., a desire to find a single cause for a complex process. At present, it is fully recognized that endocrine autoimmune diseases are multigenetic diseases influenced by many environmental factors, and thus the outcome of unfortunate combinations of both inborn and external factors. Of the genes involved, the most important are the MHC-linked genes, but these only confer a limited increase in the risk for disease, since other immunoregulatory genes are also involved, e.g., the CTLA-4 gene. It also becomes increasingly clear that DCs and various other subtypes of macrophages act as APC in the very early preautoimmune phases of the endocrine autoimmune diseases, and that disturbances in the function of these cells may be one of the causal factors in the initiation of the disease. Since DCs and macrophages are not only immune cells, but also cells that are able to regulate the growth and function of neighboring endocrine cells, it becomes more and more plausible that preautoimmune metabolic and growth abnormalities of the target gland underlie the attraction of the first APC to the gland, later followed by the cascade of T- and B-cell stimulation leading to the final autoimmune disease.

NOTE ADDED IN PROOF

To support the concept that immune cells and their products, e.g., cytokines are instrumental in the disturbances of growth and function of the adrenal gland, a recent brief report *(179)* has appeared in which it was shown that, in a case of Cushing's syndrome owing to an adrenocortical adenoma, there was:

1. A conspicuous accumulation of lymphoid cells in and around the adenoma;
2. An in vitro responsiveness of the adenoma cells to secrete cortisol when stimulated by IL-1 (but not by ACTH); and
3. The presence of type 1 IL-1 receptor protein in the adenoma cells.

ACKNOWLEDGMENTS

The author wants to thank T. M. van Os for the preparation of the figures, and Petra Assems for her excellent typographical help in preparing the manuscript. Work on dendritic cells and macrophages in endocrine autoimmunity is supported by NWO-Medical Sciences (903-40-167; 903-43-089) and the Dutch Diabetic Fund.

REFERENCES

1. Addison T. Anaemia: disease of the supra-renal capsules. Lond Med Gazette 1849;43:517.
2. Addison T. On the constitutional and local effects of disease of the suprarenal capsules. In: A Collection of the Published Writings of the Late Thomas Addison, MD, Physician to Guy's Hospital, London New Sydenham Society, London, 1868. Reprinted in Med Classics 1937;2:244–293.
3. Mulligan TM, Sowers JR. Hyperpigmentation, vitiligo and Addison's disease. Cutis 1985;36:317–318.
4. Tuck ML, Stern N. Adrenal diseases. In: Hershman JM, ed. Endocrine Pathophysiology. Lea & Febiger, Philadelphia, 1988, pp. 77–125.
5. Kannan CR. The adrenal gland. Plenum Medical, New York, 1988, pp. 504.
6. Gilliland PF. Endocrine emergencies. Adrenal crisis, myxedema coma, and thyroid storm. Postgrad Med 1983;74:215–220.
7. Stuart-Mason A, Meade TW, Lee JAH, Morris JN. Epidemiological and clinical picture of Addison's disease. Lancet 1968;2:744–747.
8. Kong MF, Jeffcoate W. Eighty-six cases of Addison's disease. Clin Endocrinol 1988;41:757–761.
9. Zelissen PM, Bast EJ, Croughs RJ. Associated autoimmunity in Addison's disease. J Autoimmunity 1995;8:121–130.
10. Nerup J. Addison's disease. Thesis, Olaf Mollers, Copenhagen, 1974.
11. Mooij P, Drexhage HA. Autoimmune thyroid disease. Clin Lab Med 1993;13:683–697.
12. Sommers SC. Adrenal glands. In: Kissane JM, ed. Anderson's Pathology. C.V. Mosby, St. Louis, MO, 1985, pp. 1429–1450.
13. Bigazzi PE. Autoimmunity of the adrenals. In: Volpe R, ed. Autoimmunity and Endocrine Disease. Marcel Dekker, New York, 1985, pp. 345–374.

14. Kiefer H. Addisonsche erkrankung infolge chronischer nebennierendystrophie mit adenomartigen regeneraten. Virchows Arch Pathol Anat 1927;265:472–480.
15. Saphir O, Binswanger HF. Suprarenal cortical insufficiency and cytotoxic contraction of the suprarenals. JAMA 1930;95:1007–1011.
16. Guttman PH. Addison's disease. A statistical analysis of five hundred and sixty-six cases and a study of the pathology. Arch Pathol 1930;10:742.
17. Ruppell V, Noltenius H. Sogenannte zytotoxische Schrumpfnebennieren. Med Welt 1969;24: 1397–1402.
18. Sloper JC, Fox B. The adrenal glands. In: Symmers, WSC, ed. Systemic Pathol, 2nd ed., Churchill Livingstone, New York, 1978, pp. 1913–1974.
19. Neville AM, O'Hare MJ. The Human Adrenal Cortex, Springer Verlag, New York, 1982, pp. 252.
20. Teding van Berkhout F, Croughs RJM, Kater L, Schuurman HJ, Gmelig Meyling FJH, et al. Familial Cushing's syndrome due to nodular adrenocortical dysplasia. A putative receptor-antibody disease? Clin Endocrinol 1986;24:299–310.
21. Young WF, Carney JA, Musa BV, Wulffraat NM, Lens JW, Drexhage HA. 1989; Familial Cushing's syndrome due to primary pigmented nodular adrenocortical disease. Reinvestigation 50 years later. N Engl J Med 321:1659–1664.
22. Bohm N, Lippman-Grob B, von Petrykowski W. Familial Cushing's syndrome due to pigmented multinodular adrenocortical dysplasia. Acta Endocrinol (Copenh) 1983;102:428–435.
23. Petri M, Nerup J. Addison's adrenalitis. Studies on diffuse lymphocytic adrenalitis (idiopathic Addison's disease) and focal lymphocytic infiltration in a control material. Acta Pathol Microbiol Scand 1971;79:381–388.
24. Hayashi Y, Hiyoshi T, Takemura T, Kurashima C, Hirokawa K. Focal lymphocytic infiltration in the adrenal cortex in the elderly: Immunohistological analysis of infiltrating lymphocytes. Clin Exp Immunol 1989;77:101–105.
25. Wulffraat NM. Adrenal autoimmunity. Thesis, Free University Press, Amsterdam, 1987.
26. Kooistra HS, Rijnberk A, van den Ingh TS. Polyglandular deficiency syndrome in a boxer dog: thyroid hormone and glucocorticoid deficiency. Vet Q 1995;17:59–63.
27. McNichol AM. Histopathology of the adrenal gland in Addison's disease. In: Bhatt HR, James VHT, Besser GM, Bottazzo GF, Keen H, eds. Advances in Thomas Addison's diseases, vol. 2. Journal of Endocrinology Ltd, Bristol, 1994, pp. 5–12.
28. Weetman AP. The potential immunological role of the thyroid cell in autoimmune thyroid disease. Thyroid 1994;4:493–399.
29. Hill JA, Welch WR, Faris HMP, Anderson DJ. Induction of class II major histocompatibility complex antigen expression in human granulosa cells by interferon gamma: a potential mechanism contributing to autoimmune ovarian failure. Am. J Obstet Gynecol 1990;162:534–540.
30. Jackson R, McNicol AM, Farquharson M, Foulis AK. Class II MHC expression in normal adrenal cortex and cortical cells in autoimmune Addison's disease. J Pathol 1988;155:113–120.
31. Eisenbarth GS. Autoimmune endocrine disorders. In: DeGroot LS, ed. Endocrinology. W.B. Saunders, Philadelphia, 1989, pp. 2632–2648.
32. Schmidt MB. Eine biglandulate Erkrankung (Nebennieren und Schildruse) bei Morbus Addisonii Verh Dtsch Ges Pathol 1926;21:212.
33. Carpenter CC, Solomon N, Silverberg S. Schmidt's syndrome (thyroid and adrenal insufficiency). A review of the literature and a report of 15 new cases including 10 instances of co-existent diabetes mellitus, Medicine (Baltimore) 1964;43:153–180.
34. MacLaren NK, Blizzard RM. Adrenal autoimmunity and autoimmune polyglandular syndrome. In: Rose NL, MacKay I eds. The Autoimmune Diseases. Academic, New York, 1985, pp. 202–225.
35. Ahonen P, Mylarniemi S, Sipila I, Perheentupa J. Clinical variations of autoimmune polyendocrinopathy-candidiasis-ectodermal dystrophy (APECED) in a series of 68 patients. N Engl J Med 1990; 322:1829–1836.
36. Green A, Gale EA, Patterson CC. Incidence of childhood-onset insulin-dependent diabets mellitus: EURODIAB ACE Study. Lancet 1992;339:905–909.
37. MacLaren NK, Riley WJ. Autoimmune endocrinopathies. In: Samter M, Talmage DW, Frank MM, et al., eds. Immunological Diseases. Little, Brown, Boston 1988, pp. 1737–1746.
38. Napolitano G, Mirakian R, Bottazzo GF. Thyroid and its diseases framed in the autoimmune polyendocrine syndrome. In: Monaco F, Satta MA, Shapiro B, Troncone L, eds. Thyroid Diseases: Clinical Fundamentals and Therapy. CRC, Boca Raton, FL, 1993, pp. 565–572.

39. Anderson JR, Goudie RB, Gray KG, Timbury GC. Auto-antibodies in Addison's disease. Lancet 1957;1:1123–1124.
40. Blizzard RM, Chandler RW, Kyle MA, Hung W. Adrenal antibodies in Addison's disease. Lancet 1962;2:901–903.
41. Betterle C, Pedini B, Presotto F. Serological markers in Addison's disease. In: Bhatt R, James VHT, Besser GM, Bottazzo GF, Keen H, eds. Advances in Thomas Addison's Diseases. Journal of Endocrinology Ltd, Bristol, 1994, pp. 67–84.
42. Brown FM, Kamalesh M, Adri S, Rabinowe SL. Anti-adrenal medullary antibodies in IDDM subjects and subjects at high risk of developing IDDM. Diabetes Care 1988;11:30–33.
43. Zanone MM Peakman M, Purewal T, et al. Autoantibodies to nervous tissue structures and associated with autonomic neuropathy in type 1 (insulin-dependent) diabetes mellitus. Diabetologia 1993;36:564–569.
44. Scherbaum WA Mogel H, Boehm BO, Hedderich U, Gluck M, Schernthauer G, Bottazzo GF, Pfeiffer. Autoantibodies to adrenal medullary and thyroid calcitonin cells in type 1 diabetes mellitus. A prospective study. J Autoimmunity 1988;1:219–230.
45. Betterle C, Scalici C, Presotto F, et al. The natural history of adrenal function in autoimmune patients with adrenal autoantibodies. J Endocrinol 1988;117:467–475.
46. Betterle C, Zanette F, Zanchetta R, Pedini B, Trevisan A, Mantero F, Rigon F. Complement-fixing adrenal autoantibodies as a marker for predicting onset of idiopathic Addison's disease. Lancet 1983;1:1238–1241.
47. Betterle C, Volpato M. Adrenal and ovarian autoimmunity. Eur J Endocrinol 1998;138:16–25.
48. De Bellis A, Bizzarro A, Rossi R, Amoresano Paglionico V, Criscuolo T, Lombardi G, et al. Remission of subclinical adrenocortical failure in subjects with adrenal autoantibodies. J Clin Endocrinol Metab 1993;76:1002–1007.
49. Anderson JR, Goudie RB, Gray K, Stuarth Smith DA. Immunological features of idiopathic Addison's disease: an antibody to cells producing steroid hormones. Clin Exp Immunol 1968;3:107–117.
50. Sotsiou F, Bottazzo GF, Doniach D. Immunofluorescence studies on autoantibodies to steroid-producing cells, and to germline cells in endocrine diesae and infertility. Clin Exp Immunol 1980;39:97–111.
51. Finer N, Fogelman I, Bottazzo GF. Pregnancy in a woman with premature ovarian failure. Postgrad Med J 1985;61:1079–1080.
52. Betterle C, Rossi A, Dalla Pria S, Artifoni A, Pedini B, Gauasso S, Caretto A. Premature ovarian failure: autoimmunity and natural history. Clin Endocrinol 1993;39:35–43.
53. Smith BR, Furmaniak J. Adrenal and gonadal autoimmune diseases [Editorial]. J Clin Endocrinol Metab 1995;80:1502–1505.
54. Winqvist O, Karlsson FA, Kämpe O. 21-hydroxylase, a major autoantigen in idiopathic Addison's disease. Lancet 1992;339:1159–1562.
55. Baumann-Antczak A, Wedlock N, Bednarek J., Kiso Y, Krishnan H, Fowler S, et al. Autoimmune Addison's disease and 21-hydroxylase [Letter]. Lancet 1992;340:429–430.
56. Krohn K, Uibo R, Aavik E, Peterson P, Savilahti K. Identification by molecular cloning of an autoantigen associated with Addison's disease as steroid 17-α-hydroxylase. Lancet 1992;339:770–773.
57. Winqvist O, Gustafsson J., Rorsman F, Karlsson FA, Kämpe O. Two different cytochrome p450 enzymes are the adrenal antigens in autoimmune polyendocrine syndrome type 1 and Addison's disease. J Clin Invest 1993;92:2377–2385.
58. Uibo R, Perheentupa J., Ovod V, Krohn KJE. Characterization of adrenal autoantigens recognized by sera from patients with autoimmune polyglandular syndrome (APG) type 1. J Autoimmunity 1994;7:399–411.
59. Vello LA, Winqvist O, Gustafsson J, Kämpe O, Karlsson FA. Autoantibodies against a novel 51 kDa islet antigen and glutamate decarboxylase isoforms in autoimmune polyendocrine syndrome type 1. Diabetologia 1994;37:61–69.
60. Chen S, Sawicka S, Betterle C, Powell M, Prentice L, Volpato M, et al. Autoantibodies to steroidogenic enzymes in autoimmune polyglandular syndrome. Addison's disease and premature ovarian failure. J Clin Endocrinol Metab 1996;81:1871–1876.
61. Peterson P, Uibo R, Peränen J, Krohn K. Immunoprecipitation of steroidogenic enzyme autoantigens with autoimmune polyglandular syndrome type I (APS I) sera; further evidence for humoral imunity to p450 c17 and p450 21. Clin Exp Immunol 1997;107:335–340.
62. Song Y-H, Connor E, Muir A, She JX, Zorovich B, Derovanesian D, et al. Autoantibody epitope mapping of the 21-hydroxylase antigen in autoimmune Addison's disease. J Clin Endocrinol Metab 1994;78:1108–1112.

63. Arif S, Vallian S, Farzaneh F, Zanone MM, James SL, Pietropaolo M, et al. Identification of 3β-hydroxysteroid dehydrogenase as a novel target of steroid cell autoantibodies: association of autoantibodies with endocrine autoimmune disease. J Clin Endocrinol Metab 1996;81:4439–4445.
64. Husebye ES, Gebre-Medhin G, Tuomi T, Perheentupa J, Landin-Olsson M, Gustafsson J, et al. Autoantibodies against aromatic L-amino acid decarboxylase in autoimmune polyendocrine syndrome type I. J Clin Endocrinol Metab 1997;82:147–150.
65. Colls J, Betterle C, Volpato M, Rees Smith B, Furmaniak J. A new immunoprecipitation assay for autoantibodies to steroid 21-hydroxylase in Addison's disease. Clin Chem 1995;41:375–380.
66. Falorni A, Nikoshkov A, Laureti S, Grenbäck E, Hulting AL, Casucci G, et al. High diagnostic accuracy for idiopathic Addison's disease with a sensitive radiobinding assay for autoantibodies against recombinant human 21-hydroxylase. J Clin Endocrinol Metab 1995;80:2752–2755.
67. Tanaka H, Perez M, Powell M, Sauders JF, Sawicka J, Chen S, Prentice L, Asawa T, Betterle C, Volpato M, Smith BR, Furmaniak J. Steroid 21-hydroxylase autoantibodies: measurements with a new precipitation assay. J Clin Endocrinol Metab 1997;82:1440–1446.
68. Winqvist O, Söderbergh A, Kämpe O. The autoimmune basis of adrenocortical destruction in Addison's disease. Mol Med Today 1996;2:282–289.
69. Falorni A, Laureti S, Nikoshkov A, Picchio ML, Hallengren B, Vandewalle CL, et al. 21-hydroxylase autoantibodies in adult patients with endocrine autoimmune diseases are highly specific for Addison's disease. Clin Exp Immunol 1997;107:341–346.
70. Furmaniak J, Kominami S, Asawa T, Wedlock N, Colls J, Rees Smith B. Autoimmune Addison's disease: evidence for a role of steroid 21-hydroxylase autoantibodies in adrenal insufficiency. J Clin Endocrinol Metab 1994;79:1517–1521.
71. McNatty KP, Short RV, Barnes EW, Irvine WJ. The cytotoxic effect of serum from patients with Addison's disease and autoimmune ovarian failure on human granulosa cells in culture. Clin Exp Immunol 1975;22:378–384.
72. Wheatcroft NJ, Toogood A, Li TC. Detection of antibodies to ovarian antigens in women with premature ovarian failure. Clin Exp Immunol 1994;26:122–128.
73. Prabhakar BS, Fan J-L, Seetharamaiah GS. Thyrotropin-receptor-mediated diseases: a paradigm for receptor autoimmunity. Immunol Today 1997;18:437–442.
74. Graus YM, De Baets MH. Myasthenia gravis: an autoimmune response against the acetylcholine receptor. Immunol Res 1993;12:78–100.
75. Drexhage HA, Bottazzo GF, Bitensky L, et al. Evidence for thyroidgrowth stimulating immunoglobulins in some goitrous thyroid diseases. The Lancet 1981;1:287–291.
76. Steel NR, Weightman DR, Taylor J, Kendall-Taylar P. Blocking activity to action of thyroid stimulating hormone in serum from patients with primary hypothyroidism. Br Med J 1984;288:1559–1562.
77. Flier JS, Kah CR, Roth J. Receptors, antireceptor antibodies and mechanism of insulin resistance. N Engl J Med 1979;300:413–419.
78. Kendall-Taylor P, Lambert A, Mitchell R, Robertson WR. Antibody that blocks stimulation of cortisol secretion by adrenocorticotrophic hormone in Addison's disease. Br Med J 1988;296:1489–1492.
79. Wulffraat NM, Drexhage HA, Bottazzo GF, Wiersinga WM, Jeucken P, van der Gaag RD. Immunoglobulins of patients with idiopathic Addison's disease block the in vitro action of ACTH. J Clin Endocrinol Metab 1989;69:231–238.
80. Chayen J, Loveridge N, Daly JR. A sensitive bioassay for adrenocorticotrophic hormone in human plasma. Clin Endocrinol 1972;1:219–233.
81. Drexhage HA. Autoimmunity and thyroid growth. Where do we stand? Eur J Endocrinol 1996;135:39–45.
82. Wardle CA, Weetman AP, Mitchell R, et al. Adrenocorticotropic hormone receptor-blocking immunoglobulins in serum from patients with Addison's disease: a reexamination. J Clin Endocrinol Metab 1993;77:750–753.
83. Nerup J, Bendixen G. Anti-adrenal hypersensitivity in Addison's disease. 2. Correlation with clinical and serological findings. Clin Exp Immunol 1969;5:341–353.
84. Volpé, R. ed. Autoimmunity in the Endocrine System. Springer-Verlag, Berlin, 1981, pp. 149–175.
85. Nerup J, Anderson V, Bendixen G. Anti-adrenal cellular hypersensitivity in Addison's disease. IV. n vivo and in vitro investigations on the mitochondrial fraction. Clin Exp Immunol 1970;6:733–739.
86. Freeman M, Weetman AP. T and B cell reactivity to adrenal antigens in autoimmune Addison's disease. Clin Exp Immunol 1992;88:275–279.

87. Mosmann TR, Cerwinski H, Bond MW, Giedlin MA, Coffman RL. Two types of murine helper T cell clone. I. Definition according to profiles of lymphokine activities and secreted proteins. J Immunol 1986;136:2348–2357.
88. Mosmann TR, Coffman RL. Th1 and Th2 cells: Different patterns of lymphokine secretion lead to different functional properties. Ann Rev Immunol 1989;7:145–173.
89. Romagnani S. Human Th1 and Th2 subsets: regulation of differentiation and role in protection and immunopathology. Int Arch Allergy Immunol 1989;98:279–285.
90. Scott P. IL–12: initiation cytokine for cell-mediated immunity. Science 1993;260:496–497.
91. Moore KV, O'Garra A, de Waal Malefyt R, Vieira P, Mosmann TR. Interleukin 10. Ann Rev Immunol 1993;11:165–190.
92. d'Andrea A, Aste-Amezaga M, Valiante NM, Ma X, Kubin M, Trinchieri G. Interleukin 10 (IL–10) inhibits human lymphocyte interferongamma-production by suppressing natural killer cell stimulatory factor/IL-12 synthesis in accessory cells. J Exp Med 1993;178:1041–1048.
93. Powrie F, Menon S, Coffman RL. Interleukin-4 and interleukin-10 synergize to inhibit cell-mediated immunity *in vivo*. Eur J Immunol 1993;23:2223–2229 (published erratum appears in Eur J Immunol 1994;24:785).
94. Betz M, Fox BS. Prostaglandin E2 inhibits production of Th1 lymphokines but not of Th2 lymphokines. J Immunol 1991;146:108–113.
95. Day MJ, Tse AG, Puklavec M, Simmonds SJ, Mason DW. Targeting autoantigen to B cells prevents the induction of a cell mediated autoimmune disease in rats. J Exp Med 1992;175:655–659.
96. Liblau R, Singer S, McDevitt H. Th1 and Th2 CD4+ T cells in the pathogenesis of organ-specific autoimmune diseases. Immunol Today 1995;16:34–38.
97. Powrie F, Coffman RL. Cytokines regulation of T cell function: potential for therapeutic intervention. Immunol Today 1993;14:270–274.
98. O'Garra A, Murphy K. T cell subsets in autoimmunity. Curr Opinion Immunol 1993;5:880–886.
99. O'Garra A, Steinman L, Gijbels K. CD4+ T cell subsets in autoimmunity. Curr Opinion Immunol 1997; 9:872–883.
100. Groux H, O'Garra A, Bigler M, Rouleau M, Antonenko S, de Vries J, Roncarolo MG. A CD4+ T cell subset inhibits antigen-specific T cell responses and prevents colitis. Nature 1997;389:737–742.
101. Chen Y, Kuchroo VK, Inobe J-I, Hafler DA, Weiner HL.; Regulatory T cell clones induced by oral tolerance: suppression of autoimmune encephalytis. Science 1994265:1237–1240.
102. Fairchild RS, Schimke RN, Abdou NI. Immunoregulation abnormalities in familial Addison's disease. J. Clin Endocrinol Metab. 1980;51:104–1077.
103. Verghese MW, Ward FE, Eisenbarth GS. Decreased suppressor cell activity in patients with polyglandular failure. Clin Res 1980;28:270A.
104. Volpé, R. The immunoregulatory disturbance in autoimmune thyroid disease. Autoimmunity 1988;2:55–72.
105. Tomer Y, Shoenfeld Y. The significance of T suppressor cells in the development of autoimmunity. Autoimmunity 1989;2:739–758.
106. Ludwig H, Schernthaner G. Multi organ spezifizienz autoimmunität bei idiopathishcher nebennierenrinde insuffizienz. Wien Klin Wochenschr 1978;90:736–741.
107. Rabinowe SL, Jackson RA, Dluhy RG, Williams GH. Ia-positive T lymphocytes in recently diagnosed idiopathic Addison's disease. Am J Med 1984;77:597–601.
108. Jackson RA, Haynes BF, Burch WM, Shimizu K, Bowring MA, Eisenbarth GS. Ia+ T cells in new onset Graves' disease. J Clin Endocrinol Metab 1984;59:187–190.
109. Jackson RA, Morris MA, Haynes B, Eisenbarth GS. Increased circulating Ia-antigen bearing T cells in type I diabetes mellitus. N Engl J Med 1982;306:785–788.
110. Mathison J, Schreiber RD, La Forest AC, Ulevitch RJ. Suppression of ACTH-induced steroidogenesis by supernatants from LPS-treated peritoneal exudate macrophages. J Immunol 1983;130:2757–2762.
111. Kennedy RL, Jones TH. Cytokines in endocrinology: their roles in health and in disease. J Endocrinol 1991;129:167–178.
112. Winter JSD, Gow KW, Perry YS, Greenberg AH. A stimulatory effect of interleukin-1 on adrenocortical cortisol selection mediated by prostaglandins. Endocrinology 1990;127:1904–1909.
113. Woloski BMRNJ, Smith EM, Meyer WJ, Fuller GM, Blalock JE. Corticotrophin-releasing activity of monokines. Science 1985;230:1035–1037.
114. Milgrom F, Bigazzi PE. Adrenals. In: Miescher PA, Muller-Eberhard HJ, eds. Textbook of Immunopathology, 2nd ed. Grune & Stratton, New York, 1976, pp. 831–839.

115. Thomsen M, Platz P, Anderson OO, Christy M, Nerup J, Rassmusseu K, Ryder LP, Nielsen LS, Svejgaard A. MLC typing in juvenile diabetes mellitus and idiopathic Addison's disease. Transplant Rev 1975;22:125–147.
116. Latinne D, Vandeput Y, De Bruyere M, Bottazzo GF, Sokal G, Crabbe J. Addisons' disease:immunological aspects. Tissue Antigens 1987;30:23–24.
117. MacLaren NK, Riley WR. Inherited susceptibility to autoimmune Addison's disease is linked to human leucocyte antigens-DR3 and/or DR4, except when associated with type I autoimmune polyglandular syndrome. J Clin Endocrinol Metab 1986;62:455–459.
118. Weetman AP, Zhang L, Tandon N, Edwards OM. HLA associations with autoimmune Addison's disease. Tissue Antigens 1991;38:31–33.
119. Betterle C, Volpato M, Greggio AN, Presotto F. Type 2 polyglandular autoimmune disease. J Pediatr Endocrinol Metab 1996;9:113–123.
120. Foulis AK, Bottazzo GF. Insulitis in the human pancreas. In: Lefebvre PJ, Pipeleers DG, eds. The Pathology of the Endocrine Pancreas in Diabetes. Springer-Verlag, Berlin, 1988, pp. 41–52.
121. Ahonen P, Koskimies S, Lokki ML, Tiilikainen A, Perheentupa J. The expression of autoimmune polyglandular disease type I appears associated with several HLA-A-DR. J Clin Endocrinol Metab 1988;66:1152–1157.
122. Nagamine K, Peterson P, Scott HS, Kudoh J, Minoshima S, Heino M, et al. Positional cloning of the APECED gene. Nature Genet 1997;17 393–398.
123. The Finnish-German APECED Consortium. An autoimmune disease, APECED, caused by mutations in a novel gene featuring two PHD-type zinc-finger domains. Nature Genet 1997;17:399–403.
124. Betterle C, Greggio NA, Volpato M. Clinical review: autoimmune polyglandular syndrome type 1. J Clin Endocrinol Metab 1998;83:1049–1055.
125. Donner H, Rau H, Walfish PG, Braun J, Siegmund T, Finke R, et al. CTLA4 alanine-17 confers genetic susceptibility to Graves' disease and to type 1 diabetes mellitus. J Clin Endocrinol Metab 1997;82:143–146.
126. Donner H, Braun J, Seidl C, Rau H, Finke R, Ventz M, et al. Codon 17 polymorphism of the cytotoxic T lymphocyte antigen 4 gene in Hashimoto's thyroiditis and Addison's disease. J Clin Endocrinol Metab 1997;82:4130–4132.
127. Freudiger U. Die nebennierenrinden-insuffizienzen beim Hund. Dtsch Tieraerztl Wochenschr 1966;72:60–64.
128. Willard MD, Schall WD, McCaw DE, Nachreiner RF. Canine hypoadrenocorticism: report of 37 cases and review of 39 previously reported cases. J Am Vet Med Assoc 1982;180:59–62.
129. Freudiger U. Literuturubersicht uber nebennierenrinden-erkrankungen der Katze und Beschreibung eines Falles von primarer Nebennierenrinden-Insuffizienz. Schweiz Arch Tierheilk 1986;128:221–230.
130. Peterson ME, Greco DS, Orth DN. Primary hypoadrenocorticism in ten cats. J Vet Int Med 1989;3:55–58.
131. Barnett EV, Dumonde DC, Glynn LE. Induction of autoimmunity to adrenal gland. Immunology 1963;6:382–402.
132. Lewis M, Rose NR. Experimental models in autoimmune endocrine disease. In: Volpe R, ed. Autoimmunity and Endocrine Disease. Marcel Dekker, New York, 1985, pp. 39–92.
133. Andrada JA, Skelton FR, Andrada EC, Milgrom F, Witebsky E. Experimental autoimmune adrenalitis in rats. Lab Invest 1968;19:460–465.
134. Irino T, Grollman A Induction of adrenal insufficiency in the rat by sensitization with homologous tissue. Metabolism 1968;17:717–724.
135. Taguchi O, Nishizuka Y, Sakakura T, Kojima A. Autoimmune oophoritis in thymectomized mice: detection of circulation antibodies against oocytes. Clin Exp Immunol 1980;40:540–553.
136. Miyake T, Taguchi O, Ikeda H, Sato Y, Takeuchi S, Nishizuka Y. Acute oocyte loss in experimental autoimmune oophoritis as a possible model of premature ovarian failure. Am J Obstet Gynecol 1988;158:186–192.
137. Tung KS, Smith S, Teuscher C, Cook C, Anderson RE. Murine autoimmune oophoritis, epididymoorchitis, and gastritis induced by day 3 thymectomy. Am J Pathol 1987;126:293–302.
138. Taguchi O, Nishizuka Y. Autoimmune oophoritis in the thymectomized mice: T cell requirement in the adoptive cell transfer. Clin Exp Immunol 1980;42:324–331.
139. Sakaguchi S, Takahashi T, Nishizuka Y. Study on cellular events in postthymectomy autoimmune oophoritis in mice. 1. Requirement of Lyt-1 effector cells for oocytes damage after adoptce transfer. J Exp Med 1982;156:1565–1576.

140. Smith H, Sakamoto Y, Kasai K, Tung KSK. Effector and regulatory cells in autoimmune oophoritis elicited by neonatal thymectomy. J Immunol 1991;147:2928–2933.
141. Smith H, Lou YH, Lacy P, Tung KS. Tolerance mechanism in experimental ovarian and gastric autoimmune diseases. J Immunol 1992;149:2212–2218.
142. Smith H, Chen IM, Kubo R, Tung KS. Neonatal thymectomy results in a repertoire enriched in T cells deleted in adult thymus. Science 1989;245:749–752.
143. Sakaguchi S, Sakaguchi N. Organ-specific autoimmune disease induced in mice by elimination of T cell subsets. V. Neonatal administration of cyclosporin A causes autoimmune disease. J Immunol 1989;142:471–480.
144. Wick G, Brezinschek HP, Hala K, Dietrich H, Wolf H, Kroemer G. The obese strain of chickens: an animal model with spontaneous autoimmune thyroiditis. Adv Immunol 1989;47:433–500.
145. Voorbij HA, van der Gaag RD, Jeucken PH, Bloot AM, Drexhage HA. The goitre of the BB/O rat: an animal model for studying the role of immunoglobulins stimulating the growth of thyroid cells. Clin Exp Immunol 1989;76:290–295.
146. Many MC, Maniratunga S, Varis I, Dardenne M, Drexhage HA, Denef JF. Two-step development of Hashimoto-like thyroiditis in genetically autoimmune prone non-obese diabetic mice: effects of iodine-induced cell necrosis. J Endocrinol 1995;147:311–320.
147. Peters JH Gieseler R, Thiele B, Steinbach F. Dendritic cells: from ontogenetic orphans to myelomonocytic descendants. Immunol Today 1996;17:273–278.
148. Leenen PJM, Campbell PA Heterogeneity of mononuclear phagocytes. An interpretive review. In: Horton MH, ed. Blood Cell Biochemistry, vol. 5. Plenum, New York, 1993, pp. 29–84.
149. Kabel PJ, Voorbij HA, de Haan M, van der Gaag RD, Drexhage HA. Intrathyroidal dendritic cells. J Clin Endocrinol Metab 1988;65:199–207.
150. Hala K, Malin G, Dietrich H, Loesch U, Boeck G, Wolf H, et al. Analysis of the initiation period of spontaneous autoimmune thyroiditis (SAT) in obese strain (OS) of chickens. J Autoimmunity 1996;9: 129–138.
151. Voorbij HAM, Jeucken PHM, Kabel PJ, de Haan M, Drexhage HA. Dendritic cells and scavenger macrophages in the pancreatic islets of prediabetic BB rats. Diabetes 1989;38:1623–1629.
152. Jansen A, Homo-Delarche F, Hooijkaas H, Leenen PJM, Dardenne M Drexhage HA. Immunohistochemical characterization of monocytes-macrophages and dendritic cells involved in the initiation of the insulitis and β cell destruction in NOD mice. Diabetes 1994;43:667–675.
153. Voorbij HA, Kabel PJ, de Haan M, Jeucken PH, van der Gaag RD, de Baets MH, et al. Dendritic cells and class II MHC expression on thyrocytes during autoimmune thyroid disease of the BB rat. Clin Immunol Immunopathol 1990;55:9–22.
154. Shimizu J, Carrasco-Marin E, Kanagawa O, Unanue ER. Relationship between beta cell injury and antigen presentation in NOD mice. J Immunol 1995;155:4095–4099.
155. Clare-Salzler M, Mullen Y. Marked dendritic cell-T cell cluster formation in the pancreatic lymph node of the non-obese diabetic mouse. Immunology 1992;76:478–484.
156. Yoon JW. The role of viruses and environmental factors in the induction of diabetes. Curr Top Microbiol Immunol 1990;164:95–123.
157. Onodera T, Awaya A. Anti-thyroglobulin antibodies induced with recombinant reovirus infection in Balb/c mice. Immunology 1990;71:581–585.
158. Charlton B, Bacelj A, Slattery RM, Mandel TE. Cyclophosphamide-induced diabetes in NOD/WEHI mice. Evidence for suppression in spontaneous autoimmune diabetes mellitus. Diabetes 1989;38: 441–447.
159. Mooij P. The thyroid, iodine and autoimmunity. Thesis, Erasmus University, Rotterdam, 1993.
160. Hoek A, Allaerts W, Leenen PJM, Schoemaker J, Drexhage HA. Dendritic cells and macrophages in the pituitary and the gonads. Evidence for their role in the fine regulation of the reproductive endocrine response. Eur J Endocrinol 1997;136:8–24.
161. Allaerts W, Jeucken PHM, Debets R, Hoefakker S, Claassen E, Drexhage HA. Heterogeneity of pituitary folliculo-stellate cells: implications for interleukin-6 production and accessory function in vitro. J Neuroendocrinol 1997;9:43–53.
162. Allaerts W, Salomon B, Leenen PJM, van Wijngaardt S, Jeucken PHM, Ruuls S, et al. A population of interstitial cells in the anterior pituitary with a hematopoietic origin and a rapid turnover: a relationship with folliculo-stellate cells? J Neuroimmunol 1996;78:184–197.
163. Simons PJ, Delemarre FGA, Drexhage HA. Antigen-presenting dendritic cells as regulators of the growth of thyrocytes: a role of interleukin-1β and interleukin-6. Endocrinology 1998;139:3148–3156.

164. Truden JL, Sundick RA, Levine S, Rose NR. The decreased growth rate of obese strain chicken thyroid cells provides in vitro evidence for a primary target organ abnormality in chickens susceptible to autoimmune thyroiditis. Clin Immunol Immunopathol 1983;29:294–304.
165. Simons PJ, Delemarre FGA, Jeucken PHM, Drexhage HA. Pre-autoimmune thyroid abnormalities in the biobreeding diabetes-prone (BB-DP) rat: a possible relation with the intrathyroid accumulation of dendritic cells and the initiation of the thyroid autoimmune response. J Endocrinol 1998;157:43–51.
166. Jansen A, Rosmalen JGM, Homo-Delarche F, Dardenne M, Leiter EH, Drexhage HA. Effect of prophylactic insulin treatment on the number of ER-MP23$^+$ macrophages in the pancreas of NOD mice. Is the prevention of diabetes based on β-cell rest? J Autoimmunity 1996;9:341–348.
167. Serreze DV, Gaedeke JW, Leiter EH. Hematopoietic stem-cell defects underlying abnormal macrophage development and maturation in NOD/lt mice: defective regulation of cytokine receptors and protein kinase C. Proc Natl Acad Sci USA 1993;90:9625–9629.
168. Delemarre FGA, Drexhage HA. Dendritic cells of the BB-DP rat are deficient accessory cells, particularly for CD8$^+$ and RT6$^+$ T cells ("suppressor cells"). Exp Clin Endocrinol Diabetes 1997;105:5,6.
169. Greiner DL, Handler ES, Nakono K, Mordes JP, Rossini AA. Absence of the RT-6 T cell subset in diabetes-prone BB/W rats. J Immunol 1986;136:148–151.
170. Tas MPR, de Haan-Meulman M, Kabel PJ, Drexhage HA. Defects in monocyte polarization and dendritic cell clustering in patients with Graves disease. A putative role of a nonspecific immunoregulatory factor related to retroviral p15E. Clin Endocrinol 1991;34:441–448.
171. Jansen A, van Hagen M, Drexhage HA. Defective maturation and function of antigen presenting cells in type 1 diabetes. The Lancet 1995;345:491–492.
172. Chung YH, Juns HS, Kang Y, Hirasawa K, Lee BR, Van Rooijen N, et al. Role of macrophages and macrophage-derived cytokines in the pathogenesis of Kilham rat virus-induced autoimmune diabetes in diabetes-resistant BioBreeding rats. J Immunol 1997;159:466–471.
173. Ciampolillo A, Marini V, Mirakian R, Buscema M, Schulz T, Pujol-Borrell R, et al. Retrovirus-like sequences in Graves' disease: implications for human autoimmunity. Lancet 1989;1:1096–1100.
174. Wick G, Grubeck-Löbenstein B, Trieb K, Kalischnig G, Aguzzi A. Human foamy virus antigens in thyroid tissue of Graves' disease patients. Int Arch Allergy Immunol 1992;99:153–156.
175. Yokoi K, Kawai H, Akaike M, Mine H, Saito S. Presence of human T-lymphotropic virus type II-related gens in DNA of peripheral leukocytes from patients with autoimmune thyroid diseases. J Med Virol 1995;45:392–398.
176. Schweizer M, Turek R, Hahn H, Schliephake A, Netzer KO, Eder G, et al. Markers of foamy virus infections in monkeys, apes, and accidently infected humans: appropriate testing fails to confirm suspected foamy virus prevalence in humans. AIDS Res Hum Retroviruses 1995;11:161–170.
177. Metcalfe RA, Ball G, Kudesia G, Weetman AP. Failure to find an association between hepatitis C virus and thyroid autoimmunity. Thyroid 1997;7:421–424.
178. Tominaga T, Katamine S, Namba H, Yokoyama N, Nakamura S, Morita S, Yamashita S, et al. Lack of evidence for the presence of human immunodeficiency virus type 1-related sequences in patients with Graves' disease. Thyroid 1991;1:307–314.
179. Willenberg HS, Stratakis CA, Marx C, Ehrhart-Bornestein M, Chrousos GP, Bornstein SR. Aberrant interleukin-1 receptors in a cortisol-secreting adrenal adenoma causing Cushing's syndrome. NEJM 1998;339:27–31.

14 Autoimmune Hypophysitis

Shereen Ezzat, MD, FRCP(C), and Robert G. Josse, MD, FRCP(C)

CONTENTS
INTRODUCTION
PATHOLOGICAL FEATURES
PATHOGENETIC MECHANISMS
CLINICAL FEATURES
MANAGEMENT
CONCLUSIONS
REFERENCES

INTRODUCTION

Lymphocytic hypophysitis is a rare inflammatory lesion of the pituitary gland. More than 100 cases have been described since the original report of the entity in 1962 *(1)*. The disease shows a striking female predilection of approx 8:1. Hypophysitis commonly affects young women during late pregnancy or in the postpartum period. Many reports strongly support the original suggestion of an autoimmune pathogenesis of this lesion and associate it with other autoimmune disorders, primarily thyroiditis and adrenalitis, and less commonly atrophic gastritis and lymphocytic parathyroiditis *(1–19)*.

Clinically, lymphocytic hypophysitis may have an acute onset and occasionally leads to severe complications, even a lethal outcome. In addition, the clinical presentation and radiographic findings may mimic pituitary adenoma. The diagnosis can only be clearly established by histologic examination.

In this chapter, we describe our experience and compare it with the literature on the basis of histologically proven cases of lymphocytic adenohypophysitis. The clinicopathologic features are analyzed and compared with those of other forms of pituitary pathology.

PATHOLOGICAL FEATURES

Gross Findings

The histologic features of autoimmune hypophysitis appear to be fairly uniform (Figs. 1 and 2). Grossly, the gland may be enlarged or atrophic. This may represent, like in other autoimmune endocrinopathies, a spectrum of disease from diffuse enlargement with inflammatory infiltrate to an atrophic fibrotic gland.

From: *Contemporary Endocrinology: Autoimmune Endocrinopathies*
Edited by: R. Volpe © Humana Press Inc., Totowa, NJ

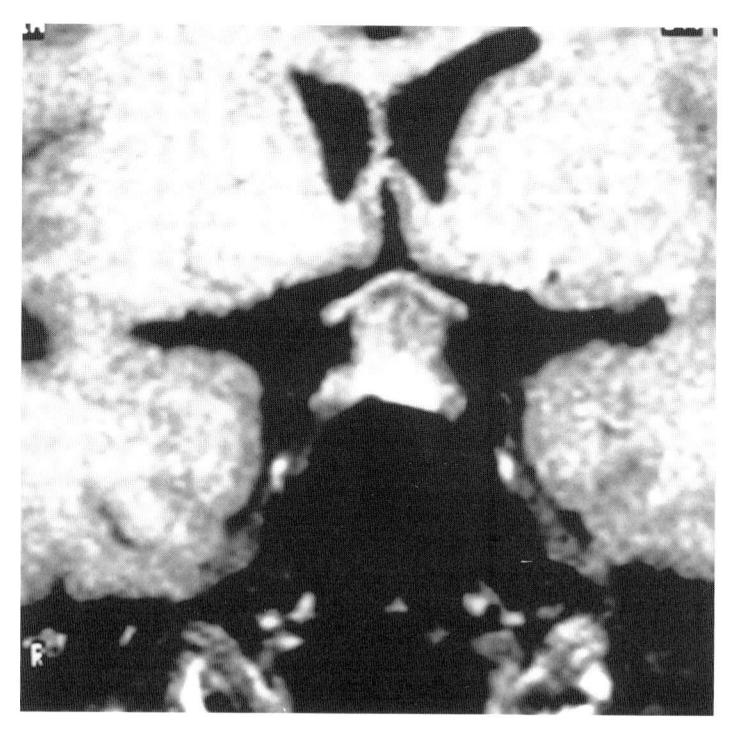

Fig. 1. Radiographic features of the pituitary in lymphocytic hypophysitis. Preoperative MRI scan reveals a large intrasellar mass with significant suprasellar and cavernous sinus extension closely mimicking a primary pituitary adenoma. Reproduced from ref. *(20)* with permission.

Light Microscopic Features

Light microscopy shows marked diffuse changes in the anterior lobe of the pituitary. There is extensive infiltration consisting chiefly of lymphocytes, but also plasma cells and on occasion eosinophils. Lymphoid follicles with germinal centers are often seen. The reticulin framework of the acini is usually intact with few regions of focal disruption and collapse. The involved gland shows various degrees of destruction, but foci of uninvolved pituitary tissue are morphologically normal. The distinctive absence of granulomata distinguishes this condition from the granulomatous hypophysitis seen in association with tuberculosis, syphilis, sarcoidosis, and giant-cell granuloma. Neurohypophysial tissue previously thought to be uninvolved can be infiltrated with inflammatory cells, but this is much less common.

Immunohistochemical Features

Immunocytochemically, the presence of immunoreactive prolactin (PRL), growth hormone (GH), adrenocorticotrophic hormone (ACTH), follicle-stimulating hormone (FSH), leuteinizing hormone (LH), and thyrotropin-stimulating hormone (TSH) within surviving adenohypophysial cells can be demonstrated. The number of cells immunopositive for each hormone varies depending on the degree of gland destruction. In cases of autoimmune hypophysitis associated with pregnancy or occurring in the postpartum period, immunohistochemical staining reveals pituitary cell cords containing predominantly PRL cells surrounded by the inflammatory infiltrate. The inflammatory cells are

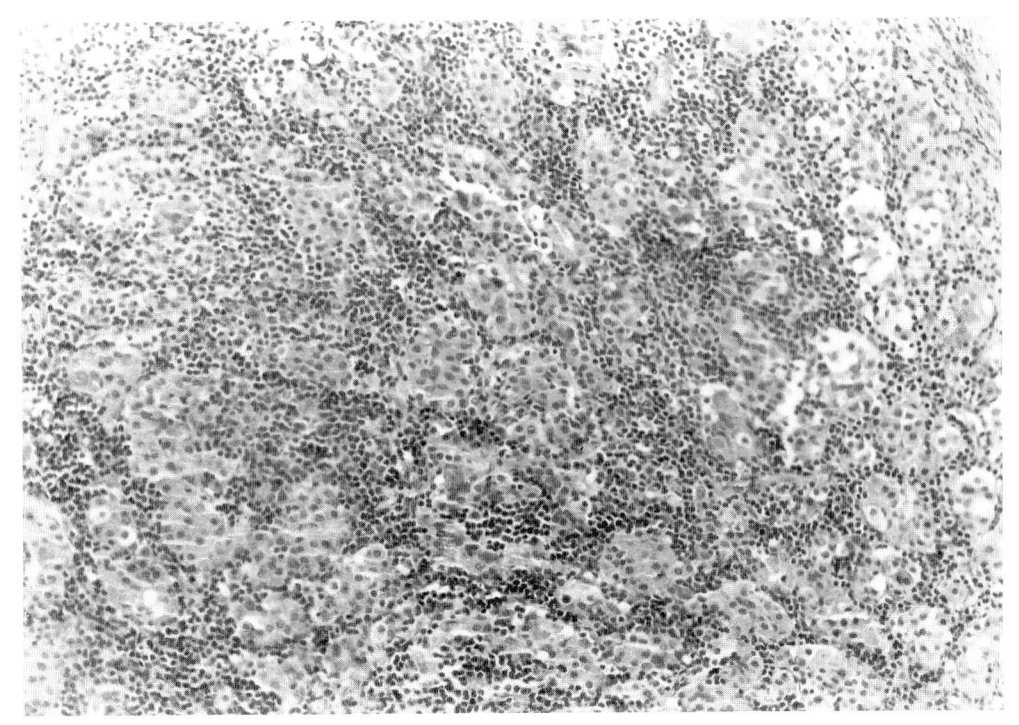

Fig. 2. Light microscopic features of the anterior pituitary in lymphocytic hypophysitis. The lesion is characterized by a lymphoplasmacytic infiltrate that surrounds areas of residual pituitary cells, which exhibit abundant granular eosinophilic cytoplasm, indicative of oxyphilic change. Reproduced from ref. *(20)* with permission.

a polyclonal population of T and B cells with positivity for leukocyte common antigen (LCA), L-26, UCHL-1, and κ/λ light chains.

Electron Microscopic Features

Electron microscopic features reveal adenohypophysial cells infiltrated by various inflammatory cells, including plasma cells, lymphocytes, macrophages, and less commonly eosinophils and neutrophils (Fig. 3). In the areas of most dense inflammatory cell infiltration, pituitary cells show interdigitation, with activated lymphocytes at the common interface. Some of these pituitary cells show oncocytic transformation. In general, the morphologic features of hypophysitis resemble those of other autoimmune endocrinopathies.

PATHOGENETIC MECHANISMS

The pathogenesis of lymphocytic hypophysitis has been suspected to be autoimmune in origin from the time of its original description *(1)*. Indeed, several lines of evidence support this hypothesis.

Antipituitary Antibodies

Circulating autoantibodies are a hallmark component of autoimmune disorders. Antipituitary antibodies, however, have been difficult to detect and have thus far been isolated in a minority of patients with the disease *(7,10,20)*. The association of lymphocytic

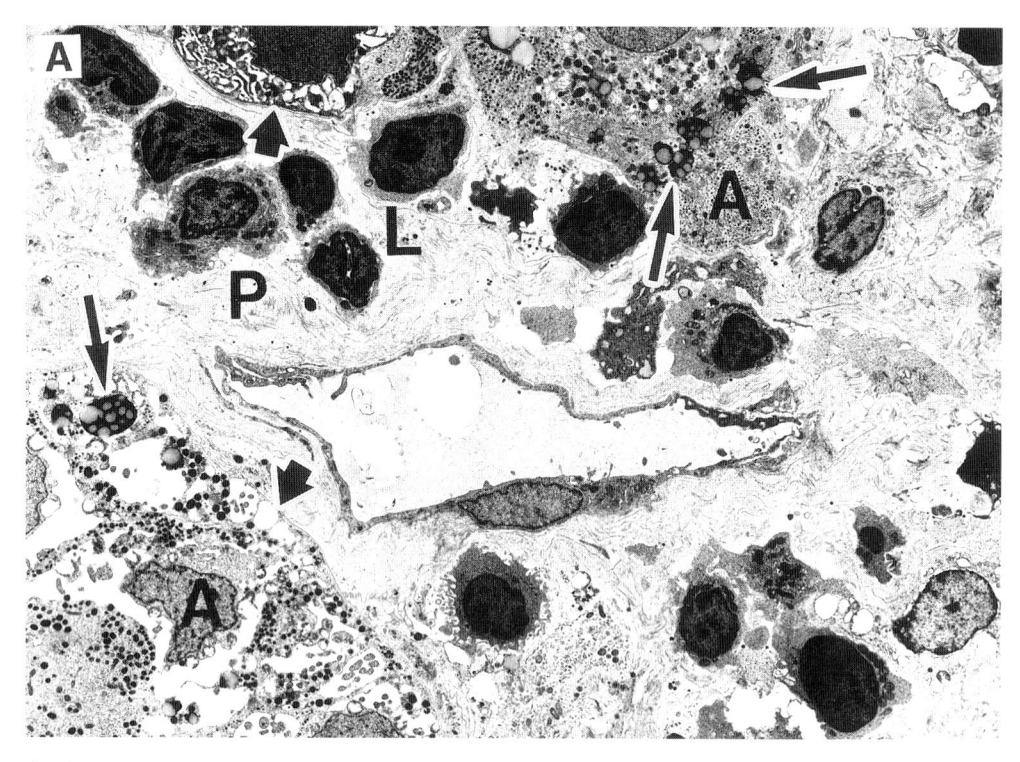

Fig. 3. Electron microscopic features of lymphocytic hypophysitis. (**A**) The pituitary is infiltrated by lymphocytes (L) and plasma cells (P) with stromal fibrosis, particularly surrounding a capillary. The adjacent adenohypophysial cells (A) show degeneration with swelling and vacuolation of organelles (short arrows), and accumulation of lysosomes (long arrows).

hypophysitis with pregnancy has been explained by the documentation of antibodies that react with nonhormonal antigens in hyperplastic lactotrophs *(21)*. Antipituitary antibodies have also been detected in patients with other pituitary disorders, including the "empty sella syndrome"*(22)*, idiopathic GH deficiency *(23)*, Cushing's syndrome *(24)*, as well as different autoimmune poly-endocrinopathies without hypophysitis *(21)*. In an isolated case of ACTH deficiency, the presence of antibodies to corticotroph antigens was detected in secretory granules that contained neither ACTH nor other pro-opiomelanocortin (POMC)-derived peptides *(25)*. These findings suggest that the antigen in question could well be a cell-specific factor required for POMC processing.

The different methods for detection and quantitation of circulating antipituitary antibodies used in various studies do not permit firm conclusions *(23,26)*. The earliest reports used a complement fixation technique. Reactivity was identified in approx 20% of postpartum patients. The clinical features of these patients were not detailed, bringing in to question their clinical relevance. In the 1970s, immunofluorescence was developed using freshly frozen human hypophysectomy tissue. Nearly 6% of 300 patients with polyglandular autoimmune disease were found to have reactive antibodies using this technique *(27,28)*. However, low titers of antipituitary antibodies by immunofluorescence are rarely associated with clinical pituitary insufficiency *(27)*. Pituitary tissue derived from other species, including rat, guinea pig, mouse, and fetal tissue, has also been utilized with similar results *(28,29)*. More recently, immunoblotting approaches have been adopted in the identification and measurement of antipituitary antibodies (Fig. 4). Using

Chapter 14 / Autoimmune Hypophysitis

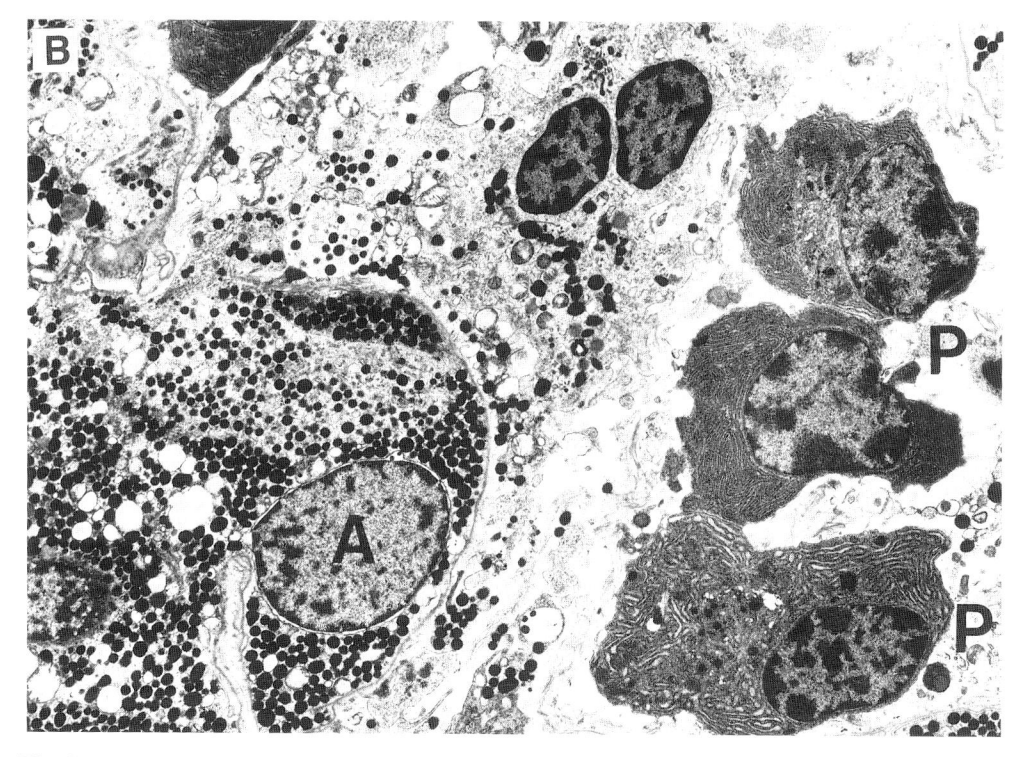

Fig. 3. (Continued). (**B**) The plasma cells (P) intimately associated with adenohypophysial cells (A) exhibiting varying degrees of degenerative change. Reproduced from ref. *(20)* with permission.

autopsy pituitary gland as substrate, cytosolic autoantigens can be identified. Sera examined from patients with proven hypophysitis reveal proteins of 49- and 40-kDa species *(29a)*. The exact nature of the autoantigen is not known, since reactivity of the 49-kDa protein is found in other tissues, including brain, adrenal, thyroid, liver, and spleen *(27)*. The current major problem with immunoblotting, as with other approaches, is specificity. Sera from patients with other autoimmune diseases, including Hashimoto's thyroiditis, Graves' disease, and pituitary adenomas, are also reactive to these antigens. In many of these latter cases, greater serum dilutions often abrogates immunoreactivity. Collection of samples before treatment or surgery may avoid some of the potential causes for false positivity. Furthermore, high titers of pituitary autoantibodies by immunoblotting are strongly compatible with, but not pathognomonic of hypophysitis. The nature of the antigen/antibodies identified thus far and their exact role in the pathogenesis of lymphocytic hypophysitis remain to be determined.

HLA Typing and Autoimmune Hypophysitis

Specific subtypes of the major histocompatibility complex (MHC) human leukocyte antigens (HLA) can be correlated with a number of autoimmune endocrine disorders. Most HLA antigens have been detected in patients with lymphocytic hypophysitis by some investigators *(5,10,12,30–34)*. Others, using immunohistochemistry, did not identify MHC class II-positive antigens on pituitary cells from patients with lymphocytic hypophysitis *(35)*. It is likely that HLA-DR genes are not responsible for the genesis of the autoimmune response *per se*, but may be closely related, in some subjects, with the genes directly responsible.

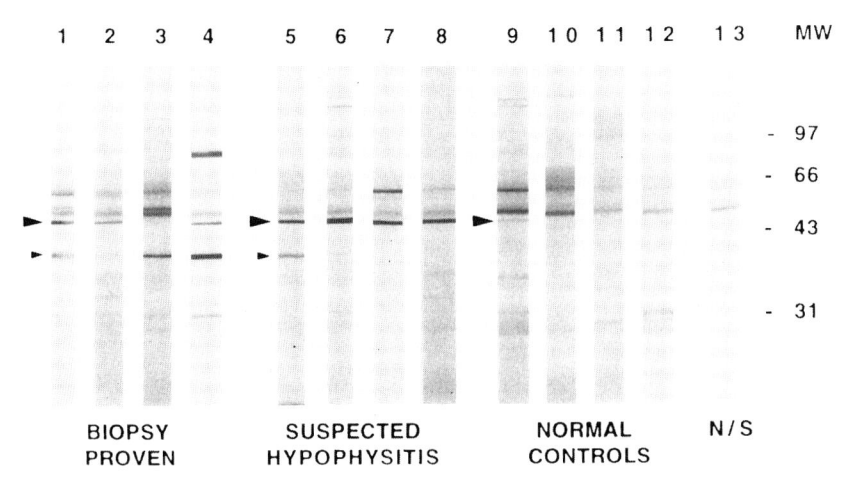

Fig. 4. Western blotting analysis of serum from patient with lymphocytic hypophysitis. Reproduced from ref. *(29a)* with permission.

Experimental Model of Hypophysitis

Experimentally, subcutaneous injections of human anterior pituitary gland homogenates in Freund's adjuvant produce a disease histologically similar to lymphocytic hypophysitis, characterized by focal lymphoid aggregates and diffuse mononuclear cell infiltration of the pituitary. Interestingly, this adenohypophysitis was found to be more pronounced in pregnant and lactating rats *(36)*. Similar results have been obtained by immunization of rabbits with homologous pituitary tissue in complete Freund's adjuvant *(37)*. Although induction of hypophysitis in hamsters is associated with the development of antipituitary antibodies, passive transfer of these antibodies does not propagate the disease *(38)*.

CLINICAL FEATURES

Patient Profiles

From a literature review of the first 100 patients, nearly 85% of subjects affected were females. The mean age at presentation was approx 30 yr compared with 40 yr in males. At least two-thirds of cases have been associated with pregnancy, nearly half presenting during the second or third trimester and the other half during the first 6 mo following delivery *(12,20,39)*.

Presenting Complaints

The clinical presentation of patients with lymphocytic hypophysitis involves four categories of symptoms. Those resulting from mass effects, such as headache and visual field impairment, have been reported in nearly 60% of patients *(12,20,31,40–44)*. Double vision arising from extension of the inflammatory mass into the cavernous sinuses has been noted in 6% of patients with lymphocytic hypophysitis *(31,40)*.

Hyperprolactinemia

Hyperprolactinemia is a feature of nearly 40% of patients with lymphocytic hypophysitis *(10,12,17,20,45,45a)*. Although PRL hypersecretion is a physiologic feature of pregnancy and the postpartum period, this observation only partially explains the PRL

Table 1
Clinical Presentation
of Patients with Lymphocytic Hypophysitis

Finding	Frequency
Female gender	90%
Pituitary enlargement	80%
Mass effects	60%
(headache, visual fieldl defect)	
Hyperprolactinemia	40%
Pituitary insufficiency	
Anterior	65%
Diabetes Insipidus	20%
Associated autoimmune disorders	25%

excess noted in this condition. Indeed lactotroph hyperplasia demonstrated by electron microscopy in some patients may represent an alternative explanation (20). However, of the nearly 20 cases in the literature with reported hyperprolactinemia, several have been in males (20,30,31,43,46), and at least half were females who were not pregnant or breast-feeding at the time of diagnosis (35,40,42,47–49). In many of these patients, elevated PRL levels may represent an endocrine marker of the disease. Several possibilities have been proposed to explain these findings. Stalk compression resulting in reduced dopamine delivery to the anterior pituitary (stalk phenomenon) represents a feasible possibility. This theory most likely accounts for hyperprolactinemia associated with suprasellar masses. Alternatively, the inflammatory process may directly alter dopaminergic receptors and the inhibitory effect of dopamine on PRL release. An autoimmune mechanism involving the production of stimulating antibodies by plasma cells may lead to increased hormone secretion, analogous to the pathophysiologic mechanisms implicated in Graves' disease of the thyroid. Finally, diffuse destruction by the inflammatory process may in some cases result in escape of hormone into the systemic circulation. These latter possibilities may account for PRL hypersecretion in some patients and, possibly, the GH or GH and PRL excess documented in others (20,50,51).

Anterior Pituitary Insufficiency

Symptoms resulting from partial or complete anterior hypopituitarism are noted in 65% of patients (10,20,30,43,46,52) (Table 1).

Selective loss of adenohypophysial cells is likely to be the result of a targeted autoimmune attack. The absence of corticotrophs histologically correlates well with the clinical presentation of cortisol deficiency. This finding is often based on biopsy specimens and, therefore, needs to be interpreted with caution, since it may not indicate total absence of corticotrophs in the entire pituitary. Even though isolated ACTH deficiency is rare, it represents the most common isolated type of anterior pituitary hormone deficiency encountered in patients with proven or suspected lymphocytic hypophysitis (2,13,15,16,25). Isolated TSH or gonadotropin deficiency has also been described (53).

Posterior Pituitary Insufficiency

Neurohypophysial involvement manifesting as diabetes insipidus is encountered in 20% of patients (6,20,42,54). Neurohypophysial dysfunction may be attributed either to direct inflammatory invasion, destruction, and/or compression of the posterior lobe or pituitary stalk.

Associated Autoimmune Dysfunction

A review of previously published reports indicates that nearly 20% of patients present with a history of other autoimmune conditions. Among these, primary hypothyroidism owing to chronic lymphocytic thyroiditis represents the most common finding. A similar frequency of 25% was identified in our recent series *(20)*. In addition, transient lymphocytic thyroiditis *(7,15)*, parathyroiditis, adrenalitis, atrophic gastritis *(5,12,19)*, and autoimmune polyglandular failure have also been reported *(53,55)*.

Other endocrinological findings included hypercalcemia in a minority of patients. Although this has occasionally been associated with parathyroid hyperplasia *(20,56)*, it is more commonly attributed to coexisting hypocortisolism.

Radiographic Features

Computer tomography (CT) or magnetic resonance imaging (MRI) reveals pituitary enlargement or a sellar mass similar to a pituitary tumor in almost 80% of cases (Fig. 1). In many instances, suprasellar extension cannot be easily distinguished from a pituitary adenoma *(57–59)*. Recent reports, however, point to some possible unusual features, which may be more specific to hypophysitis. These include loss of the hyperintense "bright spot" signal of the normal posterior pituitary on sagittal views, thickening of the pituitary stalk, and actual enlargement of the posterior pituitary *(60–62)*. These radiographic features, however, still require prospective validation. Occasionally, only a stalk lesion can be detected, whereas in others, the examination may be unremarkable.

Differential Diagnosis of Hypophysitis

There is an ongoing debate that some of the cases reported earlier as Sheehan's syndrome may have represented lymphocytic hypophysitis *(63)*. The other main form of hypophysitis is granulomatous hypophysitis *(64–66)*. The latter condition is characterized histologically by the presence of necrosis and giant-cell granulomata *(65–68)*. Lymphocytic infiltration can also be seen in the same pathologic specimen. This raises the question concerning whether the two conditions represent different ends of the same spectrum. Clinically, granulomatous hypophysitis has been reported to occur more commonly in postmenopausal women *(69,70)*. Other biochemical and radiographic features, however, are more difficult to distinguish from lymphocytic hypophysitis.

MANAGEMENT

Management of patients with suspected lymphocytic hypophysitis must be evaluated against the background of the natural history of this condition. Progressive severe and permanent hypopituitarism reflective of the degree of destruction of pituitary cells has resulted in a fatal outcome in almost 20 subjects *(20)*. In contrast, spontaneous recovery of pituitary function with near resolution of the pituitary mass has been described in several cases with histologically proven hypophysitis *(7,17,71,72)*. In some of these cases, the hypopituitarism may have been due to hypophysial edema, rather than to cell necrosis. The majority of patients, however, require active treatment. Although the administration of bromocriptine can improve visual field deficits and lower the hyperprolactinemia, the beneficial impact of this agent on the course of the disease is unproven. Glucocorticoid therapy has been advocated to reduce inflammation, and has been temporally effective in some patients *(40,41,71)*. The true efficacy of corticosteroids in this condition, however, also remains uncertain.

Transsphenoidal surgery should be performed in cases associated with progressive compressive features or those in whom radiographic and/or clinical progression occurs during conservative medical management *(73,74)*. Additionally, transsphenoidal surgery is both diagnostic and therapeutic. Amelioration of symptoms associated with a sellar mass effect is rapidly reversed *(20,73,74)*. Similarly, the hyperprolactinemia *(9,40,75)* and pituitary insufficiency *(71,72)* resolve following pituitary surgery in most cases. We have documented gradual and total recovery of pituitary dysfunction in two cases following transsphenoidal biopsy *(20)*. In rare instances, surgical intervention has been associated with further deterioration of the visual field deficit *(10)* and/or the associated hypopituitarism *(10,41,75,76)*. These latter complications highlight the importance of early suspicion of the diagnosis and conservative management in patients with nonprogressive disease.

In the event that surgery is contemplated, we propose that in cases of suspected hypophysitis, a frozen section should be obtained to confirm the diagnosis to avoid aggressive resection of potentially viable pituitary tissue.

CONCLUSIONS

Lymphocytic hypophysitis should be considered in the differential diagnosis of pituitary masses in women, especially during the latter half of pregnancy and in the first 6 mo postpartum, as well as those patients in whom pituitary hormone deficiency is noted in association with a coexisting autoimmune disorder. Other patients who should be suspected of harbouring such lesions include those who present with rapidly growing pituitary masses, and those whose PRL levels decline marginally or show modest therapeutic responses to bromocriptine. Owing to the lack of specificity of any of the other markers of the disease, the diagnosis can only be currently confirmed with histologic examination. Nevertheless, because of the potentially transient endocrine and compressive features of this condition in many instances, conservative management on the basis of clinical suspicion may eliminate the need for aggressive pituitary surgery.

REFERENCES

1. Goudie RB, Pinkerton PH. Anterior hypophysitis and Hashimoto's disease in a young woman. J Pathol Bacteriol (Lond) 1962;83:584–585.
2. Richtsmeier AJ, Henry RA, Bloodworth JMB Jr, Ehrlich EN. Lymphoid hypophysitis with selective adrenocorticotropic hormone deficiency. Arch Intern Med 1980;140:1243–1245.
3. Sobrinho-Simoes M, Brandao A, Paiva ME, Vilela B, Fernandes E, Carneiro-Chaves F. Lymphoid hypophysitis in a patient with lymphoid thyroiditis, lymphoid adrenalitis and idiopathic retroperitoneal fibrosis. Arch Pathol Lab Med 1985;109:230–233.
4. Ludwig H, Schernthaner G. Multiorganspezifische Autoimmunität bei idiopathischer Nebennierenrindeninsuffizienz. Weiner Klinische Wochenschrift 1978;90:736–741.
5. Pholsena M, Young J, Couzinet B, Schaison G. Primary adrenal and thyroid insufficiencies associated with hypopituitarism: A diagnostic challenge. Clin Endocrinol (Oxford) 1994;40:693–695.
6. Paja M, Estrada J, Ojeda A, Ramon y Cajal S, Garcia-Uria J, Lucas T. Lymphocytic hypophysitis causing hypopituitarism and diabetes insipidus, and associated with autoimmune thyroiditis, in a nonpregnant woman. Postgrad Med J 1994;70:220–224.

7. Ozawa Y, Shishiba Y. Recovery from lymphocytic hypophysitis associated with painless thyroiditis: clinical implications of circulating antipituitary antibodies. Acta Endocrinol (Copenh) 1993;128:493–498.
8. Hume R, Roberts GH. Hypophysitis and hypopituitarism: report of a case. Br Med J 1967;2:548–550.
9. Mazzone T, Kelly W, Ensinck J. Lymphocytic hypophysitis associated with antiparietal cell antibodies and vitamin B_{12} deficiency. Arch Int Med 1983;143:1794–1795.
10. Pestell RG, Best JD, Alford FP. Lymphocytic hypophysitis. The clinical spectrum of the disorder and evidence for an autoimmune pathogenesis. Clin Endocrinol (Oxford) 1990;33:457–466.
11. Lack EE. Lymphoid "hypophysitis" with end organ insufficiency. Arch Pathol 1975;99:215–219.
12. Asa SL, Bilbao JM, Kovacs K, Josse RG, Kreines K. Lymphocytic hypophysitis of pregnancy resulting in hypopituitarism: a distinct clinicopathologic entity. Ann Inter Med 1981;95:166–171.
13. Gal R, Schwartz A, Gukovsky-Oren S, Peleg D, Goldman J, Kessler E. Lymphocytic hypophysitis associated with sudden maternal death: report of a case and review of the literature. Obstet Gynecol 1986;41:619–621.
14. Ishihara T, Nakatsu S, Hino M, Hattori N, Moridera K, Ikekubo K, et al. A case of pregnancy-induced lymphocytic adenophypophysitis complicated by postpartum painless thyroiditis. Nippon Naibunpi Gakkai Zasshi-Foli Endocrinol Jp (Kyoto)al Med 1991;67:222–229.
15. Bevan JS, Othman S, Lazarus JH, Parkes AB, Hall R. Reversible adrenocorticotropin deficiency due to probable autoimmune hypophysitis in a woman with postpartum thyroiditis. J Clin Endocrinol Metab (Baltimore) 1992;74:548–552.
16. Escobar-Morreale H, Serrano-Gotarredona J, Varela C. Isolated adrenocorticotropic hormone deficiency due to probable lymphocytic hypophysitis in a man. J Endocrinol Invest (Milano) 1994;17:127–131.
17. Ober KP, Elster A. Spontaneously resolving lymphocytic hypophysitis as a cause of postpartum diabetes insipidus. The Endocrinologist 1994;4:107–111.
18. Jensen MD, Handwerger BS, Scheithauer BW, Carpenter PC, Mirakian R, Banks PM. Lymphocytic hypophysitis with isolated corticotropin deficiency. Ann Intern Med 1986;105:200–203.
19. Roosens B, Maes E, van Steirteghem A, Vanhaelst L. Primary hypothyroidism associated with secondary adrenocortical insufficiency. J Endocrinol Invest (Milano) 1982;5:251–254.
20. Thodou E, Asa SL, Kontogeorgos G, Kovacs K, Horvath E, Ezzat S. Lymphocytic hypophysitis: Clinicopathological findings. J Clin Endocrinol Metab (Baltimore) 1995;80:2302–2311.
21. Bottazzo GF, Pouplard A, Florin-Christensen A, Doniach D. Autoantibodies to prolactin-secreting cells of human pituitary. Lancet (Lond) 1975;ii:97–101.
22. Komatsu M, Kondo T, Yamauchi K, Yokokawa N, Ichikawa K, Ishihara M, et al. Antipituitary antibodies in patients with the primary empty sella syndrome. J Clin Endocrinol Metab (Baltimore) 1988;67:633–638.
23. Crock P, Salvi M, Miller A, Wall J, Guyda H. Detection of anti-pituitary autoantibodies by immunoblotting. J Immunol Methods 1993;162:31–40.
24. Scherbaum WA, Schrell U, Glück M, Fahlbusch R, Pfeiffer EF. Autoantibodies to pituitary corticotropin-producing cells: Possible marker for unfavourable outcome after pituitary microsurgery for Cushing's disease. Lancet (Lond) 1987;i:1394–1398.
25. Sauter NP, Toni R, McLaughlin CD, Dyess EM, Kritzmanm J, Lechan RM. Isolated adrenocorticotropin deficiency associated with an autoantibody to corticotroph antigen that is not adrenocorticotropin or other proopiomelanocortin-derived peptides. J Clin Endocrinol Metab (Baltimore) 1990;70:1391–1397.
26. Pouplard A. Pituitary autoimmunity. Hor Res (Basel) 1982;16:289–297.
27. Parent AD, Cruse JM, Smith EE. Lymphocytic hypophysitis—autoimmune reaction? Adv Biosci 1988;69:465–469.
28. Pour PM, Lepinard V, Luxembourger R, Rohmer V, Berthclot J, Bigorgne JC. Circulating pituitary autoantbodies against cells secreting luteinzing and follicle stimulating hormones in children with cryptochidism. Lancet (Lond) 1984;ii:631–632.
29. Sugiura M, Hashimoto A, Shizawa M, Tsukasda M, Maruyama S, Ishido T, et al. Heterogeneity of anterior pituitary cell antibodies detected in insulin-dependent diabetes mellititis and adrenoctoricotrophic hormone defficiency. Diabetes Res 1986;3:111–114.
29a. Crock PA. Cytosolic autoantigens: lymphocytic hypophysitis. J Clin Endocrinol Metab (Baltimore) 1998;83:609–618.
30. Guay AT, Agnello V, Tronic BC, Gresham DG, Freidberg SR. Lymphocytic hypophysitis in a man. J Clin Endocrinol Metab (Baltimore) 1987;64:631–634.
31. Supler ML, Mickle JP. Lymphocytic hypophysitis: Report of a case in a man with cavernous sinus involvement. Surg Neurol 1992;37:472–476.

32. Feigenbaum SL, Martin MC, Wilson CB, Jaffe RB. Lymphocytic adenohypophysitis: a pituitary mass lesion occurring in pregnancy. Proposal for medical treatment. Am J Obstet Gynecol 1991;164:1549–1555.
33. Meichner RH, Riggio S, Manz HJ, Earll JM. Lymphocytic adenohypophysitis causing pituitary mass. Neurology (Cleveland) 1987;37:158–161.
34. Miyamoto M, Sugawa H, Mori T, Hashimoto N, Imura H. A case of hypopituitarism due to granulomatous and lymphocytic adenohypophysitis with minimal pituitary enlargement: a possible variant of lymphocytic adenohypophysitis. Endocrinol Jp (Tokyo) 1988;35:607–616.
35. McCutcheon IE, Oldfield EH. Lymphocytic adenohypophysitis presenting as infertility. J Neurosurg (Baltimore) 1991;74:821–826.
36. Levine S. Allergic adenohypophysitis: new experimental disease of the pituitary gland. Science 1967;158:1190–1190.
37. Klein I, Kraus KE, Martines AJ, Weber S. Evidence for cellular mediated immunity in an animal model of autoimmune pituitary disease. Endocr Res Commun 1982;9:145–153.
38. Yoon JW, Choi DS, Liang HC, et al. Induction of an organ-specific autoimmune disease, lymphocytic hypophysitis, in hamsters by recombinant rubella virus glycoprotein and prevention of disease by neonatal thymectomy. J Virol 1992;66:1210–1214.
39. Josse RG. Autoimmune hypophysitis. In: Volpé R, ed. Autoimmune Diseases of the Endocrine System. CRC, Boca Raton, FL, 1990, pp. 331–351.
40. Nussbaum CE, Okawara S-H, Jacobs LS. Lymphocytic hypophysitis with involvement of the cavernous sinus and hypothalamus. Neurosurgery (Baltimore) 1991;28:440–444.
41. Stelmach M, O'Day J. Rapid change in visual fields associated with suprasellar lymphocytic hypophysitis. J Clin Neuro-Ophthalmol 1991;11:19–24.
42. Ludmerer KM, Kissane JM. Headaches, diabetes insipidus, and hyperprolactinemia in a woman with an enlarged pituitary gland. Am J Med 1993;95:332–339.
43. Lee J-H, Laws ER, Jr., Guthrie BL, Dina TS, Nochomovitz LE. Lymphocytic hypophysitis: occurrence in two men. Neurosurgery (Baltimore) 1994;34:159–162.
44. Scully RE, Mark EJ, McNeely WF, McNeely BU. Case 25–1195. N Engl J Med 1995;33:441–447.
45. Parent AD. Lymphoid hypophysitis. In: Wilkins RH, Rengachary SS, eds. Neurosurgery Update, vol. 1. McGraw-Hill, New York, 1990, pp. 3–8.
45a. Ezzat S, Josse RG. Autoimmune hypophysitis. Trends Endocrinol Metab 1997;81:74–80.
46. Puchner MJA, Lüdecke DK, Saeger W. The anterior pituitary lobe in patients with cystic craniopharyngiomas: Three cases of associated lymphocytic hypophysitis. Acta Neurochirurgica (Wien) 1994;126:38–43.
47. Portocarrero CJ, Robinson AG, Taylor AL, Klein I. Lymphoid hypophysitis. An unusual cause of hyperprolactinemia and enlarged sella turcica. J Am Med Assoc 1981;246:1811–1812.
48. McConnon JK, Smyth HS, Horvath E. A case of sparsely granulated growth hormone cell adenoma associated with lymphocytic hypophysitis. J Endocrinol Invest (Milano) 1991;14:691–696.
49. Masana Y, Ikeda H, Fujimoto Y, Matsumura I, Kawakami F, Mori S, et al. Lymphocytic adenohypophysitis: Case report. Neurologia Medico-Chirurgica 1990;30:853–857.
50. Hughes JM, Harris BS, Ellsworth C Lymphocytic hypophysitis masquerading as acromegaly. The Endocrine Society 76th Annual Meeting (Program & Abstracts), 1993, p. 69.
51. Hughes HM, Ellsworth CA, Harris BS. Clinical Case Seminar: A 33-year-old women with a pituitary mass and panhypopituitarism. J Clin Endocrinol Metab (Baltimore) 1995;80:1521–1525.
52. Cosman F, Post KD, Holub DA, Wardlaw SL. Lymphocytic hypophysitis. Report of 3 new cases and review of the literature. Medicine 1989;68:240–256.
53. Barkan AL, Kelch RP, Marshall JC. Isolated gonadotrope failure in the polyglandular autoimmune syndrome. N Engl J Med 1985;312:1535–1540.
54. Koshiyama H, Sato H, Yorita S, Koh T, Kanatsuna T, Nishimura K, et al. Lymphocytic hypophysitis presenting with diabetes insipidus: Case report and literature review. Endocr J 1994;41:93–97.
55. Kojima I, Nejima I, Ogata E. Isolated adrenocorticotropin deficiency associated with polyglandular failure. J Clin Endocrinol Metab (Baltimore) 1982;54:182–186.
56. Vasikaran SD, Tallis GA, Braund WJ. Secondary hypoadrenalism presenting with hypercalcemia. Clin Endocrinol (Oxford) 1994;41:261–264.
57. Quencer RM. Lymphocytic adenohypophysitis: Autoimmune disorder of the pituitary gland. Am J Neuroradiol 1980;1:343–345.

58. Mayfield RK, Levine JH, Gordon L, Powers J, Galbraith RM, Rawe SE. Lymphoid adenohypophysitis presenting as a pituitary tumor. Am J Med 1980;69:619–623.
59. Hungerford GD, Biggs PJ, Levine JH, Shelley BE Jr, Perot PL, Chambers JK. Lymphoid adenohypophysitis with radiologic and clinical findings resembling a pituitary tumor. Am J Neuroradiol 1982;3: 444–446.
60. Imura H, Nakao K, Shimatsu A, Ogawa Y, Sando T, Fujisawa I, et al. Lymphocytic infundibuloneurohypophysitis as a cause of central diabetes insipidus. N Engl J Med 1993;329:683–689.
61. Abe T, Matsumoto K, Sanno N, Osamura Y. Lymphocytic hypophysitis: Case report. Neurosurgery (Baltimore) 1995;36:1016–1019.
62. Ahmadi J, Meyers GS, Segall HD, Sharma OP, Hinton Dr. Lymphocytic adenohypophysisits: contrast enhanced MRI imaging in five cases. Radiology (Easton, PA) 1995;195:30–34.
63. Ushio Y, Arita N, Yoshimine T, Nagatani M, Mogami H. Glioblastoma after radiotherapy for craniopharyngioma: case report. Neurosurgery (Baltimore) 1987;21:33–38.
64. Rickards AD, Harvey PW. Giant-cell granuloma and the other pituitary granulomata. Q J Med 1989; 23:425–439.
65. Scanarini M, d'Ercole AJ, Rotilio A, Kitromilis N, Mingrino S. Giant-cell granulomatous hypophysitis: a distinct clinicopathological entity. J Neurosurg (Baltimore) 1989;71:681–686.
66. Scully RE, Mark EJ, McNeely BU. Case records of the Massachusetts General Hospital: Case 5–1985. N Engl J Med 1993;312:297–305.
67. Albini CH, MacGillvray MHFJE, Woorhess ML, Klein DM. Triad of hypopituitarism, granulomatous hypophysitis, and ruptured Rathk's cleft cyst. Neurosurgery 1988;22:133–136.
68. Chanson P, Timsit J, Kujas M, Violante A, Guillausseau PJ, Derome PJ, et al. Pituitary granuloma and pyoderma gangrenosum. J Endocrinol Invest 1990;13:677–681.
69. Oeckler RCT, Bise K. Non-specific granulomas of the pituitary: report of six cases treated surgically. Neurosurg Rev 1991;14:185–190.
70. Taylon C, Duff TA. Giant cell granuloma involving the pituitary gland. J Neurosurg (Baltimore) 1980; 52:584–587.
71. Bitton RN, Slavin M, Decker RE, Zito J, Schneider BS. The course of lymphocytic hypophysitis. Surg Neurol 1991;36:40–43.
72. McGrail KM, Beyerl BD, Black PM, Klibanski A, Zervas NT. Lymphocytic adenohypophysitis of pregnancy with complete recovery. Neurosurgery (Baltimore) 1987;20:791–793.
73. Prasad A, Madan VS, Sethi PK, Prasad ML, Buxi TBS, Kanwar CK. Lymphocytic hypophysitis: Can open exploration of the sella be avoided? Br J Neurosurg 1991;5:639–642.
74. Nishioka H, Ito H, Miki T, Akada K. A case of lymphocytic hypophysitis with massive fibrosis and the role of surgical intervention. Surg Neurol 1994;42:74–78.
75. Levine SN, Benzel EC, Fowler MR, Shroyer JVI, Mirfakhraee M. Lymphocytic hypophysitis: clinical, radiological and magnetic resonance imaging characterization. Neurosurgery (Baltimore) 1988;22: 937–941.
76. Reusch JE-B, Kleinschmidt-De Masters BK, Lillehei KO, Rappe D, Gutierrez-Hartmann A. Preoperative diagnosis of lymphocytic hypophysitis (adenohypophysitis) unresponsive to short course dexamethasone: case report. Neurosurgery (Baltimore) 1992;30:268–272.

15 The Polyglandular Autoimmune Syndromes

Marc Maes, MD, PhD, and George S. Eisenbarth, MD, PhD

Contents

INTRODUCTION
AUTOIMMUNE PRIMER
APS TYPE I
AUTOIMMUNE POLYGLANDULAR SYNDROME TYPE II (APS-II)
ORGAN-SPECIFIC AUTOANTIBODIES
CELL-MEDIATED AUTOIMMUNITY
SUMMARY
ACKNOWLEDGMENTS
REFERENCES

The polyglandular autoimmune syndromes are a rare constellation of autoimmune disorders characterized by more than one endocrine gland failure occurring in individuals and their families. In addition to endocrine glands, other nonendocrine organs may be targeted by the immune system, resulting in hypofunction as well as hyperfunction of the affected organs.

The specific aims of the present chapter are to review the clinical presentation, the treatment, the genetics, and the pathogenesis of the two major autoimmune polyglandular syndromes, namely autoimmune polyglandular syndromes Type I (APS-I) and Type II (APS-II) *(1–4)*.

INTRODUCTION

The two major autoimmune endocrine syndromes, APS-I and APS-II, share distinct as well as common features (Table 1). Both have Addison's disease as a common and prominent component *(5–7)* (*see also* Chapter 13). The familial clustering of these syndromes over several generations suggests the contribution of genetic factors to the development of these disorders. However, chronic mucocutaneous candidiasis and hypoparathyroidism are uniquely associated with APS-I. Also, the genes involved in these two are distinct: APS-I is associated with mutations of the autoimmune regulatory gene

From: *Contemporary Endocrinology: Autoimmune Endocrinopathies*
Edited by: R. Volpe © Humana Press Inc., Totowa, NJ

Table 1
Comparison of APS-I and APS-II

Type I	Type II
Addison's disease: 60–72%	Addison's disease: 70%
Autosomal recessive	Polygenic inheritance
Autoimmune regulator gene (AIRE) on chromosome 21q22.3	(some disease components associated with DQ2/DQ8)
Equal sex incidence	Female preponderance
Onset in infancy	Peak incidence ages 20–60
Mucocutaneous candidiasis	No mucocutaneous candidiasis
Hypoparathyroidism common	Hypoparathyroidism rare
Type 1 diabetes mellitus: lifetime frequency: 14%	Type 1 diabetes mellitus: ≈50%

(AIRE) located on the tip of the long arm of chromosome 21, *(8–10)* whereas some of the disease components of APS-II are associated with immune response genes located in the major histocompatibility complex of the short arm of chromosome 6, namely, human leukocyte antigens (HLA). APS type I is usually manifested in infancy, whereas type II has its peak incidence in middle age. Female preponderance is found in APS-II, but in APS-I, males as well as females are equally affected. In both syndromes, clinical expression of component diseases is preceded by circulating autoantibodies against endocrine and nonendocrine cells. The detection of these autoimmune markers is clinically useful, since they allow early diagnosis and appropriate therapy prior to potential morbidity and mortality. Some authors have attempted to subdivide further APS-II on the basis of the association of specific component diseases (i.e., association of autoimmune thyroid disease with an autoimmune disorder other than Addison's disease). However, this is debatable, since little information is gained by adding this subdivision in terms of understanding pathogenesis or predicting the development of future disorders in affected individuals and their relatives.

AUTOIMMUNE PRIMER *(11,12)*

The evidence supporting the autoimmune nature of the component diseases of the APS is compelling:

1. Affected organs demonstrate a characteristic mononuclear infiltrate consisting namely of B and T lymphocytes (helper CD4+ and cytotoxic-CD8+ T cells).
2. The presence of circulating organ-specific autoantibodies preceding diagnosis.
3. Cell-mediated immune defects.
4. Association of some component diseases of APS-II with specific HLA alleles.

The major determinants of autoimmune endocrine diseases are CD4+ and CD8+ T lymphocytes and autoantibodies produced by B lymphocytes. Although multiple effector pathways leading to cellular destruction by T lymphocytes are characterized (e.g., Fas-FasLigand, CD8 direct cytoxicity, lymphokine production), fundamental questions, such as what triggers autoimmunity, remain unanswered. The current hypothesis is that the genetic background predisposes to autoimmunity, which in turn is triggered or dampened by environmental factors, and can lead to progressive glandular destruction and finally overt disease. The most clearly established genetic association with autoimmune predisposition is that related to HLA alleles. HLA alleles may affect predisposition by several mechanisms that are not mutually exclusive, including shaping of the T-cell receptor repertoire, peptide selection, and presentation. However, the HLA haplotype *per se* is insufficient for development of autoimmune diseases as shown by the fact that that these haplotypes are also found in perfectly normal individuals. Therefore, other genes, linked and not linked to HLA, have to be discovered. Environmental agents may trigger autoimmunity through molecular mimicry, where memory T-cell clones primed by the initial antigen would recognize a structurally similar, but unrelated antigenic molecule in the affected organ, thereby leading to its destruction. Other possible mechanisms include the release of sequestered antigens or the alteration of self-antigens by environmental factors to which the immune system was previously tolerant, leading to the loss of self-tolerance. The expression of viral or bacterial superantigens by endocrine cells that activate a broad spectrum of T cells is still another proposed mechanism for the breakdown of self-tolerance. Why multiple different endocrine organs are affected by the autoimmune process in APS remains unknown. One possible explanation may be that peptides originating from different glands with related sequences may trigger the activation of additional autoreactive T cells, since recognition of an antigen by T cells requires as few as three properly spaced amino acids of a linear sequence of nine.

APS TYPE I

Clinical Presentation

APS-I, also known as APECED or autoimmune polyendocrinopathy-candidiasis-ectodermal dystrophy (MIM number 240300) syndrome, is an autosomal-recessive disorder classically characterized by the triad of chronic mucocutaneous candidiasis, autoimmune hypoparathyroidism, and adrenal insufficiency *(5–7)*. Only two of the manifestations in the index case and only one in the siblings are required for establishing the diagnosis.

Chronic mucocutaneous candidiasis is often the first manifestation detected, followed by hypoparathyroidism and Addison's disease. In addition, other endocrine and nonendocrine manifestations may be present (Table 2). Decades may elapse between the development of one disorder and the onset of another in the same individual. Consequently, lifelong follow-up is important to allow the early detection of additional components. Males and females are equally affected.

APS-I may occur sporadically as well as in families, and large cohorts of patients have been reported in Finland *(6,7)*, Israel *(13)*, and the US *(5)*. In the Finnish series of 72 patients reported initially by Ahonen et al. *(6)* and later by Perheentupa *(7)*, all patients had chronic candidiasis, 79% experienced hypoparathyroidism, 72% acquired Addison's disease, and 57% had all three of these classic components. Deficiencies of cortisol and aldosterone do not necessarily appear together, but may be separated as much as 3 to 5 yr and in random order *(6,7)*.

Hypogonadism was present in 60% of female patients ≥13 yr old and in 14% of male patients ≥16 yr old *(6,7)*. Most often, gonadal failure presents as total or partial failure of pubertal development. In some women, however, ovarian failure is not complete, and the patient may first complain of infertility or irregular menses later in life *(14)*. Type 1 diabetes mellitus appeared in 14% of the patients and for 60% of them, the diabetes occurs before 21 yr of age *(6,7)*. Primary hypothyroidism of the atrophic type was less

Table 2
Component Disorders of the APS-1

Component disorders	
Endocrine	Addison's disease
	Hypoparathyroidism
	Hypothyroidism
	Primary hypogonadism
	Type 1 diabetes mellitus
Dermatologic	Chronic mucocutaneous candidiasis
	Alopecia
	Vitiligo
Gastrointestinal	Fat malabsorption
	Chronic active hepatitis
Hematologic	Pernicious anemia
	Pure red cell hypoplasia
Ectodermal	Dental enamel hypoplasia
	Nail dystrophy
	Tympanic membranes calcification
Other manifestations	Asplenism
	Keratopathy
	Progressive myopathy

frequent and was present only in 4% of the patients. Many other patients remained euthyroid despite high titers of circulating antithyroid antibodies.

Other nonendocrine organ diseases included alopecia (29%), vitiligo (13%), pernicious anemia (13%), and autoimmune hepatitis (12%) *(6,7)*. Chronic hepatitis was present in all but two patients, who died from fulminant hepatitis. Other rare manifestations of autoimmunity include dermal vasculitis, rheumatoid disease, and pure cell red aplasia *(7)*.

Recurrent candidiasis commonly affects the oral mucosa and nails, and less frequently, the skin and the esophagus. Ectodermal dystrophy is manifested by pitted nails, keratopathy, and most frequently by enamel hypoplasia, and is not thought to be immune mediated. Also, pitted nails appeared to be unrelated to candidiasis. Calcified tympanic membranes were detected in one-third of the patients and were unrelated to middle ear infections. Intermittent malabsorption with steatorrhea may be owing to bacterial and fungal overgrowth or hypoparathyroidism. In contrast to the Finnish patients, hypoparathyroidism (96%) was the most frequent finding in 23 Jewish patients from 19 families of Iranian origin, candidiasis (17%) was less frequently found, and keratopathy was absent *(13)*. Sporadic cases are more frequent and share common clinical manifestations with familial cases.

Immunogenetics

APS-I is unique among autoimmune endocrine disorders, in that it is not associated with class II HLA alleles *(15)*. APS-I is inherited as an autosomal-recessive disorder, with a 25% recurrence risk for siblings of affected individuals. The genetic locus responsible for the disease has been mapped to the long arm of chromosome 21 (21q22.3) with DNA markers by Aaltonen et al. *(8)*. Studies of linkage disequilibrium increased the informativeness of the analyses and helped locate the gene to a 500-kb segment. Björses et al. *(16)* found that the Persian-Jewish disorder mapped to the same region of 21q22.3.

Furthermore, haplotype analysis of the APS-I chromosomes in the 21 non-Finnish, non-Jewish families provided independent evidence for linkage to the same chromosomal region and revealed no evidence of locus heterogeneity. The haplotype analysis suggested that APS-I in different populations is owing to a number of different mutations in a gene on chromosome 21. This gene has recently been identified and named AIRE or autoimmune regulator, which encodes a putative nuclear protein containing motifs suggestive of a transcription factor, including two zinc-finger motifs, expressed in different tissues, but in particular in the thymus *(9,10)*.

Immunopathogenesis

The mechanism(s) whereby mutations in a putative transcription factor leads to the protean manifestations of the APS-I with variable penetrance among affected individuals remains at present unknown. As speculated for other autoimmune diseases, participation of environmental agents or of alterations of other immune response-related genes, as well as nonidentity in immune repertoires created by the stochastic process of T-cell receptor or immunoglobulin gene segment assembly may be additional mechanisms that could explain the variable penetrance as well as the variety of organs affected.

Therapy

Hormonal substitution therapy remains the cornerstone of therapy for the different endocrine organ failures and is not different from those prescribed for individual organ failures with the caveat that malabsorption may complicate treatment.

Mucocutaneous candidiasis is treated with antifungal drugs, such as fluconazole and ketoconazole *(17,18)*. Because ketoconazole is a global P-450 cytochrome inhibitor, patients must be monitored for potential decompensation of marginal adrenal insufficiency. Also, these antifungal drugs can cause transient elevation of liver enzymes and occasionally hepatitis for which patients have to be monitored. Immune hepatitis is usually treated with immunosuppressive therapy.

Screening of affected individuals as well as their relatives for new disorders before overt symptoms develop is necessary to avoid mortality and morbidity. Assessment of autoantibodies, electrolytes, calcium and phosphorus levels, thyroid and liver functions, blood smears, and vitamin B_{12} levels is recommended. Individuals at risk for adrenal insufficiency should be screened by measuring basal corticotropin adrenocorticotropic hormone (ACTH), plasma renin levels, and dynamic cortisol testing as appropriate. Whether preventive therapy may be effective in this condition remains to be determined.

AUTOIMMUNE POLYGLANDULAR SYNDROME TYPE II (APS-II)

Clinical Presentation

APS-II is the most common of the immunoendocrinopathies, occurs two to three times more frequently in females than in males, and is commonly diagnosed between 20 and 40 yr of age. APS-II is usually defined by the occurrence in the same individual of two or more of the following: primary adrenocortical insufficiency, autoimmune thyroid disease, and Type 1 diabetes mellitus. Thyroid disease may manifest itself as chronic lymphocytic thyroiditis with goiter and/or hypothyroidism or Graves'disease. The association of thyroiditis and Addison's disease was first described by Schmidt in 1926, *(19)*, whereas Carpenter et al. extended the syndrome in 1964 to include insulin-dependent

Table 3
Component Disorders of APS-II

Component disorders	
Endocrine	Addison's disease
	Hypothyroidism
	Graves' disease
	Type 1 diabetes mellitus
	Primary hypogonadism
	Late-onset hypoparathyroidism
	Hypohysitis
Gastrointestinal	Celiac disease
Dermatologic	Alopecia
	Vitiligo
	Dermatitis herpetiformis
Hematologic	Pernicious anemia
	Idiopathic thrombocytopenic purpura
Neurologic	Myasthenia gravis
	Pernicious anemia
	Stiff Man syndrome
	Parkinson's disease
Other manifestations	IgA deficiency
	Serositis
	Idiopathic heart block
	Goodpasture's syndrome

diabetes mellitus (20). It was not until 1956 that the autoimmune pathogenesis of these disorders began to be documented with the discovery of circulating precipitating autoantibodies to thyroglobulin in patients with Hashimoto's thyroiditis by Roitt et al. (21). Other endocrine and nonendocrine diseases include primary hypogonadism (22,23), myasthenia gravis (24,25), and celiac disease (23,26). Vitiligo (27), alopecia, serositis (28), and pernicious anemia (29) also occur with increased frequency in individuals with this syndrome and in their family members (Table 3).

Among 244 patients reported by Neufeld et al. (5) the onset of the syndrome is heralded by adrenal insufficiency about half of the time. In these patients, Type 1 diabetes mellitus (52%) and autoimmune thyroid disease (69%) were the most frequent coexisting conditions. The detection of diabetes or chronic thyroiditis may be concurrent with the diagnosis of adrenalitis or may be delayed up to 20 yr. Less common features included vitiligo (5%) and gonadal failure (4%). Among patients with Type 1 diabetes mellitus, thyroid autoimmunity and celiac disease coexist with sufficient frequency to justify screening. Thyroid peroxidase autoantibodies are present in 10% of children with Type 1 diabetes, and this frequency increases with age (30). However, thyroid autoantibodies may be present for many years without progression to overt thyroid disease. Thus, annual measurement of thyroid-stimulating hormone (TSH) levels is recommended as cost-effective in patients with Type 1 diabetes mellitus.

Approximately 2–3% of patients with Type 1 diabetes mellitus have celiac disease (30–32), and screening can be performed by measuring antiendomysial autoantibodies (33). If antiendomysial autoantibodies are present, a small bowel biopsy is warranted to determine whether celiac disease has developed. Although a gluten-free diet should be

Table 4
Predominant HLA Association with Component Disorders of APS-II

Disease	HLA association DRB	DQA/DQB	Comment
Addison's disease	0404	0301/0302	DR3/DR4 with
	0301	0501/0201	DRB1*0404 is the
	0501	0501/0301	predominant genotype
Celiac disease	0301	0501/0201	DR3 or DR5/DR7 in *trans*
		0501/0202	
Type 1 diabetes mellitus	0301	0501/0201	
	0401,02,04	0301/0302	
Graves' disease	0301	0501/0201	
Myasthenia gravis	0301	0501/0201	Idiopathic
		0201/0202	
Stiff Man syndrome	0301	0501/0201	Penicillamine-induced

prescribed in symptomatic patients, introduction of such a diet in asymptomatic patients is being debated. However, osteopenia *(34)* and increased risk of gastrointestinal lymphoma have been described in untreated patients with celiac disease *(35)*.

Hypoparathyroidism is rare in APS-II in contrast to APS-I. If hypocalcemia occurs in a patient with the type II syndrome, celiac disease is more likely than primary hypoparathyroidism. Nevertheless, hypoparathyroidism has been described in several elderly patients with APS-II where antibodies suppressing parathyroid function were present *(36)*.

Immunogenetics

Although APS-II and its component disorders tend to aggregate in families, there is no discernible pattern of inheritance. Susceptibility is probably determined by multiple genetic loci (with HLA having the strongest effect) that interact with environmental factors. Only for celiac disease has an environmental antigen, dietary gliadin, been identified.

Many of the disorders of APS-II are associated with an HLA-extended haplotype formed by HLA-A1, HLA-B8, HLA-DR3, DQA1*0501, DQB1*0201 (DQ2) *(37–45)*. These include Graves' disease, atrophic thyroiditis, Type 1 diabetes mellitus (also HLA-DR4 associated), Addison's disease (also DR4 associated), myasthenia gravis, celiac disease, selective IgA deficiency, and dermatitis herpetiformis (Table 4).

Mclaren and Riley found that autoimmune Addison's disease was strongly associated with HLA-DR3 and HLA-DR4: relative risks were 6.0, 4.6, and 26.5 for DR3, DR4, and DR3/DR4, respectively *(40)*. In our studies, approx 50% of patients with Addison's disease are DR3/DR4 heterozygotes (genotype DQ2/DQ8) in comparison to 2.3% of the general population. What is particularly interesting concerning this haplotype is that it is also a high-risk genotype for Type 1 diabetes mellitus. In addition, Yu et al. *(41)* in our laboratory demonstrated recently that among patients with DR4, Addison's disease was strongly associated with a specific DRB1 subtype: DRB1*0404 (11/12 patients from 6 families in contrast to 109/408 DR4 Type 1 diabetes patients without Addison's disease having DRB1*0404; $p < 10^{-5}$) (Fig. 1). The association of DRB1*0404 with the haplotype DQ2/DQ8 is likely to account for a significant portion of the association between Addison's disease and Type 1 diabetes mellitus. The haplotype DQA1*0102, DQB1*0602 appears to provide dominant protection against Type 1 diabetes mellitus even in the

B = DRB1*0404, DQA1*0301, DQB1*0302
a,c,d,e,h = DRB1*0301, DQA1*0501, DQB1*0201

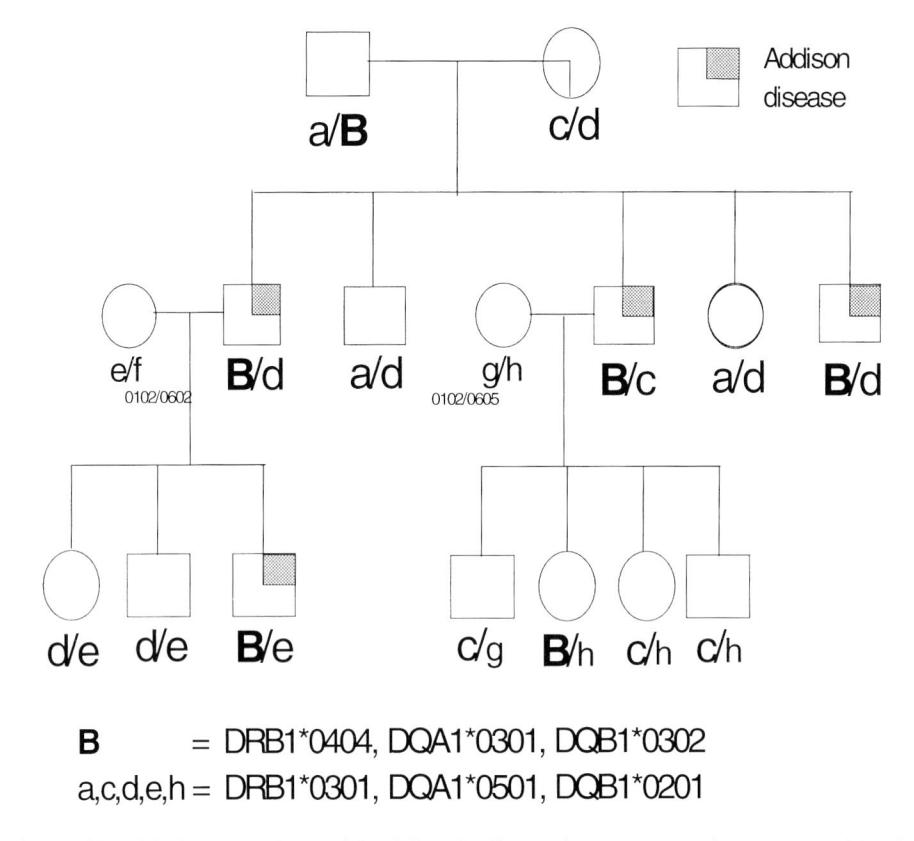

Fig. 1. Family with three members with addison's disease in two generations. None of the family members have diabetes or anti-islet antibodies. Multiple members have thyroid autoimmunity or vitiligo. All members with addison's disease have a DR3/DR4 genotype with DRB1*0404. This unusual genotype with DRB1*0404 appears to be a major genotype of addison's disease. Note that multiple DR3 haplotypes (d,c,e) are present in affected patients along with the DR4 haplotype introduced once into the family.

presence of anti-islet autoantibodies, since approx 7% of first-degree relatives of diabetic patients who express anti-islet autoantibodies have DQA1*0102, DQB1*0602, and the great majority of such individuals do not progress to diabetes *(46)*. In a similar manner, patients with 21-hydroxylase autoantibodies and DRB1*0401 and DRB1*0402 appear less often to progress to Addison's disease *(41)*.

Celiac disease occurs primarily in individuals expressing HLA-DQ2 (DQA1*0501, DQB1*0201) either in *cis* (with both alleles on the same chromosome 6) or in *trans* (DQA1*0501 from DR5 on one chromosome 6 and DQB1*0202 from DR7 on the other chromosome 6). Although for celiac disease the HLA contribution may be limited to the DQ molecules for Type 1 diabetes mellitus and several other component diseases of APS-II, other HLA genes in addition to DQ appear to contribute to susceptibility. Thirty-five percent of the individuals who acquire Type 1 diabetes are heterozygous for the high-risk combination HLA-DR3 (DQA1*0501, DQB1*0201) and HLA-DR4 (DQA1*0301, DQB1*0302) haplotypes compared to 2–3% of the US population *(47)*. Component disorders of APS-II that are not associated with HLA-DR3 *(48,49)*, include pernicious anemia, goitrous thyroiditis, and vitiligo. It is likely that there are genes outside the HLA region or tightly linked to HLA that influence immune function and contribute to the multiple organs to which tolerance is lost. At present, the identity of these genes is largely unknown despite possible candidate loci identified by genome-wide scan in selected diseases, such as Type 1 diabetes mellitus *(50,51)*.

Therapy

The clinical management of APS-II patients includes early diagnosis of associated disorders. Since the number of associated disorders that will develop and their age of appearance are clinically unpredictable, long-term follow-up is necessary.

Associated disorders are then treated as they are diagnosed, keeping in mind that certain disease combinations require specific management. Thyroxine therapy for hypothyroidism can precipitate life-threatening adrenal insufficiency in a patient with untreated adrenal insufficiency. Decreasing insulin requirement or the increasing occurrence of hypoglycemia in a patient with Type 1 diabetes can be one of the earliest indications of adrenocortical failure. Hypocalcemia is more likely because of celiac disease rather than the rare hypoparathyroidism. Finally, it is possible that thyroxine therapy may favorably alter the course of Graves' disease, but prospective randomized trials are needed *(52)*.

ORGAN-SPECIFIC AUTOANTIBODIES

The identification of circulating organ-specific autoantibodies provided the earliest and strongest evidence for the autoimmune pathogenesis of the APSs. Although their pathogenic relevance remains unclear, their importance as diagnostic indicators and predictive markers of future disease is well established. Initially, these autoantibodies were detected by indirect immunofluorescence using human endocrine tissue as substrate. More recently, more standardized and sensitive assays have been developed using the identified recombinant antigen where the antigen–autoantibody complex is detected by enzyme-linked immunosorbent assays, immunoinhibition, and most often with immunoprecipitation.

The antigens to which these autoantibodies react appear to fit into four groups:

1. Enzymes associated with differentiated endocrine function.
2. Hormones or protein products of the gland.
3. Receptor or surface proteins.
4. Proteins associated with secretory granules (Table 5).

It has been suggested that the intracellular enzymes may be displayed on the cell surface during hormone synthesis and that thereby some antienzyme antibodies may be functionally significant.

There is much debate about whether most of these autoantibodies initiate or maintain the autoimmune process. Autoantibodies reactive to cell-surface proteins, such as thyroid-stimulating immunoglobulins or thyroid-blocking autoantibodies, are clear effectors of disease, since the transplacental passage of these autoantibodies results in transient clinical disease in the neonate. However, except for these few exceptions, most of these autoantibodies have no pathogenic role and probably reflect tissue damage secondary to inflammation.

Thyroid Autoantibodies

The predictive values of autoantibodies vary greatly. The least predictive are autoantibodies against thyroid peroxidase or thyroglobulin, since they can be present for long

Table 5
Autoantibodies in APS

Disease	Autoantigens
Type 1 diabetes mellitus	ICA, IAA, GAD65, ICA512/IA-2, etc.
Atrophic thyroiditis	Thyroid peroxidase, thyrogloblin
Vitiligo	Tyrosinase
Graves' disease	Thyroid peroxidase, thyrogloblin, TSH receptor
Pernicious anemia	H/K-ATPase, intrinsic factor
Chronic active hepatitis	P450 c IA2
Celiac disease	Transglutaminase
Gonadal failure	Cholesterol side-chain cleavage enzyme, 17-hydroxylase
Addison's disease	21-Hydroxylase, 17-hydroxylase
Hypoparathyroidism	Ca-sensing receptor

periods without progression to overt hypothyroidism. The reason for the frequent discordance between thyroid autoimmunity and disease is not known. The human TSH receptor (TSHR) is the primary antigenic target of autoimmune hyperthyroidism: thyroid-stimulating autoantibodies to the TSHR elicit hyperthyroidism in Graves' disease by mimicking the ability of TSH to bind to the TSHR, thereby inducing a chronic overproduction of thyroid hormones *(53)*. Conversely, blocking antibodies to the TSHR may result in atrophic thyroiditis, which is often accompanied by hypothyroidism *(54)*.

Adrenal Autoantibodies

In contrast to thyroid autoantibodies, adrenal autoantibodies (ACA) measured by immunofluorescence are associated with risk of Addison's disease. Indeed in 92% of patients with APS-I, adrenal autoantibodies were observed before adrenocortical failure in contrast to 22% of patients who maintained normal adrenal function *(55)*. However, some of these patients may have a preclinical or a compensated phase of adrenal insufficiency identified by a decreased response to adrenocorticotrophic hormone (ACTH) with increased ACTH and plasma renin activity levels. ACA have also been found in 1–2% of individuals with autoimmune diseases other than adrenal insufficiency, such as Type 1 diabetes *(56,57)*. The frequency is higher among adults with premature ovarian failure (8.9%) and in children with hypoparathyroidism (48%) *(56)*.

The major autoantigen of ACA is the steroidogenic enzyme P450c21 or 21-hydroxylase (*see* Chapter 8). Between 80 and 100% of patients positive for ACA are positive for 21-hydroxylase autoantibodies. These autoantibodies have been documented in 90–100% of patients with APS-II and Addison's disease and 92% of patients with APS-I and Addison's disease *(58,59)*. As for ACA, 21-hydroxylase autoantibodies correlate with progression to adrenal insufficiency. Therefore, it is recommended that patients with organ-specific autoimmunity should be screened yearly for the presence of these autoantibodies. When present, evaluation of adrenal function should be performed to allow early diagnosis and treatment.

Steroid Cell Autoantibodies

Autoimmune gonadal failure is associated with the presence of autoantibodies that recognize antigens in several steroid-producing cells, such as the testicular Leydig cell, the ovarian luteal cell, and the syncythiotrophoblast of the placenta *(60)*. Recently the steroidal autoantigens were identified as the cytochrome enzymes P450 scc (side-chain cleavage involved in cholesterol synthesis) and P450c17 (17-hydroxylase) in patients with APS-I and gonadal failure *(55,61)*. When detected, these "steroidal cell" autoantibodies carry a high risk (approx 40%) for future gonadal failure in women (see Chapter 16). In men, these autoantibodies do not seem to increase the risk of hypogonadism *(62)*.

Anti-islet Autoantibodies

Expression of a single anti-islet autoantibody (of insulin, GAD65 and ICA512/ IA-2) is associated with only a small increase in the risk of Type 1 diabetes mellitus. The risk of progression to diabetes when only one of these autoantibodies is present is only 15% in first-degree relatives of diabetics *(63)*. The risk of Type 1 diabetes in patients with APS-I or APS-II and GAD65 autoantibodies appears to be even lower *(64)*. In APS-I, 41% of 39 nondiabetic patients were found to have GAD65 autoantibodies. In these patients, fasting plasma C-peptide levels and first-phase insulin response to iv glucose administration were lower than in patients without autoantibodies *(7)*. This suggests that many patients may have a subclinical nonprogressive insulitis. Progression to diabetes in these patients may be heralded by contribution of additional unknown genes or exposure to ill-defined environmental factors. In Type II APS, high titers of GAD autoantibodies are associated with a low risk of progression to diabetes. It has been demonstrated that these autoantibodies react only with the B cells of rat islets and fail to react with mouse islets, and are therefore called restrictive or selective. This unusual form of autoantibodies confers a lower risk of Type 1 diabetes as compared to nonrestricted autoantibodies for both APSs' patients and relatives of patients with Type 1 diabetes *(65,66)*.

Autoantibodies reactive with a novel islet 37-kDa antigen are a better predictor of progression to Type 1 diabetes in APS-II patients compared to cytoplasmic ICA *(67)*. The 37-kDa molecule and the related 40-kDa molecule are now sequenced, and are identified as ICA512/IA-2 *(67,68)* and Phogrin/IA-2b *(69,70)* members of a family of the tyrosine phosphatase-like proteins. Similar to relatives of patients with diabetes with Type 1 diabetes, the best predictor of progression to diabetes appears to be expression of multiple autoantibodies. Five of six APS II patients progressing to diabetes expressed ≥ 2 of GAD65, insulin, or ICA512 autoantibodies *(63)*.

Celiac Disease Autoantibodies

In patients with celiac disease, IgA autoantibodies against gliadin, reticulin, or endomysium are present *(71–73)*. Antiendomysial autoantibodies correlate best with gliadin ingestion and with intestinal pathology. A recent study has demonstrated that the major autoantigen of antiendomysial autoantibodies is the molecule tissue transglutaminase *(74)*. This enzyme catalyzes the crosslinking of proteins through glutamylysine bonds leading to the hypothesis that gliadin may become crosslinked to transglutaminase and thereby create a novel epitope responsible for the immune response to the self-protein transglutaminase. Testing for transglutaminase autoantibodies will likely replace the other antibody assays. Approximately 10% of patients with Type 1 diabetes express transglutaminase autoantibodies with a high risk of celiac disease on biopsy.

Other Autoantibodies

Recently, the extracellular domain of the calcium-sensing receptor has been identified as the target of autoantibodies associated with hypoparathyroidism *(75)*. Patients with autoimmune gastritis and pernicious anemia have autoantibodies that react with the H/K-ATPase, the proton pump of gastric parietal cells *(76)*. Autoantibodies against the hepatic cytochrome P450-1A2 are associated with chronic active hepatitis in patients with autoimmune hepatitis and APS-I *(77)*.

CELL-MEDIATED AUTOIMMUNITY

Significant cellular immune dysfunction, which may predispose to candidiasis and life-threatening infections, has been described in patients with APS-I *(78,79)*. Also, peripheral cellular GAD65 reactivity has been demonstrated in some patients with Type 1 diabetes and APS-I *(7)*. However, T cell-mediated immunity is more difficult to study than humoral autoimmunity, since the consistent demonstration of specifically activated T cells in the circulation has been difficult to reproduce. Therefore, more sensitive and specific T-cell assays are needed before they can be clinically useful.

SUMMARY

The APS-I and APS-II syndromes have and continue to contribute to our understanding of autoimmunity. With the cloning of the gene for APS-I (AIRE), major efforts are under way to understand how mutations of this gene lead to multiple autoimmune disorders. With expression of AIRE message in the thymus, a site of T cell development, it is likely that abnormalities of T-cell selection will underlie susceptibility. Of note, in this syndrome, HLA alleles appear not to contribute to susceptibility or protection from disease. Thus, AIRE mutations may bypass the normal influence of HLA molecules on T-cell selection.

In contrast to APS-I, APS-II is strongly HLA-associated. Non-HLA genes in APS-II probably influence the maintenance of tolerance to multiple tissues. In both syndromes, the specific disorders that develop in an individual are not "predictable." This may be owing to the interaction of environmental factors, but we believe it is more likely that "chaotic" or random events will underlie these differences.

Clinically, many of the disorders associated with APS-I and APS-II can be readily treated. For example, the administration of vitamin B_{12} in a patient with pernicious anemia prevents neuropathies, which in untreated patients can become irreversible. Patients with celiac disease are treated with diets lacking wheat proteins. Such diets are reported to decrease the risk of fatal gastrointestinal malignancies. As immunogenetic and immunologic disease prediction improves, early therapy becomes likely and, in the long-term, trials for disease prevention.

ACKNOWLEDGMENTS

This work was supported by a grant from the Foundation St. Luc (U.C.L.) and from the ESPE (M.M) and by an NIH grant (R37DK32083, R01DK32493, R01DK450979, R01DK55969) and Clinical Research Units for adults (5M01RR00051) and children (M01RR00069).

REFERENCES

1. Muir A, Schatz DA, Maclaren NK. Polyglandular failure syndromes. In: DeGroot LJ, Besser M, Burger HG, Jameson JL, eds. Endocrinology. W.B. Saunders, Philadelphia, 1995, pp. 3013–3024.

2. Garg SK, Kligensmith GJ, Eisenbarth GS. Autoimmune polyendocrine syndromes. In: Eisenbarth GS, Lafferty KG, eds. Type 1 Diabetes Mellitus: Molecular, Cellular, and Clinical Immunology. Oxford University Press, Oxford, 1996, pp. 153–171.
3. Brosman P, Riley WJ. Autoimmune polyglandular syndromes. In: Sperling MA, ed. Pediatric Endocrinology. W.B. Saunders, Phiadelphia, 1996, pp. 509–522.
4. Verge CF, Eisenbarth GS. Immunoendocrinopathy syndromes. In: Wilson JD, Foster DW, eds. Williams Textbook of Endocrinology, 9th ed. W. B. Saunders, Philadelphia, 1997, pp. 1651–1662.
5. Neufeld M, Maclaren NK, Blizzard RM. Two types of autoimmune Addison's disease associated with different polyglandular autoimmune (PGA) syndromes. Medicine 1981;60:355–362.
6. Ahonen P, Myllarniemi S, Sipila I, Perheentupa J. Clinical variation of autoimmune polyendocrinopathy-candidiasis-ectodermal dystrophy (APECED) in a series of 68 patients. N Engl J Med 1990;322:1829–1836.
7. Perheentupa J. Autoimmune polyendocrinopathy-candidiasis-ectodermal dystrophy (APECED). Horm Metab Res 1996;28:353–356.
8. Aaltonen J, Bjorses P, Sandkuijl L, Perheentupa J, Peltonen L. An autosomal locus causing autoimmune polyglandular disease type I assigned to chromosome 21. Nat Genet 1994;8:83–87.
9. Nagamine K, Peterson P, Scott H, et al. Positional cloning of the APECED gene. Nat Genet 1997;17:393–398.
10. The Finnish-German APECED consortium. An autoimmune disease, APECED, caused by mutations in a novel gene featuring two PHD-type zinc-finger domains. Nat Genet 1997;17:399–403.
11. Theofilopoulos AN. The basis of autoimmunity: part I: Mechanisms of aberrant self-recognition. Immunol Today 1995;16:90–98.
12. Theofilopoulos AN. The basis of autoimmunity: part II: Genetic predisposition. Immunol Today 1995;16:150–159.
13. Zlotogora J, Shapiro MS. Polyglandular autoimmune syndrome type I among Iranian jews. J Med Genet 1992;29:824–826.
14. Belvisi L, Bombelli F, Sironi L, Doldi N. Organ specific autoimmunity in patients with premature ovarian failure. J Endocrinol Invest 1993;16:889–892.
15. Ahonen P, Koskimies M, Lokki M-L, Tilikainen A, Perheentupa J. The expression of autoimmune polyglandular disease type I appears associated with several HLA-A antigens but not with HLA-DR. J Clin Endocrinol Metab 1988;66:1152–1157.
16. Bjorses P, Aaltonen J, Vikman A, et al. Genetic homogeneity of autoimmune polyglandular disease type I. Am J Med Genet 1996;879–886.
17. Como JA, Dismukes WE. Oral azole drugs as systemic antifungal therapy. N Engl J Med 1994;330:263–272.
18. Ahonen P, Myllarniemi S, Kahanpaa A, et al. Ketoconazole is effective against the chronic mucocutaneous candidiasis of the autoimmune polyendocrinopahy-candidiasis-ectodermal dystrophy (APECED). Acta Med Scand 1986;220:333–339.
19. Schmidt MB. Eine biglandulare erkrankung (nebennieren und schilddrusse) bei morbus Addisonii. Verh Dtsch Ges Pathol Ges 1926;21:212–221.
20. Carpenter CCJ, Solomon N, Silverberg SG, et al. Schmidt's syndrome (thyroid and adrenal insufficiency): a review of the litterature and a report of fifteen new cases inckuding 10 instances of coexistent diabetes mellitus. Medicine 1964;43:153–180.
21. Roitt IM, Doniach D, Campbell PN, et al. Autoantibodies in Hashimoto's disease (lymphadenoid goitre). Lancet 1956;2:820–821.
22. Turkington RW, Lebowitz HE. Extra-adrenal endocrine deficiencies in Addison's disease. Am J Med 1967;43:499–507.
23. Zelissen PM, Bast EJEG, Croughs RJM. Associated autoimmunity in Addison's disease. J Autoimmunity 1995;8:121–130.
24. Dumas P, Archambeaud-Mouveroux F, Vallat JM. Myasthenia gravis associated with adrenocortical insufficiency. Report of two cases. J Neurol 1985;232:354–356.
25. Okada T, Kawamura T, Tamura T, et al. Myasthenia gravis associated with Addison's disease. Intern Med 1994;33:686–688.
26. Hooft C, Roels H, Devos E. Diabetes and coeliac disease. Lancet 1969;ii:1192.
27. Peserico A, Rigon F, Semsenzato G, et al. Vitiligo and polyglandular autoimmune disease with autoantibodies to melanin-producing cells. A new syndrome? Arch Dermatol 1981;117:751–752.
28. Tucker WS, Niblack GD, McLean RH, Alspaugh MA, Wyatt RJ, Jordan SC, et al. Serositis with autoimmune endocrinopathy: clinical and immunogenetic features. Medicine 1987;66:138–147.

29. Irvine WJ, Davies SH, Delamore IW, et al. Immunological relationship between pernicious anemia and thyroid disease. Br Med J 1962;5302:454–456.
30. Verge CF, Howard NJ, Rowley MJ, et al. Anti-glutamate decarboxylase and other antibodies at the onset of childhood IDDM: a population-based study. Diabetologia 1994;37:1113–1120.
31. Savilahti E, Simell O, Koskimies K, et al. Celiac disease in inslulin-dependent diabetes mellitus. J Pediatr 1986;108:690–693.
32. Barera G, Bianchi C, Calisti L, et al. Screening of diabetic children for coeliac disease with antigliadin antibodies and HLA typing. Arch Dis Child 1991;66:491–494.
33. Ferreira M, Davies SL, Buttler M, et al. Endomysial antibody: is it the best screening test for coeliac disease? Gut 1992;33:1633–1637.
34. Mora S, Weber G, Barera G, et al. Effect of a gluten-free diet on bone mineral content in growing patients with coeliac disease. Am J Clin Nutr 1993;57:224–228.
35. Holmes GKT, Prior P, Lane MR, et al. Malignancy in coeliac disease-effect of a gluten-free diet. Gut 1989;30:333–338.
36. Posillico JT, Worstman J, Srikanta S, et al. Parathyroid cell surface autoantibodies that inhibit parathyroid hormone secretion from dispersed human parathyroid cells. Bone Miner Res 1986;5:475–485.
37. Eisenbarth GS, Wilson P, Ward F, et al. HLA type and disease occurence in familial polyglandular failure. N Engl J Med 1978;298:92–94.
38. Partanen J, Peterson P, Westman P, et al. Major Histocompatibilty Complex Class I and II in Addison's disease. Hum Immunol 1994;41:135–140.
39. Badenhoop K, Walfish PG, Rau H, et al. Susceptibility and resistance alleles of human lucocyte antigen (HLA) DQA1 and HLA DQB1 are shared in autoimmune disease. J Clin Endocrinol Metab 1995; 80:2112–2117.
40. Maclaren NK, Riley WJ. Inherited susceptibility to autoimmune Addison's disease is linked to human leucocyte antigens DR3 and/or DR4 except whe associated with type I autoimmune polyglandular syndrome. J Clin Endocrinol Metab 1986;62:455–459.
41. Yu L, Brewer K, Gates S, et al. Immunogenetic determinants of Addison's disease among patients with 21-hydroxylase autoantiodies. J Clin Endocrinol Metab 1999Jan;84(1):328–335.
42. Faas S, Trucco M. Major Histocompatibility Locus and other genes that determine the risk of development of insulin-dependent diabetes mellitus. In: Leroith D, Taylor SI, Olefsky JM, eds. Diabetes Mellitus. Lippincott-Raven, Philadelphia, 1996, pp. 326–333.
43. Fisfalen M-E, DeGroot LJ. Graves' disease and autoimmune thyroiditis. In: Weintraub B, ed. Molecular Endocrinology. Raven Press, New York, 1995, pp. 319–370.
44. Volonakis JE, Zhu Z, Schaffer FM, et al. Major Histocompatibilty Class II genes and susceptibility to immunoglobulin A deficiency and common variable immunodeficiency. J Clin Invest 1992;89: 1914–1922.
45. Reijonen H, Ilonen J, Knip M, et al. Insulin-dependent diabetes mellitus associated with dermatitis herpetiformis: evidence for heterogeneity of HLA-associated genes. Tissue Antigens 1991;37:94–96.
46. Baisch JM, Weeks T, Gilles R, et al. Analysis of HLA-DQ genotypes and susceptibility in insulin-dependent diabetes mellitus. N Engl J Med 1990;322:1836–1841.
47. Thomson G, Robinson WP, Kuhner MK, et al. Genetic heterogeneity, modes of inheritance, and risk of estimates for a joint study of Caucasians with insulin-dependent diabetes mellitus. Am J Hum Genet 1988;43:799–816.
48. Santamaria P, Barbosa JJ, Lindstrom AL, et al. HLA-DQB1-associated susceptibility that distinguishes Hashimoto's thyroiditis from Graves' disease in Type 1 diabetic patients. J Clin Endocrinol Metab 1994;878–883.
49. Inoue D, Sato K, Sugawa H, et al. Apparent genetic difference between hypothyroid patients with blocking type thyrtropin receptor antibody and those without, as shown by restriction fragment length polymorphism analyses of HLA-DP loci [see comments]. J Clin Endocrinol Metab 1993;77:606–610.
50. Bennett ST, Lucassen AM, Gough SCL, et al. Susceptibilty to human type I diabetes mellitus at IDDM2 is determined by tandem repeat variation at the insulin gene minisatellite locus. Nat Genet 1995;9:284–292.
51. McLachlan SM. The genetic basis of autoimmune thyroid disease: time to focus on chromosomal loci other than the histocompatibity complex (HLA in man) [editorial]. J Clin Endocrinol Metab 1995;77:605a–605c.
52. Hershman JM. Does thyroxine therapy prevent recurrence of Graves' hyperthyroidism [editorial]? J Clin Endocrinol Metab 1995;80:1479–1480.
53. McGregor AM. Autoantibodies to the TSH receptor in patients with autoimmune thyroid disease. Clin Endocrinol 1990;33:683–685.

54. Valente WA, Vitti P, Yavin Z, Yavin E, Rotella CM, Grollman EF, et al. Monoclonal antibodies to the thyrotropin receptor: stimulating and blocking antibodies derived from lymphocytes of patients with Graves' disease. Proc Natl Acad Sci USA 1982;79:6680–6684.
55. Uibo R, Perheentupa J, Ovod V, Krohn KJE. Characterization of adrenal autoantigens recognized by sera from patients with autoimmune polyglandular syndrome type I. J Autoimmun 1994;7:399–441.
56. Betterle C, Volpato M, Smith BR, et al. Adrenal cortex and steroid 21-hydroxylase autoantibodies in children with organ-specific autoimmune diseases: markers of high progression to clinical Addison's disease. J Clin Endocrinol Metab 1997;82:939–942.
57. Falorni A, Laureti S, Nikoshkov A, et al. 21-hydroxylase autontibodies in adult patients with endocrine autoimmune diseases are highly specific for Addison's disease. Clin Exp Immunol 1997;107:341–346.
58. Tanaka H, Perez MS, Powell M, et al. Steroid 21-hydroxylase autoantibodies: measurements with a new immunoprecipitation assay. J Clin Endocrinol Metab 1997;82:1440–1446.
59. Chen S, Sawicka J, Betterle C, et al. Autoantibodies to steroidogenic enzymes in autoimmune polyglandular syndrome, Addsion's disease, and premature ovarian failure. J Clin Endocrinol Metab 1996;81:1871–1876.
60. Anderson JR, Goudie RB, Gray K, et al. Immunological features of idiopathic Addison's disease: an antibody to cells producing steroid hormones. Clin Exp Immunol 1968;3:107–117.
61. Uibo R, Aavik E, Peterson P, Perheentupa J, Aranko S, Pelkonen P, et al. Autoantibodies to cyochrome P450 enzymes P450scc, P450c17, and P450c21 in autoimmune polyglandular disease type I and II and in isolated Addison's disease. J Clin Endocrinol Metab 1994;78:323–328.
62. Betterle C, Rossi A, Dalla Pria S, et al. Premature ovarian failure: autoimmunity and natural history. Clin Endocrinol 1993;39:35–43.
63. Verge CF, Giannani R, Kawasaki E, et al. Prediction of Type 1 diabetes mellitus in first degree relatives using a combination of insulin, glutamic acid decarboxylase and ICA512bdc/IA2 autoantibodies. Diabetes 1996;45:926–933.
64. Wagner R, Genovese S, Bosi E, et al. Slow metabolic deterioration towards diabetes in islet cell antibody positive patients with autoimmune polyendocrine disease. Diabetologia 1994;37:365–371.
65. Gianani R, Pugliese A, Bonner-Weir S, et al. Prognostically significant heterogeneity of cytoplasmic islet cell antibodies in relatives of patients with Type 1 diabetes. Diabetes 1992;41:347–353.
66. Genovese S, Bonifacio E, McNally JM, et al. Distinct cytoplasmic islet cell antibodies with different risks for type I (insulin-dependent) diabetes mellitus. Diabetologia 1992;35:385–388.
67. Christie MR, Genovese S, Cassidy D, et al. Antibodies to islet 37k antigen, but not to glutamate decarboxylase, discriminate rapid progression to IDDM in endocrine autoimmunity. Diabetes Metab Rev 1994;43:1254–1259.
68. Rabin DU, Peasic SM, Shapiro JA, et al. Islet cell antigen 512 is a diabetes-specific islet autoantigen related to protin tyrosine phosphatases. J Immunol 1994;152:3183
69. Wasmeier C, Hutton J. Molecular cloning of phogrin, a homologue localized to insulin secretory granule membranes. J Biol Chem 1996;71:18,161–18,170.
70. Kawasaki E, Eisenbarth GS, Wasmeier C, Hutton JC. Autoantibodies to protein tyrosine phosphatase-like proteins in type I diabetes: overlapping specificities to phogrin and ICA512/IA-2. Diabetes Metab Rev 1996;45:1344–1349.
71. Berger R, Schmidt G. Evaluation of six anti-gliadin antibody assays. J Immunol Methods 1996;191:77–86.
72. Chan KN, Phillips AD, Mirakian R, Walker-Smith JA. Endomysial antibody screening in children. J Pediatr Gastroenterol Nutr 1994;18:316–320.
73. Karsaka K, Tuckova L, Steiner L, Tlaskalova-Hogenova H, Michalak M. Calreticulin-he potential autoantigen in celiac disease. Biochem Biophys Res Commun 1995;209:597–605.
74. Dietrich W, Ehnis T, Bauer M, Donner P, Volta U, Riecken EO, et al. Identification of tissue transglutaminase as the autoantigen of celiac disease. Nature Med 1997;3:797–801.
75. Li Y, Song YH, Rais N, Connor E, Schatz D, Muir A, et al. Autoantibodies to the extracellular domain of the calcium sensing receptor in patients with acquired hypoparathyroidism. J Clin Invest 1996;97:910–914.
76. Toh B-H, Van Driel IR, Gleeson PA. Pernicious anemia. N Engl J Med 1997;337:1441–1448.
77. Clemente MG, Obermayerstraub P, Meloni A, Strassburg CP, Arangino V, Tukey RH, et al. Cytochrome P450 1A2 is a hepatic autoantigen in autoimmune polyglandular syndrome Type 1. J Clin Endocrinol Metab 1997;82:1353–1361.
78. Fairchild RS, Schimke RN, Abdou NI. Immunoregulation abnormalities in familial Addison's disease. J Clin Endocrinol Metab 1980;51:1074–1077.
79. Kaffe S, Petigrow CS, Cahill LT, et al. Variable cell-mediated immune defects in a family with "Candida endocrinopathy syndrome." Exp Clin Immunogenetics 1975;20:397–401.

16 Autoimmune Endocrinopathies in Female Reproductive Dysfunction

Antonio R. Gargiulo, MD, and Joseph A. Hill, MD

CONTENTS

> INTRODUCTION
> DISORDERS OF GONADAL STEROIDOGENESIS AND GAMETOGENESIS
> DISORDERS OF IMPLANTATION AND PLACENTATION
> HORMONE-DEPENDENT CONDITIONS
> SUMMARY
> REFERENCES

INTRODUCTION

Reproductive medicine is a discipline that deals with a peculiar set of organ systems whose concerted action is essential to species perpetuation. This discipline thrives on the intellectual contributions of biomedical researchers with diverse backgrounds. Reproductive endocrinology and reproductive immunology are two closely related fields of reproductive medicine that study the role of the endocrine and the immune systems in reproduction. The close association between these two specialties is further underlined by the practical consideration that currently many clinical reproductive immunologists have a background in either internal medicine or obstetrics and gynecology.

Many features set the endocrine glands involved in reproductive processes apart. First, in the gonads, endocrine and gametogenic functions coexist and are deeply intertwined. Therefore the clinician approaching ovarian and testicular endocrinopathies must be cognizant of the correlated reproductive dysfunctions. Second, some pivotal reproductive endocrine glands, such as the dominant ovarian follicle, the corpus luteum, and the placenta, are ephemeral structures. These transitory organs have an intrinsic dynamism as they proceed through a well timed ontogeny. Finally, as a teleologic corollary to the concept that reproduction is not essential to the individual's survival, failure of reproductive endocrine functions does not generally translate into life-threatening disease.

Several aspects of immune physiology within reproductive organs are also unique. Prime examples are the survival of the semiallogenic conceptus in an immune-competent woman, and the development within immunologic sanctuaries of male gametes bearing new antigenic surface molecules long after the establishment of self from nonself. Both

From: *Contemporary Endocrinology: Autoimmune Endocrinopathies*
Edited by: R. Volpe © Humana Press Inc., Totowa, NJ

of these are active and dynamic processes whose derangement may result in reproductive failure.

This chapter will discuss the clinical endocrinologic and rheumatologic applications of reproductive immunology. In particular, we will focus on those hormonal and hormone-dependent conditions contributing to reproductive failure through an autoimmune mechanism. Conversely, alloimmune causes of reproductive failure, comprising a number of highly controversial issues with scarce endocrinologic implications, will not be discussed here.

In consideration of the interdependence of endocrine and gametogenic function within the gonads, our discussion will include autoimmune factors that may affect both, thereby impairing steroidogenesis and fertility. Premature ovarian failure will be presented as a prime example of autoimmune gonadal derangement.

Failure to achieve or maintain the pregnant state during the reproductive years may also in certain cases be viewed as a derangement of female endocrine physiology. Indeed, the feto-placental unit clearly fulfills the characteristics of a classic endocrine gland. Therefore, autoimmune issues potentially contributing to abnormal implantation or placentation will also be presented. However, in keeping with the highly specialized context of this chapter, our coverage of nonendocrine autoimmune causes of infertility, as well as that of strictly obstetrical issues, will be limited.

Finally, we will describe the controversial role of autoimmunity in endometriosis, which is dependent on ovarian endocrine function, and which in turn may be a factor in reproductive failure and decreased ovarian reserve.

In summary, this chapter proposes to offer a scientific overview of a few major concepts of reproductive immunology of potential practical use to the clinical endocrinologist and rheumatologist. As clinical reproductive endocrinologists, we have intended this review as a tool to foster effective clinical cooperation with our medical colleagues. The sections of this chapter are arranged according to the facets of reproductive function being affected:

1. Steroidogenesis/gametogenesis and fertilization.
2. Implantation/placentation.
3. Other hormone-dependent conditions.

For each section, fundamentals of reproductive physiology and their immunologic correlates are briefly reviewed, followed by clear nosologic definitions, and by the available evidence for an autoimmune etiology. Finally, a critical review of the specific therapeutic interventions is offered, concluding with our current management recommendations.

DISORDERS OF GONADAL STEROIDOGENESIS AND GAMETOGENESIS

Premature Ovarian Failure (POF)

Hypergonadotropic hypogonadism is a physiologic state in women when it presents as persistent secondary amenorrhea occurring at the median age of 51 yr *(1)*. The onset of menopause at age 43 lies 2 standard deviations below the mean. According to conventional medical statistics, 2.5% of women will experience cessation of ovarian function before age 43, which is labeled as abnormal. However, the classic definition of POF is even more conservative: the unphysiologic cessation of menses between puberty and age 40 *(2)*. A more modern description of the condition suggests that the onset of gonadal failure can precede or usher puberty, thereby presenting as primary amenorrhea *(3)*.

The estimated incidence of POF defined by these criteria is approx 1% *(4)*. Several pathophysiologic mechanisms can lead to the end result of untimely follicular exhaustion, with resulting anovulatory infertility and hypoestrogenism. These include chromosomal, genetic, enzymatic, iatrogenic, infectious, and immunologic factors *(5)*.

The association of POF with several autoimmune diseases has been discussed since the 1950s, with an average reported frequency of 17% *(6)*. Currently, several lines of evidence indicate that in some cases, idiopathic POF is the result of an autoimmune process directed against the hormone-secreting cells of the ovarian follicles, much in the same way as other destructive autoimmune endocrinopathies, such as Addison's disease or type 1 diabetes mellitus. Two distinct clinical scenarios can be identified for which different levels of evidence pointing at an autoimmune etiology are available: (1) idiopathic POF associated with manifestations of adrenal autoimmunity; and (2) idiopathic POF with exclusive manifestations of ovarian autoimmunity.

IDIOPATHIC POF WITH MANIFESTATIONS OF ADRENAL AUTOIMMUNITY

Addison's disease results from hypofunction of the adrenal gland occurring when more than 90% of the adrenal cortex is destroyed by an infectious, neoplastic, or autoimmune process. In developed countries, the prevalence is 3–6/100,000 with the autoimmune etiology accounting for over 80% of cases *(7)* (*see* Chapter 13).

Clearly, isolated autoimmune Addison's disease represents the exception rather than the rule. More often, the condition is found in association with other endocrinopathies as well as other organ damage owing to autoimmunity. Such multiorgan autoimmune syndromes are known as autoimmune polyglandular syndromes (APGS) of which two distinct forms are currently recognized (*see* Chapter 15). APGS type 1, also known as Blizzard's syndrome, or autoimmune polyendocrinopathy-candidiasis-ectodermal dystrophy (APECED), is an extremely rare autosomal-recessive disorder. Major components of this syndrome are chronic mucocutaneous candidiasis (73–100%), Addison's disease (72–100%), and hypoparathyroidism (79–76%). Premature ovarian failure is the most common of the other associated endocrinopathies (17–60%) *(8,9)*. APGS type 2, originally termed Schmidt's syndrome, describes Addison's disease (100%) in association with autoimmune thyroid disease (69%), type 1 diabetes mellitus (52%), gonadal failure (4%), and other rarer autoimmune features *(9,10)*. APSG type 2 is an autosomal-dominant disorder with incomplete penetrance, in which affected siblings often display different components of the syndrome.

Approximately one fourth of women with idiopathic Addison's disease develop amenorrhea in the course of the disease, and 10% have POF *(11,12)*. Conversely, when POF is studied as the index disorder, 2–10% of cases are associated with idiopathic Addison's and/or serologic evidence of adrenal autoimmunity *(6)*.

A very important step in the characterization of idiopathic Addison's disease as an autoimmune disease has been the discovery that peripheral serum from these individuals contains immunoglobulins that specifically bind antigens on human adrenal cortex, as identified on cryostat sections by indirect immunofluorescence assays (IIF). Two varieties of binding activity have been identified: adrenal autoantibodies (AA) with exclusive specificity for the adrenal cortex, and steroid cell autoantibodies (SCA), which cross-react with other steroidogenic tissues, namely, placental syncytiotrophoblast,

Leydig areas of testis, and the theca interna/granulosa layers of ovarian follicles *(12–14)*. SCA seropositivity has only been found if AA were also present.

More recently, some of the molecular targets of AA and SCA have been characterized through immunoblotting techniques as microsomal enzymes catalyzing key steps of steroid hormone synthesis. Particularly, cytochrome p450 enzyme 21 hydroxylase, an adrenal-specific antigen, appears as the natural target responsible for the AA binding observed with IIF *(15,16)*. Other microsomal components that are also present in gonads and placenta, such as cytochrome p450 17-α-hydroxylase and cytochrome p450 side-chain cleavage enzyme, probably represent the main SCA targets *(17–19)* (*see* Chapter 8). More recently, Arif et al. screened an adrenal complementary DNA expression library using SCA-positive serum from a patient with idiopathic POF and no evidence of Addison's disease *(20)*. They identified recombinant 3β-hydroxysteroid dehydrogenase (3βOHSD) as the target of SCA in this patient, which was confirmed by loss of SCA detectability after absorption of the SCA-positive serum with recombinant 3βOHSD. The authors then tested SCA-negative sera from another 47 patients with idiopathic POF and no evidence of Addison's, and found that autoantibodies to 3βOHSD were detected by immunoblot in 21% of these women compared to 5% of healthy controls ($P = 0.002$). The study also tested small groups of patients with known autoimmune endocrinopathies (AA-positive Addison's, autoimmune thyroiditis, and type 1 diabetes mellitus) and found evidence of autoantibodies to 3βOHSD in 0, 17, and 23% of patients in these three groups, respectively. The authors concluded that their study had identified 3βOHSD as the target of SCA, which has been typically associated with POF. However, in women with idiopathic POF not associated with Addison's, as was the case in this study, SCA is rarely positive *(21)*. In fact, the autoantibody identified in this study was associated with idiopathic POF, but not with SCA: only 1 out of 10 patients in whom the 3βOHSD autoantibody was detected by immunoblot also had detectable SCA activity as detected with IIF. This would imply that molecular biology techniques are proving to be more accurate and sensitive tools than IIF to define the nature of autoantibody targets in steroid-secreting cells. Eventually, terms like SCA and AA are likely to be abandoned in favor of more specific panels of antibodies to steroidogenic cell antigens. Further studies are needed to correlate the presence of such specific autoantibodies to autoimmune conditions. Data accumulated thus far with SCA support the hypothesis of an autoimmune etiology for a number of cases of idiopathic POF, and provide important prognostic information *(22)*. However, SCA are not good markers of POF as such, although when POF is associated with Addison's disease, the frequency of SCA is very high (60–80% of subjects) *(14,22,23)*. The presence of SCA is therefore a marker for the association of Addison's disease and POF. In the few SCA-positive POF patients without adrenal insufficiency, longitudinal observation reveals a high risk of progression to adrenal insufficiency *(24,25)*. Thus, close observation of adrenal function in these individuals over the years is warranted to allow early diagnosis of autoimmune adrenocortical failure. The progression of multiglandular failure in these women is generally slow. A recent study in which 119 women with idiopathic POF underwent a one-time screening for adrenal, thyroid, and pancreatic islet function could not identify any cases of subclinical adrenal failure *(26)*.

The reciprocal is also true; SCA-positive Addison's patients without POF are at high risk for developing ovarian failure, although the latency period is substantial *(25,27,28)*. The long latency period from the appearance of circulating autoantibodies (SCA) and the clinically apparent condition (POF) is typical of the natural history of autoimmune conditions: this observation further supports the autoimmune nature of some cases of idiopathic POF.

Because of the fact that ovarian biopsies should not be performed, studies of ovarian histopathology in patients with idiopathic POF are primarily historical. Moreover, the poorly predictable progression of the disease makes it difficult to obtain ovarian tissue during acute exacerbations. Nonetheless, the available data in SCA-positive POF patients indicate that lymphocytic oophoritis is a consistent finding (for a complete review of published pathology case series, *see* ref. 29). $CD4^+$ and $CD8^+$ T lymphocytes are the primary immune cells infiltrating the ovary in these patients. Plasma cells also abound, but B lymphocytes and antigen-presenting cells are less common. T lymphocytes and plasma cells surround virtually all follicles that are beyond the primordial stage, and increase in number around more mature and active steroid-secreting follicles *(30–32)*. Most interestingly, granulosa cells of patients with POF have been shown to respond in vitro to interferon γ (IFN-γ) with *de novo* surface expression of class II major histocompatibility complex (MHC) molecules *(33)*. One can therefore hypothesize that in vivo the Th1 subset of $CD4^+$ T cells infiltrating the ovarian cortex induce, via paracrine secretion of IFN-γ, the expression of MHC class II on granulosa cells. MHC class II molecules allow the granulosa cells to act as antigen-presenting cells to the T lymphocytes, thereby potentiating the local autoimmune response.

Several animal models of experimental autoimmune oophoritis exist, which even with the limitations of interspecies data extrapolation, have provided strong support to the hypothesis of an autoimmune etiology of POF in SCA-positive patients. Two of these models in particular, neonatal thymectomy in mice and thymocyte transfer to athymic nude mice, have highlighted a significant relationship between the thymus gland and reproductive function. In the murine neonatal thymectomy model, organ-specific autoimmune derangement, including oophoritis, is observed when thymectomy is performed between days 2 and 5 of life *(34–36)*. Observations of ovarian follicle depletion in athymic girls *(37)* and in newborn rhesus monkeys thymectomized *in utero (38)* indicate that the murine models may have functional correlates in primates. The current hypothesis proposes that autoimmunity is avoided in euthymic animals by active production of $CD4^+$ thymic lymphocytes with suppressor activity, which counteract the effect of naturally occurring effector autoimmune $CD4^+$ T cells. The thymus generates and exports T cells of both suppressor and effector types. However, the former type appears later in fetal life. Early thymectomy may therefore create an unbalanced state in which the suppressor/effector T-cell ratio is severely decreased. This altered balance is also demonstrated by the induction of autoimmune oophoritis in mice that are recipients of circulating $CD4^+$ T cells from thymectomized donors *(39,40)*. Very significant is the constant appearance of circulating ovarian, although not adrenal, autoantibodies in this animal model. Such autoantibodies, which include steroid-secreting cell antibodies, eventually become undetectable in some animals once ovarian atrophy has been established *(34–36)*. Extrapolation of these findings to the human suggests that depending on the time in the course of the disease in which the patient with POF presents to medical attention, SCA may not be detectable despite an autoimmune etiology. In keeping with the lack of adrenal antibodies, there is no histologic evidence of adrenal autoimmunity in the mice neonatal thymectomy model. Otherwise, the pattern of lymphocyte infiltration at the level of the ovary is strikingly similar to that described in SCA-positive women with POF. Identical histologic findings are described in the model of thymocyte transfer to athymic nude mice, in which CD4+/CD8− thymocytes from normal mice are transferred to athymic mice, causing autoimmune oophoritis in 50–75% of the recipients *(41)*.

Assessing genetic susceptibility in POF patients with associated adrenal autoimmunity is complicated by the separate susceptibility for the adrenal component (and potentially for other components of APGS). The gene responsible for APGS type 1 has been mapped to chromosome 21 *(42)* and may soon be identified.

In conclusion, several lines of evidence support the hypothesis that POF, when associated with serological or clinical evidence of adrenal autoimmunity, is an autoimmune endocrinopathy. The presence of autoantibodies *per se* is not a major factor in support of this model, since it does not prove causality. However, the epidemiological and pathological data, and the observations on the time-course of autoimmune oophoritis in available animal models together suggest that such antibodies against key steroidogenic enzymes of the adrenal and/or ovary may be involved in the pathogenesis of the disease.

IDIOPATHIC POF WITH EXCLUSIVE MANIFESTATIONS OF OVARIAN AUTOIMMUNITY

The majority of women with presumed autoimmune ovarian failure (90–98%) neither have Addison's disease nor SCA *(6)*. The pathogenesis of these cases remains uncertain. One major issue that would argue against the involvement of autoimmunity in these cases is the fact that the aforementioned lymphocytic infiltration is consistently absent. Follicular atrophy is a distinctive histologic feature in 60% of cases, but some residual follicular presence is observed in the remainder. In about 10% of cases of idiopathic POF not associated with Addison's disease, numerous ovarian follicles remain. These cases are probably best classified as secondary forms of the resistant ovary syndrome (ROS), a heterogeneous clinical syndrome of hypergonadotropic amenorrhea in karyotypically normal women with identifiable ovarian follicles and relative insensitivity to ovulation induction with exogenous gonadotropins *(43)*. Autoimmunity is one of several proposed etiologies for ROS, none of which has been adequately substantiated to date.

Lack of lymphocytic infiltration and atrophy do not by themselves exclude the possibility of prior autoimmune damage leading to functional loss extending beyond the acute phase: in fact, evidence in favor of an autoimmune component even in this group of patients exists.

Even in the absence of an association with Addison's disease, antibodies to other endocrine and systemic antigens are found in some of these patients *(6)*. In particular, thyroid autoantibodies and autoimmune thyroid disease have been described in 14% of patients without adrenal autoimmunity.

Autoantibodies against ovarian steroid-secreting cells (SCA), however, are typically absent in these women when assessed with IIF *(14,23,28)*. However, more sensitive and specific detection assays have demonstrated in controlled studies that ovarian autoantibodies may be a feature of a substantial number of patients with isolated POF, as in the case of anti-3β OHSD activity *(20)*. In the absence of a classic histological picture of oophoritis, circulating antibodies may be the consequence rather than the cause of the disease.

Ovarian autoantibodies described in association with isolated POF are not limited to classic steroid-secreting cell antibodies or antibodies toward microsomal cytochrome enzymes. Antibodies against antigens of the zona pellucida surrounding the oocyte may also occur and be a factor in reproductive difficulty. ZP3 in particular is a sulfated glycoprotein antigen that functions as the primary sperm receptor at fertilization in the human *(44,45)*. Purified ZP3 antigens induce ovarian failure owing to follicular depletion in experimental murine autoimmune oophoritis, one of the few animal models potentially supporting the autoimmune nature of isolated idiopathic POF *(46,47)*. ZP3 is highly conserved among mammalian species *(46)*, and can be spread as a potentially sensitizing epitope throughout the individual life during the process of follicular atresia.

Blocking autoantibodies to gonadotropin receptors has been proposed as an autoimmune etiologic factor in isolated POF and in ROS. The data are inconclusive because most of the studies have employed binding assays with nonhuman tissue as the substrate, although recent data indicate poor interspecies overlap in gonadotropin receptor specificity *(48,49)*. The only study employing human recombinant luteinizing hormone (LH) and follicle-stimulating hormone (FSH) receptors as the substrate to test interference of hypothetic circulating autoantibodies could not demonstrate any binding in POF patients or in controls *(50)*.

Finally, in the absence of histologic evidence of immune cell involvement in the autoimmune processes potentially leading to isolated POF, several studies have compared peripheral levels of leukocytes between these patients and healthy volunteers to test the hypothesis that a cellular immune abnormality may be associated with the disease (reviewed in *29*). Studies on peripheral leukocytes have several intrinsic limitations that impair the interpretation of the data. In the specific case of POF, for example, the observed increase in activated peripheral T cells has been subsequently attributed to a stimulatory effect of hypoestrogenemia in these patients *(51)*.

Overall the data are somewhat suggestive of an autoimmune etiology in selected cases of isolated POF and ROS. Several important issues, however, remain unanswered, such as the role of peripheral leukocyte abnormalities and autoantibodies against gonadotropin receptors. Likewise, data derived from immunogenetic studies have been inconsistent: to date, no clear association has been demonstrated between POF and any specific human leukocyte antigen (HLA) haplotypes (the products of MHC class I and class II genes) *(52)*.

THERAPEUTIC CONSIDERATIONS

Ovum donation is the treatment of choice for infertility in women with POF. However, autoimmune ovarian failure is a waxing and waning disease susceptible to spontaneous remissions and occasional conceptions *(53)*. Thus, it is important to counsel patients that spontaneous conceptions can occur. Likewise, recognizing the autoimmune nature of ROS can be important in dictating the level of aggressiveness in the planning of infertility treatment, considering that complete follicular exhaustion may follow in time. Autoimmune ovarian failure may be amenable to treatment with immunomodulating agents *(54,55)*. However, these studies are controversial and did not address the possibility of spontaneous remissions. Finally, periodic screening for other autoimmune endocrinopathies should be considered in patients with idiopathic POF.

DISORDERS OF IMPLANTATION AND PLACENTATION

Autoantibodies in Recurrent Pregnancy Loss

In the singular self-limited physiologic state of pregnancy, an ephemeral endocrine gland, the placenta, forms at the maternal–fetal interface, whose target organ is the maternal organism. Placental hormones cause profound physical, biochemical, immunological, and neuropsychological modifications in the maternal host that are necessary for successful gestation. Unique to human pregnancy is the formidable increase in the level of circulating gonadal steroids following the luteal–placental shift owing to the high synthetic rates of placental syncytiotrophoblast. The secretory rate of estradiol-17β and progesterone in near-term pregnancy is 200 times higher than that observed during a normal menstrual cycle. Such massive placental steroidogenesis relies on the continued supply of precursors from the fetus and the mother for estrogen and progesterone production, respectively *(56)*. Human placentation is of the hemochorioendothelial type. This implies that maternal blood, carried to the placental intervillous space by the decidual spiral arteries, directly bathes the syncytiotrophoblast. Conversely, fetal blood is confined within the capillaries of the fetal villous syncytiotrophoblast at least until approx the 15th wk of gestation, when the vasculosyncytial membrane porosity allows maternal IgG antibodies to cross into the fetal circulation. Data have accumulated over the past 40 plus years characterizing the cellular and molecular basis of the maternal recognition of pregnancy. The discipline of reproductive immunology was founded with the first proposed conceptual analogy of the fetus as an allograft *(57)*. A comprehensive review of gestational immunology is beyond the scope of this chapter. Instead, the controversial clinical issue of recurrent pregnancy loss and evidence supporting a role for circulating autoantibodies in the pathophysiology of this condition will be presented.

Recurrent spontaneous abortion (RSA), classically defined as three or more consecutive pregnancy losses before 20 wk of gestation, affects 1–3% of couples/yr in the United States *(58)*. This definition of RSA has been challenged recently, since most clinicians currently recommend diagnostic evaluation following two consecutive spontaneous abortions. Given the high incidence of sporadic spontaneous abortion in the general population (occurring in 12% of pregnant women below age 20, and in 26% of those over age 40 *(59)*), it is important to consider that the incidence of RSA in our species is higher than that expected based on the spontaneous abortion rate *(60,61)*. This suggests that specific causes of repeated pregnancy failure exist. It is clear that RSA is not a specific disease, but rather a symptom that can be observed in association with several potential abortifacient conditions (reviewed in *(62)*). Particularly abundant are the proposed etiologic hypotheses involving immunologic mechanisms, which can be broadly grouped into autoimmune (immunity of the female partner against self-antigens) and alloimmune theories (immunity of the female partner against nonself antigens) *(63)*.

ANTIPHOSPHOLIPID ANTIBODIES

Of the proposed autoimmune etiologies for RSA that involves antiphospholipid antibodies is the only one to be substantiated by several lines of adequately controlled studies. The term antiphospholipid antibodies is highly generic, since the majority of these autoantibodies have no association with human disease. The pathogenesis of pregnancy failure in women with antiphospholipid antibodies has not been elucidated unequivocally. Thus, all current therapeutic interventions are based on hypothetic rationales and are therefore empirical.

Antiphospholipid antibodies are circulating autoantibodies of the IgG, IgM, and IgA classes whose epitopes bind negatively charged phospholipids. Approximately 2–4% of healthy individuals have some type of antiphospholipid antibody detectable in their blood. Testing for every isotype of every antibody will result in unacceptably high rates of false-positive findings *(64)*. This is because of the unstandardized nature of most of the antiphospholipid antibody assays. Many use 2.5 SD above the mean to represent a positive value that may occur in 5% of the general population. By definition, the probability that a test is positive in a certain patient by chance alone is $1-(0.95)^n$, where the power n is the number of independent tests performed. In the hypothetical case where the power is 1, the probability is 0.05. However, when several tests are performed on a single individual, the multiplicative rule of probability for independent events applies. For example, the calculated probability that an individual tested for 3 isotypes of 8 autoantibodies (24 tests total) will display positive levels of one of them by chance alone is 0.71. Even if we concede that positive results for the three isotypes of a given autoantibody are not independent events, but on the contrary, they are mutually inclusive events, the power of 8 tests at our arbitrary cutoff level will still result in a positive test being found in 34% of individuals by chance alone. This numerical phenomena should be kept in mind when reading the medical literature where this type of fatal flaw abounds. It also serves to highlight the fact that failure to include normal fertile controls drastically reduces the clinical relevance of any published series looking at prevalence of autoantibodies in a particular group of patients. Finally, it stresses the fundamental issues of test standardization and clinical laboratory quality *(65,66)*.

Antiphospholipid antibodies can be found in normal women. However, it is also possible that some of these antibodies may be associated with human disease. Primary antiphospholipid syndrome (APS) is a chronic condition that is by definition not associated with any rheumatologic disease, and is characterized clinically by:

1. Pregnancy loss;
2. Arterial or venous thrombosis;
3. Autoimmune thrombocytopenia; and
4. Biochemically by the presence of antiphospholipid autoimmunity, in the form of sustained moderate to high titers of anticardiolipin antibodies (aCL) or evidence of lupus anticoagulant activity (LA) *(67)*.

At least one clinical and one laboratory feature must be present to configure APS *(67)*. When systemic lupus erythematosus (SLE) or other less common rheumatologic conditions are also present, the condition is referred to as secondary APS *(68,69)*.

The frequent association of antiphospholipid antibodies with other less specific autoantibodies suggests that they may arise either as consequence of a generalized B-cell activation rather than as a response to a specific antigenic stimulus, or simply as an epiphenomenon, since there is no direct evidence for generalized B-cell activation. The ELISA for the detection of aCL and the clotting assays screening for LA measure closely related antibodies. Evidence suggests that these two tests are separating two distinct entities *(70,71)*. Since these two tests are not 100% concordant in the same patient, the current recommendation is to perform both when APS is suspected. A lupus anticoagulant test (LA) is either positive when clotting is prolonged beyond 2 SD above the control mean, or negative. Tests most commonly employed to screen for LA are the activated partial thromboplastin time (aPTT) or the more sensitive dilute Russell viper venom time (dRVVT) *(72)*. A positive result should be confirmed to rule out a specific clotting factor deficiency and to confirm the phospholipidic nature of the anticoagulant target. Only IgG and IgM isotypes are tested in standardized aCL ELISA. Titers should always be reported as negative, low-positive, medium-positive, or high-positive. This is of the utmost importance owing to recent evidence that only the last two have clinical significance *(73)*. Patients should not be labeled as APS and treated on the basis of low-positive IgM or IgG titers, or because of borderline positive LA. Other antiphospholipid antibodies, such as antiphosphatidylserine and antiphosphatidylethanolamine, have been described as possible factors in abnormal placentation *(74,75)*, but their association with pregnancy loss is not currently supported by clinical studies *(76)*, and their routine evaluation is not recommended outside of the research setting.

Conversely, a link between a positive LA (or moderate to high levels of aCL) and the clinical correlates of APS has been established by numerous retrospective studies. Patients with positive antiphospholipid antibodies are at high risk for thrombotic events, both venous and arterious in nature, which tend to occur in young patients and in relatively unusual locations *(68,77–79)*. The issue is particularly germane to reproductive medicine, because more than half of such vascular accidents occur during pregnancy and other hyperestrogenic states, such as early postpartum or in women on combination oral contraceptives *(80)*. APS in the setting of SLE is a particularly high-risk condition for vascular accidents with an estimated risk of 14 and 8% annually for venous and arterial thrombosis, respectively *(81)*.

Several appropriately controlled prospective and retrospective case series comparing the prevalence of LA and aCL IgG in normal women and in women with recurrent pregnancy loss have shown a significant association of these autoimmune markers with embryonic and fetal loss *(82–85)*. Overall it appears that second-trimester fetal loss, rather than early spontaneous abortion, is the condition most often associated with these autoantibodies *(86)* and that a high titer of IgG aCL is the best predictor of fetal loss *(87)*. Antiphospholipid antibodies are an infrequent cause of RSA (3% in the published series from the Center for Reproductive Medicine at Brigham and Women's Hospital *[88]*). Despite the rarity of the condition, screening for antiphospholipid antibodies in patients with RSA is important, because of the significant medical implications of the antiphospholipid syndrome and because the condition is potentially treatable *(64)*. On the contrary, the role of autoimmune factors in sporadic fetal loss is not supported by available studies *(89,90)*.

The pathophysiological mechanism underlying adverse pregnancy outcome in women with APS remains ill defined. The theory that microthrombotic events occur within the spiral arteries of the pregnant uterus is appealing because of the thrombophylic character of this condition. Indeed, in some patients with evidence of LA activity, deposition of aCL of the IgG subfraction has been demonstrated in decidual vessels by immunofluorescence *(91)*.

Damage on the placental side is also possible owing to the hemochorioendothelial architecture where maternal blood is in direct contact with trophoblastic villi. This is an early occurring event, since the feto-placental circulation is established by the end of the 5th wk of gestation. Antiphospholipid antibodies may theoretically disrupt a pregnancy even before this stage by acting on the delicate endometrial-trophoblastic paracrine milieu of the implantation-stage embryo. Placental thrombosis and infarction have been described, but their severity does not correlate with obstetrical outcome *(92,93)* Recent investigation suggests that several circulating plasma proteins can bind phospholipids. These lipoprotein complexes appear to represent the actual target of antiphospholipid antibodies, and may act as important cofactors in endothelial recognition and vascular damage *(94–97)*.

Maternal autoantibodies of the IgG class gain access to the fetal circulation after 15 wk of gestation *(98)*. Although not directly demonstrated in the fetal circulation, it is conceivable that endothelial cell activation by maternal antiphospholipid antibodies may initiate a thrombotic process in much the same way as described in the adult circulation *(99)*.

In the absence of a clearly defined etiologic factor, therapeutic recommendations have been based on data derived from empirically designed clinical trials. Anticoagulants, anti-inflammatory agents, and even iv immunoglobulin have been employed in various combinations. Many of these trials have lacked a control group, and very few were properly randomized. Another limitation hindering understanding of the disease process is that study populations may significantly differ by a factor that may not as yet have been determined. Recent evidence indicates that patients with low positive titers of antiphospholipid antibodies have similar prognosis as women without these antibodies *(73)*. However, several studies to date have included an unspecified number of this group of patients. This evidently constitutes a problem when comparing treatment groups within a study and between different studies.

Data derived from prospective controlled studies, with or without randomization, may guide us in the choice of the least harmful and most effective empirical treatment available to prevent fetal loss in women with primary or secondary APS.

The best evidence to date favors the use of sc heparin with low-dose oral ASA as an effective and overall safe protocol: low-dose ASA alone, however, does not appear to be protective *(100–103)*. Heparin has also been shown to bind aCL in vitro, which may be a factor in the observed drop of maternal aCL titers in many pregnancies proceeding to term *(103a)*. Our current therapeutic recommendations consist of chronic use of 81 mg of aspirin/d (for prevention of thromboembolic events), followed by 10,000–20,000 U of sc heparin/d once pregnancy is established. Alternatively, low- mol-wt (LMW) heparin 2500–5000 U once daily should be considered owing to the reduced dosing and the potential decreased osteoporosis risk *(104)*. An additional advantage of heparin over prednisone is that of providing protection against thrombotic events. Anticoagulation should be monitored by weekly assessment of aPTT until fine adjustment of the dose is reached, and pregnancies continuing beyond the first trimester should be followed by a maternal–fetal medicine specialist. Incidence of heparin-induced osteoporosis can also be limited by adopting a few general measures, such as an aerobic exercise routine and an adequate intake of calcium and vitamin D supplements. The empiric use of anticoagulants without evidence of the antiphospholipid syndrome is unjustified and potentially dangerous *(73)*. A matter of debate is the management of the primigravida with positive antiphospholipid antibodies. In addition to the need for periodic platelet counts to rule out autoimmune thrombocytopenia and aggressive monitoring of fetal well-being starting at the end of the second trimester *(105)*, there is no specific recommendation at this time. One could argue that in the presence of high-positive aCL IgG, some form of treatment could be sparing these patients the tragic experience of a fetal loss. As long as potential side effects are clearly discussed, heparin plus low-dose acetylsalicylate (ASA) should be considered.

Oral prednisone plus low-dose ASA has been shown by a recent study to be comparable to placebo in patients with two or more fetal losses, LA, and medium-high titers of aCL IgG *(106)*. If these results should be confirmed by a different group, then this protocol should become obsolete.

At this time, no compelling scientific data exist to indicate that intravenous immune globulins (IVIG) are effective in preventing fetal loss in patients with APS. The current literature offers only case reports and a small noncontrolled trials *(107–109)*. There are three randomized double-blind trials designed to assess the efficacy of IVIG in preventing unexplained recurrent pregnancy loss *(110–112)*, all of which were limited by insufficient statistical power, which would have allowed for a meaningful recommendation. Only one of these studies suggested that IVIG improved subsequent successful pregnancy *(111)*. The mechanism by which high iv doses of pooled foreign antibodies should modulate immune function also remains obscure. In light of the insufficient quality of evidence, the occasional severe medical complications *(113,114)*, and the formidable costs, there is currently no place for IVIG treatment in APS outside of a formal well-designed clinical trial.

OTHER AUTOANTIBODIES

Subclinical autoimmunity is a nebulous diagnosis that should imply that the affected patient has either serological evidence of an autoimmune response in the absence of a pathologic condition or a disease mimicking classic autoimmune conditions in the absence of serum markers of autoimmunity. In a rather improper way, however, it is sometime used to label patients with RSA in which circulating autoantibodies are detected. This is a different situation from both APS and the issue of nulliparous patients with antiphospholipid antibodies described previously. One of the main differences for example is the fact that 10–15% of normal pregnant women have detectable antinuclear antibodies (ANA), a number comparable to women with RSA *(115)*. Moreover, in the same study, the rate of pregnancy loss in the subsequent pregnancy was not different in the RSA group with higher ANA titers compared with the RSA group with negative ANA. In strict analogy, a large case-control study demonstrated that among patients with two consecutive antiphospholipid-negative unexplained spontaneous abortions, the 17.3% ANA-positive patients had a lower subsequent abortion rate compared with ANA-positive individuals *(116)*. When less strict criteria of titer cutoff are employed, up to 20% of healthy pregnant women will be ANA-positive *(117)*. More recently, a large case-control study reported a similar incidence of sporadic spontaneous abortion in ANA-positive women and matched controls *(118)*.

Other studies have reported an association between pregnancy loss and the presence of autoantibodies. Two such studies in particular have contributed to the myth of subclinical autoimmunity and should be mentioned. The study by Gleicher et al. *(119)* was a small uncontrolled descriptive study in which 33 separate autoantibody tests were performed. If one remembers how the multiplicative rule of probability for independent variables applies, the probability that at least one of the 33 tested variables would be positive by chance alone in a given subject could be as high as 0.82. The authors, however, speculated that polyclonal B cell activation may be causally related to recurrent pregnancy loss. A more recent, and even more controversial, study by Kwak et al. *(76)* suggested that the rate of pregnancy loss in women with autoantibodies could be significantly decreased by a regimen, including heparin, low-dose ASA, and prednisone. Not only was that study not randomized, but a high percentage of patients in the treatment groups also had antiphospholipid antibodies, which could explain the effectiveness of a treatment, including heparin and ASA. In summary, testing for ANA is a test of unacceptably low specificity in the absence of clear stigmata of connective tissue disorders. Prescribing corticosteroids or heparin on the basis of such nonspecific findings is a practice not supported by scientific evidence and appears unnecessarily hazardous in the absence of the APS. As far as more radical, and more costly, types of immunotherapy are concerned, the same considerations made for IVIG use in patients with APS apply here. Furthermore, there is evidence that paternal leukocyte immunization (PLI), a highly controversial and invasive immunotherapy practice without a scientific rationale (for review, *see 120,121*), significantly decreases successful pregnancy rates in patients with autoantibodies and therefore should be doubly contraindicated in these women *(122)*.

Antithyroglobulin and antithyroid-microsomal antibodies, commonly found in patients with Hashimoto's thyroiditis and Graves' disease, may be increased in women with a history of RSA, as indicated by some prospective studies *(123–125)*. One of the limitations of such studies, however, is the fact that other potential factors associated with RSA were not eliminated. It is possible that these antibodies are secondary to a generalized autoimmune status, although their presence in patients with recurrent pregnancy loss was higher compared to nonorgan-specific antibodies *(126)*. In consideration of the limited evidence of antithyroid antibody causality in RSA, and the lack of specific treatment, the current rationale to obtain antithyroid antibodies in RSA patients would be to screen for a subgroup at risk of developing hypothyroidism during a future pregnancy or postpartum. Of interest, thyroid function tests in RSA patients with positive antithyroid antibodies are generally normal *(125)*.

Autoantibodies in Unexplained Infertility

Infertility is a retrospective diagnosis based on a probabilistic rationale. According to the seminal epidemiologic work by Guttmacher on conception rate in a known fertile population, 85% of couples who conceived did so within 12 mo and 93% within 24 mo *(127)*. For clinical purposes, infertility has been conventionally defined as the failure to conceive over 12 mo of unprotected intercourse. A diagnostic evaluation to identify risk factors associated with infertility is performed, much in the same way as for couples with RSA. Unexplained infertility is a diagnosis of exclusion and one that is much less clearly delineated than that of infertility. Conceptually, in order to define unexplained infertility, all known factors possibly associated with infertility have to be eliminated. This means that, as new diagnostic tools become available and others become obsolete, the patient population identified and studied may vary. A prime example is the inclusion of diagnostic laparoscopy in the first-line diagnostic armamentarium of infertility specialists, which has gone in and out of vogue over the years. Another confounder in defining unexplained infertility is the duration of infertility in the given couple. Couples with unexplained infertility with fewer than 3 yr of duration have an 83% spontaneous pregnancy rate over the subsequent 24 mo, whereas couples whose period of infertility extends beyond 5 yr only have a 30% chance to conceive subsequently over the same period of time *(128)*. Therefore, comparable length of infertility between patient groups is a key factor in the design of any study involving patients with unexplained infertility.

The role of autoantibodies as a potential cause of unexplained infertility is particularly controversial. As described above, antiphospholipid antibodies have been convincingly associated with recurrent pregnancy loss and also, more specifically, with RSA. A very popular concept over recent years has been that the disruptive effect of such autoantibodies may affect the embryo in the preimplantion stage or in the early phases of implantation. As a consequence, preclinical implantation failure would occur despite successful fertilization, and a picture of unexplained infertility rather than RSA would result *(119)*. Moreover, this pathophysiological mechanism could not be overcome by current assisted reproduction technologies (ART), thereby affecting pregnancy rates in some patients. Studies assessing the role of antiphospholipid and other autoantibodies are broadly categorized into circumstantial observational evidence and evidence from

ART-related studies. An observational study that tested women's serum levels for IgG, IgM, and IgA autoantibodies to 11 separate self-antigens reported an 88% positivity of at least one test in the 26 patients with unexplained infertility *(119)*.

In addition to the statistical considerations examined before, the interpretation of this study is rendered difficult by the lack of appropriate controls. Taylor et al. *(53)* compared serum levels of IgG, IgM, and IgA autoantibodies against smooth muscle, nuclear, and phospholipid antigens: all of these were significantly greater in women with unexplained infertility. The quality of their control group, however, was questionable, being composed of women volunteers sampled during pregnancy. Finally, a recent uncontrolled study performed a battery of 21 separate tests on a small and heterogeneous group of patients with unexplained infertility *(129)*. These tests included, in addition to antiphospholipid antibodies, antithyroid antibodies, systemic $CD56^+$ cells, and embryotoxicity of peripheral serum. Among the 25 patients with unexplained infertility, 71% had at least one positive test result, a result clearly predictable by chance alone.

Studies on patients undergoing in vitro fertilization (IVF) and intrauterine embryo transfer (ET) have the potential to offer a much better model to study factors affecting the periimplantation phase of development. Recent studies attempting to correlate autoantibody status with pregnancy rates from ART cycles abound *(130–137)*. Of the studies including patients with unexplained infertility, only one retrospective series reported a significant correlation between the presence of at least one of seven autoantibodies and poor implantation rate per embryo transferred *(134)*. Limitations of this small study are the inclusion of a control group of unproven fertility and the lack of information regarding the distribution of fundamental IVF parameters other than implantation rate in the study groups.

Preliminary data from a prospective study including 166 infertile women undergoing IVF, 158 healthy fertile controls, and 50 women with APS provide more useful information *(138)*. The authors tested serum samples in a blinded fashion for the presence of seven distinct antiphospholipid antibodies, using assay-specific standards and very strict criteria of normalcy (>99th percentile of 169 blood bank controls). The study confirmed that the incidence of antiphospholipid antibodies was similar in infertile patients undergoing IVF and in fertile women. Moreover, no difference in the embryo implantation rate was seen between seropositive and seronegative patients undergoing IVF (61 vs 55%; $P = 0.46$).

Overall, available data indicate that polyclonal B-cell activation is not a significant factor in determining the pregnancy rate of couples undergoing ART cycles. Similarly, previous IVF procedures do not appear to be causally linked to the induction of autoantibodies *(130,139)*.

Despite the lack of evidence of causal autoantibody involvement in the pathophysiology of infertility, clinical trials have been conducted to evaluate the efficacy of various empirical treatments in improving IVF pregnancy rates in these patients *(131,132,140)*. None of these trials were randomized, and none included appropriate controls (i.e., antibody-positive treated vs antibody-positive untreated, or antibody-negative treated vs antibody-negative untreated). Only one of these studies concluded that empiric treatment improves IVF pregnancy rates in patients with antiphospholipid antibodies *(140)*. These authors screened an unselected group of women undergoing IVF for the presence of a battery of 18 separate antiphospholipid antibodies. They observed that infertile women with organic pelvic pathology (pelvic inflammatory disease, iatrogenic abdominopelvic adhesions, and endometriosis) had a significantly higher prevalence of seropositivity compared to women with unexplained infertility or other infertility factors. They also observed that there was no difference in pregnancy rates between seropositive and seronegative women. The authors selectively assigned some of the seropositive patients to receive heparin, 5000 IU sc twice a day and ASA 81 mg po daily, starting with gonadotropin treatment. A smaller number of seropositive patients were not treated and served as a control group. Overall comparisons indicated that 49% of treated seropositive women achieved a subsequent clinical pregnancy vs 16% of untreated seropositive controls, a statistically significant difference. When analysis within subgroups with a certain pelvic pathology was performed, however, the differences were no longer significant. The final outcome of the clinical pregnancies was not reported. The authors concluded that patients with known pelvic pathology undergoing ART cycles should be screened for antiphospholipid antibodies, and treated with heparin/ASA if seropositivity were detected. The potential for selection bias, inclusion of patients with any detectable level of antibody into the seropositive group, and high number of independent antiphospholipid antibody determinations ($n = 18$) per patient are only a few of the serious methodological flaws of this study.

Currently, there is no treatment of proven efficacy in improving clinical pregnancy rates in patients with autoantibodies having IVF for unexplained infertility or for any other reason.

Autoimmune Factors in Ectopic Implantation

Ectopic pregnancy is a significant cause of maternal mortality worldwide, and its incidence has steadily increased throughout the second half of this century *(141)*. One of the main risk factors for this condition is a prior pelvic infection *(142)*. Most women with ectopic pregnancy do not offer such a history: nevertheless, in half of the cases where an ectopic pregnancy is found, evidence of tubal damage related to pelvic adhesions exists *(141)*. *Chlamydia trachomatis* is the major pathogen considered capable of producing silent salpingitis, and adequately controlled studies have shown an excess of chlamydia seropositivity in women with ectopic pregnancies *(143)*.

A hypothesis has been proposed whereby *C. trachomatis* infection could induce tubal damage by an antigen-specific immunopathologic mechanism accompanied by a host inflammatory response. Studies have reported that 41–50% of patients with ectopic pregnancy have high titers of circulating antibodies to a 57-kDa triton X-extractable protein antigen of *C. trachomatis*, a significantly higher prevalence than that found in matched controls *(144,145)*. This chlamydial hypersensitivity antigen is capable of inducing delayed inflammatory responses in the lamina propria of immunologically primed animals *(146,147)*. The 57-kDa triton X-extractable *C. trachomatis* antigen has high sequence homology with human heat-shock protein 60 *(148)*. Therefore, autoimmunity triggered by this antigen may be a feature of chlamydial immunopathology. This hypothesis awaits verification.

HORMONE-DEPENDENT CONDITIONS

The Role of Autoimmunity in Endometriosis

Ectopic (extrauterine) growth of endometrial glands and stroma defines endometriosis, a frequently occurring nonneoplastic condition in women of reproductive age, with protean clinical and pathological manifestations. The overall prevalence of this enigmatic disorder is estimated at 5–15% *(149)*, but is remarkably higher in women with infertility or pelvic pain *(150)*. Despite the fact that concentration of estrogen and progesterone receptors is lower in endometriotic lesions than in eutopic endometrium *(151,152)*, endometriosis is a hormone-dependent condition. Estrogen is the primary mitogenic stimulus in the development of endometriosis *(153)*, which constitutes the rationale for its current medical management *(154)*. Although it is evident that endometriotic lesions thrive on an estrogenic milieu, endometriosis still eludes clear nosologic classification, and the histogenesis of this disorder remains speculative. Menstrual dissemination of endometrial tissue into the pelvic cavity, the original etiologic hypothesis proposed *(155)*, still holds as that most experimentally favored. According to this model, eutopic endometrium is shed in retrograde fashion through the fallopian tubes onto pelvic peritoneal surfaces where autologous transplantation eventually occurs. Retrograde menstruation has been described in 76–95% of women during menses *(156,157)*. Retrograde endometrial shedding appears to occur with the same frequency in women with and without endometriosis *(156–158)*. Why then do not all women develop endometriosis? Furthermore, if endometriosis arises from autologous endometrial transplantation, why is it associated with inflammation and immune cell activation? Recent investigation suggests that an aberrant immune response may be crucial in the pathophysiology of this disease. The main hypothesis to explain successful ectopic implantation of endometrium in selected patients is that abnormal immunologic defense results in impaired peritoneal clearance of endometrial cells shed during retrograde menstruation *(159–162)*. A corollary of this assumption is that excessive retrograde shedding, or a particularly high intrinsic implantation potential of the endometrium in some women can override an otherwise functional peritoneal clearance system. According to this model, in women without endometriosis, peritoneal monocytes suppress implantation of endometrial cells, whereas natural killer (NK) cells, activated macrophages, and cytotoxic T lymphocytes perform immunologic clearance of ectopic endometrium. Conversely, in women with endometriosis, ectopic endometrial implantation may be allowed or even stimulated by abnormal monocyte function, but cytotoxic peritoneal immune cell functions are suppressed. Once successful ectopic endometrial transplantation is permitted, activated macrophages may still recognize the tissue as modified or senescent self-antigens and may therefore originate, or perpetuate, a cytokine-driven activatory cascade of T cells and eventually of B cells. B cells would then differentiate into plasma cells with the ultimate effect of specific antibody secretion against endometrial cell-derived antigens.

In summary, many believe today that endometriosis is a true autoimmune disease, and some of the available data seem to support this hypothesis. However, the autoimmune nature of this condition is far from being ascertained.

First and foremost the speculation that endometriosis develops only in women with altered cellular immunity and impaired peritoneal clearance of endometrial cells assumes that endometrial cells, either eutopic or ectopic, are antigenic. This assumption, however, has never been unequivocally proven. Several studies over the last decade have reported a significant incidence of abnormal autoantibodies, including antiendometrial antibodies, in women with endometriosis *(163–170)*. Nevertheless, flaws in the design of these studies limit their usefulness, such as inclusion of heterogeneous study groups, inappropriate choice of controls, and unspecified timing of laparoscopy when biopsies of the disease were obtained. Particularly problematic is the comparison of data between studies, owing to lack of standardization of the specimens studied and the autoantibody assay techniques employed. Female prevalence and familial occurrence of endometriosis are epidemiologic considerations often cited to support the theory of an autoimmune etiology. Although endometriosis clearly runs in families *(171)*, it is not associated to a specific HLA haplotype *(172,173)*, unlike other autoimmune disorders. With the exception of rare case reports of urinary tract endometriosis in male patients on high doses of exogenous estrogen *(174)(175)*, pelvic endometriosis is by definition a disease of the menstruating woman. Invoking female prevalence as an epidemiologic indicator of autoimmune etiology seems therefore quite inappropriate.

In addition to abnormalities in humoral immunity, specific functional changes in cell-mediated immunity have also been reported in women with endometriosis. Although the number and ratio of circulating immune cell subsets do not differ between normal women and women with endometriosis *(176)*, decreased recognition of autologous endometrial antigens by peripheral blood lymphocytes, as indicated by in vitro proliferation assays, has been described in the latter group *(159,177)*. Similarly, cytotoxicity studies employing nonstandardized autologous endometrial cells and peripheral cytotoxic T lymphocytes from subfertile women have shown decreased activity in those patients with endometriosis *(161,162,178)*. The caveat here is that data derived from functional studies on peripheral lymphocytes may not necessarily reflect actual cell behavior in specific tissue sites. Moreover, interpretation of data from circulating leukocytes in normal adults may be limited by external variables not always accounted for, such as smoking, some medications, and exercise. The nonstandardized endometrial cells employed in these studies also raise the question of between-study and between-patient differences in target cell sensitivity.

Reports of decreased NK cell activity in association with endometriosis have been previously reviewed and challenged *(179)*. Particularly, recent data from carefully designed in vivo studies in the baboon endometriosis model have provided persuading evidence that NK and cytotoxic T-lymphocyte activity are unlikely to be causally related to this disease *(180,181)*.

Although an etiologic role of autoimmunity in endometriosis is not ascertained, there are good data to suggest that local immunologic mechanisms may contribute to the maintenance of the inflammatory state and the progression of the disease once endometriosis is established. Most of the experimental evidence implicates the peritoneal monocyte/macrophage system as the main player in this setting. Peripheral blood monocytes are attracted to the peritoneal cavity in response to local irritation associated with retrograde menstrual flow where they give rise to peritoneal macrophages. These cells, together with NK cells and the complement system, represent the main mediators of innate immunity and contribute to the nonspecific defense mechanism of inflammation through the secretion of cytokines. Macrophages are increased in concentration and activation status in peritoneal fluid obtained from women with endometriosis compared to normal controls *(182–185)*. Peritoneal macrophages in women with endometriosis suppress endometrial cell proliferation, as demonstrated in coculture systems of immune and endometrial cells *(186)*. Macrophages, however, are able to attract other immune and inflammatory cells into the peritoneal fluid milieu through secretion of several chemokines, such as complement-component 3, RANTES, and interleukin (IL-8) *(187–189)*.

Once *in situ*, these cells can secrete a wide range of modulatory cytokines with potential to enhance the progression of endometriotic foci. By far the most promising of these inflammatory cytokines is tumor necrosis factor-α (TNF-α). This polypeptide, mainly derived from activated mononuclear phagocytes, is a pleiotropic factor with a variety of cytotoxic and proinflammatory effects *(190)*. TNF-α is currently considered a major mediator of endometrial cell dyscohesion and apoptosis processes during the late secretory and menstrual phases, in response to estrogen withdrawal *(191–193)*. Peritoneal fluid concentrations of TNF-α have been shown to be significantly increased in fertile and infertile patients with endometriosis compared to matched controls, employing both immunoassay and bioassay techniques *(194,195)*. More recent data have confirmed the above findings and have demonstrated significant suppression of TNF-α in the peritoneal fluid of women with endometriosis after treatment with danazol or a gonadotropin-releasing hormone (GnRH) analog *(196)*. Finally, a recent in vitro study has shown that physiological levels of TNF-α significantly enhance adhesion of endometrial stromal cells onto a mesothelial cell layer *(197)*. Together, these data suggest that abnormal local production of TNF-α by macrophages and activated lymphocyes may be a facilitatory factor in the peritoneal implantation of endometrial debris.

Moreover, given the physiologic role of TNF-α in endometrial dyscohesion, one could also hypothesize that a more generalized dysfunction involving this cytokine could allow untimely retrograde shedding of basalis endometrium, a pluripotent tissue with higher implantation potential. The finding that expression of the steroidogenic enzyme aromatase is increased in ectopic and eutopic endometrium of patients with endometriosis *(198)* further supports the above hypotheses, owing to the fact that endometrial and intralesional synthesis of estrogen could enhance the net local effect of TNF-α through enhancement of its receptor synthesis *(199)*.

In conclusion, rigorously derived data currently do not support a classic antibody-mediated autoimmune etiology for endometriosis. Likewise, the concept that endometriosis may originate from defective cell-mediated immunity and resulting impaired clearance of retrograde endometrial shedding remains speculative. Although definitive data are still lacking, the hypothesis that local peritoneal inflammatory cells may contribute to the histogenesis and maintenance of endometriotic lesions appears more promising.

SUMMARY

Several endocrine and endocrine-dependent organs and tissues can be potentially affected by a faulty recognition of self by the immune system. The many facets of autoimmune endocrinopathy in human reproduction have been examined in a systematic fashion. Particular attention has been given to idiopathic premature ovarian failure, recurrent spontaneous abortion, and endometriosis. Current evidence strongly supports the role of an autoimmune response, either cell-mediate or humoral, in the pathophysiology of idiopathic POF associated with serologic evidence of autoimmune Addison's disease. For the majority of cases of idiopathic POF, however, the association with abnormal immune response is more tenuous, and more investigation will be needed in order to identify that subset of patients in which autoimmunity is causally relevant. The accurate and early diagnosis of autoimmune POF may have fundamental prognostic and therapeutic implications for these women. Some of these, like immunomodulatory therapies, have been discussed; other exciting possibilities will likely be offered in the near future through gamete micromanipulation techniques and in vitro maturation of oocytes.

The role of autoantibodies, either to phospholipid or other tissue ligands, in bringing about failure of implantation and placentation has been critically reviewed with a clear emphasis on the many pitfalls of study design and interpretation in the clinical setting of recurrent pregnancy loss and unexplained infertility. The antiphospholipid syndrome, be it primary or secondary, is a potentially fatal condition that typically affects women during the reproductive years and is particularly incident in pregnancy. The autoimmune nature of this syndrome is well characterized, although its exact pathophysiology currently eludes detection. Empirical treatment regimens have been proposed, none of which are highly effective or completely innocuous, and larger controlled randomized clinical trials are needed before a therapeutic standard can be established. Important questions remain, such as the best management for asymptomatic nulliparous patients with serological evidence of APS. Laboratory standardization and limiting the number of antibodies tested is the key to avoiding gross overestimation of the condition in the general patient population. At present, consideration should be given to obtaining aCL IgG and IgM, and LA. Minidose aspirin and anticoagulation with subcutaneous heparin should be offered to patients with the antiphospholipid syndrome. There is no place for costly and potentially harmful immunotherapies in the prevention of autoimmune pregnancy loss. Likewise, there is no place for immunotherapy or anticoagulation in the setting of infertility associated with autoantibodies.

Finally, recent data indicate that the perpetuation of the exquisitely estrogen-dependent pelvic endometriotic lesions might have its explanation in a dysregulation of the peritoneal leukocytes responsible for innate immunity. The implications of any breakthrough discovery on the role of the immune system in this setting would have enormous therapeutical implication potential, by opening nonhormonal treatment avenues that could potentially avoid the untoward effects of iatrogenic hypoestrogenemia.

REFERENCES

1. McKinlay SM, Brambilla DJ, Posner JG. The normal menopause transition. Maturitas 1992;14:103–115.
2. de Moraes-Ruehsen M, Jones GS. Premature ovarian failure. Fertil Steril 1967;18:440–461.
3. Rebar RW, Connolly HV. Clinical features of young women with hypergonadotropic amenorrhea. Fertil Steril 1990;53:804–810.
4. Coulam CB, Adamson SC, Annegers JF. Incidence of premature ovarian failure. Obstet Gynecol 1986;67:604–606.
5. Nelson LM, Anasti JN, Flack MR. Premature ovarian failure. In: Adashy EY, Rock JA, Rosenwaks Z, eds. Reproductive Endocrinology, Surgery, and Technology, 1st ed., vol. 2. Lippincott-Raven, Philadelphia, PA, 1996, pp. 1393–1410.
6. La Barbera AR, Miller MM, Ober C, Rebar RW. Autoimmune etiology in premature ovarian failure. Am J Reprod Immunol Microbiol 1988;16:115–122.
7. Weetman AP. Autoimmunity to steroid-producing cells and familial polyendocrine autoimmunity. Baillieres Clin Endocrinol Metab 1995;9:157–174.
8. Ahonen P, Myllarniemi S, Sipila I, Perheentupa J. Clinical variation of autoimmune polyendocrinopathy-candidiasis-ectodermal dystrophy (APECED) in a series of 68 patients. N Engl J Med 1990;322:1829–1836.
9. Neufeld M, Maclaren NK, Blizzard RM. Two types of autoimmune Addison's disease associated with different polyglandular autoimmune (PGA) syndromes. Medicine (Baltimore) 1981;60:355–362.
10. Papadopoulos KI, Hallengren B. Polyglandular autoimmune syndrome type II in patients with idiopathic Addison's disease. Acta Endocrinol (Copenh) 1990;122:472–478.
11. Turkington RW, Lebovitz HE. Extra-adrenal endocrine deficiencies in Addison's disease. Am J Med 1967;43:499–507.
12. Irvine WJ, Chan MM, Scarth L, Kolb FO, Hartog M, Bayliss RI, et al. Immunological aspects of premature ovarian failure associated with idiopathic Addison's disease. Lancet 1968;2:883–887.
13. Blizzard RM, Chee D, Davis W. The incidence of adrenal and other antibodies in the sera of patients with idiopathic adrenal insufficiency (Addison's disease). Clin Exp Immunol 1967;2:19–30.

14. Sotsiou F, Bottazzo GF, Doniach D. Immunofluorescence studies on autoantibodies to steroid-producing cells, and to germline cells in endocrine disease and infertility. Clin Exp Immunol 1980;39:97–111.
15. Winqvist O, Karlsson FA, Kampe O. 21-Hydroxylase, a major autoantigen in idiopathic Addison's disease [*see* comments]. Lancet 1992;339:1559–1562.
16. Baumann-Antczak A, Wedlock N, Bednarek J, Kiso Y, Krishnan H, Fowler S, et al. Autoimmune Addison's disease and 21-hydroxylase [letter; comment]. Lancet 1992;340, 429–430.
17. Krohn K, Uibo R, Aavik E, Peterson P, Savilahti K. Identification by molecular cloning of an autoantigen associated with Addison's disease as steroid 17 alpha-hydroxylase [*see* comments]. Lancet 1992;339:770–773.
18. Winqvist O, Gustafsson J, Rorsman F, Karlsson FA, Kampe O. Two different cytochrome P450 enzymes are the adrenal antigens in autoimmune polyendocrine syndrome type I and Addison's disease. J Clin Invest 1993;92:2377–2385.
19. Uibo R, Aavik E, Peterson P, Perheentupa J, Aranko S, Pelkonen R, et al. Autoantibodies to cytochrome P450 enzymes P450scc, P450c17, and P450c21 in autoimmune polyglandular disease types I and II and in isolated Addison's disease. J Clin Endocrinol Metab 1994;78:323–328.
20. Arif S, Vallian S, Farzaneh F, Zanone MM, James SL, Pietropaolo M, et al. Identification of 3 beta-hydroxysteroid dehydrogenase as a novel target of steroid cell autoantibodies: association of autoantibodies with endocrine autoimmune disease. J Clin Endocrinol Metab 1996;81:4439–4445.
21. Mignot MH, Schoemaker J, Kleingeld M, Rao BR, Drexhage HA. Premature ovarian failure. I: The association with autoimmunity. Eur J Obstet Gynecol Reprod Biol 1989;30:59–66.
22. Betterle C, Rossi A, Dalla Pria S, Artifoni A, Pedini B, Gavasso S, et al. Premature ovarian failure: autoimmunity and natural history. Clin Endocrinol (Oxford) 1993;39:35–43.
23. Elder M, Maclaren N, Riley W. Gonadal autoantibodies in patients with hypogonadism and/or Addison's disease. J Clin Endocrinol Metab 1981;52:1137–1142.
24. Betterle C, Zanette F, Zanchetta R, Pedini B, Trevisan A, Mantero F, et al. Complement-fixing adrenal autoantibodies as a marker for predicting onset of idiopathic Addison's disease. Lancet 1983;1:1238–1241.
25. Betterle C, Scalici C, Presotto F, Pedini B, Moro L, Rigon F, et al. The natural history of adrenal function in autoimmune patients with adrenal autoantibodies. J Endocrinol 1988;117:467–475.
26. Kim TJ, Anasti JN, Flack MR, Kimzey LM, Defensor RA, Nelson LM. Routine endocrine screening for patients with karyotypically normal spontaneous premature ovarian failure. Obstet Gynecol 1997;89:777–779.
27. Betterle C, Presotto F, Pedini B, Moro L, Slack RS, Zanette F, et al. Islet cell and insulin autoantibodies in organ-specific autoimmune patients. Their behaviour and predictive value for the development of type 1 (insulin-dependent) diabetes mellitus. A 10-year follow-up study. Diabetologia 1987;30:292–297.
28. Ahonen P, Miettinen A, Perheentupa J. Adrenal and steroidal cell antibodies in patients with autoimmune polyglandular disease type I and risk of adrenocortical and ovarian failure. J Clin Endocrinol Metab 1987;64:494–500.
29. Hoek A, Shoemaker J, Drexage HA. Premature ovarian failure and ovarian autoimmunity. Endocr Rev 1997;18:107–134.
30. Bannatyne P, Russell P, Shearman RP. Autoimmune oophoritis: a clinicopathologic assessment of 12 cases. Int J Gynecol Pathol 1990;9:191–207.
31. Sedmak DD, Hart WR, Tubbs RR. Autoimmune oophoritis: a histopathologic study of involved ovaries with immunologic characterization of the mononuclear cell infiltrate. Int J Gynecol Pathol 1987;6:73–81.
32. Gloor E, Hurlimann J. Autoimmune oophoritis. Am J Clin Pathol 1984;81:105–109.
33. Hill JA, Welch WR, Faris HM, Anderson DJ. Induction of class II major histocompatibility complex antigen expression in human granulosa cells by interferon gamma: a potential mechanism contributing to autoimmune ovarian failure. Am J Obstet Gynecol 1990;162:534–540.
34. Tung KS, Smith S, Teuscher CCC, Anderson RE. Murine autoimmune oophoritis, epididymo-orchitis, and gastritis induced by day 3 thymectomy. Am J Pathol 1987;126:293–302.
35. Miyake T, Taguchi O, Ikeda H, Sato Y, Takeuchi S, Nishizuka Y. Acute oocyte loss in experimental autoimmune oophoritis as a possible model of premature ovarian failure. Am J Obstet Gynecol 1988;158:186–192.
36. Taguchi O, Nishizuka Y, Sakakura T, Kojima A. Autoimmune oophoritis in thymectomized mice: detection of circulating antibodies against oocytes. Clin Exp Immunol 1980;40:540–553.
37. Miller ME, Chatten J. Ovarian changes in ataxia teleangectasia. Acta Paediatr Scand 1967;56:559–561.

38. Healy DL, Bacher J, Hodgen GD. Thymic regulation of primate fetal ovarian-adrenal differentiation. Biol Reprod 1985;32:1127–1133.
39. Smith H, Sakamoto Y, Kasai K, Tung KSK. Effector and regulatory cells in autoimmune oophoritis elicited by neonatal thymectomy. J Immunol 1991;147:2928–2933.
40. Sakaguchi S, Takahashi T, Nishizuka Y. Study on cellular events in postthymectomy autoimmune oophoritis in mice. 1. Requirement of Lyt–1 effector cells for oocytes damage after adoptive transfer. J Exp Med 1982;156:1565–1576.
41. Smith H, Lou YH, Lacy P, Tung KS. Tolerance mechanism in experimental ovarian and gastric autoimmune diseases. J Immunol 1992;149:2212–2218.
42. Aaltonen J, Bjorses P, Sandkuijl L, Perheentupa J, Peltonen L. An autosomal locus causing autoimmune disease: autoimmune polyglandular disease type I assigned to chromosome 21. Nat Genet 1994;8:83–87.
43. Dewhurst CJ, de Koos EB, Ferreira HP. The resistant ovary syndrome. Br J Obstet Gynaecol 1975;82:341–345.
44. Kamada M, Daitoh T, Mori K, Maeda N, Hirano K, Irahara M, et al. Etiological implication of autoantibodies to zona pellucida in human female infertility. Am J Reprod Immunol 1992;28:104–109.
45. Dean J. Biology of mammalian fertilization: the role of the zona pellucida. J Clin Invest 1992;89:1055–1059.
46. Rhim SH, Millar SE, Robey F, Luo AM, Lou YH, Yule T, et al. Autoimmune disease of the ovary induced by ZP3 peptide from the mouse zona pellucida. J Clin Invest 1992;89:28–35.
47. Lou Y, Tung KS. T cell peptide of a self-protein elicits autoantibody to the protein antigen. Implications for specificity and pathogenetic role of antibody in autoimmunity. J Immunol 1993;151:5790–5799.
48. Tilly JL, Aihara T, Nishimori K, Jia XC, Billig H, Kowalski KI, et al. Expression of recombinant human follicle-stimulating hormone receptor: species-specific ligand binding, signal transduction, and identification of multiple ovarian messenger ribonucleic acid transcripts. Endocrinology 1992;131:799–806.
49. Jia XC, Oikawa M, Bo M, Tanaka T, Boime I, Hsueh AJ. Expression of human luteinizing hormone receptor: interaction with LH and chorion gonadotropin from human, but not equine, rat, and ovine species. Mol Endocrinol 1991;5:759–768.
50. Anasti JN, Flack MR, Froelich J, Nelson LM. The use of human recombinant gonadotropin receptors to search for immunoglobulin G-mediated premature ovarian failure. J Clin Endocrinol Metab 1995;80:824–828.
51. Ho PC, Tang GWK, Lawton JW. Lymphocyte subsets and serum immunoglobulins in patients with premature ovarian failure before and after oestrogen replacement. Hum Reprod 1993;8:714–716.
52. Anasti JN, Adams S, Kimzey LM, Defensor RA, Zachary AA, Nelson LM. Karyotypically normal spontaneous premature ovarian failure: evaluation of association with class II major histocompatibility complex. J Clin Endocrinol Metab 1994;78:722–723.
53. Taylor PV, Campbell JM, Scott JS. Presence of autoantibodies in women with unexplained infertility [*see* comments]. Am J Obstet Gynecol 1989;161:377–379.
54. Blumenfeld Z, Halachmi S, Peretz BA, Shmuel Z, Golan D, Makler A, et al. Premature ovarian failure—the prognostic application of autoimmunity on conception after ovulation induction. Fertil Steril 1993;59:750–755.
55. Corenblum B, Rowe T, Taylor PJ. High-dose, short-term glucocorticoids for the treatment of infertility resulting from premature ovarian failure. Fertil Steril 1993;59:988–991.
56. Albrecht ED, Pepe GJ. Placental steroid hormone biosynthesis in primate pregnancy. Endocr Rev 1990;11:124.
57. Medawar PB. Some immunological and endocrinological problems raised by the evolution of viviparity in vertebrates. Academic, New York, 1953, Society for Experimental Biology, vol. 7.
58. U.S. Department of Health and Human Services. Reproductive impairment among married couples. US vital and health statistics. Hyattsville,MD: National Center for Health Statistics series 23, 11, 1992, pp. 5–31.
59. Harlop S, Shiono PH, Ramcharan S. A life table of spontaneous abortions and the effects of age, parity and other variables. In: Porter IH, Hook EB, eds. Human Embryonic and Fetal Death. Academic, New York, 1980, p. 145.
60. Regan L. Recurrent miscarriage. Br Med J 1991;302:543–544.
61. Regan L. Recurrent early pregnancy failure. Curr Opinion Obstet Gynaecol 1992;4:220–228.

62. Hill JA. Sporadic and recurrent spontaneous abortion. Curr Prob Obstet Gynecol Fertil 1994;17: 114–162.
63. Hill JA. Immunologic factors in spontaneous abortion. In: Bronson RA, Alexander NJ, Anderson DJ, Branch DW, Kutteh WH, eds. Reproductive Immunology. Blackwell Science, Cambridge, MA, 1996, pp. 433–442.
64. Lockshin DW. Answers to the antiphospholipid antibody syndrome? N Engl J Med 1995;332: 1025–1027.
65. Peaceman AM, Silver RK, MacGregor SN, Socol ML. Interlaboratory variation in antiphospholipid antibody testing [see comments]. Am J Obstet Gynecol 1992;166, 1780–1784; discussion 1784–1787.
66. Harris EN. Special report. The Second International Anti-cardiolipin Standardization Workshop/the Kingston Anti-Phospholipid Antibody Study (KAPS) group. Am J Clin Pathol 1990;94:476–484.
67. Asherson RA, Khamashta MA, Ordi-Ros J, Derksen RH, Machin SJ, Barquinero J, et al. The "primary" antiphospholipid syndrome: major clinical and serological features. Medicine (Baltimore) 1989;68: 366–374.
68. Harris EN, Gharavi AE, Boey ML, Patel BM, Mackworth-Young CG, Loizou S, et al. Anticardiolipin antibodies: detection by radioimmunoassay and association with thrombosis in systemic lupus erythematosus. Lancet 1983;2:1211–1214.
69. Fort JG, Cowchock FS, Abruzzo JL, Smith JB. Anticardiolipin antibodies in patients with rheumatic diseases. Arthritis Rheum 1987;30:752–760.
70. Exner T, Sahman N, Trudinger B. Separation of anticardiolipin antibodies from lupus anticoagulant on a phospholipid-coated polystyrene column. Biochem Biophys Res Commun 1988;155:1001–1007.
71. Chamley LW, Pattison NS, McKay EJ. Separation of lupus anticoagulant from anticardiolipin antibodies by ion-exchange and gel filtration chromatography. Haemostasis 1991;21:25–29.
72. Clifford K, Rai R, Watson H, Regan L. An informative protocol for the investigation of recurrent miscarriage: preliminary experience of 500 consecutive cases. Hum Reprod 1994;9:1328–1332.
73. Silver RM, Porter TF, van Leeuween I, Jeng G, Scott JR, Branch DW. Anticardiolipin antibodies: clinical consequences of "low titers." Obstet Gynecol 1996;87:494–500.
74. Klinman HJ, Feinman MA, Strauss JFI. Differentiation of human cytotrophoblasts into syncytiotrophoblasts in culture. Trophoblast Res 1987;2:407–421.
75. Lyden TW, Ng AK, Rote NS. Modulation of phosphatidylserine epitope expression by BeWo cells during forskolin treatment. Placenta 1993;14:177–186.
76. Kwak JY, Gilman-Sachs A, Beaman KD, Beer AE. Reproductive outcome in women with recurrent spontaneous abortions of alloimmune and autoimmune causes: preconception versus postconception treatment. Am J Obstet Gynecol 1992;166:1787–1795; discussion 1795–1788.
77. Lechner K, Pabinger-Fasching I. Lupus anticoagulants and thrombosis. A study of 25 cases and review of the literature. Haemostasis 1985;15:254–262.
78. Brey RL, Hart RG, Sherman DG, Tegeler CH. Antiphospholipid antibodies and cerebral ischemia in young people. Neurology 1990;40:1190–1196.
79. Ferro D, Quintarelli C, Rasura M, Antonini G, Violi F. Lupus anticoagulant and the fibrinolytic system in young patients with stroke. Stroke 1993;24:368–370.
80. Branch DW, Silver RM, Blackwell JL, Reading JC, Scott JR. Outcome of treated pregnancies in women with antiphospholipid syndrome: an update of the Utah experience. Obstet Gynecol 1992; 80:614–620.
81. Glueck HI, Kant KS, Weiss MA, Pollak VE, Miller MA, Coots M. Thrombosis in systemic lupus erythematosus. Relation to the presence of circulating anticoagulants. Arch Intern Med 1985;145: 1389–1395.
82. Petri M, Golbus M, erson R, Whiting OKQ, Corash L, Hellmann D. Antinuclear antibody, lupus anticoagulant, and anticardiolipin antibody in women with idiopathic habitual abortion. A controlled, prospective study of forty-four women. Arthritis Rheum 1987;30:601–606.
83. Parke AL, Wilson D, Maier D. The prevalence of antiphospholipid antibodies in women with recurrent spontaneous abortion, women with successful pregnancies, and women who have never been pregnant. Arthritis Rheum 1991;34:1231–1235.
84. Parazzini F, Acaia B, Faden D, Lovotti M, Marelli G, Cortelazzo S. Antiphospholipid antibodies and recurrent abortion. Obstet Gynecol 1991;77:854–858.
85. Out HJ, Bruinse HW, Christiaens GC, van Vliet M, Meilof JF, de Groot PG, et al. Prevalence of antiphospholipid antibodies in patients with fetal loss. Ann Rheum Dis 1991;50:553–557.
86. Oshiro BT, Silver RM, Scott JR, Yu H, Branch DW. Antiphospholipid antibodies and fetal death. Obstet Gynecol 1996;87:489–493.

87. Lockshin MD, Druzin ML, Goei S, Quamar T, Magid MS, Jovanovic L, et al. Antibody to cardiolipin predicts placental insufficiency in pregnant patients with systemic lupus erythematosus. N Engl J Med 1985;313:152–156.
88. Hill JA, Polgar K, Harlow BL, Anderson DJ. Evidence of embryo- and trophoblast-toxic cellular immune response(s) in women with recurrent spontaneous abortion. Am J Obstet Gynecol 1992; 166:1044–1052.
89. Infante-Rivard C, David M, Gauthier R, Rivard GE. Lupus anticoagulants, anticardiolipin antibodies, and fetal loss. A case-controlled study. N Engl J Med 1991;325:1063–1066.
90. Haddow JE, Rote NS, Dostal-Johnson D, et al. Lack of an association between late fetal death and antiphospholipid antibody measurements in the second trimester. Am J Obstet Gynecol 1991;165: 1308–1312.
91. Peaceman AM, Rehnberg KA. The effect of immunoglobulin G fractions from patients with lupus anticoagulant on placental prostacyclin and thromboxane production. Am J Obstet Gynecol 1993;169: 1403–1406.
92. De Wolf F, Carreras LO, Moerman P, Vermylen J, Van Assche A, Renaer M. Decidual vasculopathy and extensive placental infarction in a patient with repeated thromboembolic accidents, recurrent fetal loss, and a lupus anticoagulant. Am J Obstet Gynecol 1982;142:829–834.
93. Erlendsson K, Steinsson K, Johannsson JH, Geirsson RT. Relation of antiphospholipid antibody and placental bed inflammatory vascular changes to the outcome of pregnancy in successive pregnancies of 2 women with systemic lupus erythematosus. J Rheumatol 1993;20:1779–1785.
94. McNeil HP, Simpson RJ, Chesterman CN, Krilis SA. Anti-phospholipid antibodies are directed against a complex antigen that includes a lipid-binding inhibitor of coagulation: beta 2-glycoprotein I (apolipoprotein H). Proc Natl Acad Sci USA 1990;87:4120–4124.
95. Roubey RA. Autoantibodies to phospholipid-binding plasma proteins: a new view of lupus anticoagulants and other "antiphospholipid" autoantibodies [*see* comments]. Blood 1994;84:2854–2867.
96. Galli M, Comfurius P, Maassen C, Hemker HC, de Baets MH, van Breda-Vriesman PJ, et al. Anticardiolipin antibodies (ACA) directed not to cardiolipin but to a plasma protein cofactor [*see* comments]. Lancet 1990;335:1544–1547.
97. Fleck RA, Rapaport SI, Rao LV. Anti-prothrombin antibodies and the lupus anticoagulant. Blood 1988;72:512–519.
98. Katano K, Aoki K, Ogasawara M, Sasa H, Hayashi Y, Kawamura M, et al. Specific antiphospholipid antibodies (aPL) eluted from placentae of pregnant women with aPL-positive sera. Lupus 1995;4: 304–308.
99. Del Papa N, Guidali L, Sala A, Buccellati C, Khamashta MA, Ichikawa K, et al. Endothelial cells as target for antiphospholipid antibodies. Human polyclonal and monoclonal anti-beta 2-glycoprotein I antibodies react in vitro with endothelial cells through adherent beta 2-glycoprotein I and induce endothelial activation. Arthritis Rheum 1997;40:551–561.
100. Cowchock FS, Reece EA, Balaban D, Branch DW, Plouffe L. Repeated fetal losses associated with antiphospholipid antibodies: A collaborative randomized trial comparing prednisone with low dose heparin treatment. Am J Obstet Gynecol 1992;166:1318–1323.
101. Kutteh WH. Antiphospholipid antibody-associated recurrent pregnancy loss: treatment with heparin and low-dose aspirin is superior to low-dose aspirin alone. Am J Obstet Gynecol 1996;174:1584–1589.
102. Kutteh WH, Ermel LD. A clinical trial for the treatment of antiphospholipid antibody-associated recurrent pregnancy loss with lower dose heparin and aspirin. Am J Reprod Immunol 1996;35:402–407.
103. Cohen RRH, Regan MDL. Randomized controlled trial of aspirin and aspirin plus heparin in pregnant women with recurrent miscarriage associated with phospholipid antibodies (or antiphospholipid antibodies). Br Med J 1997;314:253–257.
103a. Ermel LD, Marshburn PB, Kutteh WH. Interaction of heparin with antiphospholipid antibodies (APA) from the sera of women with recurrent pregnancy loss (RPL). Am J Reprod Immunol 1995;33:14–20.
104. Hunt BJ, Boughty HA, Majumdar G, Copplestone A, Kerslake S, Buchanan N, et al. Thromboprophylaxix with low molecular weight heparin (Fragmin) in high risk pregnancies. Thromb Haemost 1997;77: 39–43.
105. Druzin ML, Lockshin M, Edersheim TG, Hutson JM, Krauss AL, Kogut E. Second-trimester fetal monitoring and preterm delivery in pregnancies with systemic lupus erythematosus and/or circulating anticoagulant. Am J Obstet Gynecol 1987;157:1503–1510.
106. Laskin CA, Bombardier C, Hannah ME, Mandel FP, Ritchie JW, Farewell V, et al. Prednisone and aspirin in women with autoantibodies and unexplained recurrent fetal loss [*see* comments]. N Engl J Med 1997;337:148–153.

107. Kaaja R, Julkunen H, Ammala P, Palosuo T, Kurki P. Intravenous immunoglobulin treatment of pregnant patients with recurrent pregnancy losses associated with antiphospholipid antibodies. Acta Obstet Gynecol Scand 1993;72:63–66.
108. Scott JR, Branch DW, Kochenour NK, Ward K. Intravenous immunoglobulin treatment of pregnant patients with recurrent pregnancy loss caused by antiphospholipid antibodies and Rh immunization. Am J Obstet Gynecol 1988;159:1055,1056.
109. Wapner RJ, Cowchock FS, Shapiro SS. Successful treatment in two women with antiphospholipid antibodies and refractory pregnancy losses with intravenous immunoglobulin infusions. Am J Obstet Gynecol 1989;161:1271,1272.
110. Group TGRI. Intravenous immunoglobulin in the prevention of recurrent miscarriage. Br J Obstet Gynaecol 1994;101:1072–1077.
111. Coulam CB, Krysa L, Stern JJ, Bustillo M. Intravenous immunoglobulin for treatment of recurrent pregnancy loss. Am J Reprod Immunol 1995;34:333–337.
112. Christiansen OB, Mathiesen O, Husth M, Rasmussen KL, Ingerslev HJ, Lauritsen JG, et al. Placebo-controlled trial of treatment of unexplained secondary recurrent spontaneous abortions and recurrent late spontaneous abortions with i.v. immunoglobulin. Hum Reprod 1995;10:2690–2695.
113. Ratko TA, Burnett DA, Foulke GE, Matuszewski KA, Sacher RA. Recommendations for off-label use of intravenously administered immunoglobulin preparations. University Hospital Consortium Expert Panel for Off-Label Use of Polyvalent Intravenously Administered Immunoglobulin Preparations [see comments]. J Am Med Assoc 1995;273:1865–1870.
114. Schiff RI. Transmission of viral infections through intravenous immune globulin [editorial; comment] [see comments]. N Engl J Med 1994;331:1649–1650.
115. Harger JH, Rabin BS, Marchese SG. The prognostic value of antinuclear antibodies in women with recurrent pregnancy losses: a prospective controlled study. Obstet Gynecol 1989;73:419–424.
116. Ogasawara M, Aoki K, Kajiura S, Yagami Y. Are antinuclear antibodies predictive of recurrent miscarriage [letter]? Lancet 1996;347:1183,1184.
117. Rosenberg AM, Bingham MC, Fong KC. Antinuclear antibodies during pregnancy. Obstet Gynecol 1986;68:560–562.
118. Kiuttu J, Hartikainen AL, Makitalo R, Ruuska P. The outcome of pregnancy in antinuclear antibody-positive women. Gynecol Obstet Invest 1994;37:160–163.
119. Gleicher N, el-Roeiy A, Confino E, Friberg J. Reproductive failure because of autoantibodies: unexplained infertility and pregnancy wastage. Am J Obstet Gynecol 1989;160:1376–1380; discussion 1380–1375.
120. Hill JA, Anderson DJ. Blood transfusions for recurrent abortion: is the treatment worse than the disease [letter]? Fertil Steril 1986;46:152–154.
121. Hill JA. Immunotherapy for recurrent pregnancy loss: "Standard of care or buyer beware." J Soc Gynecol Invest 1997;4:267–273.
122. Gleicher N. Introduction—the worldwide collaborative observational study and MULTI-analysis on allogeneic leukocyte immunotherapy for recurrent abortion [editorial; comment]. Am J Reprod Immunol 1994;32:53,54.
123. Stagnaro-Green A, Roman SH, Cobin RH, el-Harazy E, Alvarez-Marfany M, Davies TF. Detection of at-risk pregnancy by means of highly sensitive assays for thyroid autoantibodies [see comments]. J Am Med Assoc 1990;264:1422–1425.
124. Glinoer D, Soto MF, Bourdoux P, Lejeune B, Delange F, Lemone M, et al. Pregnancy in patients with mild thyroid abnormalities: maternal and neonatal repercussions. J Clin Endocrinol Metab 1991;73:421–427.
125. Singh A, Dantas ZN, Stone SC, Asch RH. Presence of thyroid antibodies in early reproductive failure: biochemical versus clinical pregnancies. Fertil Steril 1995;63:277–281.
126. Pratt D, Novotny M, Kaberlein G, Dudkiewicz A, Gleicher N. Antithyroid antibodies and the association with non-organ-specific antibodies in recurrent pregnancy loss [see comments]. Am J Obstet Gynecol 1993;168:837–841.
127. Guttmacher AF. Factors affecting normal expectancy of conception. J Am Med Assoc 1956;161:855–860.
128. Hull MG, Glazener CM, Kelly NJ, Conway DI, Foster PA, Hinton RA, et al. Population study of causes, treatment, and outcome of infertility. Br Med J (Clin Res Ed) 1985;291:1693–1697.
129. Roussev RG, Stern JJ, Thorsell LP, Thomason EJ, Coulam CB. Validation of an embryotoxicity assay. Am J Reprod Immunol 1995;33:171–175.

130. Birdsall MA, Lockwood GM, Ledger WL, Johnson PM, Chamley LW. Antiphospholipid antibodies in women having in-vitro fertilization [*see* comments]. Hum Reprod 1996;11:1185–1189.
131. Kutteh WH, Yetman DL, Chantilis SJ, Crain J. Effect of antiphospholipid antibodies in women undergoing in-vitro fertilization: role of heparin and aspirin. Hum Reprod 1997;12:1171–1175.
132. Birkenfeld A, Mukaida T, Minichiello L, Jackson M, Kase NG, Yemini M. Incidence of autoimmune antibodies in failed embryo transfer cycles. Am J Reprod Immunol 1994;31:65–68.
133. el-Roeiy A, Gleicher N, Friberg J, Confino E, Dudkiewicz A. Correlation between peripheral blood and follicular fluid autoantibodies and impact on in vitro fertilization. Obstet Gynecol 1987;70:163–170.
134. Geva E, Amit A, Lerner-Geva L, Azem F, Yovel I, Lessing JB. Autoimmune disorders: another possible cause for in-vitro fertilization and embryo transfer failure. Hum Reprod 1995;10:2560–2563.
135. Gleicher N, Liu HC, Dudkiewicz A, Rosenwaks Z, Kaberlein G, Pratt D, et al. Autoantibody profiles and immunoglobulin levels as predictors of in vitro fertilization success [*see* comments]. Am J Obstet Gynecol 1994;170:1145–1149.
136. Kowalik A, Vichnin M, Liu HC, Branch W, Berkeley AS. Midfollicular anticardiolipin and antiphosphatidylserine antibody titers do not correlate with in vitro fertilization outcome. Fertil Steril 1997;68:298–304.
137. Nip MM, Taylor PV, Rutherford AJ, Hancock KW. Autoantibodies and antisperm antibodies in sera and follicular fluids of infertile patients; relation to reproductive outcome after in- vitro fertilization. Hum Reprod 1995;10:2564–2569.
138. Porter TF, Hatasaka HH, Branch DW, Silver RM, Cramer DW, Hill JA. Antiphospholipid antibodies in women undergoing in vitro fertilization. Society for Gynecologic Investigation—45th Annual Meeting. Atlanta, GA, Elsevier, 1998, p. 88A.
139. Fisch B, Fried S, Manor Y, Ovadia J, Witz IP, Yron I. Increased antiphospholipid antibody activity in in-vitro fertilization patients is not treatment-dependent but rather an inherent characteristic of the infertile state. Am J Reprod Immunol 1995;34:370–374.
140. Sher G, Feinman M, Zouves C, Kuttner G, Maassarani G, Salem R, et al. High fecundity rates following in-vitro fertilization and embryo transfer in antiphospholipid antibody seropositive women treated with heparin and aspirin. Hum Reprod 1994;9:2278–2283.
141. Chow WH, Daling JR, Cates W, Greenberg RS. Epidemiology of ectopic pregnancy. Epidemiol Rev 1987;9:70–94.
142. Marchbanks PA, Annegers JF, Coulam CB, Strathy JH, Kurland LT. Risk factors for ectopic pregnancy. A population-based study. J Am Med Assoc 1988;259:1823–1827.
143. Chow JM, Yonekura ML, Richwald GA, Greenland S, Sweet RL, Schachter J. The association between Chlamydia trachomatis and ectopic pregnancy. J Am Med Assoc 1990;263:3164–3167.
144. Brunham RC, Peeling R, Maclean I, Kosseim ML, Paraskevas M. Chlamydia trachomatis-associated ectopic pregnancy: serologic and histologic correlates. J Infect Dis 1992;165:1076–1081.
145. Wagar EA, Schachter J, Bavoil P, Stephens RS. Differential human serologic response to two 60,000 molecular weight *Chlamydia trachomatis* antigens. J Infect Dis 1990;162:922–927.
146. Morrison RP, Belland RJ, Lyng K, Caldwell HD. Chlamydial disease pathogenesis. The 57-kD chlamydial hypersensitivity antigen is a stress response protein. J Exp Med 1989;170:1271–1283.
147. Morrison RP, Lyng K, Caldwell HD. Chlamydial disease pathogenesis. Ocular hypersensitivity elicited by a genus-specific 57-kD protein. J Exp Med 1989;169:663–675.
148. Cerrone MC, Ma JJ, Stephens RS. Cloning and sequence of the gene for heat shock protein 60 from Chlamydia trachomatis and immunological reactivity of the protein. Infect Immun 1991;59:79–90.
149. Guzick DS. Clinical epidemiology of endometriosis and infertility. Obstet Gynecol Clin North Am 1989;16:43–59.
150. Koninckx PR, Meuleman C, Demeyere S, Lesaffre E, Cornillie FJ. Suggestive evidence that pelvic endometriosis is a progressive disease, whereas deeply infiltrating endometriosis is associated with pelvic pain [*see* comments]. Fertil Steril 1991;55:759–765.
151. Prentice A, Randall BJ, Weddell A, McGill A, Henry L, Horne CH, et al. Ovarian steroid receptor expression in endometriosis and in two potential parent epithelia: endometrium and peritoneal mesothelium. Hum Reprod 1992;7:1318–1325.
152. Bergqvist A, Ferno M. Oestrogen and progesterone receptors in endometriotic tissue and endometrium: comparison of different cycle phases and ages. Hum Reprod 1993;8:2211–2217.
153. Bergqvist IA. Hormonal regulation of endometriosis and the rationales and effects of gonadotropin-releasing hormone agonist treatment: a review. Hum Reprod 1995;10:446–452.

154. Gargiulo AR, Hornstein MD. The role of GnRH agonists plus add-back therapy in the treatment of endometriosis. Semin Reprod Endocrinol 1997;15:273–284.
155. Sampson JA. Peritoneal endometriosis due to menstrual dissemination of endometrial tissue into the pelvic cavity. Am J Obstet Gynecol 1927;14:422–469.
156. Blumenkrantz MJ, Gallagher N, Bashore RA, Tenckhoff H. Retrograde menstruation in women undergoing chronic peritoneal dialysis. Obstet Gynecol 1981;57:667–670.
157. Halme J, Hammond MG, Hulka JF, Raj SG, Talbert LM. Retrograde menstruation in healthy women and in patients with endometriosis. Obstet Gynecol 1984;64:151–154.
158. Koninckx PR, Ide P, Vanderbroucke W, Brosens IA. New aspects of the pathophysiology of endometriosis and associated fertility. J Reprod Med 1980;24:257–260.
159. Dmowski WP, Steele RW, Baker GF. Deficient cellular immunity in endometriosis. Am J Obstet Gynecol 1981;141:377–383.
160. Hill JA. Immunology and endometriosis. Fact, artifact, or epiphenomenon? Obstet Gynecol Clin North Am 1997;24:291–306.
161. Oosterlynck DJ, Cornillie FJ, Waer M, Vandeputte M, Koninckx PR. Women with endometriosis show a defect in natural killer activity resulting in a decreased cytotoxicity to autologous endometrium. Fertil Steril 1991;56:45–51.
162. Vigano P, Vercellini P, Di Blasio AM, Colombo A, Candiani GB, Vignali M. Deficient antiendometrium lymphocyte-mediated cytotoxicity in patients with endometriosis. Fertil Steril 1991;56:894–899.
163. Chihal HJ, Mathur S, Holtz GL, Williamson HO. An endometrial antibody assay in the clinical diagnosis and management of endometriosis. Fertil Steril 1986;46:408–411.
164. Confino E, Harlow L, Gleicher N. Peritoneal fluid and serum autoantibody levels in patients with endometriosis. Fertil Steril 1990;53:242–245.
165. Garza D, Mathur S, Dowd MM, Smith LF, Williamson HO. Antigenic differences between the endometrium of women with and without endometriosis. J Reprod Med 1991;36:177–182.
166. Kennedy SH, Nunn B, Cederholm-Williams SA, Barlow DH. Cardiolipin antibody levels in endometriosis and systemic lupus erythematosus [*see* comments]. Fertil Steril 1989;52:1061–1062.
167. Kilpatrick DC, Haining RE, Smith SS. Are cardiolipin antibody levels elevated in endometriosis? Fertil Steril 1991;55:436,437.
168. Mathur S, Garza DE, Smith LF. Endometrial autoantigens eliciting immunoglobulin (Ig)G, IgA, and IgM responses in endometriosis. Fertil Steril 1990;54:56–63.
169. Switchenko AC, Kauffman RS, Becker M. Are there antiendometrial antibodies in sera of women with endometriosis [*see* comments]. Fertil Steril 1991;56:235–241.
170. Wild RA, Shivers CA, Medders D. Detection of antiendometrial antibodies in patients with endometriosis: methodological issues. Fertil Steril 1992;58:518–521.
171. Malinak LR, Buttram VC Jr, Elias S, Simpson JL. Heritage aspects of endometriosis. II. Clinical characteristics of familial endometriosis. Am J Obstet Gynecol 1980;137:332–337.
172. Maxwell C, Kilpatrick DC, Haining R, Smith SK. No HLA-DR specificity is associated with endometriosis. Tissue Antigens 1989;34:145–147.
173. Simpson JL, Malinak LR, Elias S, Carson SA, Radvany RA. HLA associations in endometriosis. Am J Obstet Gynecol 1984;148:395–397.
174. Oliker AJ, Harris AE. Endometriosis of the bladder in a male patient. J Urol 1971;106:858.
175. Schrodt GR, Alcorn MO, Ibanez J. Endometriosis of the male urinary system: a case report. J Urol 1980;124:722–723.
176. Gleicher N, Dmowski WP, Siegel I, Liu TL, Friberg J, Radwanska E, et al. Lymphocyte subsets in endometriosis. Obstet Gynecol 1984;63:463–466.
177. Steele RW, Dmowski WP, Marmer DJ. Immunologic aspects of human endometriosis. Am J Reprod Immunol 1984;6:33–36.
178. Oosterlynck DJ, Lacquet FA, Waer M, Koninckx PR. Lymphokine-activated killer activity in women with endometriosis. Gynecol Obstet Invest 1994;37:185–190.
179. Hill JA. Immunology and endometriosis. Fertil Steril 1992;58:262–264.
180. D'Hooghe TM, Scheerlinck JP, Koninckx PR, Hill JA, Bambra CS. Anti-endometrial lymphocytotoxicity and natural killer cell activity in baboons (Papio anubis and Papio cynocephalus) with endometriosis. Hum Reprod 1995;10:558–562.
181. D'Hooghe TM, Hill JA. Killer cell activity, statistics, and endometriosis [letter; comment]. Fertil Steril 1995;64:226–228.

182. Halme J, Becker S, Hammond MG, Raj MH, Raj S. Increased activation of pelvic macrophages in infertile women with mild endometriosis. Am J Obstet Gynecol 1983;145:333–337.
183. Halme J, Becker S, Wing R. Accentuated cyclic activation of peritoneal macrophages in patients with endometriosis. Am J Obstet Gynecol 1984;148:85–90.
184. Halme J, Becker S, Haskill S. Altered maturation and function of peritoneal macrophages: possible role in pathogenesis of endometriosis. Am J Obstet Gynecol 1987;156:783–789.
185. Badawy SZ, Cuenca V, Marshall L, Munchback R, Rinas AC, Coble DA. Cellular components in peritoneal fluid in infertile patients with and without endometriosis. Fertil Steril 1984;42:704–708.
186. Braun DP, Muriana A, Gebel H, Rotman C, Rana N, Dmowski WP. Monocyte-mediated enhancement of endometrial cell proliferation in women with endometriosis. Fertil Steril 1994;61:78–84.
187. Isaacson KB, Galman M, Coutifaris C, Lyttle CR. Endometrial synthesis and secretion of complement component-3 by patients with and without endometriosis. Fertil Steril 1990;53:836–841.
188. Khorram O, Taylor RN, Ryan IP, Schall TJ, Landers DV. Peritoneal fluid concentrations of the cytokine RANTES correlate with the severity of endometriosis. Am J Obstet Gynecol 1993;169:1545–1549.
189. Ryan IP, Tseng JF, Schriock ED, Khorram O, Landers DV, Taylor RN. Interleukin-8 concentrations are elevated in peritoneal fluid of women with endometriosis. Fertil Steril 1995;63:929–932.
190. Le J, Vilcek J. Tumor necrosis factor and interleukin 1: cytokines with multiple overlapping biological activities. Lab Invest 1987;56:234–248.
191. Tabibzadeh S, Kong QF, Satyaswaroop PG, Zupi E, Marconi D, Romanini C, et al. Distinct regional and menstrual cycle dependent distribution of apoptosis in human endometrium. Potential role of T cells and TNF-alpha. Endocr J 1994;2:87–95.
192. Tabibzadeh S, Kong QF, Sun XZ. Regulatory roles of TNF-alpha on transepithelial migration of leukocytes and epithelial dyscohesion. Endocr J 1993;1:417–425.
193. Philippeaux MM, Piguet PF. Expression of tumor necrosis factor-alpha and its mRNA in the endometrial mucosa during the menstrual cycle. Am J Pathol 1993;143:480–486.
194. Mori H, Sawairi M, Nakagawa M, Itoh N, Wada K, Tamaya T. Peritoneal fluid interleukin-1 beta and tumor necrosis factor in patients with benign gynecologic disease. Am J Reprod Immunol 1991;26: 62–67.
195. Eisermann J, Gast MJ, Pineda J, Odem RR, Collins JL. Tumor necrosis factor in peritoneal fluid of women undergoing laparoscopic surgery. Fertil Steril 1988;50:573–579.
196. Taketani Y, Kuo TM, Mizuno M. Comparison of cytokine levels and embryo toxicity in peritoneal fluid in infertile women with untreated or treated endometriosis. Am J Obstet Gynecol 1992;167: 265–270.
197. Zhang RJ, Wild RA, Ojago JM. Effect of tumor necrosis factor-alpha on adhesion of human endometrial stromal cells to peritoneal mesothelial cells: an in vitro system. Fertil Steril 1993;59:1196–1201.
198. Noble LS, Simpson ER, Johns A, Bulun SE. Aromatase expression in endometriosis. J Clin Endocrinol Metab 1996;81:174–179.
199. Ininns EK, Gatanaga M, Cappuccini F, Dett CA, Yamamoto RS, Granger GA, et al. Growth of the endometrial adenocarcinoma cell line AN3 CA is modulated by tumor necrosis factor and its receptor is up-regulated by estrogen in vitro. Endocrinology 1992;130:1852–1856.

17 Immunotherapy and Prevention of Autoimmune Endocrinopathies

*Parth Narendran, BSc, MRCP,
Edwin A. M. Gale, MA, FRCP,
and Colin M. Dayan, PhD, FRCP*

CONTENTS

INTRODUCTION
NONDISEASE-SPECIFIC IMMUNOTHERAPY AND RELATED APPROACHES
TOWARD AN ORGAN-SPECIFIC APPROACH TO THE MANAGEMENT
  OF AUTOIMMUNE ENDOCRINOPATHIES
CONCEPTS UNDERLYING ANTIGEN-SPECIFIC IMMUNOTHERAPY
ANIMAL STUDIES IN INVOLVING ANTIGEN-SPECIFIC IMMUNOTHERAPY
POTENTIAL PROBLEMS WITH ANTIGEN-SPECIFIC IMMUNOTHERAPY
HUMAN STUDIES INVOLVING ANTIGEN-SPECIFIC IMMUNOTHERAPY
SUMMARY AND CONCLUSIONS
REFERENCES

INTRODUCTION

Most autoimmune endocrinopathies result in hormone deficiency and are treated by hormone replacement: Type 1 diabetes is managed with insulin, Hashimoto's thyroiditis with thyroxine, and Addison's disease with steroids. Perfectly regulated substitution of endogenous hormone secretion is, however, not possible, and as a result outcomes, although generally good for thyroid or adrenal deficiency, are unsatisfactory for diabetes. Some 30% of patients with Type 1 diabetes still develop nephropathy and 50% are likely to require laser therapy for retinopathy, complications that could in theory be prevented by near-physiological glucose control (1). An additional challenge is Graves' (thyroid) ophthalmopathy, which unlike other manifestations of autoimmune thyroid disease is not generally improved by treatment of the endocrine disturbance. In general, hormone replacement does not affect the underlying immune process in these diseases.

Where clinical outcomes are unsatisfactory, immunotherapy would be a rational alternative provided it confers a better result for the patient overall. Safety is a key issue here, and generalized immunosuppression, as used in such conditions as rheumatoid arthritis or systemic lupus erythematosus, has side effects that would be unacceptable for most

From: *Contemporary Endocrinology: Autoimmune Endocrinopathies*
Edited by: R. Volpé © Humana Press Inc., Totowa, NJ

autoimmune endocrinopathies. Alternative approaches are therefore required to improve the balance between the benefits of preserving or restoring endogenous hormone production, and the side effects of therapy. Autoimmune endocrinopathies, particularly Type 1 diabetes, therefore provide a strong incentive to develop antigen-specific immunomodulation. This implies the ability to downregulate the immune response to one or a group of proteins (antigens) without compromising the immune system as a whole—a long-sought-after goal in the field of immunotherapy.

This chapter will outline the successes and failures of attempted immunotherapy of the autoimmune endocrinopathies, concentrating mainly on Type 1 diabetes. We will first describe nonselective immunotherapy and other approaches that do not modulate the immune response in an organ-specific manner. Following this, we will outline the principles underlying current approaches to antigen-specific immunotherapy, and present data from animal and human studies to show the promise of these techniques.

NONDISEASE-SPECIFIC IMMUNOTHERAPY AND RELATED APPROACHES

Type 1 (Insulin-Dependent) Diabetes

BACKGROUND

Type 1 diabetes results from autoimmune destruction of the insulin-producing β cells within the pancreatic islets. It is a polygenic disorder with a major contribution from the major histocompataibility complex (MHC) region; other gene regions involved include the variable number of tandem reports (VNTR) region adjacent to the insulin gene on chromosome 11 *(2)*. The incidence of childhood diabetes has risen steadily in genetically stable populations *(3)*, an observation that has suggested that environmental influences encountered *in utero* or soon after birth may play an important part in the disease process. For whatever reason, circulating islet autoantibodies may appear soon after birth, and are usually established by about the age of three in most children at risk for diabetes *(4)*. At a later stage in the disease process, activated T lymphocytes directed against islet constituents may be detected in the circulation, and a declining first-phase insulin response to IV glucose may provide the first evidence of target organ failure (*see* Chapter 12).

Autoimmune diabetes is thought to represent a disease spectrum. For example, human leukocyte antigen (HLA) DR3/DR4 heterozygotes are heavily overrepresented in early-onset Type 1 diabetes, but are much less apparent in adult-onset disease *(5)*. Insulitis is characteristic in post-mortem pancreatic specimens from children who die soon after diagnosis of diabetes, but is infrequently detected in deaths after the age of 15 yr *(6)*. Insulin autoantibodies (IAA) and antibodies to tyrosine phosphatase/IA-2 (IA2 Ab) are characteristic of early-onset disease, but are less commonly present with advancing age of onset *(7)*. In contrast, islet cell antibodies (ICA) and antibodies to glutamic acid decarboxylase (GADA) are present in some 5–10% of all patients presenting with diabetes after the age of 40, and are considered predictive of β-cell failure and insulin dependency *(8)*.

One major limitation of attempts to understand the natural history of the disease process is that islet tissue is for practical purposes unobtainable. Events in the pancreas must therefore be inferred from changes in circulating markers. A useful animal model, the nonobese diabetic (NOD) mouse, has however allowed the evolution of the disease process to be studied in detail, and interventions to be tested. Valuable though this model is, it provides little more than an analogy for human β-cell destruction, and lessons learned in the laboratory can be difficult and laborious to apply to the human situation *(9)*.

STRATEGIES OF INTERVENTION

An understanding—although incomplete—of the natural history of the disease is fundamental to planning types of intervention. Three potential levels of intervention are recognized. Primary prevention would be therapy aimed at preventing initiation or development of islet autoimmunity. This form of treatment, for example, by removal of environmental risk factors would need to be introduced early in life, ideally before circulating autoantibodies had appeared in the circulation. Secondary prevention refers to treatment aimed at an established, but still subclinical autoimmune process, and recruitment relies on risk analysis based mainly on circulating humoral markers. Tertiary prevention in this context refers to intervention after clinical diagnosis, in the attempt to salvage residual β cells.

Safety is of paramount importance in planning an intervention in Type 1 diabetes. In the first place, only a small proportion of those exposed to any form of primary intervention would be expected to develop childhood diabetes. The balance of risk-to-benefit is therefore firmly tilted against any intervention that is not relatively innocuous. More hazardous therapy may be applied for tertiary prevention, which has 100% efficiency in identifying disease, but risks of treatment need to be considered in the light of a disease for which a safe and well-established form of hormone-replacement therapy is available. The role of efficacy is in contrast sometimes overemphasized. A safe treatment with relatively low efficacy that could be widely applied for primary prevention would, for example, prevent far more cases of diabetes than a more potent, but more hazardous therapy for secondary prevention *(9)*.

THERAPIES FOR PRIMARY PREVENTION

The Milk Hypothesis. This developed from three observations. The first was that prolonged breast-feeding is mildly protective against later development of Type 1 diabetes; second, addition or removal of dietary cows' milk modulated diabetes development in the BioBreeding (BB) rat, a model of autoimmune diabetes, and third, patients with newly diagnosed diabetes had increased levels of antibodies to milk constituents *(10)*. The issue remains highly controversial, in that early studies favored an effect of introduction of cows' milk into the diet before 4 mo of age, but subsequent studies failed to confirm this *(11)*. T-cell proliferative responses to β casein constituents of cows' milk are reportedly high in newly diagnosed patients *(12)*, suggesting that crossreactivity between islet cell proteins and β casein might underlie this association, but this report has yet to be confirmed. A pilot study of cows' milk avoidance in infancy has been carried out in 20 infants of mothers with diabetes, randomized to either standard formula or a casein hydrolysate formula. No difference in antibody levels was seen, and one child in the casein hydrolysate group developed Type 1 diabetes at 14 mo, preceded by the appearance of ICA, IAA, and GADA in the circulation *(13)*. At present, it is uncertain whether larger trials of this type will be undertaken.

The Viral Hypothesis. A number of studies have implicated enteroviral infection in the causation of Type 1 diabetes *(14)*. The role of such infection remains unclear, but if confirmed would make some forms of primary prevention feasible. For example, congenital rubella predisposes to later development of Type 1 diabetes, but this rare variant has now been eliminated by rubella vaccination in the female population. Maternal Coxsackie B infection has been reported to increase the risk of diabetes in the offspring *(15)* and, if confirmed, would allow a similar vaccination program to be undertaken.

SECONDARY PREVENTION

Predicting Diabetes. The central aim of secondary prevention is to identify individuals at high risk of progression to Type 1 diabetes and to intervene to lower this risk. Circulating autoantibodies remain the mainstay of disease prediction. Genetic markers are at present too nonspecific to identify high levels of risk, but a first-degree family history of diabetes provides a simple surrogate for genetic risk. For example, siblings are some 15 times more likely to develop childhood diabetes than a child from the background population *(16)*. Family members are in addition highly motivated to take part in clinical studies.

Family studies show that islet autoantibodies may precede the onset of disease by many years, suggesting a slow smouldering disease prodrome during which screening for risk can be undertaken and interventions tested. Prospective studies from birth suggest that evidence of an established autoimmune response is usually present by 3 yr of age and often earlier than this *(4,17)*; family studies suggest that antibody levels are relatively stable over the age of 5. A high risk of progression is associated with young age and the presence of multiple islet autoantibodies. Autoantibodies to 3/4 of the standard markers, ICA, GADA, IA-2-Ab, and IAA are associated with a >80% risk of progression to insulin therapy within 10 yr in first-degree relatives *(18,19)*, and promise to be almost equally predictive in the general population. Progression to target organ failure can be monitored by measurement of the first-phase insulin response to the intravenous glucose tolerance test (IVGTT) *(20)*, which provides a useful indication of time to onset of the disease. Not everyone with antibodies to islet antigens will progress to Type 1 diabetes, however, and slow or nonprogression is associated with age >40 yr, the presence of single (rather than multiple) antibody types, and the presence of protective alleles, such as DQB1*0602 *(21)*.

End Points for Secondary Intervention. The major practical problem associated with secondary prevention is that very large numbers of first-degree relatives need to be screened in order to recruit the numbers needed to achieve adequate statistical power. Further, at present, the only useful end point to such a study is diabetes development. This means that trials must not only be large, but also long. For example, the European Nicotinamide Diabetes Intervention Trial (ENDIT) has needed to screen some 40,000 first-degree relatives in order to identify 528 study entrants and is likely to run for 5 yr *(see below)*. Smaller studies risk overoptimistic outcomes or may discard useful treatment effects. Valid surrogate end points would greatly simplify evaluation of treatment in prediabetes, but are not available as yet.

TERTIARY PREVENTION

Postmortem studies suggest that β-cell destruction is far from complete at clinical onset. Comparison with studies in baboons suggests that even when the first-phase insulin response is undetectable, some 40–50% of the β-cell mass remains viable *(22)*. Follow-up studies in humans with C-peptide stimulation tests suggest that the remaining β cells are usually destroyed within a few years of diagnosis, although residual insulin secretion may persist in some over many years. A diagrammatic plot of β-cell mass over time is shown in Fig. 1.

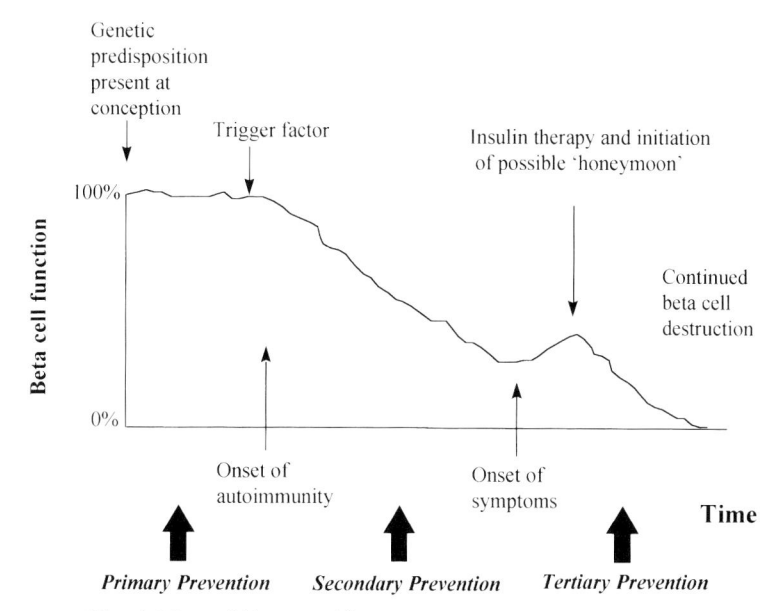

Fig. 1. Natural history of β-cell function in Type 1 diabetes.

The main practical advantages of intervention after clinical diagnosis are that all those treated are affected by the disease, and that it offers a convenient means of testing therapies for efficacy. For this reason, all earlier trials with relatively toxic agents focused on newly diagnosed individuals. Proof of effect at this stage of the disease would provide a powerful incentive for attempted secondary prevention. The potential disadvantage is that some therapies might prove effective at an earlier stage of the disease, but ineffective in its terminal stages, and thus be discarded unnecessarily.

End Points for Tertiary Intervention. Many individuals show some improvement of metabolic control associated with falling insulin requirements in the months following diagnosis, but the concept of "remission" of Type 1 diabetes remains poorly defined. Treatment protocols vary, and it is difficult to distinguish between the strategy of management (amount of insulin used, degree of glycemic control achieved) and the underlying pathophysiology (recovery of residual insulin secretion). Few patients achieve full independence from insulin associated with near-normoglycaemic control, and evaluation of response therefore rests largely on measurement of stimulated C-peptide secretion. Standard criteria for evaluation have been agreed *(23)*, but many published studies do not follow these and are therefore difficult to evaluate.

THERAPIES FOR SECONDARY AND TERTIARY PREVENTION

The principles of therapy do not differ for these two stages of the disease, and they will therefore be considered together.

Cyclosporin A. Cyclosporin is a fungal metabolite that suppresses the proliferative potential of the whole T-lymphocyte repertoire by actions on interleukin 2 (IL-2) and cyclophilin *(24)*. Two major placebo-controlled trials in the 1980s showed that it has the potential to slow the progression of β-cell destruction in newly diagnosed patients *(25,26)*. In these studies, it was administered orally at starting doses of 5–10 mg/kg as opposed to the standard starting dose of 10–15 mg/kg for suppression of transplant rejection—its

Table 1
Trials of Immunotherapy in Human Type 1 Diabetes Involving Cyclosporin A[a]

Study	Trial design	Outcome
Feutren et al. (25) 122 recently diagnosed subjects Age 15–40	7.5 mg/kg/d Follow-up for 9 mo Double-blind, placebo-controlled trial	More remissions recorded in the treated group; differences between 2 groups first noted at 6 mo
Canadian-European randomized trial group (26) 188 recently diagnosed subjects Age 10–35	Initial dose of 20 mg/kg/d adjusted to trough concentrations Follow-up for 1 yr Double-blind, placebo-controlled trial	Greater number of remissions and higher stimulated C peptide in the treated group; benefits greater in most recently diagnosed subjects
DeFilippo et al. (128) 83 newly diagnosed subjects Average age 10	7.2 mg/kg/d Average duration of therapy was 18 mo Subjects followed up for 6 yr in total Control population obtained from another study	Treated group sustained twice the number of remissions and recorded twice the stimulated C peptide as the untreated group; however, this difference was only significant over the first 4 yr
Chase et al. (129) 43 newly diagnosed subjects Age 9–24	Initial dose of 10 mg/kg/d adusted to blood levels Therapy continued for 4 mo Placebo-controlled	No difference in stimulated C peptide, glycosylated hemoglobin, or insulin doses between treatment subjects

[a]*See also* register of published immune intervention trials in Type 1 diabetes (127).

more common clinical use. It should be noted though that the maintenance doses of cyclosporin used in the studies were broadly similar to those used in transplant rejection. Use of cyclosporin resulted in a marked increase in insulin-independent remissions in these studies, a response that was most evident in those with the highest trough levels of the drug. The benefits of cyclosporin were, however, transient and were largely lost within 2 yr of diagnosis. A small pilot study in prediabetes suggested that cyclosporin treatment delayed the development of diabetes (in comparison with historical controls), but four of the six patients receiving treatment developed diabetes in the course of follow-up (27). Some of these studies are summarized in Table 1.

Many smaller, less-well-controlled studies have also been performed with cyclosporin, which have at the very least contributed to our knowledge of the side effects of therapy with this drug. The main side effect of cyclosporin, other than immunosuppression, is dose-related nephrotoxicity and therefore serum levels need to be monitored carefully. Renal biopsies in 192 patients treated for autoimmune diseases with a mean cyclosporin dose of 8.2 ± 2.8 mg/kg/d showed that 41 had nephropathic changes (28), although these usually resolve on stopping the drug (29). The risk of these side effects is minimized by using doses no greater than 5 mg/kg/d, and by stopping the drug if serum creatinine shows a >30% increase from baseline. Occasional patients have shown apparent striking benefit

Table 2
Trials of Immunotherapy in Human Type 1 Diabetes Involving Azathioprine[a]

Study	Trial design	Outcome
Harrison et al. (138) 24 recently diagnosed subjects Age 15–40	2 mg/kg/d Therapy for 12 mo Randomized study	Treated group had higher basal and stimulated C peptide and more remissions (7/13 vs 1/11)
Cook et al. (31) 49 recently diagnosed subjects Age 2–20	2 mg/kg/d Therapy for 12 mo Double-blind control study	Significant improvement in stimulated C peptide with therapy at 3–6 mo but this was not sustained; no improvement in remission rates
Silverstein et al. (32) 46 newly diagnosed subjects Age 4–33	Oral prednisone 2 mg/kg/d reducing to nil over 10 wk Azathioprine 2 mg/kg/d Therapy for 1 yr Unblinded study	Lower insulin requirements and higher stimulated C peptide in treated group; steroids caused transient cushinoid appearance; mild azathioprine associated side effects in three patients

[a]*See also* register of published immune intervention trials in Type 1 diabetes (127).

—one remains insulin-independent 7 yr after diagnosis (30), but for practical purposes, cyclosporin is generally considered too toxic for use in Type 1 diabetes.

Azathioprine. Azathioprine is a cytotoxic agent that is commonly used as an immunosuppressant. Like cyclosporin, it is usually given for the prevention of transplant rejection, but azathioprine has also been used to treat conditions, such as inflammatory bowel disease and rheumatoid arthritis. Azathioprine has been used only for tertiary prevention in Type 1 diabetes. A placebo-controlled trial in 49 children showed no effect on the remission period (31). In contrast, a controlled trial of azathioprine plus prednisolone in 23 newly diagnosed patients showed some benefit in terms of residual insulin secretion, and 3 remained insulin-independent at 2 yr (32)—see Table 2. Once again, the potential for side effects, including myelosuppression and hepatotoxicity, has limited the further use of this agent.

Nicotinamide. Nicotinamide, a soluble B-group vitamin, is a precursor of nicotinamide adenine dinucleotide (NAD), a coenzyme involved in a wide range of energy-transfer processes within the cell. Its β-cell protective effects were first described in 1947 in the alloxan-induced rat model of this disease and, subsequently, in streptozotocin-treated animals. Nicotinamide is moderately protective against spontaneous diabetes in the NOD mouse, and has been shown to have β-cell sparing effects in a variety of other in vitro and in vivo models of damage (33).

Its effects may be mediated in three possible ways. It is a free radical scavenger, it inhibits the intranuclear repair enzyme poly-ADP-ribose polymerase (PARP), and also replenishes intracellular levels of NAD. Work by Heller et al. (34) has suggested that inhibition of PARP is the most important of these properties.

High-dose nicotinamide has been used for tertiary prevention in a number of trials, with conflicting results. Meta-analysis of these studies has, however, suggested a weak yet significant effect on insulin secretory reserve. Its use has appeared more promising in secondary prevention, particularly because of a relative lack of side effects. Elliott and Chase treated 14 children at high risk of diabetes *(35)*. Follow-up of this cohort showed that by 30 mo, 5/14 had developed diabetes, as opposed to 8/8 historical controls *(36)*. Elliott extended this work by setting up a large diabetes prevention trial using nicotinamide in ICA-positive schoolchildren, suggesting that a population of children screened for ICA and offered treatment if strongly positive had a reduced incidence of diabetes compared to an unscreened comparison group *(37)*.

Based on these results, two randomized control trials were started in ICA-positive first-degree relatives. The first of these, a German national study, was discontinued when equal numbers (7 vs 6) developed diabetes on nicotinamide or placebo. This study was, however, designed to detect an 80% treatment effect—much greater than that reported in pilot studies—and was therefore relatively underpowered. The second, ENDIT, is still under way. This multinational trial has screened in excess of 40,000 first-degree relatives for ICA; those with confirmed levels > 20 Juvenile Diabetes Foundation (JDF) units and aged 5–40 yr have been randomized to high-dose nicotinamide or placebo. The recruitment target of 528 was reached toward the end of 1997, and the study is expected to be reported in 2002.

Insulin. Administration of subcutaneous insulin to the BB rat and NOD mouse slows progression of the autoimmune process and delays the onset of diabetes *(38,39)*. Since insulin is given to all newly diagnosed patients with Type 1 diabetes, it is difficult to evaluate as a means of tertiary prevention. In one influential study, newly diagnosed patients were treated with carefully titrated doses of intravenous insulin by Biostator for 2 wk in order to obtain optimal blood sugar control. This intervention alone was sufficient to result in higher C-peptide levels and better glucose control for up to a year *(40)*. This study has never been convincingly replicated. Based on this study and the animal data, 12 high-risk prediabetics were offered insulin prophylaxis involving intermittent iv insulin and twice-daily sc insulin. Seven refused treatment, and all developed diabetes within 3 yr. Of five who accepted treatment, only one developed diabetes within the same period *(41)*.

Metabolically active β cells have been proposed to offer more of a target to the immune system *(42)*, and it was hypothesized that insulin might work by inducing "β-cell rest." This hypothesis remains unproven, however, and it seems unlikely that the insulin doses used are sufficient to suppress C-peptide production. Alternatively, the iv insulin used as part of the regimen might have a role in tolerance induction (*see* Concepts Underlying Antigen-Specific Immunotherapy), but the true mechanism is uncertain. Hypoglycemia apart, insulin is a safe therapy, and has formed the basis of the first major US trial known as Diabetes Prevention Trial 1 (DPT1). DPT1, sponsored by the National Institute of Health, began recruitment in 1994 and has set out to screen 60,000 first-degree relatives *(43)*. Those judged to be at high risk of developing diabetes (>50% over the next 5 yr) on the basis of high-titer ICA plus metabolic testing are randomized to a combination of intermittent iv and regular sc insulin or to a no-treatment arm. The end point will be the development of disease. A second arm of the study, based on the concept of oral tolerance, is described later in this chapter.

Bacille Colmette-Gúerin (BCG). The use of BCG vaccination as immunotherapy is based on the observation that hyperactivation of the immune system (either with BCG or complete Freunds' adjuvant [CFA]) in NOD mouse model of Type 1 diabetes retards the development of disease *(44)*. In a pilot study, administration of a standard BCG vaccination dose to newly diagnosed patients resulted in more insulin-independent remissions than in unvaccinated patients *(45)*. This finding was not however confirmed in a later trial of 72 newly diagnosed patients, in whom the effect of BCG plus nicotinamide was compared with that of nicotinamide alone; addition of BCG did not influence the outcome *(46)*.

Therapy with Cytokines and Monoclonal Antibodies (MAbs). Many other non-organ-specific immunotherapies have been attempted on animal models of Type 1 diabetes with varying degrees of success. Many them act through the manipulation of T cells without regard for their receptor specificity. These have been extensively reviewed in previous articles *(47,48)*. These therapeutic approaches have been slow to be taken forward to human studies because of their nonspecific mode of action and side-effect profile.

Thyroid Disease

Autoimmune thyroid disease is a spectrum of diseases encompassing Graves' disease, primary myxoedema, and Hashimoto's and postpartum thyroiditis *(49)*. In addition, there is a very large body of subclinical disease, particularly in the female population *(50)*. The central antigens in all these diseases are thyroglobulin (Tg), the thyroid stimulating hormone (TSH) receptor (TSHR), and thyroid peroxidase (TPO), previously known as the thyroid microsomal antigen (*see* Chapter 9).

Since satisfactory therapies exist for controlling both hyper- and hypothyroidism, conventional immunosuppressive therapy has not been used to treat autoimmune thyroid disease. However, the commonly used antithyroidal drugs methimazole, carbimazole, and propylthiouracil may act partly via an immunosuppressive effect. In vitro thyroid antibody production by cultured lymphocytes is reduced by the addition of methimazole or carbimazole *(51)*, and lymphocyte proliferation is suppressed in the presence of propyl thiouracil or methimazole *(51)*. In vivo, approx 50% of Graves' patients treated with these drugs go into remission after 18 mo of therapy *(52)*. However, only historical controls prior to the introduction of these drugs are available for comparison to the spontaneous remission rate. Furthermore, it is difficult to control for any effects of the reduced thyroid hormone production induced by these drugs (*53,54*; *see* Chapter 9 for comment on this point).

In contrast to hyper- and hypothyroidism, satisfactory treatments are not available for the orbitopathy associated with autoimmune thyroiditis—thyroid eye disease (TED). In its severer forms, TED can progress to exposure keratitis, disfigurement of appearance, persistent diplopia, and occasionally blindness from retro-orbital optic nerve compression. A variety of immunotherapies have therefore been applied in TED. However, the natural course of the condition is very hard to predict, and spontaneous remissions are common. Therefore, favorable results in uncontrolled studies need to be interpreted with caution (*see* Chapter 10).

In the active phase, TED has been shown to respond to high-dose steroids given orally with or without cyclosporine *(55)*. In this study, side effects were common particularly because of the doses used; of the 40 patients, 4 developed a derangement of liver function tests, 4 developed hypertension, and 1 developed a Klebsiella pneumonia. High-dose immunoglobulin treatment appears to be as effective as high-dose steroid treatment, but without the side effects. It has also been tried in the management of pretibial myxoedema *(56)*; results have been favorable with a reduction in affected skin thickness and lymphocytic infiltration when compared with steroids. However, immunoglobulin therapy is expensive, iv administration necessitates repeated daily hospital admissions compared with the simple oral administration of steroids, and past use has been complicated by viral contamination. Present unlicensed use is therefore recommended only when standard approaches have failed. In recent years, low-dose orbital radiotherapy has been used for TED with or without adjunctive lower-dose steroids and azathioprine. Results are not available from a controlled trial, but uncontrolled studies look promising with low toxicity at least in the short term and good final outcomes *(57)*. It seems unlikely that radiation therapy will prove applicable to other autoimmune endocrinopathies.

Polyglandular Autoimmunity Plus Gonadal Autoimmunity

Autoimmune oophritis may account for as much as 30% of the cases of premature ovarian failure *(58)*. There are reports of a recurrence of menses with steroid therapy *(59,60)*. In all cases, the patient had polyglandular autoimmunity with associated Addison's disease, and it was for this reason that 5-10 mg steroid replacement was started. However, this small dose is unlikely to cause significant immunosuppression. The mechanism may be related to the correction of any salt imbalance associated with Addison's disease. (*See* Chapters 15 and 16.)

Adrenal Autoimmunity (Addison's Disease)

Addison's disease is usually managed by steroid replacement, with increases in dosage during intercurrent stress. Few studies of immunotherapy have been conducted in this area. In a Chinese study *(61)*, cadaveric adrenal tissue from fetuses over 5 mo of age was transplanted into 13 Addisonian patients. Rejection was controlled with hydrocortisone in combination with either cyclosporin or azathioprine. Though 11 of these patients did not require steroid replacement, they received it as part of the general immunosuppressive protocol for an average for 4 yr. One patient developed baldness as a complication of azathioprine (*See* Chapter 13.)

TOWARDS AN ORGAN-SPECIFIC APPROACH TO THE MANAGEMENT OF AUTOIMMUNE ENDOCRINOPATHIES

The above trials suggest that nonspecific immunosuppression may be of limited use because of poor efficacy and high risk of side effects. In human Type 1 diabetes, this may partly be owing to the suboptimal doses utilized in order to limit potential side effects. As a result, there has been increasing interest in more organ-specific approaches over the past 10 yr.

It was demonstrated as early as 1911 by Wells that guinea pigs fed hen egg lysosyme had a reduced immune response to subsequent challenge with this protein, but retained normal responses to other antigens *(62)*. This is often referred to as the induction of antigen-specific tolerance, to distinguish it from treatments that cause generalized immunosuppression. Exploitation of this phenomenon to generate organ-specific tolerance would clearly represent an ideal approach to treating endocrine autoimmunity.

There is now little doubt that such antigen-specific tolerance can be induced in animal models. However, the immune mechanisms underlying this phenomenon and the optimal protocol for tolerance induction in adult animals have only recently begun to be elucidated. Furthermore, the application of these techniques to spontaneous autoimmune diseases in which the immune response appears to have multiple antigenic targets, and

Chapter 17 / Autoimmune Endocrinopathies 403

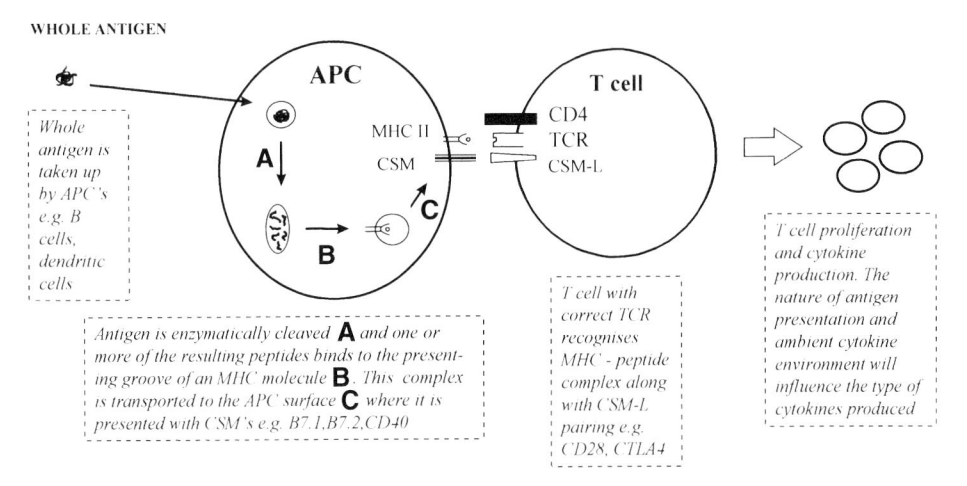

Fig 2. CD4 T-cell recognition of antigen. Abbreviations: APC, antigen presenting cell; CSM, costimulatory molecule; CSM-L, CSM ligand; MHC, major histocompatibility antigen; TCR, T-cell receptor.

in which the immune process has already begun at the time of tolerance induction, poses additional problems.

Current approaches to developing organ-specific immunotherapy are described in this section. The concepts and mechanisms underlying immune tolerance induction will first be reviewed to provide a framework for understanding developments in this area. This will be followed by a summary of progress in animal studies. Though human trials in autoimmune endocrinopathies are ongoing, none have as yet been completed. However, data from other human autoimmune diseases will be summarized before assessing future prospects in this area.

CONCEPTS UNDERLYING ANTIGEN-SPECIFIC IMMUNOTHERAPY

Mechanisms of Antigen-Specific Tolerance

T CELLS: THE "GATEKEEPERS" OF THE IMMUNE RESPONSE

T cells play a pivotal role in the initiation and control of an immune response *(63)*. Helper (CD4) T-cell activation is the first step in generating both a high-affinity antibody response (via T cell–B cell collaboration) and for a CD8 T-cell-mediated cytotoxic response (via T cell–T cell collaboration). T-cell activation is initiated by the interaction of the antigen-specific T-cell receptor on the T-cell surface with a combination of a peptide fragment of the antigen and the MHC molecule complexed together on the surface of an antigen-presenting cell (*see* Fig. 2). Activation results in T-cell proliferation and cytokine production. T cells are also thought to play a key role in regulating the immune response and suppressing unwanted immune reactions though the mechanisms involved are still unclear. (*See* Chapter 1.)

THE ROLE OF THE THYMUS: "CENTRAL" VS "PERIPHERAL" TOLERANCE

T cells are required to pass through the thymus gland in order to develop to functional maturity. Over 95% *(64)* of T-cell precursors die within the thymus itself and are not released into the circulation. Recent studies confirm that developing T cells that recognize self-antigen in the thymus with high affinity are destroyed *(65)*. Therefore, the failure of most individuals to react to their own self-proteins is partly the result of intrathymic deletion of T cells able to mount such an immune response. This mechanism is referred to as "central tolerance." It should be distinguished from "peripheral tolerance" in which mature, circulating T cells already released from the thymus are "tolerized" to self-antigen either by anergy or deletion. Mechanisms for inducing peripheral tolerance are of particular interest to immunotherapists, since this approach can be applied to older children or adults in whom the majority of T cells have already emerged from the thymus.

Peripheral Tolerance: A Dynamic Process Maintained Through Different Mechanisms—Deletion, Anergy, Suppression

The T-cell response to a given antigen can be abolished in one of three ways. First, all T cells able to react to the antigen could be destroyed or "deleted." Second, these T cells could be functionally silenced rather than actually deleted. Here, the T cell remains viable, but can no longer respond to further challenge with the target antigen by proliferation or initiation of other arms of the immune response. Such refractory T cells are referred to as being in a state of "anergy" *(66)*. Third, T cells can be rendered into a state in which, like anergy, they are still viable, but behave differently on further challenge with antigen. Unlike the anergic state, these T cells can respond by releasing cytokines that are able to suppress cellular immune responses in bystander T cells. Such cells are often referred to as "regulatory" T cells. Recent studies confirm that T cells can indeed change the profile of cytokines they produce in such a way as to promote or suppress immune responses *(67)*.

Th1 vs Th2 Cells: Immune Deviation

In 1986 Mossman reported in mouse studies that on receiving an antigenic stimulus, T-helper cells (Th), which carry the surface marker CD4, can differentiate into one of two cell types producing different cytokine profiles *(68)*. Th1 cells predominantly secrete interferon γ (IFN-γ) and interleukin 2 (IL-2), and generate cell-mediated immunity *(69)*, but Th2 cells secrete IL-4, IL-10, and transforming growth factor β (TGF-β), and promote humoral immunity *(70)*. The direction of differentiation is decided partly by the ambient cytokine milieu *(71)*; the presence of IFN-γ encourages maturation down the Th1 pathway, whereas IL-4 promotes the formation of Th2 cells. Therefore, production of one type of T cells in an immune response tends to be self-perpetuating, since their cytokine products provide the milieu for more of the same Th type of cells to develop. Note that T cells specific for the same antigen can have different cytokine profiles.

In murine studies, it appears that the majority of immune responses are polarized to either a Th1- or a Th2-type response. In humans, the picture is less clear–cut, but most cell-mediated autoimmune endocrinopathies, such as Type 1 diabetes and autoimmune thyroiditis, appear to feature a Th1-type response *(72,73)*. Studies in mouse models indicate that interventions able to change the Th1- to a Th2-type response are associated with prevention or amelioration of the autoimmune damage. Therefore, this represents a potential approach to immunotherapy. The conversion of an immune response from Th1 to a Th2 type (or vice versa) is referred to as "immune deviation."

Th2 cells specific for antigens in the target tissue can potentially act as "suppressor cells" in autoimmune endocrinopathies. If such T cells home to the target organ owing to their antigenic specificity, reactivation by self-antigens in the target tissue will cause them to release IL-4 and related Th2 cytokines (particularly IL-10) into the local environ-

Chapter 17 / Autoimmune Endocrinopathies

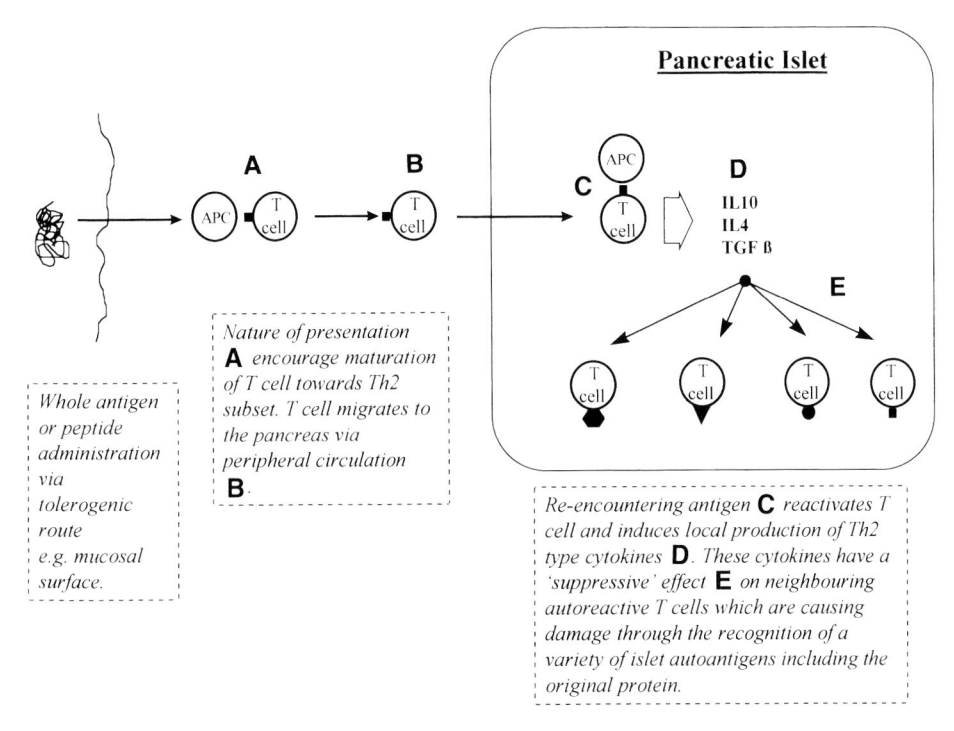

Fig 3. An example of bystander suppression in the pancreatic beta cell.

Figure labels:
- Whole antigen or peptide administration via tolerogenic route e.g. mucosal surface.
- Nature of presentation **A** encourage maturation of T cell towards Th2 subset. T cell migrates to the pancreas via peripheral circulation **B**.
- Re-encountering antigen **C** reactivates T cell and induces local production of Th2 type cytokines **D**. These cytokines have a 'suppressive' effect **E** on neighbouring autoreactive T cells which are causing damage through the recognition of a variety of islet autoantigens including the original protein.

ment. This will slow the surrounding Th1-type response, downregulating the activity of nearby Th1 cells. Since all T cells in the immediate vicinity will be affected, this phenomenon is often referred to as "bystander suppression" *(74)* (*see* Fig. 3). This mechanism differs from that of classical "suppressor T cells" in two ways: first, the regulatory Th2 cells are of CD4 rather than CD8 phenotype, and second, their action is not strictly antigen-specific. This latter property carries the advantage that at least in theory, the immune response to all organ-specific autoantigens could be downregulated by the presence of Th2 cells with only a single specificity.

Identifying Disease-Specific Autoantigens: The Problem of Identifying T-Cell Epitopes

Restricting immunotherapy to an organ requires the prior identification of antigenic targets on that organ. In the last 12 yr, studies of circulating autoantibodies have identified one or more target antigens in the majority of autoimmune endocrinopathies, including autoimmune thyroiditis, Type 1 diabetes, and autoimmune adrenalitis (*see* Chapter 8). A major exception is thyroid ophthalmopathy in which the antigen that links this condition to Graves' disease has been elusive, although the TSHR remains a strong candidate *(75)*.

Unfortunately, there is no guarantee that B-cell autoantigens (those recognized by autoantibodies) will be the same as T-cell autoantigens. As we have seen, tolerance induction is almost entirely a T-cell-dependent phenomenon, making this more than an academic issue. Studying autoantigen responses by T cells is significantly more difficult than studying autoantibody levels. T-cell assays are less sensitive, less reproducible, and if performed on peripheral blood, may miss the majority of autoreactive T cells, which will be concentrated in the target organ. Such data as are available *(76–78)* appear to support the view that T and B cells recognize similar self-proteins in autoimmunity. However, in contrast to autoantibody responses, it is common to have similar T-cell responses in both affected individuals and controls *(79)*, emphasizing that the presence of self-reactive T cells in the peripheral blood is not sufficient alone to result in autoimmune disease.

Note also that even where T cells and B cells recognize the same protein, individual T cells recognize short linear peptides (epitopes), whereas B cells tend to recognize aspects of the three-dimensional configuration of a protein. Therefore, for any given protein, the epitopic regions recognized by B and T cells can be different.

Techniques of Antigen Administration That Promote T-Cell Tolerance

In the original studies of Wells *(62)*, administration of antigen by the oral route was found to induce tolerance, in contrast to conventional routes of immunization. Since that time, considerable effort has been devoted to developing ways of administering antigen in order to induce tolerance in a more effective manner.

EFFECT OF ROUTE OF EXPOSURE

Antigens entering the body by different routes encounter different types of lymphoid cells and antigen-processing pathways. In general, delivery of antigen to mucosal surfaces by oral or intranasal administration results in tolerance *(80,81)*, whereas administration via the sc route usually results in immunization. Intraperitoneal (ip) and iv antigen administration of antigen also tend to result in tolerance rather than immunization.

EFFECT OF ADJUVANT

Antigen in particulate form, e.g., complexed with aluminum hydroxide or suspended in oil in the presence of mycobacteria CFA, enhances the immune response induced. In contrast to immunization with adjuvant, the administration of antigen in soluble form or in oil alone (incomplete Freund's adjuvant) appears to promotes tolerance induction.

EFFECT OF DOSE ADMINISTERED

The importance of antigen dose in inducing tolerance when given to neonatal animals or intravenously to adult animals is well recognized *(82)*. Recent work with transgenic mice given antigen via a mucosal route has shown that the dose of antigen also influences the mechanism by which tolerance is induced. Using the oral route, high doses were found to cause deletion of antigen-specific T cells in the lymphoid tissue of the gut, the Peyer's patches. At lower doses, deletion was not seen, but rather an increase in the production of the Th2-type cytokines, IL-4, and IL-10, by antigen-specific T cells suggesting immune deviation *(83–85)* .

EFFECT OF WHOLE ANTIGEN VS EPITOPE

Th cell (CD4) epitopes are typically 10–12 amino acids long. Just as exposure to the whole antigen can downregulate an immune response when given under the appropriate conditions, so can exposure to the T-cell epitope of that antigen alone *(86)*. Recent experiments suggest that engineering analogs of the peptide epitope that bind to the MHC class II molecule with altered affinity can increase their "tolerogenicity" *(87)*, possibly through immune deviation *(88)*. Using peptides also has the added advantage of minimizing the risk of B cell epitopes on whole protein, thus enhancing autoreactive antibody production.

Table 3
Successful Antigen Specific Immunotherapeutic Interventions
in the NOD Mouse Model of Type 1 Diabetes: Year and Reference to Studies

	Autoantigen used for tolerization	
	GAD	Insulin
Treatment before onset of insulitis	1993 *(91)*, 1994 *(89)*	1996 *(130)*
Treatment after onset of insulitis	1994 *(131)*, 1996 *(132)*	1996 *(93,130)*
Ag administration via the oral route	1995 *(133)*	1991 *(130,94)*
Ag administration via the sc route	ND[a]	1995 *(92)*, 1996 *(96)*
Ag administration via the ip route	1995 *(134)*, 1996 *(97)*	ND
Ag administration via the iv route	1993 *(91)*	1995 *(135)*
Ag administration via the intranasal route	1996 *(95)*	1996 *(93,96)*
T-cell epitope as therapeutic agent	1996 *(95)*	1996 *(136)*, 1997 *(137)*

[a] ND, not published to our knowledge.

ANIMAL STUDIES IN INVOLVING ANTIGEN-SPECIFIC IMMUNOTHERAPY

Type 1 Diabetes

Studies of antigen-specific immunotherapy in Type 1 diabetes have largely been conducted in the NOD mouse model. The antigens predominantly used to induce tolerance have been glutamic acid decarboxylase (GAD) and insulin, although only the latter is truly islet cell-specific.

Table 3 summarizes the variety of approaches used. Successful techniques include ip administration of soluble antigen at birth *(89)*, intrathymic injection of antigen at 3 wk of age *(90)*, iv injection of antigen at 3 wk of age *(91)*, sc injections in incomplete Freund's adjuvant at 1 mo of age *(92)*, intranasal administration after 4 wk *(93)*, and oral administration of whole antigen *(94)*.

Peptide immunotherapy with the T-cell target epitopes of GAD and insulin have also been successfully conducted, the former being administered via the nasal route *(95)* and the latter effective both via the nasal as well as the sc route *(96)*.

Note therefore that this tolerogenic approach can be effective when administered in a variety of antigenic forms, through a variety of routes and at different stages of disease. The therapy has been beneficial when administered as late as 3 mo *(97)*, an age at which lymphocytic infiltration into pancreatic β cells is well established in a standard NOD mouse colonies. However, the studies suggest that early therapy provides better results.

Animal models other than the NOD mouse have also been effectively treated: transgenic mice expressing the viral nucleoprotein of the lymphocytic choriomeningitis virus (LCMV) under control of the rat insulin promoter develop Type 1 diabetes on infection with LCMV. Disease incidence can be reduced by 1 mg oral insulin twice a week either before or after virus infection, i.e., before or after onset of disease *(98)*.

The mechanism of tolerance induction has not been elucidated for every technique used. Evidence for immune deviation has been obtained following a single intranasal or ip administration of GAD at 3 wk *(95,97)* and weekly oral administration of porcine insulin *(94)*. Dose appeared critical in this latter study: oral tolerance was achieved with a 1-mg dose of insulin, but not with 500 μg or 5 mg. In several studies, protection against diabetes could be passed to naive recipients by the transfer of CD4 T cells, consistent with immune deviation and bystander suppression. Note, however, that if antigen-specific Th2 cells are transferred along with Th1-type cells, protection is not conferred on the recipient *(99)*.

Two other antigens have been used to form the basis of antigen-specific immunotherapy in NOD mice. Subcutaneous injection of a T-cell epitope of the 65-kDa heat-shock protein (hsp65), which has been shown to be an autoantigen in NOD mouse diabetes, in incomplete Freund's adjuvant is effective at treating disease when given as late as 4–12 wk of age *(100,101)*. Therapy was associated with a switch in the secretion of Th1-type cytokines toward that of Th2. Furthermore, the investigators also showed that the response to islet antigens other than hsp65 was downregulated, whereas responses to control antigens were unaffected *(102)*, suggesting that mechanisms of anergy and immune deviation can be activated with identical protocols. Transgenic expression of the insulin precursor proinsulin in the thymus has also been shown to prevent diabetes in the NOD mouse *(103)*.

The ability to prevent disease with a range of antigens is important. This suggests that it is not necessary to select one dominant antigen for this approach to immunotherapy to be successful.

Thyroid

A murine model of Hashimoto's disease, experimental autoimmune thyroiditis (EAT), can be produced by immunization of susceptible mice with Tg. This results in the typical histological changes, as well as evidence of T- and B-cell immunity to thyroidal antigens *(104)*. Feeding Tg to such mice either before or after disease induction reduces the histological grade of thyroiditis along with a reduction in T cell proliferation and antibody titers to Tg *(105,106)*. This effect was best seen with a dose of 500 µg/d. As with the tolerogenic therapies in the NOD mouse, better results were obtained by feeding before the induction of disease rather than after. In this study, splenic T cell secretion of IL-2 and IFN-γ was reduced, but secretion of IL-4 and TGF-β was increased, providing evidence of immune deviation in this model. In support of this, intrathyroidal injection of IFN-γ has been shown to induce disease, whereas ip injection of IL-10 ameliorated it *(107,108)*. Successful treatment of EAT has also been achieved by iv administration of TG *(109)*.

The study of Graves' disease has been hampered by the lack of animal models. Previous approaches to the creation of a Graves' disease model have involved the xenografting of human thyroid tissue into immunodeficient mice. The resulting models have not had a sufficient strength or duration of thyroid-stimulating activity for effective study *(110)*.

POTENTIAL PROBLEMS WITH ANTIGEN-SPECIFIC IMMUNOTHERAPY

Immunization rather than tolerization is always a risk with antigen-specific immunotherapy, since the protocols used are sometimes not very different from those used to induce disease. However, in the published studies, worsening of disease has not been reported once an effective protocol has been established.

Tolerization techniques that rely on immune deviation run the particular risk of inducing an exaggerated humoral (Th2) immune response, resulting in antibody-mediated organ damage. Although no such effects have been reported in models of autoimmune endocrinopathies, pathology resulting from immune deviation has recently been described in a primate model of multiple sclerosis. Genain et al. *(111)* reported that treatment with soluble antigen resulted in a shift toward a Th2-like pattern of cytokine production in this model associated with an initial reduction in clinical and pathological disease scores. However, after cessation of treatment, a severe hyperacute disease developed that was worse than that in untreated controls. The exacerbation of disease was associated with an elevated antibody titer to the target autoantigen.

Recently, the transfer of Th2 cells from either NOD mice or mice with experimental autoimmune encephalitis (an animal model of multiple sclerosis) to immunocompromised mice has been shown to result in disease *(112,113)*. Although this is slower in onset, histologically it is worse than that in untreated animals. These studies suggest that under certain conditions immune deviation can be hazardous and underline the fact that our understanding of antigen-specific tolerization is still incomplete *(114)*.

HUMAN STUDIES INVOLVING ANTIGEN-SPECIFIC IMMUNOTHERAPY

Although no studies have yet been completed in the human autoimmune endocrinopathies, several trials of antigen-specific immunotherapy are in progress in this field, and some have been completed in other cell-mediated autoimmune diseases. In almost all cases, tolerization via the oral route has been used. These are described below.

Type 1 Diabetes

DPT1, presently ongoing in the US, was designed to determine if intervention with insulin-based therapies could delay or prevent the clinical onset of disease in subjects at risk of Type 1 diabetes *(43)*. It has two arms, each administering antigen through different routes. The parenteral arm, described earlier, is based on the observation that sc insulin can reduce the progression to disease. The mechanism underlying this was originally thought to be "β-cell rest," though it may ultimately be shown to be immunomodulatory.

The second arm began more recently and is based on the concept of oral tolerance. Relatives of Type 1 diabetic subjects judged to be at intermediate risk of disease (i.e., 26–50% risk of disease onset within the next 5 yr) will be given 7.5 mg of oral recombinant insulin in capsules or sprinkled on food. The trial will be double-blinded and placebo-controlled. Subjects screened for the original parenteral protocol arm will be used, and randomization for this arm began in September 1996.

The study end point will be the development of Type 1 diabetes, though there will be six monthly glucose tolerance tests to evaluate β-cell function and exclude the development of insulin dependence.

The study commenced in February 1994, and screening is expected to continue for more than 4 yr. Interim results may be available before then.

There is also an Australian tolerization study in progress looking at the effect of nasally administered insulin on progression to disease in subjects at risk for diabetes. More than 30 subjects are being assessed in a double-blind, placebo-controlled crossover trial *(115)*. Results are awaited with interest.

Multiple Sclerosis (MS)

MS is an inflammatory disease of the central nervous system of presumed autoimmune etiology *(116)*. The major targets are thought to be myelin basic protein (MBP) and proteolipid protein (PLP). Oral administration of these proteins has been shown to suppress disease in two different animal models of MS *(84,117,118)*

An oral tolerization study of 30 patients with the relapsing remitting form of MS has been conducted by Weiner et al. *(119)*. Fifteen subjects were treated with 300 mg of oral bovine myelin/d for 1 yr; 15 age- and disease-matched controls were treated with powdered bovine milk product. Treated subjects showed no improvement in their disease scores or their requirement for steroids. However, subgroup analysis revealed a small improvement in males and in subjects carrying the HLA susceptibility allele for MS, HLA DR2. Short-term T-cell lines derived from myelin-treated subjects revealed a higher frequency of TGF-β-secreting myelin-specific T cells as compared with nontreated subjects *(120)*. This change was found to be antigen-specific, providing evidence for immune deviation. There was no change in IFN-γ-secreting antigen-specific T cells.

A larger 515-patient placebo-controlled trial on relapsing remitting MS patients using oral bovine myelin has recently been conducted by the same team. This showed no difference between treated and untreated groups in relapse rates, though there was a high placebo effect *(81)*.

Rheumatoid Arthritis (RA)

RA is an autoimmune synovial disease in which Type II collagen is a candidate autoantigen. Tolerization with collagen has been shown to ameliorate disease in animal studies *(121)*. Two human trials with oral collagen have been published. Trentham et al. conducted a study of 60 patients given 0.1 mg/d of type II collagen for 1 mo followed by 0.5 mg/d for 2 mo. A significant reduction in the number of swollen joints and joint tenderness scores compared to placebo-treated controls was reported *(122)*. Interestingly, the serum from those subjects treated showed no change in anticollagen antibodies or in rheumatoid factor concentrations.

The same group has, however, recently completed a 360-patient placebo-controlled phase II trial using a much lower dose of 60 µg of oral collagen, and preliminary results appear to show no difference between treated and placebo groups *(81)*. Similar negative results have been obtained by another group using 1–10 mg/d of bovine collagen given orally for 12 wk *(123)*.

Uveitis

Anterior uveitis, in animal models of eye disease, has been shown to involve an autoimmune response against retinal proteins, including the retinal S antigen, and to respond to treatment with oral S antigen *(124,125)*. Oral tolerance in humans using this antigen has therefore been attempted in a small trial of 10 patients treated initially with 30 mg of bovine S antigen 3 times a week for the first 8 wk, reducing to just once a week for the rest of the 1-yr follow up *(126)*. No significant improvement in time to recurrence of inflammation was seen in comparison with placebo-treated controls, although there was a (nonsignificant) trend in the treated group toward a reduction in requirement for immunosuppressive therapy.

Comments on Human Studies

In contrast to animal models, studies of antigen-specific immunotherapy in humans have so far been disappointing. However, several points need to be taken into account. First, the human subjects studied represent a genetically more diverse population treated at a later stage in the autoimmune process. Second, only the oral route of tolerization has so far been studied, using whole-antigen rather than peptide epitopes or modified peptide epitopes. Third, the number of subjects studied in some cases was small, and important effects may be missed in placebo-controlled studies owing to the natural variation in the course of many autoimmune diseases. Finally, studies in animal models have suggested that the dose of antigen used for oral tolerization can be critical. The success of 0.1–0.5 mg of oral collagen, but not 60 µg or 1–10 mg in treating RA may represent such an effect.

It does seem that more powerful protocols will need to be devised for use in human disease. The intranasal route and the use of modified peptide epitopes may be particularly valuable. In addition, targeting of treatment to subgroups of patients at earlier stages in disease is likely to be important. In this latter respect, it is particularly encouraging that no significant adverse effects have been reported from any of the studies to date.

SUMMARY AND CONCLUSIONS

In keeping with the persistently high long-term morbidity levels in Type I diabetes, efforts at immunotherapy in autoimmune endocrinopathies have concentrated on this disease. Initial results of nonantigen-specific immunosuppression with cyclosporin were promising, but longer-term data have been disappointing with the majority of remissions being short-lived. More success has been obtained with general immunosuppression in Graves' opthalmopathy, a disease that spontaneously remits in the majority of cases. Remarkably, very few side effects from generalized immunosuppression, such as opportunistic infection and neoplasia, were seen in these trials, but the lack of long-term success has resulted in attention switching in the last decade to alternative forms of immunotherapy.

Large trials are currently under way in diabetes using therapies, such as nicotinamide and insulin. The exact immunomodulatory role of some parts of these therapies remains uncertain, but the outcome of these trials is awaited with interest.

Immunologists have focused their efforts on the development of antigen-specific immunotherapies that do not result in generalized immunosuppression. The identification of candidate target autoantigens is a prerequisite for developing such therapies, and great progress has been made in this area. Using a combination of immunization routes, antigen doses, and formulations, considerable success has been achieved in treating animal models of endocrine autoimmune disease with antigen-based therapy. In particular, such studies have indicated that administration of a single antigen can ameliorate disease known to involve a variety of autoantigenic targets. Immune deviation with a switch to Th2-type cytokine production in the target organ has been invoked to explain such "bystander suppression." In addition, antigen-specific immunotherapy has been successful in some cases even when administered after the onset of disease. Both of these observations augur well for the success of this treatment approach in humans.

To date, however, the results of oral tolerization studies conducted in humans with nonendocrine autoimmune disease have been disappointing, although thankfully free from deleterious side effects. Animal studies are now suggesting improved techniques, including intranasal dosing and the use of modified T-cell target peptides, rather than whole antigen to improve efficacy. The possibility that antigen-specific immunotherapy might result in exacerbation of disease needs to be borne in mind. In this respect, newly diagnosed Type 1 diabetic subjects would be one of the safest groups to study, since the natural history of the disease is progression to complete β-cell destruction, and at worst, this process would be accelerated.

Our understanding of immune tolerance induction is improving rapidly, and further trials of a variety of protocols for antigen-based immunotherapy in humans are likely in the near future. There is little doubt that progress in this area is urgently required to improve the outcome in Type I diabetes, particularly in view of the increasing incidence of this disease in children under 5 yr of age *(3)*. Improved treatment for Graves' opthalmopathy is also needed.

In diabetes, successful immunotherapy is likely to be the only method of ultimately relieving the burden of monitoring and daily insulin therapy, which most patients with Type I diabetes feel. When one 15-yr-old diabetic who had had to endure extensive dental work was asked which she hated more—her diabetes or the dentist—she had no hesitation in replying, "my diabetes." Comments such as this should remind us that despite its complexities, the goal of immunotherapy is well worth pursuing.

REFERENCES

1. DCCT Study Group. The effect of intensive treatment of diabetes on the development and progression of long-term complications in insulin-dependent diabetes-mellitus. N Engl J Med. 1993;329:977–986.
2. Bennett ST, Wilson AJ, Cucca F, Nerup J, Pociot F, Mckinney PA, et al. IDDM 2-VNTR-encoded susceptibility to Type 1 diabetes—dominant protection and parental transmission of alleles of the insulin gene-linked minisatellite locus. J Autoimmunity 1996;9:415–421.
3. Gardner SG, Bingley PJ, Sawtell PA, Weeks S, Gale EAM. Rising Incidence of insulin dependent diabetes in children aged under 5 years in the Oxford region: time trend analysis. BMJ 1997;315:713–717.
4. Roll U, Christie MR, Fuchtenbusch M, Payton MA, Hawkes CJ, Ziegler AG. Perinatal autoimmunity in offspring of diabetic parents—the German Multicenter BABY-DIAB study—detection of humoral immune-responses to islet antigens in early childhood. Diabetes 1996;45:967–973.
5. Caillat-Zucman S, Garchon HJ, Timsit J, Assan R, Boitard C, Djilalisaiah I, et al. Age dependent HLA genetic heterogeneity of Type 1 insulin dependent diabetes mellitus. J Clin Invest 1992:90:2242–2250.
6. Foulis AK, Liddle CN, Farquharson MA, Richmond JA, Weir RS. The histopathology of the pancreas in Type 1 (insulin dependent) diabetes mellitus: a 25 year review of deaths in patients under 20 years of age in the United Kingdom. Diabetologia 1986;29:267–274.
7. Karjalainen J, Salmela P, Ilonen J, Surcel HM, Knip M. A comparison of childhood and adult Type 1 diabetes-mellitus. N Engl J Med 1989;320:881–886.
8. Turner R, Stratton I, Horton V, Manley S, Zimmet P, Mackay IR, et al. UKPDS 25: autoantibodies to islet-cell cytoplasm and glutamic acid decarboxylase for prediction of insulin requirement in Type 2 diabetes. Lancet 1997;350:1288–1293.
9. Gale EAM, Bingley PJ. Can we prevent IDDM. Diabetes Care 1994;17:339–344.
10. Scott FW, Norris JM, Kolb H. Milk and Type 1 diabetes—examining the evidence and broadening the focus. Diabetes Care 1996;19:379–383.
11. Ellis TM, Atkinson MA. Early infant diets and insulin dependent diabetes. Lancet 1996;347:1464–1465.
12. Cavallo MG, Fava D, Monetini L, Barone F, Pozzilli P. Cell mediated immune response to beta-casein in recent onset insulin dependent diabetes—implications for disease pathogenesis. Lancet 1996;348: 926–928.
13. Martikainen A, Saukkonen T, Kulmala PK, Reijonen H, Ilonen J, Teramo K, et al. Disease associated antibodies in offspring of mothers with IDDM. Diabetes 1996;45:1706–1710.
14. Graves PM, Norris JM, Pallansch MA, Gerling IC, Rewers M. The role of enteroviral infections in the development of IDDM -limitations of current approaches. Diabetes 1997;46:161–168.
15. Dahlquist G, Frisk G, Ivarsson SA, Svanberg L, Forsgren M, Diderholm H. Indications that maternal coxsackie B virus-infection during pregnancy is a risk factor for childhood onset IDDM. Diabetologia 1995;38:1371–1373.
16. Bingley PJ, Bonifacio E, Gale EAM. Can we really predict IDDM? Diabetes 1993;42:213–220.
17. Roll U, Christie MR, Hillebrand B, Rabl W, Ziegler AG. On the appearance of islet associated autoimmunity in offspring of diabetic mothers—a prospective study from birth. Diabetologia 1993;36:A 58.
18. Bingley PJ, Christie MR, Bonifacio E, Bonfanti R, Shattock M, Fonte MT, et al. Combined analysis of autoantibodies improves prediction of IDDM in islet cell antibody positive relatives. Diabetes 1994;43:1304–1310.

19. Verge CF, Gianani R, Kawasaki E, Yu LP, Pietropaolo M, Jackson RA, et al. Production of Type 1 diabetes in first degree relatives using a combination of insulin, GAD and ICA512/IA-1 autoantibodies. Diabetes 1996;45:926–933.
20. Bingley PJ, Bonifacio E, Williams AJK, Genovese S, Bottazzo GF, Gale EAM. Prediction of IDDM in the general population—strategies based on combinations of autoantibody markers. Diabetes 1997; 46:1701–1710.
21. Pugliese A, Gianani R, Moromisato R, Awdeh ZL, Alper CA, Erlich HA, et al. HLA-DQB1*0602 is associated with dominant protection from diabetes even among islet cell antibody positive first-degree relatives of patients with IDDM. Diabetes 1995;44:608–613.
22. Mcculloch DK, Koerker DJ, Kahn SE, Bonnerweir S, Palmer JP. Correlations of invivo beta cell function tests with beta cell mass and pancreatic insulin content in streptozocin administered baboons. Diabetes 1991;40:673–679.
23. Kolb H, Bach JF, Eisenbarth GS, Harrison LC, Maclaren NK, Pozzilli P, et al. Criteria for immune trials in Type 1 diabetes. Lancet 1989;2:686.
24. Schreiber SL. Chemistry and biology of the immunophilins and their immunosuppressive ligands. Science 1991;251:283–287.
25. Feutren G, Assan R, Karsenty G, Durostu H, Sirmai J, Papoz L, et al. Cyclosporin increases the rate and length of remissions in insulin-dependent diabetes of recent onset—results of a multicenter double-blind trial. Lancet 1986;2:119–124.
26. Dupre J, Kolb H. Cyclosporin induced remission of IDDM after early intervention—association of 1 yr of cyclosporin treatment with enhanced insulin secretion. Diabetes 1988;37:1574–1582.
27. Carel JC, Boitard C, Eisenbarth G, Bach JF, Bougneres PF. Cyclosporine delays but does not prevent clinical onset in glucose intolerant pre-Type 1 diabetic children. J Autoimmunity 1996;9:739–745.
28. Feutren G, Mihatsch MJ. Risk-factors for cyclosporine induced nephropathy in patients with autoimmune diseases. N Engl J Med 1992;326:1654–1660.
29. Assan R, Timsit J, Feutren G, Bougneres P, Czernichow P, Hannedouche T, et al. The kidney in cyclosporine A treated diabetic patients—a long-term clinicopathological study. Clin Nephrol 1994; 41:41–49.
30. Koivisto VA, Leirisalorepo M, Ebeling P, Tuominen JA, Knip M, Turunen U, et al. Seven years of remission in a type 1 diabetic patient. Diabetes Care 1993;16:990–995.
31. Cook JJ, Hudson I, Harrison LC, Dean B, Colman PG, Werther GA, et al. Double blind controlled trial of azathioprine in children with newly diagnosed type 1 diabetes. Diabetes 1989;38:779–783.
32. Silverstein J, Maclaren N, Riley W, Spillar R, Radjenovic D, Johnson S. Immunosuppression with azathioprine and prednisone in recent onset insulin dependent diabetes mellitus. N Engl J Med 1988; 319:599–604.
33. Mandruppoulsen T, Reimers JI, Andersen HU, Pociot F, Karlsen AE, Bjerre U, et al. Nicotinamide treatment in the prevention of insulin dependent diabetes mellitus. Diabetes Metab Rev 1993;9: 295–309.
34. Heller B, Wang ZQ, Wagner EF, Radons J, Burkle A, Fehsel K, et al. Inactivation of the poly (ADP-ribose) polymerase gene affects oxygen radical and nitric oxide toxicity in islet cells. J Biol Chem 1995;270:11,176–11,180.
35. Elliott RB, Chase HP. Prevention or delay of type-1 (insulin-dependent) diabetes mellitus in children using nicotinamide. Diabetologia 1991;34:362–365.
36. Gale EAM. Theory and practice of nicotinamide trials in pretype 1 diabetes. J Pediatr Endocrinol Metab 1996;9:375–379.
37. Elliott RB, Pilcher CC, Fergusson DM, Stewart AW. A population based strategy to prevent insulin-dependent diabetes using nicotinamide. J Pediatr Endocrinol Metab 1996;9:501–509.
38. Gotfredsen CF, Buschard K, Frandsen EK. Reduction of diabetes incidence of BB Wistar rats by early prophylactic insulin treatment of diabetes prone animals. Diabetologia 1985;28:933–935.
39. Atkinson MA, Maclaren NK, Luchetta R. Insulitis and diabetes in NOD mice reduced by prophylactic insulin therapy. Diabetes 1990;39:933–937.
40. Shah SC, Malone JI, Simpson NE. A randomized trial of intensive insulin therapy in newly diagnosed insulin dependent diabetes mellitus. N Engl J Med 1989;320:550–554.
41. Keller RJ, Eisenbarth GS, Jackson RA. Insulin prophylaxis in individuals at high risk of type 1 diabetes. Lancet 1993;341:927–928.
42. Hao W, Li LS, Mehta V, Lernmark A, Palmer JP. Functional state of the beta-cell affects expression of both forms of glutamic acid decarboxylase. Pancreas 1994;9:558–562.

43. DPT-1 Study group. The Diabetes Prevention Trial—Type I diabetes (DPT1): implementation of screening and staging of relatives. Transplantation Proc 1995;27:3377
44. McInerney MF, Pek SB, Thomas DW. Prevention of insulitis and diabetes onset by treatment with complete freunds adjuvant in NOD mice. Diabetes 1991;40:715–725.
45. Shehadeh N, Calcinaro F, Bradley BJ, Bruchlim I, Vardi P, Lafferty KJ. Effect of adjuvant therapy on development of diabetes in mouse and man. Lancet 1994;343:706–707.
46. Pozzilli P. BCG vaccine in insulin-dependent diabetes mellitus. Lancet 1997;349:1520–1521.
47. Bach JF. Strategies in immunotherapy of insulin-dependent diabetes mellitus. Ann NY Acad Sci 1993; 696:364–376.
48. Ramiya VK, Maclaren NK. Immunotherapies in diabetes. Trends Endocrinol Metab 1996;7:252–257.
49. Dayan CM, Daniels GH. Chronic autoimmune-thyroiditis. N Engl J Med 1996;335:99–107.
50. Dayan CM. The natural history of autoimmune thyroiditis: how normal is autoimmunity? Proc R Coll Physicians Edinburgh 1996;26:419–433.
51. McGregor AM, Peterson MM, McLachlan SM, Rooke P, Smith BR, Hall R. Carbimazole and the autoimmune response in Graves disease. N Engl J Med 1980;303:302–307.
52. Weetman AP, Ratanachaiyavong S, Middleton GW, Love W, John R, Owen GM, et al. Prediction of outcome in Graves-disease after carbimazole treatment. Q J Med 1986;59:409–419.
53. Weetman AP, McGregor AM, Hall R. Are antithyroid drugs immunosuppressive. Br Med J 1984; 288:1004
54. Weetman AP, McGregor AM, Hall R. Evidence for an effect of antithyroid drugs on the natural history of Graves disease. Clin Endocrinol 1984;21:163–172.
55. Kahaly G, Schrezenmeir J, Krause U, Schweikert B, Meuer S, Muller W, et al. Cyclosporin and prednisone Vs prednisone in treatment of Graves ophthalmopathy—a controlled, randomized and prospective study. Eur J Clin Invest 1986;16:415–422.
56. Antonelli A, Navarranne A, Palla R, Alberti B, Saracino A, Mestre C, et al. Pretibial myxoedema and high dose intravenous immunoglobulin treatment. Thyroid 1994;4:399–408.
57. Claridge KG, Ghabrial R, Davis G, Tomlinson M, Goodman S, Harrad RA, Potts MJ. Combined radiotherapy and medical immunosuppression in the management of thyroid eye disease. Eye 1997;11: 717–722.
58. Coulam CB, Kempers RD, Randall RV. Premature ovarian failure—evidence for the autoimmune mechanism. Fertil Steril 1981;36:238–240.
59. Finer N, Fogelman I, Bottazzo G. Pregnancy in a woman with premature ovarian failure. Postgrad Med J 1985;61:1079–1080.
60. Cowchock FS, Mccabe JL, Montgomery BB. Pregnancy after corticosteroid administration in premature ovarian failure (polyglandular endocrinopathy syndrome). Am J Obstet Gynecol 1988;158: 118–119.
61. Yan ZB, Bing ZX, Yang WR, Long WL. A study of cadaveric fetal adrenal used for adrenal transplantation to treat Addisons disease—13 cases reported. Transplantation Proc 1990;22:280–282.
62. Wells H Studies on the chemistry of anaphylaxis. III Experiments with isolated proteins, especially those of hens eggs. J Infect Dis 1911;9:147–151.
63. Janeway CA, Travers P. Basic concepts in immunology. In: Immunobiology. Anonymous. Garland, New York, 1998, pp. 1:1–1:32.
64. Scollay R, Butcher EC, Weissman IL. Thymus cell migration. Quantitative aspects of cellular traffic from the thymus to the periphery in mice. Eur J Immunol 1980;10:210–218.
65. Ashtonrickardt PG, Bandeira A, Delaney JR, Vankaer L, Pircher HP, Zinkernagel RM, et al. Evidence for a differential avidity model of T cell selection in the thymus. Cell 1994;76:651–663.
66. Lafferty KJ, Gill RG. The maintenance of self tolerance. Immunol Cell Biol 1994;6:407–413.
67. Romagnani S. The Th1/Th2 paradigm. Immunol Today 1997;18:263–266.
68. Mosmann TR, Cherwinski H, Bond MW, Giedlin MA, Coffman RL. Two types of murine helper T cell clone. 1. definition according to profiles of lymphokine activities and secreted proteins. J Immunol 1986;136:2348–2357.
69. Cher DJ, Mosmann TR. Two types of murine helper T cell clone. 2. delayed type hypersensitivity is mediated by Th1 clones. J Immunol 1987;138:3688–3694.
70. Killar L, Macdonald G, West J, Woods A, Bottomly K. Cloned, IA restricted T cells that do not produce interleukin 4(IL 4)/B cell stimulatory factor-1(BSF-1) fail to help antigen-specific B cells. J Immunol 1987;138:1674–1679.
71. Constant SL, Bottomly K. Induction of Th1 and Th2 CD4+ T cell responses: the alternative approaches. Ann Rev Immunol 1997;15:297–322.

72. Hussain MJ, Peakman M, Gallati H, Lo SSS, Hawa M, Viberti GC, et al. Elevated serum levels of macrophage derived cytokines precede and accompany the onset of IDDM. Diabetologia 1996;39: 60–69.
73. Kallmann BA, Huther M, Tubes M, Feldkamp J, Bertrams J, Gries FA, et al. Systemic bias of cytokine production toward cell mediated immune regulation in IDDM and toward humoral immunity in Graves' disease. Diabetes 1997;46:237–243.
74. Wraith DC. Antigen specific immunotherapy of autoimmune diseases: a commentary. Clin Exp Immunol 1996;103:349–352.
75. Paschke R, Vassart G, Ludgate M. Current evidence for and against the TSH receptor being the common antigen in Graves disease and thyroid associated ophthalmopathy. Clin Endocrinol 1995;42: 565–569.
76. Dayan CM, Londei M, Corcoran AE, Grubeckloebenstein B, James RFL, Rapoport B, et al. Autoantigen recognition by thyroid infiltrating T cells in Graves disease. Proc Natl Acad Sci USA 1991;88:7415–7419.
77. Lohmann T, Scherbaum WA. T cell autoimmunity to glutamic acid decarboxylase in human insulin dependent diabetes-mellitus. Hor Metab Res 1996;28:357–360.
78. Lohmann T, Halder T, Morgenthaler NG, KhooMorgenthaler UY, Seissler J, Engler J, et al. T cell responses to the novel autoantigen IA2 in IDDM patients and healthy controls. Diabetologia 1997; 40:327
79. Ota K, Matsui M, Milford EL, Mackin GA, Weiner H, Hafler DA. T cell recognition of an immunodominant myelin basic protein epitope epitope in multiple sclerosis. Nature 1990;346:183–187.
80. Metzler B, Wraith DC. Inhibition of experimental autoimmune encephalomyelitis by inhalation but not oral administration of the encephalitogenic peptide: influence of MHC binding affinity. Int Immunol 1993;5:1159–1165.
81. Weiner HL. Oral tolerance for the treatment of autoimmune diseases. Ann Rev Med 1997;48:341–351.
82. Friedman A, Weiner HL. Induction of anergy or active suppression following oral tolerance is determined by antigen dosage. Proc Natl Acad Sci USA 1994;91:6688–6692.
83. Chen YH, Inobe J, Marks R, Gonnella P, Kuchroo VK, Weiner HL. Peripheral deletion of antigen reactive T cells in oral tolerance. Nature 1995;376:177–180.
84. Bitar DM, Whitacre CC. Suppression of experimental autoimmune encephalomyelitis by the oral administration of myelin basic-protein. Cell Immunol 1988;112:364–370.
85. Gregerson DS, Obritsch WF, Donoso LA. Oral tolerance in experimental autoimmune uveoretinitis— distinct mechanisms of resistance are induced by low-dose vs high-dose feeding protocols. J Immunol 1993;151:5751–5761.
86. Metzler B, Wraith DC. Immunotherapy of autoimmune-disease with synthetic peptides. Immunol Today 1994;15:91–91.
87. Brocke S, Gijbels K, Allegretta M, Ferber I, Piercy C, Blankenstein T, et al. Treatment of experimental encephalomyelitis with a peptide analog of myelin basic-protein. Nature 1996;379:343–346.
88. Kumar V, Bhardwaj V, Soares L, Alexander J, Sette A, Sercarz E. Major histocompatibility complex binding affinity of an antigenic determinant is crucial for the differential secretion of interleukin-4/5 or interferon gamma by T cells. Proc Natl Acad Sci USA 1995;92:9510–9514.
89. Petersen JS, Karlsen AE, Markholst H, Worsaae A, Dyrberg T, Michelsen B. Neonatal tolerization with glutamic acid decarboxylase but not with bovine serum albumin delays the onset of diabetes in NOD micc. Diabetes 1994;43:1478–1484.
90. Tisch R, Yang XD, Singer SM, Liblau RS, Fugger L, Mcdevitt HO. Immune responses to glutamic acid decarboxylase correlates with insulitis in nonobese diabetic mice. Nature 1993;366:72–75.
91. Kaufman DL, Claresalzler M, Tian JD, Forsthuber T, Ting GSP, Robinson P, et al. Spontaneous loss of T cell tolerance to glutamic acid decarboxylase in murine insulin dependent diabetes. Nature 1993; 366:69–72.
92. Muir A, Peck A, Claresalzler M, Song YH, Cornelius J, Luchetta R, et al. Insulin immunization of nonobese diabetic mice induces a protective insulitis characterized by diminished intraislet interferongamma transcription. J Clin Invest 1995;95:628–634.
93. Harrison LC, DempseyCollier M, Kramer DR, Takahashi K. Aerosol insulin induces regulatory CD8 gamma delta T cells that prevent murine insulin-dependent diabetes. J Exp Med 1996;184:2167–2174.
94. Zhang JZ, Davidson I, Eisenbarth GS, Weiner HL. Suppression of diabetes in nonobese diabetic mice by the oral administration of porcine insulin. PNAS 1991;88:10,252–10,256.
95. Tian JD, Atkinson MA, Claresalzler M, Herschenfeld A, Forsthuber T, Lehmann PV, et al. Nasal administration of glutamate decarboxylase (GAD65) peptides induces Th2 responses and prevents murine insulin dependent diabetes. J Exp Med 1996;183:1561–1567.

96. Daniel D, Wegmann DR. Protection of nonobese diabetic mice from diabetes by intranasal or subcutaneous administration of insulin peptide B(9-23). Proc Natl Acad Sci USA 931996;:956–960.
97. Tian J, Claresalzler M, Herschenfeld A, Middleton B, Newman D, Mueller R, et al. Modulating autoimmune responses to GAD inhibits disease progression and prolongs islet graft survival in diabetes prone mice. Nature Med 1996;2:1348–1353.
98. Vonherrath MG, Dyrberg T, Oldstone MBA. Oral insulin treatment suppresses virus induced antigen-specific destruction of beta cells and prevents autoimmune diabetes in transgenic mice. J Clin Invest 1996;98:1324–1331.
99. Katz JD, Benoist C, Mathis D. T helper cell subsets in insulin dependent diabetes. Science 1995;268:1185–1188.
100. Elias D, Cohen IR. Treatment of autoimmune diabetes and insulitis in NOD mice with heat shock protein 60 peptide p277. Diabetes 1995;44:1132–1138.
101. Elias D, Reshef T, Birk OS, Vanderzee R, Walker MD, Cohen IR. Vaccination against autoimmune mouse diabetes with a T cell epitope of the human 65-kda heat-shock protein. Proc Natl Acad Sci USA 1991;88:3088–3091.
102. Elias D, Cohen IR. Treatment of autoimmune diabetes and insulitis in NOD mice with heat-shock-protein-60 peptide p277. Diabetes 1996;44:1132–1138.
103. French MB, Allison J, Cram DS, Thomas HE, DempseyCollier M, Silva A, et al. Transgenic expression of mouse proinsulin II prevents diabetes in nonobese diabetic mice. Diabetes 1997;46:34–39.
104. Simmon LL, Krco CJ, David CS, Kong YM. Characterization of the in vitro murine T cell proliferative responses to murine and human thyroglobulins in thyroiditis susceptible and resistant mice. Cell Immunol 1985;94:243–253.
105. Guimaraes VC, Quintans J, Fisfalen ME, Straus FH, Wilhelm K, Medeirosneto GA, et al. Suppression of development of experimental autoimmune thyroiditis by oral-administration of thyroglobulin. Endocrinology 1995;136:3353–3359.
106. Guimaraes VC, Quintans J, Fisfalen ME, Straus FH, Fields PE, Medeirosneto G, et al. Immunosuppression of thyroiditis. Endocrinology 1996;137:2199–2207.
107. Remy JJ, Salamero J, Michelbechet M, Charreire J. Experimental autoimmune thyroiditis induced by recombinant interferon-gamma. Immunol Today 1987;8:73.
108. MignonGodefroy K, Rott O, Brazillet MP, Charreire J. Curative and protective effects of IL-10 in experimental autoimmune-thyroiditis (EAT)—evidence for IL 10 enhanced cell-death in EAT. J Immunol 1995;154:6634–6643.
109. Kong YM, Okayasu I, Giraldo AA, Beisel KW, Sundick RS, Rose NR, et al. Tolerance to thyroglobulin by activating suppressor mechanisms. Ann NY Acad Sci 1982;392:191–209.
110. Volpe R. Has an experimental model for Graves' disease been established? Eur J Endocrinol 1997;136:150–152.
111. Genain CP, Abel K, Belmar N, Villinger F, Rosenberg DP, Linington C, et al. Late complications of immune deviation therapy in a nonhuman primate. Science 1996;274:2054–2057.
112. Pakala SV, Kurrer MO, Katz JD. T helper 2 (Th2) T cells induce acute pancreatitis and diabetes in immune compromised nonobese diabetic (NOD) mice. J Exp Med 1997;186:299–306.
113. Lafaille JJ, VandeKeere F, Hsu AL, Baron JL, Haas W, Raine CS, et al. Myelin basic protein specific T helper 2 (Th2) cells cause experimental autoimmune encephalomyelitis in immunodeficient hosts rather than protect them from the disease. J Exp Med 1997;186:307–312.
114. McFarland HF. Complexities in the treatment of autoimmune disease. Science 1996;274:2037.
115. Skolnick AA. First type 1 diabetes prevention trials. J Am Med Assoc 1997;278:118.
116. Mcfarlin DE, McFarland HF. Multiple-sclerosis. 1. N Engl J Med 1982:307:1183–1188.
117. Higgins PJ, Weiner HL. Suppression of experimental autoimmune encephalomyelitis by oral administration of myelin basic protein and its fragments. J Immunol 1988;140:440–445.
118. Brod SA, Alsabbagh A, Sobel RA, Hafler DA, Weiner HL. Suppression of experimental autoimmune encephalomyelitis by oral administration of myelin antigens. IV. suppression of chronic relapsing disease in the lewis rat and strain 13 guinea-pig. Ann Neurol 1991;29:615–622.
119. Weiner HL, Mackin GA, Matsui M, Orav EJ, Khoury SJ, Dawson DM, et al. Double blind pilot trial of oral tolerization with myelin antigens in multiple sclerosis. Science 1993;259:1321–1324.
120. Fukaura H, Kent SC, Pietrusewicz MJ, Khoury SJ, Weiner HL, Hafler DA. Induction of circulating myelin basic protein and proteolipid protein specific transforming growth factor beta 1 secreting Th3 T cells by oral administration of myelin in multiple sclerosis patients. J Clin Invest 1996;98:70–77.

121. Zhang ZYJ, Lee CSY, Lider O, Weiner HL. Suppression of adjuvant arthritis in lewis rats by oral administration of type II collagen. J Immunol 1990;145:2489–2493.
122. Trentham DE, Dynesiustrentham RA, Orav EJ, Combitchi D, Lorenzo C, Sewell KL, et al. Effects of oral administration of type II collagen on rheumatoid-arthritis. Science 1993;261:1727–1730.
123. Sieper J, Kary S, Sorensen H, Alten R, Eggens U, Huge W, et al. Oral type II collagen treatment in early rheumatoid arthritis—a double-blind, placebo-controlled, randomized trial. Arthritis Rheum 1996;39: 41–51.
124. Desmet MD, Yamamoto JH, Mochizuki M, Gery I, Singh VK, Shinohara T, et al. Cellular immune-responses of patients with uveitis to retinal antigens and their fragments. Am J Ophthalmol 1990; 110:135–142.
125. Nussenblatt RB. Experimental autoimmune uveitis: mechanisms of disease and clinical therapeutic indications [Proctor Lecture]. Invest Opthalmol Vis Sci 1991;32:3131–3141.
126. Nussenblatt RB, Gery I, Weiner HL, Ferris FL, Shiloach J, Remaley N, et al. Treatment of uveitis by oral administration of retinal antigens: results of a phase i/ii randomized masked trial. Am J Ophthalmol 1997;123:583–592.
127. Kolb H. Register of published immune intervention trials in type I diabetes with complete addresses of authors. In: Andreani D, Andreani H, Kolb H, Pozzilli P , eds. Immunotherapy of Type I Diabetes. John Wiley, New York, 1989, pp. 221–235.
128. DeFilippo G, Carel JC, Boitard C, Bougneres PF. Long term results of early cyclosporine therapy in juvenile IDDM. Diabetes 1996;45:101–104.
129. Chase HP, Butlersimon N, Garg SK, Hayward A, Klingensmith GJ, Hamman RF, et al. Cyclosporine A for the treatment of new onset insulin dependent diabetes mellitus. Pediatrics 1990;85:241–245.
130. Sai P, Damge C, Rivereau AS, Hoeltzel A, Gouin E. Prophylactic oral administration of metabolically active insulin entrapped in isobutylcyanoacrylate nanocapsules reduces the incidence of diabetes in nonobese diabetic mice. J Autoimmunity 1996;9:713–722.
131. Elliott JF, Qin HY, Bhatti S, Smith DK, Singh RK, Dillon T, et al. Immunization with the larger isoform of mouse glutamic-acid decarboxylase (GAD 67) prevents autoimmune diabetes in NOD mice. Diabetes 1994;43:1494–1499.
132. Tian JD, Claresalzler M, Herschenfeld A, Middleton B, Newman D, Mueller R, et al. Modulating autoimmune responses to GAD inhibits disease progression and prolongs islet graft survival in diabetes prone mice. Nature Med 1996;2:1348–1353.
133. Ramiya V, Muir A, Wasserfall C, Schott M, Schatz D, Maclaren N. Protection from diabetes by prophylactic oral insulin and GAD feedings in NOD mice. Diabetes 1995;44:A 164
134. Pleau JM, Fernandezsaravia F, Esling A, Homodelarche F, Dardenne M. Prevention of autoimmune diabetes in nonobese diabetic female mice by treatment with recombinant glutamic acid decarboxylase (GAD 65). Clin Immunol Immunopathol 1995;76:90–95.
135. Hutchings PR, Cooke A. Comparative-study of the protective effect afforded by intravenous administration of bovine or ovine insulin to young NOD mice. Diabetes 1995;44:906–910.
136. Daniel D, Wegmann DR. Intranasal administration of insulin peptide B9-23 protects NOD mice from diabetes. Ann NY Acad Sci 1996;778:371–372.
137. Polanski M, Melican NS, Zhang J, Weiner HL. Oral administration of the immunodominant B chain of insulin reduces diabetes in a co-transfer model of diabetes in the NOD mouse and is associated with a switch from Th1 to Th2 cytokines. J Autoimmunity 1997;10:339–346.
138. Harrison LC, Colman PG, Dean B, Baxter R, Martin FIR. Increase in remission rates in Type 1 diabetic subjects treated with azathioprine. Diabetes 1985;34,1306–1308.

INDEX

A

Abnormal immunoregulation, 227, 327
ACL detection,
    ELISA, 373
Acquired immunity,
    cellular and soluble mediators, 164t
Active suppression,
    T-cell tolerance breakdown, 18, 227
Adaptive immunity, 3
Addison's disease, 184, 367, 368, 402
    ACA, 358
    adrenal autoantibodies, 204t
    animal models,
        experimental allergic adrenalitis, 322, 323
        oöphoritis adrenalitis, 323, 324
        spontaneous, 322
    autoimmune thyroiditis, 219
    delayed type hypersensitivity (dth) skin tests, 320
    etiology and pathogenesis, 324–328
    family tree, 356f
    immunogenic aspects, 312–322
    macroscopic pathology, 310, 311
    major histocompatibility complex (MHC) linked genes, 321
    microscopy, 311–313
    stages, 315, 316
    steroid 17α-hydroxylase (17α-OH), 203
    steroid 21-hydroxylase (21-OH), 201
Adrenal cortex antibodies (ACA), 200–206, 314–316, 314f, 402
    adrenal autoantibodies, 204t
    APGS, 358
    autoantigens, 316, 317
    autoimmune endocrinopathies, 204t
    idiopathic POF, 367–370
    IFT, 203
    IFT and steroid 21-hydroxylase (21-OH), 201
    steroid cell antibody (St-C-Ab), 328
Adrenal gland,
    function and growth,
        blocking antibodies, 317, 318

Adrenocortical adenoma,
    Cushing's syndrome, 329
A-endorphin,
    peripheral blood lymphocytes, 36, 37
Age factors,
    AITDS incidence, 60, 219
    IDDM incidence, 59, 60
AIRE,
    APGS, 360
Allergy,
    IDDM animal models, 127, 128
Alloxan,
    IDDM, 117, 124
Androgen receptors (ARs), 171
Androgens,
    B cells, 175
    peripheral B cells, 176
    thymic size, 173
Anergy,
    T-cell tolerance breakdown, 18, 227
Animal models,
    AITDS, 63, 64
    IDDM, 62, 63, 113–129
Anterior pituitary adrenocorticotropic hormone (ACTH), 311
    Addison's disease, 309
Anterior pituitary insufficiency,
    lymphocytic adenohypophysitis, 343
Anti-CD4 Mab therapy, 103, 104
Anti-CD8 Mab therapy, 103, 104
Antigen-deprivation models,
    autoimmune endocrine disease, 49–52
Antigen presentation, 3–6, 229
Antigen presenting cells (APCs), 3, 229
    T-cell activation, 12
Antigens,
    autoimmune endocrinopathies, 183–206
    CD4 T cell recognition, 403f
    hidden, 40, 41, 43, 44
    humoral autoimmune response, 313–318
    techniques, 406
Antigen specific immunotherapy,
    animal models, 407, 408
    human studies, 409–411
    potential problems, 408, 409

underlying concepts, 403–406
Antigen-specific suppressor T(Ts) cells,
    12, 13, 228, 229
Antigen specific tolerance,
    mechanisms, 403–405
Anti-islet autoantibodies,
    APGS, 359
Antinuclear antibodies,
    AITD, 233
Antinuclear antibodies (ANA), 376
Antiphospholipid antibodies, 372–376
Antiphospholipid syndrome,
    rheumatologic disease, 373
Antithyroid microsomal antibody, 277f
APGS, see Autoimmune polyglandular
    syndrome (APGS)
APGS-I,
    clinical presentation, 351, 352
    component disorders, 352t
    immunogenetics, 352, 353
    immunopathogenesis, 353
    therapy, 353
APGS-I and APGS-II,
    comparison, 350t
APGS-II,
    clinical presentation, 353–355
    component disorders, 354t
    human leukocyte antigen (HLA)
        association, 355t
    immunogenetics, 355–357
    therapy, 357
Apoptosis,
    peripheral T-cell tolerance, 11
    T-cell tolerance breakdown, 18
APS, see Autoimmune polyglandular
    syndrome (APGS),
Aromatic L-amino acid decarboxylase
    (AADC), 205
ASA,
    low-dose oral,
        prednisone,
            oral, 375
    sc heparin, 375
Assisted reproduction technologies (ART),
    377, 378
Association studies, 65
Asymptomatic autoimmune thyroiditis,
    epidemiology, 148–150
Atrophic thyroiditis, 219
Autoantibodies, 300, 301
    APGS, 358t
    TAO, 251

thyroglobulin and TPO binding, 186
Autoantigens,
    autoimmune endocrinopathies, 183–206
    endocrine autoimmunity, 184t
    experimental autoimmune endocrine
        disease, immunoregulation, 45
    gonadal failure, 205, 206
    pituitary gland, 184, 185
Autoimmune Addison's disease, see
    Addison's disease
Autoimmune adrenocortical failure,
    309–329
Autoimmune diabetes, 394
Autoimmune diseases, 286
    age comparison, 168
    female predominance, 167, 168
    gender comparison, 168t
    hormonal modulation, 167–170
Autoimmune endocrine disease,
    antigen-deprivation models, 49–52
    experimental,
        immunoregulation, 31–54
    spontaneous remission, 41, 42
    thymectomy, 46–49, 233
Autoimmune endocrine syndromes, 271–287
Autoimmune endocrinopathies,
    autoantigens, 183–206
    female reproductive dysfunction,
        365–383
    immunotherapy and prevention, 393–412
    organ specific management approach,
        402, 403
Autoimmune factors,
    ectopic implantation, 379
Autoimmune hyperthyroidism, 218
Autoimmune hypophysitis, 337–345
Autoimmune oöphoritis,
    animal models, 369
Autoimmune polyendocrinopathy,
    Candidiasis, ectodermal dystrophy
        (APECED), 313, 367, see also
        APGS-I; Autoimmune polyglandular
        syndrome (APGS)
Autoimmune polyglandular syndrome
    (APGS), 193, 316, 317, 321, 367
    Addison's disease, 313, 314
    adrenal autoantibodies, 204t
    antigen and autoantibody groups, 357
    cell mediated autoimmunity, 360
    organ specific autoantibodies, 357–360
    steroid 17α-hydroxylase (17α-OH), 203
    steroid 21-hydroxylase (21-OH), 201

Autoimmune primer,
  APGS, 350, 351
Autoimmune thyroid disease (AITD),
    57–82, 184, 185, 186, 218f
  age-specific incidence, 60
  CTLA-4, 80, 81
  definition, 218
  development, 220, 221
  environmental influences, 97, 98, 228
  epidemiology, 141–158
  experimental models, 91–107
  familial clustering, 61
  gene mapping studies, 64–67
  genetic resistance, 91–98
    induction, 104, 105
  genetic susceptibility, 91–98
    epidemiologic evidence, 58–64
    HLA candidate genes, 67–72
  HLA linkage studies, 71
  HLA-related susceptibility, 79, 80
  immunogenetics, 220, 221
  immunological classification, 218t
  immunology, 217–236
  immunoregulation, 226, 227
  incidence, 59, 142
  induced
    thyrocyte abnormality, 225
  major histocompatibility complex
    (MHC), 219, 220
  MHC class I genes, 94, 95
  MHC class II genes, 91–94, 221
  MHC molecules,
    protective influence, 95, 96
  non-HLA candidate gene-linkage studies,
    74–76
  pathogenesis, 221, 222, 221f
    bacterial infection, 224, 225
    target cell and thyroid autoantigens,
      222, 223
    viruses, 223, 224
  pathogenic mechanisms, 102–104
    effector T-cell mechanisms, 102, 103
    immunotherapy, 103, 104
    TCR gene usage, 102
  pregnancy, 274, 275
  regulatory mechanisms, 104–107
  target cells, 226
  T cell function, specific and fundamental,
    228, 229
  TCR repertoire, 96, 97
  thyroid autoantigens and pathogenic
    peptides, 101, 102

  thyroid peroxidase, 187
  twin research, 62
  whole-genome screening, 76–78
Autoimmune thyroid dysfunction, see
    Postpartum autoimmune thyroid
    dysfunction
Autoimmune thyroiditis,
  asymptomatic,
    epidemiology, 148–150
  diagnosis, 219
  spontaneous,
    OS chickens, 45
  T cells, 227
  therapy, 235, 236
Autoimmunity, 17–20
  B-cell tolerance breakdown, 18, 19
  definition, 125
  organ-specific autoimmune disease
    hypothesis, 19, 20
  postthymectomy, 47, 48
  T-cell tolerance breakdown, 17, 18
Azathioprine,
  IDDM treatment, 399

B

Bacille Calmette-Guerin (BCG)
  IDDM, 123
  IDDM treatment, 400, 401
Bacteria,
  AITD, 224
  IDDM, 123
BALB/c mice,
  thyroiditis, 101
Basedow's disease, 218
BB rat,
  AITD, 224
  B cells, 120, 121
  colonies and lines, 121
  diet, 123, 124, 127, 128
  IDDM, 114, 117, 118, 118
  IDDM genetic predisposition, 118, 119
  insulitis, 120
  sex hormones, 124
  stress, 124
  T-cells, 122
  toxic agents, 124
B cells, see also B lymphocytes
  activation, 7, 8
  AITD, 231
  development, 167
  IDDM, 120, 121

pregnancy, 175
progesterone, 175
specific autoimmune response,
    features, 300, 301
specific T cells, 301
tolerance, 14–17
    central, 14–16
    peripheral, 16, 17
tolerance breakdown,
    autoimmunity, 18, 19
BCR gene rearrangements,
    B cell tolerance, 15
Binding stimulation index (B-S index),
    neonatal Graves' disease, 286, 287
Blizzard's syndrome, 367
B lymphocytes, 3, 350, *see also* B cells
    autoantibody production,
        T lymphocyte influence, 41
    thyroid autoantibodies,
        AITD, 231–233
Bone marrow, 175
    B cells development, 167
B-S index,
    Graves' disease, 286, 287

C

Calcium-sensing receptor (Ca-SR),
    parathyroid autoantigens, 194
Canavalia ensiformis,
    TSHR, 190
Candidate gene analysis, 66
    MODY, 66
Castration,
    B cells, 175
    peripheral B cells, 176
    thymic size, 172, 173
CD4,
    AITD T cells, 227
CD4+, 102, 103
CD8,
    AITD T cells, 227
    IDDM, 229
CD8+, 102, 103
CD154-CD40 interaction,
    T-cell activation, 7
CD28 costimulatory signal,
    T-cell activation, 6, 7
CD152 (CTLA-4), 12
CD1 molecules,
    expression, 5
CD4+ suppressor-inducer T cells, 13

CD4 T cell recognition,
    antigen, 403f
CD3 T cells, 312
CD4 T cells, 312, 319, 350, 369
CD4+ T cells, 13, 14
CD8 T cells, 312, 350, 369
CD8+T cells, 13
Celiac disease, 356, 357
Celiac disease autoantibodies,
    APGS, 359
Cell-mediated autoimmune responses,
    antigens, 318–321
Cell-mediated autoimmunity,
    APGS, 360
Central B-cell tolerance, 14–16
Central immunological tolerance, 1
Central T-cell tolerance, 8–10
Central tolerance, 403, 404
Chagas' disease, 166, 167
Chinese hamster,
    IDDM, 115
Chlorotozin,
    IDDM, 117
Cholesterol,
    subclinical hypothyroidism, 156, 157
Chorionic gonadotrophin,
    peripheral blood lymphocytes, 38
Chromosome 11p15
    IDDM, 72, 73
Chromosome 14q
    IDDM, 72, 73
Class II human leukocyte antigens (HLA)
    expression, 44, 220, 221
Clonal anergy,
    peripheral T-cell tolerance, 11
Clonal deletion,
    autoimmune endocrinopathy regulation, 43
    peripheral T-cell tolerance, 11
Clotting assay screening,
    LA measurement, 373, 374
Conserved peptides,
    Tg, 98–101
Cortical inflammatory infiltrate,
    Addison's disease, 312
Coxsackie virus P2-C protein, 197
Crohn's disease, 299
CTLA-4,
    IDDM and AITDS, 80, 81
CTLA-4 CD 152
    T-cell activation, 7
CTLA-4 gene,
    AITDS, 73

IDDM, 72, 73
Cushing's disease, 320
Cushing's syndrome, 311
    adrenocortical adenoma, 329
Cyclosporin A,
    IDDM treatment, 397–399
Cyproheptadine,
    IDDM, 117
Cytochrome P450 side-chain cleavage
        enzyme, 204, 205
Cytokines,
    IDDM treatment, 401
    TAO, 257
    thyroid cells, 229, 230
    thyroid stimulating hormone (TSH)
        stimulation, 229, 230

D

Danazol,
    endometriosis treatment, 382
    SLE, 169
Danocrine,
    SLE, 169
Datura stramonium (DSL),
    TSHR, 190
Delayed type hypersensitivity (dth) skin
        tests,
    Addison's disease, 320
Dendai virus,
    IDDM, 123
Dendritic cells,
    endocrine tissues, 325–328
Dermal fibroblasts,
    characteristics, 258t
Dermopathy, 245
Diabetes mellitus,
    type 1,
        genetic susceptibility, 57–82
Diabetes-prone rats (DP) BB rats, 114
Diet,
    IDDM, 123, 124
    IDDM animal models, 127, 128
Differential diagnosis,
    lymphocytic adenohypophysitis, 344
    postpartum destructive thyrotoxicosis,
        Graves' disease, 280t
Disease specific autoantigens,
    identification, 405, 406
DQB1, 296–298
DR2, 296–298
DR3, 296–298

DR3/4
    human leukocyte antigen (HLA), 394
DR4,
    HLA genes, 296–298
DR3/4/5 and DQB
    AITD, 220
    APGS-II, 355, 356
    human leukocyte antigen (HLA), 321
DRB1, 297, 298

E

Ectopic implantation,
    autoimmune factors, 379
ELISA,
    aCL detection, 373
Encephalomyocarditis virus variant D,
    IDDM, 123
Endocrine autoimmunity,
    autoantigens, 184t
    concepts, 40–42
    experimental models, 42–52
    simultaneous development, 40–42
Endocrine glands,
    defined, 34
    lymphokines, 36–38
    reproductive process, 365
Endocrine hormones,
    lymph nodes, 34, 35
Endocrine-immune system interaction,
    32–39
Endocrine syndromes, 271–287
Endocrine system,
    thymus, 32, 33
Endocrine tissues,
    dendritic cells, 325–328
Endometriosis, 378, 379
    altered cellular immunity, 380, 381
    autoimmunity role, 379–382
    impaired peritoneal clearance, 380, 381
    NK cell activity, 381
    treatment, 382
Enzyme autoantibodies,
    pathogenic role, 317
Epidemiology,
    definition, 141
Escherichia coli,
    thyroid peroxidase, 187
Estrogen receptors (ERs), 171
Estrogens,
    peripheral B cells, 175
    T cells, 174, 175

thymic size, 173, 174
Exophthalmos, 218, 245
Experimental allergic encephalomyelitis (EAE)
suppressor cells, 44, 45
Experimental autoimmune endocrine disease
immunoregulation, 31–54
autoantigen significance, 45
endocrine autoimmunity concepts, 40–42
experimental model regulation, 45–52
future, 52–54
immune-endocrine system interaction, 32–39
regulatory mechanisms, 42–45
Experimental autoimmune oöphoritis,
animal models, 369
Experimental autoimmune thyroiditis (EAT),
dietary iodine, 99
induction,
tolerance, 104–107
MHC class II genes, 93
MHC molecules,
protective influence, 95, 96
mouse models, 63, 64
murine model, 408
Experimentally induced IDDM, 117, 118
Experimental models,
AITDS, 91–107
endocrine autoimmunity, 42–52
Extraocular muscles,
TAO, 247, 248
Extrauterine growth, 379
Eye muscles autoantibodies,
TAO, 252, 253t
Eye muscle stimulating antibodies,
TAO, 255

F

Female reproductive dysfunction,
autoimmune endocrinopathies, 365–383
Fibroblast antibodies,
TAO, 254
Fibroblast responses,
TAO, 257
Floating regulatory force, 327
Follicle stimulating hormone (FSH), 271, 272, 371
Free T$_3$, 273
Free T$_4$, 273, 273f, 275f

Fungi,
IDDM, 123

G

Galanthus nivalis (GNL),
TSHR, 190
Gametogenesis disorder, 366–371
Gamma aminobutyric acid (GABA), 195
Gatekeepers,
immune response, 403
Gene mapping studies,
AITDS, 64–67
association studies, 65
candidate gene analysis, 66
IDDM, 64–67
linkage analysis, 65, 66
whole-genome screens, 66, 67
Genetically induced IDDM, 115–117
Genetics,
AITDS, 57–82
IDDM, 57–82
Gestational thyrotoxicosis, 272
Glandular failure,
immunopathogenic events, 326f
Glucocorticoid therapy, 345
Glutamic acid decarboxylase (GADA), 195–197, 394, 407
IA-2
IDDM, 198t, 199t
IDDM, 229
Glycoprotein, 116
Glycosylation,
TSHR, 190
Gonadal autoantigens, 200–206
Gonadal autoimmunity, 402
Gonadal failure
autoantigens, 205, 206
Gonadal steroid hormones, 170
receptors, 171t
Gonadal steroidogenesis disorder, 366–371
Gonadal steroids,
innate immunity, 171, 172
thymus, 172
Gonadotropin-releasing hormone (GnRH),
endometriosis treatment, 382
Graves' dermopathy, 218, 245
Graves' disease, 185, 282, 283, 322, 401
age-specific incidence, 60
AITD viral infections, 223
autoimmune thyroiditis, 219

binding stimulation index (B-S index), 286, 287
definition, 218
extrathyroidal manifestations, 236, 245–264
familial clustering, 61
HLA-B8, 69, 70
HLA linkage studies, 71
IL-R antagonist, 74
incidence, 146
I therapy, 234
mouse models, 64
murine model, 408
Na$^+$/I$^-$ symporter, 193
postpartum destructive thyrotoxicosis, differential diagnosis, 280t
pregnancy, 275, 275f
remissions, 233, 234
TAO, 250
T cells, 227
therapy,
  immunological aspects, 234, 235
thyroid autoantigens abnormality, 225
thyroid stimulating activities (TSA), 276, 276f
TPO gene, 74
Graves' ophthalmopathy, 218, 245
Graves' thyrotoxicosis, 231–236, 281f

H

H-2
  antigen presentation, 4
Hashimoto's disease, 185, 218
  autoimmune thyroiditis, 219
  murine model, 408
  Na$^+$/I$^-$ symporter, 193
  parathyroid autoantigens, 193, 194
  pregnancy, 275, 276
  thyroid peroxidase, 188
Hashimoto's thyroiditis (HT), 401
  age-specific incidence, 60
  CTLA-4, 322
  HLA, 70, 71
  HLA linkage studies, 71
  incidence, 59
  MHC class II genes, 92
H2Ea transgenes, 93
Heat-shock proteins (hsp), 116
Helminths *Schistosoma mansoni*, infections, 166
Hepatitis C,

AITD viral infections, 223
Hidden antigens, 40, 41, 43, 44, 49, 50
HLA-B8,
  Graves' disease, 69, 70
HLA candidate genes,
  AITDS genetic susceptibility, 67–72
  IDDM genetic susceptibility, 67–72
HLA-DR3,
  EAT, 107
HLA-DRB1 polymorphism,
  EAT susceptibility, 107
HLA-DR expressions,
  TAO, 250
HLA-related susceptibility,
  IDDM and AITDS, 79, 80, 220
Hormonal modulation,
  autoimmune diseases, 167–170
  immunity, 164–167
Hormone deficiency,
  autoimmune endocrinopathies, 393
Hormone dependent conditions, 379–382
Hormone receptors, 170, 171
Hormone replacement,
  autoimmune endocrinopathies, 393
Horror autotoxicus, 40
Human autoimmune thyroid disease (AITD),
  immunology, 217–236
Human chorionic gonadotropin (hCG), 271, 272
Human leucocyte antigen (HLA), 168, 220–224, 312,
  DR3/4, 394
  DR3/4/5 and DQB, 321
  DR expression,
    AITD, 220, 223, 224
  insulin-dependent diabetes mellitus (IDDM), 194, 195
  major histocompatibility complex (MHC), 371
Human leukocyte antigen (HLA) complex,
  antigen presentation, 4
Human leukocyte antigen (HLA) genes,
  IDDM, 296–298
Human MHC,
  antigen presentation, 4
Humoral autoimmune response,
  antigens, 313–318
Hypergonadotropic hypogonadism, 366
Hyperpigmentation, 309
Hyperprolactinemia,
  lymphocytic adenohypophysitis, 342, 343
Hyperthyroidism, 142–148, 232

incidence, 146–148
LATS, 39, 231, 232
pregnancy, 274
prevalence, 142–145
subclinical, 145, 146
Hypogonadism, 351
Hypoparathyroidism, 367
Hypopigmentation, 309
Hypothalamus,
    IL-1, 38, 39
Hypothyroidism,
    epidemiology, 150–155
    incidence, 59, 153–155
    pregnancy, 274, 275
    prevalence, 151, 152
    subclinical,
        cholesterol, 156, 157
        epidemiology, 152
        screening cost, 157

I

IA-2, 197–199
I assays,
    steroid 21-hydroxylase (21-OH), 202, 203
Iatrogenic abdominopelvic adhesions, 378, 379
IDDM animal models, 123–129
    allergy, 127, 128
    BB rat, 114
    causality vs chaotic model, 124, 125
    diabetes prediction and prevention, 128
    diet, 127, 128
    environmental influences, 123, 124
    failure of immunoregulation theory, 126, 127
    future, 128, 129
    molecular mimicry, 127
    TH1/TH2 model, 126, 127
    tolerance and autoimmunity, 125, 126
Idiopathic Addison's disease, 309–329, see also Addison's disease
Idiopathic hypoparathyroidism (IHP), 193
Idiopathic myxoedema, 218, 219, 233
Idiopathic POF, 370
    adrenal autoimmunity, 367–370
IFN-γ,
    AITD viral infections, 224, 230
IFT,
    adrenal cortex antibodies (ACA), 203
IgG,
    TAO, 255

IgG heavy-chain gene (IgH),
    AITDS, 73
Ig-H chain rearrangements,
    B-cell tolerance, 15
Ig-L chain rearrangements,
    B-cell tolerance, 15
Ignorance,
    T-cell tolerance breakdown, 18
IL-1,
    endocrine glands, 36
    hypothalamus, 38, 39
IL-10,
    POMC-derived peptides, 37
IL-2k,
    endocrine glands, 36
IL-R antagonist,
    Graves' disease, 74
IL-1R gene,
    IDDM, 72, 73
Immature B cells, 3
Immune deviation,
    TH 1 vs TH 2 cells, 404, 405
Immune-endocrine system interaction, 32–39
    anatomical associations, 34
    during development, 32, 33
    in mature structures, 34, 35
    at molecular level, 35–39
Immune physiology,
    reproductive organs, 365
Immune rebound mechanism,
    postpartum autoimmune thyroid dysfunction, 283–285, 284f
Immune response,
    lymphocyte development, 2, 3
    parasitic infections,
        hormonal modulation, 165–167
    T cells, 403
Immune system, 2–8
    antigen presentation, 3–6
    B-cell activation, 7, 8
    lymphocyte development and immune response, 2, 3
    role, 3
    T-cell activation, 6, 7
Immunoglobulin G (IgG) heavy-chain gene,
    IDDM, 72, 73
Immunological self-tolerance, see Self-tolerance
Immunopathogenic events,
    glandular failure, 326f
Immunoprecipitation assays,
    steroid 21-hydroxylase (21-OH), 201

Immunoregulation, 301, 302
  autoimmune thyroid disease (AITD), 226, 227
Implantation disorder, 371–379
Indirect IFT,
  islet cell autoantigens, 195
Indirect immunofluorecence (IIF), 314, 367
Infectious agents,
  AITD, 223–225
  IDDM, 123
Infertility,
  POF women,
    treatment, 371
  women, 378, 379
Infertility,
  unexplained,
    autoantibodies, 377–379
    tests, 378
INF-γ,
  AITD, 230
Innate immunity,
  cellular and soluble mediators, 164t
  gonadal steroids, 171, 172
  hormonal modulation, 164, 165
Insulin,
  IDDM, 199
  IDDM treatment, 400
Insulin autoantibodies (IAA), 199, 394
Insulin-dependent diabetes mellitus, 184, 322, 367, 394
  age-specific incidence, 59, 60
  animal models, 62, 63, 293–296, 407, 408
    autoimmune origin, 293–295
    effector mechanisms, 294, 295
    etiology, 296
    rupture of tolerance, 295, 296
    target antigens, 294
  antigen specific immunotherapy, 409
  autoimmune destruction, 394
  autoimmunity, 120–122
  Chinese hamster, 115
  CTLA-4, 80, 81
  epidemiology, 299, 300
  etiology and pathogenesis, 293–302
  experimentally induced, 117, 118
  familial clustering, 60, 61
  gene mapping studies, 64–67
  genetically induced, 115–117
  genetics, 118–120
  genetic susceptibility, 57–82
  epidemiologic evidence, 58–64
  HLA candidate genes, 67–72
  glutamic acid decarboxylase, IA-2, 198t, 199t
  HLA-related susceptibility, 79, 80
  human,
    autoimmune origin, 302
    genetics, 296–299
    HLA genes, 296–298
    non-HLA genes, 298
  human leucocyte antigen (HLA), 194, 195
  immune response, 120–122
    B-cell reactivity, 120, 121
    T-cell reactivity, 122
  immunotherapy, 394–402
  incidence, 58, 59
  insulin gene VNTR, 81
  intervention strategies, 395
  islet pathology, 120
  LETL rat, 114, 115
  NOD mouse, 115
  non-HLA candidate genes, 72, 73
  primary prevention therapies, 395
  research,
    twins, 62
  secondary prevention, 396
    therapy, 397–401
  tertiary prevention, 396, 397
    therapy, 397–401
  whole-genome screening, 76
Insulin gene VNTR
  IDDM, 81
Insulitis, 115, 116, 120
Intrauterine embryo transfer (ET), 378
In vitro fertilization (IVF), 378
Iodine deficiency,
  maternal hypothyroxinemia, 273
Islet cell antibodies (ICA), 394
  IDDM, 60, 61
Islet cell autoantigens, 194–200
Islet cell transplantation, 126
Isolated POF,
  adrenal autoantibodies, 204t
Isotype switching,
  B-cell activation, 7, 8
I therapy, 131f
  Graves' disease, 234
  hypothyroidism, 235t

K

51-kDa protein, 205

L

Lactate dehydrogenase virus,
  IDDM, 123
Lambs,
  autoantigens, 51, 52
LA measurement,
  clotting assay screening, 373, 374
Larval tree frog,
  autoantigens, 50
LCMV,
  IDDM, 123
Leishmania, 166, 167
LETL rat,
  IDDM, 114, 115
  insulitis, 120
Linkage analysis, 65, 66
Long-acting thyroid stimulator (LATS),
  hyperthyroidism, 39
Long-Evans Tokushima Otsuka (LETO) rat, 115
Luteinizing hormone (LH), 271, 272, 371
Lymph nodes,
  endocrine hormones, 34, 35
Lymphocyte development,
  immune response, 2, 3
Lymphocytes,
  elimination,
    autoimmune disease, 46–49
  norepinephrine, 39
  prolactin, 38
Lymphocytic adenohypophysitis,
  antipituitary antibodies, 339–341
  associated autoimmune dysfunction, 344
  clinical features, 342–344
  differential diagnosis, 344
  electron microscopic features, 339
  experimental model, 342
  histologic features, 337
  human leucocyte antigen (HLA) typing, 341
  hyperprolactinemia, 342, 343
  immunohistochemical features, 338, 339
  light microscopic features, 338
  management, 344, 345
  pathogenetic features, 339
  pathological features, 337–339
  pituitary insufficiency, 343, 344
  pregnancy, 342, 345
  radiographic features, 338f, 344
  Western blotting analysis, 342f

Lymphocytic hypophysitis, 184
Lymphokines,
  endocrine glands, 36–38
Lymphomatosen veranderung, 218

M

Maackia amurensis (MALII),
  TSHR, 190
Major histocompatibility complex (MHC), 167, 296, 327, 369, 394
  autoimmune thyroid disease (AITD), 219, 220
  human leucocyte antigen (HLA), 371
Malaria, 166, 167
Maternal hypothyroxinemia,
  iodine deficiency, 273
Maturity-onset diabetes of the young (MODY)
  candidate gene analysis, 66
MHC class I molecules,
  antigen presentation, 3, 4
Memory B cells, 3
Mengoviruses,
  IDDM, 123
12-mer Tg epitopes, 93, 94
MHC class I genes,
  AITDS, 94, 95
MHC class I (Ia) antigens,
  expression, 5, 6
MHC class II antigens,
  composition, 5, 6
  expression, 5
  organ-specific autoimmune disease, 19
MHC class I (Ib) antigens,
  expression, 5
MHC class II genes,
  AITDS, 91–94
MHC molecules,
  protective influence,
    AITDS, 95, 96
MHC region, 67, 68
MHC-transgenic mice,
  IDDM, 116
Mice,
  radiation-induced autoimmunity, 48
Microsatellite marker analysis,
  AITDS, 74–76
Microsatellite markers, 66
Milk hypothesis,
  insulin-dependent diabetes mellitus, 395

Molecular mimicry,
    IDDM animal models, 127
Monoclonal antibodies (MAbs),
    IDDM treatment, 401
Mouse hepatitis virus,
    IDDM, 123
Mouse MHC,
    antigen presentation, 4
Mouse models,
    EAT, 63, 64
    Graves' disease, 64
MTg sequencing, 107
Multiple sclerosis, 299
Multiple sclerosis (MS),
    antigen specific immunotherapy, 409, 410

N

Na^+/I^- symporter, 193
Neoantigens,
    transgenic,
        expression, 43
Neonatal Graves' disease,
    binding stimulation index (B-S index), 286, 287
Neonatal thyroid disease, 286, 287
Neonatal thyrotoxicosis,
    prediction, 287f
Nicotinamide,
    IDDM treatment, 399, 400
NK cell activity,
    endometriosis, 381
NOD mice,
    B-cells, 120, 121
    colonies and lines, 121
    diet, 123, 124, 127, 128
    IDDM, 115, 118
    IDDM genetic predisposition, 119, 120
    insulitis, 120
    sex hormones, 124
    stress, 124
    T-cells, 122
    toxic agents, 124
Non-HLA candidate gene-linkage studies,
    AITDS, 74–76
Non-HLA candidate genes, 72–76
    AITDS, 73–76
    IDDM, 72, 73
Non-MHC genes,
    dietary iodine, 98
Nonobese diabetic (NOD) mice,
    autoimmunity, 45

IDDM, 62, 63
Nonspecific suppressor T lymphocyte function, 228
Norepinephrine,
    lymphocytes, 39

O

Obese strain (OS) chickens,
    AITDS, 97, 98
    spontaneous autoimmune thyroiditis, 45
Ophthalmopathy, 70, 254
Organ-specific autoimmune disease hypothesis,
    autoimmunity, 19, 20
Ovarian autoantibodies,
    POF, 370, 371
Ovarian follicles,
    hormone secreting cells, 367
Ovaries,
    lymph draining, 35
    thymectomy, 33, 48
Ovum donation, 371
Oxazolone (OXA),
    peripheral B cells, 175, 176

P

Pancreatic β cell,
    bystander suppression, 405f
Pancreatic islet β cells,
    IDDM, 229
Parasitic infections,
    immune response,
        hormonal modulation, 165–167
    sexual dimorphism, 166t
Parathyroid autoantigens, 193, 194
Parry's disease, 218
Pelvic inflammatory disease, 378, 379
P450 enzyme, 368
P450 enzyme autoantibodies,
    pathogenic role, 317
Peptides,
    conserved,
        Tg, 98–101
Peripheral B cells, 175, 176
Peripheral B-cell tolerance, 16, 17
Peripheral blood lymphocytes,
    a-endorphin, 36, 37
    chorionic gonadotrophin, 38
Peripheral immunological tolerance, 1
Peripheral T-cell tolerance, 10–14

clonal deletion, 11
Peripheral T lymphocytes, 174, 175
Peripheral tolerance, 403, 404
Pichinde,
    IDDM, 123
Pituitary gland,
    autoantigens, 184, 185
    lesion, 337
Pituitary insufficiency,
    lymphocytic adenohypophysitis, 343, 344
Placental hormones,
    thyroid function, 271, 272
Placental syncytiotrophoblast, 367, 368
Placentation disorder, 371–379
Platelet derived growth factor (PDGF), 327
Polyclonal B-cell activators, 8
Polygenic disorder, 394
Polyglandular autoimmune syndromes,
    349–360, see also Autoimmune
    polyglandular syndrome (APGS),
Polyglandular autoimmunity, 402
Polyinosinic polycytidylic acid,
    IDDM, 117
Porcine (p) TPO,
    thyroiditis, 101
Posterior pituitary insufficiency,
    lymphocytic adenohypophysitis, 343, 344
Postpartum autoimmune diseases, 286
Postpartum autoimmune endocrine
    syndromes, 271–287
Postpartum autoimmune thyroid
    dysfunction, 276–285
    definition and classification, 276–278
    diagnosis and management, 279, 280
    immune rebound mechanism, 283–285
    long-term prognosis, 280, 281
    prevalence, 278, 279
Postpartum destructive thyrotoxicosis,
    Graves' disease,
        differential diagnosis, 280t
Postpartum Graves' disease, 282, 283
Postpartum thyroiditis (PPT), 282, 401
    epidemiology, 155, 156
Postthymectomy autoimmunity, 47, 48
Pre-B-cell receptor (pre-BCR), 14, 15
Pre-B cells, 3
Prednisone,
    oral,
        ASA,
            low-dose oral, 375
Pregnancy,
    autoimmune diseases, 168

autoimmune thyroid disease, 274, 275
bone marrow, 175
Graves' disease, 275, 275f
Hashimoto's disease, 275
hyperthyroidism, 274
loss,
    autoantibodies, 371–377
lymphocytic adenohypophysitis, 342, 345
thymic size, 174
thyroid function, 271–273, 272f
Premature ovarian failure (POF), 366, 367
Pretibial myxoedema, 218
Pretibial thyroid dermopathy, 263f
Primary myxoedema, 401
Pro-B cells, 3
Progesterone
    B cells, 175
Progesterone receptors, 171
Prolactin,
    lymphocytes, 38
Prolactin-related mRNA, 38
Pro-opiomelanocortin (POMC)-derived
    peptides,
    IL-10, 37
Pro-opiomelanocortin (POMC) mRNA,
    cytokines, 36
Pro-T cells, 2, 3
Protein tyrosin phosphatase (PTP) family, 197
Proteolytic cleavage,
    TSHR, 191

R

Radiation-induced autoimmunity,
    mice, 48
Rats,
    autoantigens, 50, 51
Recurrent pregnancy loss,
    autoantibodies, 371–377
Recurrent spontaneous abortion (RSA),
    372, 376
Regeneration nodules,
    ACTH levels, 311
Reoviruses,
    IDDM, 123
Reproductive medicine, 365
Reproductive process,
    endocrine gland, 365
Research studies,
    twins, 61, 62
Restriction fragment length polymorphisms
    (RFLP),

AITD, 220
Retrobulbar fibroblasts,
  characteristics, 258t
Rheumatoid arthritis (RA),
  antigen specific immunotherapy, 410
  gender and age ratios, 169f
RIP-LCMV model,
  IDDM, 116
Rodent models,
  AITDS, 91–107
RT-PCR,
  thyroid dermopathy, 264
Rubella,
  IDDM, 123

S

Sardinia, 299
SAT,
  dietary iodine, 99
Sc heparin,
  low-dose oral ASA, 375
Schistosoma mansoni,
  infections, 166
Schmidt's syndrome, 313, 367
Second colloid antigen, 193
Self-tolerance, 1–21
  autoimmunity, 17–20
  B-cell tolerance, 14–17
  immune system, 2–8
  T-cell tolerance, 8–14
Semiallogenic conceptus, 365
Severe combined immunodeficient
    mouse strain,
  GD, 101
Sex hormones,
  IDDM, 124
  immune responses, 163–176
Sexual dimorphism,
  gender comparison, 168t
  parasitic infections, 165, 166t
Sheehan's syndrome, 344
Somatic hypermutation,
  B-cell tolerance, 16
Spontaneous autoimmune thyroiditis,
  OS chickens, 45
Spontaneous hypothyroidism,
  incidence, 59
Steroid 17α-hydroxylase (17α-OH), 203, 204
Steroid cell antibody (St-C-Ab),
    314–316, 367
  adrenal cortex antibodies (ACA), 328

APGS, 358, 359
  autoantigens, 316, 317
Steroid 21-hydroxylase (21-OH), 200–203
Steroids,
  lympholytic effects, 36
Stiff Man Syndrome (STS), 197
Streptozotocin (STZ),
  IDDM, 117, 124
Stress,
  Graves' disease, 228
  IDDM, 124
Subacute De Quervain's thyroiditis,
  AITD viral infections, 223
Subclinical hyperthyroidism, 145, 146
Subclinical hypothyroidism,
  cholesterol, 156, 157
  epidemiology, 152
  screening,
    cost, 157
Suppressor cells,
  EAE, 44, 45
Suppressor T cells,
  AITD, 227
Susceptibility genes,
  disease induction mechanisms, 79–81
Systemic lupus erythematosus (SLE), 373
  danazol, 169
  gender and age ratios, 169f

T

Taenia crassiceps,
  infections, 166
TAP1 gene,
  IDDM, 81
T cells, *see also* T lymphocytes,
  activation, 6, 7
    APCs, 12
  AITD, 227–229
  anti-idiotype regulatory, 105
  autoimmune thyroiditis, 227
  β-cell antigens, 301
  effector,
    AITDS, 102, 103
  epitopes,
    identification, 405, 406
  genetic resistance, 105
  Graves' disease, 227
  immune response, 403
  regulatory mechanisms, 105–107
  TAO, 255–257
  tolerance, 8–14

antigen administration techniques, 406
  central, 8–10
  peripheral, 10–14
  tolerance breakdown
    autoimmunity, 17, 18
TCR genes,
  AITDS, 73
TCR signal,
  T-cell activation, 6, 7
TCR V β genes, 102
Testis,
  lymph draining, 35
Testosterone,
  peripheral B cells, 176
Therapy,
Graves' disease, 234, 235
TH 1 cells,
  vs TH 2 cells, 404, 405
Th1 concept, 320
Thymectomy,
  autoimmune endocrine disease, 46–49
  immune-endocrine interaction, 33
Thymic size,
  androgen levels, 173
  castration, 172, 173
  estrogen, 173, 174
  pregnancy, 174
Thymus,
  developing endocrine system, 32, 33
  gonadal steroids, 172
  role, 403, 404
Thymus-dependent (TD) antigen, 7
Thymus-independent (TI) antigen, 7, 8
Thyrocyte class I and II,
  AITD, 226
Thyrocyte HLA-DR expression,
  AITD viral infections, 224
Thyroglobulin, 185–187
  AITD, 226
  AITD CD8, 229
  AITD T cells, 227
  conserved peptides, 98–101
  dietary iodine, 99
  EAT tolerance induction, 104–107
Thyroglobulin autoantibodies, 59, 231, 232
Thyroid,
  murine model, 408
Thyroid acropachy, 218
Thyroid associated ophthalmopathy (TAO),
  and other thyroid disorders, 246, 247
  appearance, 246f
  classifications, 245, 246

  clinical features, 246t
  immunogenetics, 249, 250
  immunological features, 250–260
  immunomodulatory treatment, 261, 262
  management, 260t
  nongenetic factors, 250
  pathology, 247–249
  therapeutic aspects, 260–262
Thyroid autoantibodies,
  AITDS, 61
  APGS, 357, 358
  B lymphocytes,
    AITD, 231–233
  TAO, 251
Thyroid autoantibody production,
  AITD, 226
Thyroid autoantigens, 49–51, 185–193
  abnormality, 225–227
Thyroid cell membrane antigens,
  AITD bacterial infections, 224
Thyroid cells,
  cytokines, 229, 230
Thyroid dermopathy, 262–264
  treatment, 264
Thyroid disease, 286, 287, 401, 402
  central antigens, 401
  therapies, 401
Thyroid dysfunction, *see also* Postpartum
  autoimmune thyroid dysfunction,
  screening, 156–158
Thyroid eye disease (TED), 401
Thyroid follicle,
  composite diagram, 231f
Thyroid function,
  pregnancy, 271–273, 272f
Thyroiditis,
  BALB/c mice, 101
  postpartum,
    epidemiology, 155, 156
Thyroiditogenic (TCR) repertoire,
  AITDS, 96, 97
Thyroid peroxidase, 187–189
  AITD, 226
  AITD CD8, 229
  AITD T cells, 227
Thyroid peroxidase autoantibodies, 59, 233
Thyroid peroxidase (TPO), 101, 102
Thyroid stimulating activities (TSA)
  Graves' disease, 231–232, 276, 276f
Thyroid stimulating antibody (TSAb),
  218, 232t
  pregnancy, 284f

Thyroid stimulating hormone receptor
(TSHR), 101, 102, 189–192, 231–232
   AITD bacterial infections, 224
   extracellular domain, 190
   gene mutations, 189
   TAO, 259, 260
   thyroid autoantigens abnormality, 225
   thyroid dermopathy, 264
Thyroid stimulating hormone (TSH), 185, 271, 272
   antibody response, 37, 38
   EAT tolerance induction, 104–107
   stimulation,
      cytokines, 229, 230
Thyroid treatment, 234, 235
   TAO, 261
Thyrotoxicosis,
   incidence, 59, 146, 219
   prediction, 287f
Thyrotoxic periodic paralysis (TPP), 70
Thyroxine binding globulin (TBG), 273
T-lymphocyte precursors, 2, 3
T lymphocytes, *see* T cells
TNF, 382
TNF-α,
   AITD, 230
TPO gene,
   Graves' disease, 74
Transforming growth factors (TGF),
   production, 320
Transgenic diabetes models, 115–117
Transgenic neoantigen expression, 43
Tree frog,
   larval,
      autoantigens, 50
Tricioplusia ni,
   thyroid peroxidase, 188
TSH and TSHR autoantibodies (TRAb), 191, 192
   binding sites, 192
Tuberculosis, 310
Twins,
   research studies, 61, 62
Type 1 diabetes mellitus genetic susceptibility, 57–82

U

Uveitis,
   antigen specific immunotherapy, 410

V

Vaccinia,
   IDDM, 123
Vacor,
   IDDM, 117, 124
Variable number of tandem repeats (VNTR),
   IDDM, 72, 73
Viral hypothesis,
   AITD, 223
   insulin-dependent diabetes mellitus, 395, 396
Viruses,
   AITD, 223
   IDDM, 123
   triggering role, 300

W

Western blotting analysis,
   IDDM, 185
   lymphocytic adenohypophysitis, 342f
   steroid 21-hydroxylase (21-OH), 201, 202
   TSHR, 190, 191, 192
Whole-genome screening, 66, 67
   AITDS, 76–78
   IDDM, 76
Women,
   infertility, 378, 379
      treatment, 371
Woolf's formula, 65

Y

Yersinia enterocolitica,
   AITD bacterial infections, 224
Yersiniosis, 232

Z

ZP3 antigens, 371

ABOUT THE EDITOR

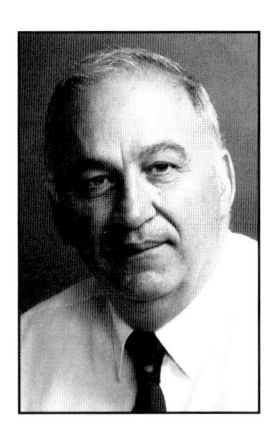

Robert Volpé, MD, FRCP(C), received his undergraduate medical education at the University of Toronto and has been a member of the Faculty of Medicine at the University of Toronto since 1957. His chief contribution has been research in autoimmune thyroid disease and other endocrine diseases. He and his staff have published over 320 articles as well as several books on endocrine disorders.

Dr. Volpé has served as President of the American Thyroid Association and President of the Canadian Society of Endocrinology and Metabolism. He has been granted a Fellowship of the Royal College of Physicians of Edinburgh and a Fellowship of the Royal College of Physicians of London. He is a member of many learned societies, including the Endocrine Society, the Association of American Physicians, and the Canadian Institute of Academic Medicine.

Dr. Volpé has won several prizes, including the Distinguished Scientist Award of the American Thyroid Association, the Novo-Nordisk Award of the Irish Endocrine Society, the Annual Visiting Lectureship of the Caledonia (Scottish) Endocrine Society, the Gold Medal of the Japan Endocrine Society, the Sandoz Award of the Canadian Society of Endocrinology and Metabolism, and the Distinguished Service Award of the Canadian Society for Clinical Investigation. Dr. Volpé's work has led to an increased understanding of the nature of Grave's disease and Hashimoto's thyroiditis.